Optum

AF731019

Clinical Validation and Documentation Integrity for Coding

Supporting ICD-10-CM and -PCS code assignments with clinical documentation

2025

optumcoding.com

Optum Notice

The *Clinical Validation and Documentation Integrity for Coding* is designed to be an accurate and authoritative source regarding coding and every reasonable effort has been made to ensure accuracy and completeness of the content. However, Optum makes no guarantee, warranty, or representation that this publication is accurate, complete or without errors. It is understood that Optum is not rendering any legal or other professional services or advice in this publication and that Optum bears no liability for any results or consequences that may arise from the use of this book. Please address all correspondence to:

Optum
2525 Lake Park Blvd.
West Valley City, UT 84120

Our Commitment to Accuracy

Optum is committed to producing accurate and reliable materials.

To report corrections, please visit email customerassistance@optum.com. You can also reach customer service by calling 1.800.464.3649, option 1.

Copyright

Made in the USA

ISBN 978-1-62254-964-1 (Softbound)
ISBN 978-1-62254-965-8 (eBook)

Acknowledgments

Marianne Randall, CPC, *Senior Product Manager*
Stacy Perry, *Manager, Desktop Publishing*
Anita Schmidt, BS, RHIA, AHIMA-approved ICD-10-CM/PCS Trainer, *Subject Matter Expert*
Laura M. Anderson, RN, BSN, CCDS, *Subject Matter Expert*
Tracy Betzler, *Senior Desktop Publishing Specialist*
Hope M. Dunn, *Senior Desktop Publishing Specialist*
Katie Russell, *Desktop Publishing Specialist*
Kate Holden, *Editor*

Subject Matter Experts

Anita Schmidt, BS, RHIA, AHIMA-approved ICD-10-CM/PCS Trainer

Ms. Schmidt has expertise in ICD-10-CM/PCS, DRG, and CPT with more than 20 years' experience in coding in multiple settings, including inpatient, observation, and same-day surgery. Her experience includes analysis of medical record documentation, assignment of ICD-10-CM and PCS codes, and DRG validation. She has collaborated with clinical documentation specialists to identify documentation needs and potential areas for physician education. Most recently she has been developing content for resource and educational products related to ICD-10-CM, ICD-10-PCS, DRG, and CPT. Ms. Schmidt is an AHIMA-approved ICD-10-CM/PCS trainer and is an active member of the American Health Information Management Association (AHIMA) and the Minnesota Health Information Management Association (MHIMA).

Laura M. Anderson, RN, BSN, CCDS

Ms. Anderson is a Registered Nurse and CDI Specialist/Educator with more than 20 years of experience in the healthcare profession. She obtained her BSN at the University of Minnesota and spent most of her bedside nursing career on Medical-Surgical care units. Her clinical documentation experience began in 2007, covering CDI specialist training, education development, and physician engagement. She has served as a CDI Team Lead and consultant, working with senior leadership to incorporate CDI work into documentation compliance and quality metrics. Ms. Anderson also has a BS degree in Biology (Winthrop University), with research experience in liver cancer and radiation-induced leukemia. She has presented at the state and national levels for the Association of Clinical Documentation Integrity Specialists (ACDIS) and has served as a co-lead for the Minnesota state chapter.

Contents

Introduction

Documentation by providers is primarily for clinical communication, with the main intent of coordinating and delivering quality care to patients. It is important that other clinicians involved in the care of the patient understand the thought processes behind decision making in order to accomplish this.

The *ICD-10-CM Official Guidelines for Coding and Reporting* state: "A joint effort between the healthcare provider and the coder is essential to achieve complete and accurate documentation, code assignment, and reporting of diagnoses and procedures. These guidelines have been developed to assist both the healthcare provider and the coder in identifying those diagnoses that are to be reported. The importance of consistent, complete documentation in the medical record cannot be overemphasized. Without such documentation, accurate coding cannot be achieved. The entire record should be reviewed to determine the specific reason for the encounter and the conditions treated."

ICD-10-CM Official Guidelines for Coding and Reporting, Section 1.A.19 states: "The assignment of a diagnosis code is based on the provider's diagnostic statement that the condition exists. The provider's statement that the patient has a particular condition is sufficient. Code assignment is not based on clinical criteria used by the provider to establish the diagnosis. If there is conflicting medical record documentation, query the provider." The rule clarifies that physician documentation of a condition is required for it to be coded. This guideline emphasizes this and places the responsibility with the physician rather than the coder to ensure complete, accurate, and appropriate documentation.

However, this guideline does not eliminate the need for coders and clinical documentation improvement (CDI) staff to communicate with physicians and work together to clarify and improve documentation issues. It does emphasize the need for a strong documentation improvement program that can provide for concurrent efforts to clarify the diagnosis and clinical indicators present in the documentation prior to coding and billing. The American Health Information Management Association (AHIMA) and Association of Clinical Documentation Integrity Specialists (ACDIS) practice brief "Guidelines for Achieving a Compliant Query Practice (2022 Update)" states:

Queries may be necessary in (but not limited to) the following instances:

- To support documentation of medical diagnoses or conditions that are clinically evident and meet the Uniform Hospital Discharge Data Set (UHDDS) requirements but without the corresponding diagnoses or conditions stated.
- To resolve conflicting diagnostic or procedural documentation between providers.
- To clarify the reason for the inpatient/outpatient encounter.
- To seek clarification when it appears a documented diagnosis is not clinically supported or is conflicting with the medical record documentation (clinical validation).
- To confirm a diagnosis documented by an independent licensed practitioner who does not meet the definition of a provider in the inpatient setting (e.g., confirmation of a pathology finding).
- To establish a cause-and-effect relationship between medical conditions.
- To establish clinically supported acuity or specificity of a documented diagnosis to avoid reporting a default or unspecified code.
- To establish the relevance of a condition documented as a "history of" to determine if the condition is active.
- To support appropriate Present on Admission (POA) indicator assignment.
- To determine if a diagnosis is ruled in or out.
- To clarify the objective and/or extent of a procedure.
- To clarify the presence or absence of a complication.
- To clarify a diagnosis on an ancillary note that has been signed but not addressed by a provider. For example, if the nutrition note states "severe malnutrition" and the note is signed by the provider, but the provider does not address the diagnosis within the documentation.

American Hospital Association (AHA) *Coding Clinic* for ICD-10, fourth quarter 2016, pages 147–149, reinforces that this guideline addresses coding, not clinical validation. It indicates that though it is linked to accurate coding, clinical validation is a separate function from the coding process and clinical skill. Codes assigned by a coding professional are based on the documentation by the physician, rather than a particular clinical definition or criteria. This guideline and the resulting advice from *Coding Clinic* stress the need for a process of validating clinical conditions prior to performing the coding process.

Medicare also has standards for clinical evidence. According to Centers for Medicare and Medicaid Services (CMS) MedLearn Matters Article SE1121, "As with all codes, clinical evidence should be present in the medical record to support code assignment."

However, the CMS Recovery Audit Contractor (RAC) Scope of Work 2013 includes this statement: "Clinical validation is an additional process that may be performed along with DRG validation. Clinical validation involves a clinical review of the case to see whether or not the patient truly possesses the conditions that were documented in the medical record. Recovery Auditor clinicians shall review any information necessary to make a prepayment or post-payment claim determination. Clinical validation is performed by a clinician (RN, CMD or therapist). Clinical validation is beyond the scope of DRG (coding) validation, and the skills of a certified coder. This type of review can only be performed by a clinician or may be performed by a clinician with approved coding credentials."

This increases the opportunity and importance of accurate, timely queries from coders and CDI staff to clarify any disconnect between physician diagnosis and other clinical documentation prior to coding and submitting the claim. Auditors are still going to validate diagnoses with clinical indicators and denials are still going to be made. It is, therefore, imperative that good query procedures and practices are in place and are followed.

Clinical validation is a key component of many audit reviews. What does this mean to a coder, to CDI staff, to physicians?

Coders are instructed to assign a diagnostic or procedure code according to physician documentation. Any discussion or questioning about what is documented as a diagnosis or procedure and the clinical evidence, or lack thereof, to support it, can often end without resolution. In the past, coders have been told not to question the physician's *clinical* judgment. Some coders believe they are not clinicians and, therefore, should not be *expected* to evaluate clinical criteria.

However, as audits from outside organizations expand, there is increasingly more emphasis on the use of the clinical criteria to support the reported codes. This emphasis is known as *clinical validation*.

For example, the Recovery Audit Contractor Program is the nationwide program created by Medicare and conducted by contracted private companies to identify and correct improper payments made to fee-for-service Medicare/Medicaid plans. The statement of work for the Recovery Audit Contractor Program includes clinical validation that is to be performed by a clinician in order to confirm that a diagnosis is supported by the clinical documentation as well as the physician documentation. In other words, the physician documentation supports the code assignment. But what supports the physician documentation? The supporting clinical validation comes from a combination of the physician's clinical experience, professional judgment, patient history, and clinical criteria, which must be found within the medical record.

Clinical criteria consist of the signs, symptoms, ancillary tests results, and subsequent therapy or treatment that define a diagnosis. In the case of procedures, it means the technical description and those components that are integral to that procedure.

Factors that affect these clinical criteria components can result in a conflict between clinical findings and a diagnostic statement. A physician may determine a diagnosis despite certain clinical results, which do not fall within the clinical confirmation range or levels. This decision-making must be documented by the physician in order to explain any inconsistencies between a physician diagnostic statement and clinical criteria.

In today's healthcare environment, it is essential that coders share the responsibility of clinical validation with CDI staff, physicians, and other qualified healthcare professionals. Coders' clinical knowledge from education and experience, in addition to critical reasoning skills, help protect from liability and fraud, the entities and people for whom they work. Their professional ethic demands integrity in coding with accuracy and conscientiousness. A coder is one of the pillars that supports compliance.

Coders and CDI staff should work together to evaluate all chart documentation and data and, when necessary, query a conflict or inconsistency, including discrepancies between clinical criteria and physician documentation.

CMS reinforces that all documentation must be consistent with other parts of the medical record. If an entry contradicts documentation found elsewhere within the record, clarification is needed. With the initiation of clinical validation denials, this now extends to a diagnostic statement and its correlating clinical criteria.

The American Hospital Association's (AHA) *Coding Clinic* for ICD-10 states coders are not to use background clinical information contained in their responses for code assignment. The AHA states this information is provided in order that a coder may make a judgment to query where there may be incomplete documentation. Coders should also not rely on *AHA Coding Clinic* responses as justification for codes from documentation that lacks clarity. To compose a clinically accurate and appropriate physician query, a coder must understand how the clinical indicators support or do not support a diagnosis or procedure and by extension, what documentation is required.

This book is an excellent way for both coders and clinical documentation improvement specialists (CDIS) to learn to apply clinical validation to enhance the quality of these query practices while complying with current regulations, medical necessity requirements, and audit programs. This book provides:

- Clinical criteria and indicators
- Official coding guidelines
- Documentation support

- Query templates
- Decision making between routine, complication, additional diagnosis, and principal diagnosis
- Descriptions of procedures to assist the user in knowing when to query

Clinical criteria can vary from adults, children, and newborns. For this reason, this book only pertains to adults.

Resources

Resources for coding and documentation advice that are common throughout this book include:

- ICD-10-CM FY 2025:
  - https://www.cdc.gov/nchs/icd/icd-10-cm/files.html?
  - https://www.cdc.gov/nchs/icd/comprehensive-listing-of-icd-10-cm-files.htm
  - https://www.cms.gov/medicare/coding-billing/icd-10-codes/2025-icd-10-cm
- ICD-10-PCS FY 2025:
  - https://www.cms.gov/medicare/coding-billing/icd-10-codes/2025-icd-10-pcs
- ICD-10-CM/PCS MS-DRG v42.0 Definitions Manual
  - https://www.cms.gov/Medicare/Medicare-Fee-for-Service-Payment/AcuteInpatientPPS/MS-DRG-Classifications-and-Software
- FY 2025 IPPS Final Rule:
  - https://www.cms.gov/medicare/payment/prospective-payment-systems/acute-inpatient-pps/fy-2025-ipps-proposed-rule-home-page
- Official ICD-10-CM and ICD-10-PCS Guidelines for Coding and Reporting 2025
- *AHA Coding Clinic* for ICD-10-CM/PCS
- *ICD-10-CM Complete Official Code Set*, 2025 Edition, Optum
- *ICD-10-PCS Complete Official Code Set*, 2025 Edition, Optum
- *DRG Expert*, 2025 Edition, Optum
- *Optum Essentials, Applying the ICD-10-CM Guidelines,* 2024 Edition, Optum
- *Optum Essentials, Applying the ICD-10-PCS Guidelines*, 2024 Edition, Optum
- *Coders' Desk Reference for ICD-10-CM Diagnosis*, 2025 Edition, Optum
- *Coders' Desk Reference for ICD-10-PCS Procedures*, 2025 Edition, Optum
- *ICD-10-CM Clinical Documentation Improvement Desk Reference*, 2024 Edition, Optum
- Medscape Reference: http://www.medscape.com/
- *The Merck Manual*
- National Center for Biotechnology Information: http://www.ncbi.nlm.nih.gov
- MLN Medicare Quarterly Provider Compliance Newsletter – Archives:
  - https://www.cms.gov/training-education/healthcare-provider-resources/mln-publications-multimedia/articles
- ICD-10-PCS Reference Manual, 2016 Edition, Centers for Medicare and Medicaid Services

Other resources are cited at the end of each section specific to the subject matter discussed within that section.

Using This Guide

The *Clinical Validation and Documentation Integrity for Coding* serves as a reference tool for multiple high-risk diagnoses and procedures that are under scrutiny from a clinical validation standpoint.

Diagnoses, listed alphabetically, are followed by procedures, which are also arranged in alphabetical order. Each diagnosis section contains a list of the ICD-10-CM codes discussed in that section, with icons noting CC, MCC, hospital-acquired condition (HAC), and/or hierarchical condition category (HCC) status. Any code followed by a dash (-) signifies a category level, or subcategory level, code that requires more characters to be a valid and complete code. Codes are followed by an in-depth discussion of criteria and pathophysiology of the disease or procedure process. Following discussion and references, a clinical criteria review is provided, referencing relevant documentation content as it relates to ICD-10-CM Official Guidelines for Coding and Reporting, Section III. Documentation should support the coding/reporting criteria for other diagnoses or additional conditions affecting patient care that requires the following:

- Physical evaluation
- Clinical evaluation

- Diagnostic procedure
- Therapeutic procedure
- Increase nursing care and/or monitoring
- Extends length of stay (LOS)

Clinical criteria and coding references are then applied to help the user understand when it is appropriate to report or not report that diagnosis in the following situations:

- Routine
- Principal diagnosis
- Comorbidity
- Complication
- Poisoning or adverse effect

Tables in each section provide a simplified clinical coding example that relates to conditions in the first column. The second column refers to the official coding guidelines (OCG) used to support the use of the diagnosis. The third and fourth columns provide appropriate documentation samples and ICD-10-CM coding advice and sequencing. Please note, not all clinical scenarios are represented and the clinical criteria are not all-inclusive. Most cases are presumed to be the initial encounter (A) unless otherwise specified.

The procedure sections are divided out by their three- or four-character prefix. Each procedure section also contains clinical narrative and valuable coding guidance on the appropriateness of reporting these procedures in the ICD-10-PCS setting.

Chapter 20, "External Causes of Morbidity," codes are not routinely included in the coding example answers as application of these codes is not the focus of the exercises.

Shaded boxes containing documentation or coding tips are provided throughout the book, which may define conditions, clarify proper code reporting, or affect reimbursement. These tips aid coders and CDI professionals with understanding the complex issues that affect code assignment.

Appendixes

Several detailed appendixes are provided to support the user by supplying valuable additional information:

Appendix A. Query Guidelines, Examples and Templates: Provides information about why and when to query and how to prepare a compliant query. Included are samples that may be used as templates and are related to the conditions and procedures discussed throughout the book.

Appendix B. ICD-10-CM Official Guidelines for Coding and Reporting: The full official ICD-10-CM conventions and guidelines for the current year are supplied with new changes in **bold** and include sections on the selection of the principal diagnosis, reporting additional diagnoses and present on admission guidelines.

Appendix C. ICD-10-PCS Official Guidelines for Coding and Reporting: Includes the full official ICD-10-PCS conventions and guidelines for the current year with new changes in **bold**. These guidelines provide instructions covering body systems, root operations, body parts, approaches, devices, obstetrics, new technology, and selection of principal procedure.

Appendix D. Abnormal EKGs: This includes information on abnormal findings on EKG reports that may indicate potential undocumented conditions that may affect patient healthcare records and impact MS-DRG reimbursement.

Appendix E. Abnormal Laboratory Values: This provides a reference range of normal laboratory values, signs/symptoms, and treatments of conditions commonly associated with abnormalities of these ranges. This information can be helpful for clinical validation and preparation of queries.

Appendix F. Pharmacology List: This reference is a comprehensive but not all inclusive list of common pharmacological agents used to treat acute and/or chronic conditions. Drugs are listed in alphabetical order by their brand and/or generic names along with their drug action and indications for which they may commonly be prescribed. Many have also been mapped to their appropriate Z code.

Appendix G. Organisms: This reference lists by specimen site normal flora and possible pathogens to aid differentiation between what is normal and what is an indication of an abnormal condition.

Appendix H. Noninvasive Diagnostic Test Outcomes: Diagnostic tests are linked with signs and symptoms as well as diagnostic outcomes to provide clinical clues that may affect code assignment.

Overview of Fundaments for Appropriate Coding and Reimbursement

Principal Diagnosis

Selection of Principal Diagnosis

ICD-10-CM Official Guidelines for Coding and Reporting, 2025

To assign an ICD-10-CM code for a principal diagnosis, criteria from official coding guidelines, Uniform Hospital Discharge Data Set (UHDDS) definition, clinical criteria, physician or other qualified healthcare professional documentation must be met.

The principal diagnosis is defined in the UHDDS as "that condition established after study to be chiefly responsible for occasioning the admission of the patient to the hospital for care."

In determining the principal diagnosis, coding conventions in the ICD-10-CM, the tabular list, and alphabetic index take precedence over the official coding guidelines.

For the complete official conventions and guidelines governing the principle diagnosis, see Appendix B, Section I.a. Conventions, and Section II. Selection of Principal Diagnosis located at the back of this book.

Other or Additional Diagnosis

To assign an ICD-10-CM code for an "other" or "additional diagnosis," comorbidity, or a complication of care, the criteria from official coding guidelines, UHDDS definition, clinical criteria, physician or other qualified healthcare professional documentation must be met.

The definition for "other diagnoses" is interpreted as additional conditions that affect patient care in terms of requiring:

- Clinical evaluation
- Therapeutic treatment
- Diagnostic procedures
- Extended length of hospital stay
- Increased nursing care and/or monitoring

The UHDDS item 11-b defines "other diagnoses" as "all conditions that coexist at the time of admission, that develop subsequently, or that affect the treatment received and/or the length of stay. Diagnoses that relate to an earlier episode which have no bearing on the current hospital stay are to be excluded."

Principal Procedure

Selection of Principal Procedure

ICD-10-PCS Official Guidelines for Coding and Reporting, 2025

The following instructions should be applied in the selection of principal procedure and clarification on the importance of the relation to the principal diagnosis when more than one procedure is performed:

1. Procedure performed for definitive treatment of both principal diagnosis and secondary diagnosis:
   a. Sequence procedure performed for definitive treatment most related to principal diagnosis as principal procedure.
2. Procedure performed for definitive treatment and diagnostic procedures performed for both principal diagnosis and secondary diagnosis:
   a. Sequence procedure performed for definitive treatment most related to principal diagnosis as principal procedure.
3. A diagnostic procedure was performed for the principal diagnosis and a procedure is performed for definitive treatment of a secondary diagnosis:
   a. Sequence diagnostic procedure as principal procedure, since the procedure most related to the principal diagnosis takes precedence.
4. No procedures performed that are related to principal diagnosis; procedures performed for definitive treatment and diagnostic procedures were performed for secondary diagnosis:
   a. Sequence procedure performed for definitive treatment of secondary diagnosis as principal procedure, since there are no procedures (definitive or nondefinitive treatment) related to principal diagnosis.

MS-DRGs

An MS-DRG is one of 773 groups (version 42.0) that classify patients into clinically cohesive groups that demonstrate similar consumption of hospital resources and length-of-stay patterns.

The MS-DRG system organizes ICD-10-CM/PCS diagnosis and procedure codes into a complex, comprehensive system based on a few simple principles. Understanding how the MS-DRG system works enables providers to recover the appropriate payment for services rendered, which is consistent with the intent of the federal government when it devised the DRG system. An MS-DRG is assigned based on specific patient attributes, such as principal diagnosis, secondary diagnoses, procedures, and discharge status.

In addition to calculating reimbursement, MS-DRGs have two major functions. The first is to help evaluate the quality of care. Not only are critical pathways designed around MS-DRGs, but benchmarking and outcomes analysis can be launched using the MS-DRG clinical framework. Quality reviews can be performed to assess clinical documentation improvement and coding practices as well as physician documentation. Ongoing education of physicians, coders, clinical documentation specialists, nurses, and utilization review personnel can be guided by the results of MS-DRG analysis.

Second, MS-DRGs assist in evaluating utilization of services. Each MS-DRG represents the average resources needed to treat patients grouped to that MS-DRG relative to the national average of resources used to treat all Medicare patients. The MS-DRG assigned to each hospital inpatient stay also relates to the hospital case mix (i.e., the types of patients the hospital treats). A hospital's Medicare population case complexity is measured by calculation of the case-mix index, which is an average of all MS-DRG relative weights for the facility during a given time period. The higher the case-mix index, the more complex the patient population and the higher the required level of resources utilized. Since severity is such an essential component of MS-DRG assignment and case-mix index calculation, documentation and code assignment to the highest degree of accuracy and specificity are of the utmost importance.

Complications and Comorbidities (MCC/CC)

Both medical and surgical classes are sometimes further defined by the presence of complications or comorbidities, which are further delineated by being classified as a complication/comorbidity (CC) or a major complication/comorbidity (MCC). These are indicated in this book by a CC or MCC icon to the far right of the code.

A complication or comorbidity diagnosis, CC condition, is defined as a significant acute disease, a significant acute manifestation of a chronic disease, an advanced or end stage chronic disease, or a chronic disease associated with systemic physiological decompensation and debility that complicates care and/or has consistently greater impact on hospital resources.

An MCC condition meets the same criteria as a CC condition but is associated with a higher acuity level; hospital resource consumption is expected to be higher than that for a CC condition. There are fewer conditions that meet the criteria as an MCC than those for a CC condition.

Hierarchical Condition Category (HCC)

Hierarchical Condition Category (HCC) coding is a risk-adjustment model developed by the Centers for Medicare and Medicaid Services (CMS) that is meant to identify patients with higher-risk complex acute or chronic conditions. Conditions that share similar cost patterns are categorized together, and include diagnoses such as depressive disorders, heart failure, diabetes, and rheumatoid arthritis. The HCC payment model is used to estimate expected risk and future annual cost of care for these patients. HCC diagnoses are indicated in this book by an HCC icon to the far right of the code.

Present on Admission (POA)

Present-on-admission (POA) indicators are required on all diagnoses and external cause-of-injury codes for all inpatient acute care hospital discharges, according to the requirement outlined in the Deficit Reduction Act of 2005, section 5001(c). The only exception is for a select group of codes that have been designated as exempt from the POA regulations. Certain facilities are also exempt from this reporting requirement and include the following:

- Critical access hospitals
- Long-term care hospitals
- Cancer hospitals
- Inpatient psychiatric hospitals
- Inpatient rehabilitation facilities
- Veterans Administration/Department of Defense hospitals
- Children's inpatient facilities
- Religious nonmedical health care institutions

The POA indicator guidelines are not intended to replace the official *ICD-10-CM Official Guidelines for Coding and Reporting*. Nor will the POA guidelines supersede the Uniform Hospital Discharge Data Set (UHDDS) definition of principal diagnosis, defined as the condition established after study to be chiefly responsible for occasioning the admission of the patient to the hospital. The definition of "additional diagnoses" also remains the same. Coders must report all conditions that coexist at the time of admission, develop subsequently, or that affect the treatment received and/or the length of stay. This significantly affects assignment of the POA indicators. Because the POA indicator should accurately reflect the patient's conditions upon admission, review of POA guidelines as well as the *ICD-10-CM Official Guidelines for Coding and Reporting* is required.

The following is a summary of the POA guidelines:

- A POA condition is defined not only as one that is clearly present at the time of admission, but also one that was clearly present but not diagnosed until after the time of admission.
- Present on admission is defined as present at the time the order for an inpatient admission is made, whether or not the patient's episode of care originated in the emergency department, ambulatory surgery area, or other outpatient area. Conditions that develop during an outpatient encounter are considered present on admission.
- A POA indicator is assigned to the principal diagnosis, secondary diagnoses, and the external cause-of-injury codes.
- The POA guidelines are not intended to replace any of the other *ICD-10-CM Official Guidelines for Coding and Reporting* guidelines.
- The intent of the POA guidelines is not to determine whether or not a condition should be coded, but rather how to apply the POA indicator.

The following reporting options, with definitions, should be used to indicate whether a condition was POA:

Y	Yes: Present at the time of inpatient admission
N	No: Not present at the time of inpatient admission
U	Unknown: Documentation is insufficient to determine if condition is present on admission
W	Clinically undetermined: Provider is unable to clinically determine whether condition was or was not present on admission

Unreported/not used—(exempt from POA reporting)—Most ICD-10-CM codes require the assignment of a POA indicator. However, some diagnoses are considered exempt from the POA reporting. For these exempt conditions, the POA field should be left blank.

Coders must review the patient record to determine whether a condition was present on admission. If POA documentation is inconsistent, missing, conflicting, or unclear, the provider should be queried. The CDI specialist can assist in obtaining clear documentation of conditions present on admission as accurate POA assignment can greatly impact the quality and final billing of the patient encounter.

Hospital-Acquired Conditions

Hospital-acquired conditions (HAC) are conditions considered reasonably preventable through the application of evidence-based guidelines. These conditions, in and of themselves, are either a CC or an MCC that as a secondary diagnosis will move the MS-DRG assignment from a lower-paying MS-DRG to a higher-paying MS-DRG. However, if these conditions are not present on admission (meaning they developed during the hospital stay), the CC or MCC designation is nullified and the case will not group to the higher-paying MS-DRG based solely upon the reporting of the HAC code. The case will be paid as though these conditions were not reported. These are indicated in this book by a HAC icon to the far right of the code.

HACs are grouped into 14 categories:

- HAC 01: Foreign Object Retained After Surgery
- HAC 02: Air Embolism
- HAC 03: Blood Incompatibility
- HAC 04: Stage III and IV Pressure Ulcers
- HAC 05: Falls and Trauma
- HAC 06: Catheter-Associated Urinary Tract Infection (UTI)
- HAC 07: Vascular Catheter-Associated Infection
- HAC 08: Surgical Site Infection – Mediastinitis After Coronary Artery Bypass Graft (CABG)
- HAC 09: Manifestations of Poor Glycemic Control
- HAC 10: Deep Vein Thrombosis (DVT)/Pulmonary Embolism (PE) with Total Knee or Hip Replacement
- HAC 11: Surgical Site Infection – Bariatric Surgery
- HAC 12: Surgical Site Infection – Certain Orthopedic Procedures of Spine, Shoulder and Elbow
- HAC 13: Surgical Site Infection (SSI) Following Cardiac Implantable Electronic Device (CIED) Procedures
- HAC 14: Iatrogenic Pneumothorax with Venous Catheterization

Query

Medical record documentation entries must be consistent with all other parts of the record. When documentation entries conflict with other data within the record, clarification must be obtained when the information is used in the assignment of diagnosis or procedure codes. The clinical data within the record and record documentation must be incorporated into a specifically stated but open-ended, or in certain cases a yes or no, formatted query to substantiate and identify why clarification is needed.

The intention of a query is to assist the physician in making a clinical interpretation of a diagnosis, condition, or procedure. Query content must be based on clinical criteria, patient past medical history and present condition, treatment rendered, evaluation performed, monitoring provided, services/resources used, official coding guidelines, coding conventions, and official references.

A physician query is appropriate to confirm a diagnosis or procedure when a conflict exists between physician documentation and clinical indicators of the diagnosis made or procedure performed. When documentation between physicians conflict or when documentation within the record is inconsistent, ambiguous, incomplete, or indicates that a higher level of specificity can be made, query for clarification from the physician who has responsibility for the final diagnosis and/or for procedures or surgeries. A query may not introduce new information or indicate a monetary relationship to the response. See appendix A for Query Guidelines, Examples and Templates.

Terminology Clarification—Postoperative and Complication

The term "post-op" or "postoperative" denotes a time period and does not convey a causal relationship between surgery and a condition. A cause-and-effect relationship must be documented, such as stating "due to," and an indication in the documentation that it is a complication, according to the official coding guideline section I.B.16. The provider is not required to specifically document the term "complication."

Conditions that occur postoperatively and are conveyed as routine, incidental or inherent to the procedure, of no clinical significance, an expected outcome, or inadvertent, are not considered complications or comorbidities and are not coded. Conditions not conveyed as routine, etc. are reportable if they meet the official coding guideline section III definition of an additional diagnosis.

Conditions that pre-exist the surgery or are exacerbated by surgery or procedure are not a complication related to the surgery. These conditions, when documented and meet official coding guidelines section III definition of an additional diagnosis and clinical criteria, may be coded as comorbidities/additional diagnoses.

As a principal diagnosis, the official coding guideline section II, "Selection of Principal Diagnosis" and section I.C "Chapter-Specific Guidelines" along with the clinical criteria and physician documentation apply. The conventions and instructions of the classification take precedence over guidelines.

The term "complication" as used in ICD-10-CM does not imply that improper or inadequate care is responsible for the condition; it is a means of classification to indicate the etiology of the condition without negative implications.

The Importance of Documentation

Accurate, complete, compliant, consistent, and timely documentation:

- Supports patient status or patient type
- Supports medical necessity
- Reduces denials
- Supports quality measures
- Promotes accountability and transparency
- Captures the level of risk and severity
- Supports accurate ICD-10-CM and ICD-10-PCS code assignment
- Supports MS-DRG assignment
- Supports hospital-acquired condition (HAC) identification
- Supports present on admission (POA) indicator
- Identifies discharge disposition
- Provides clear communication within the facility and with other providers
- Ensures efficient billing and supports proper payment

Please note that the material presented in this book is intended to assist the user in appropriate code assignment based on documentation and clinical indicators. This will discourage unwarranted "upcoding" of cases that result in improper higher reimbursement. The coding instructions presented in this book reflect official sources and guidelines with interpretation by the consensus of our authors. Questions about this product should be directed to our customer service department at 1.800.464.3649.

Diagnoses

Acidosis

E87.2Ø	**Acidosis, unspecified**	CC
E87.21	**Acute metabolic acidosis**	CC
E87.22	**Chronic metabolic acidosis**	CC
E87.29	**Other acidosis**	CC

Associated terminology: lactic acidosis; metabolic acidosis; respiratory acidosis NOS

Discussion

Acidosis is the metabolic process that results in an increased acidity of blood plasma and other tissue or alkali loss when the kidneys/lungs cannot maintain the balance. Acidemia is a component of acidosis where the arterial pH level is less than 7.35 and is not compensated by the respiratory system. Severe acidemia is a pH < 7.20. The normal pH level varies between 7.35 and 7.45. Chronic acidemia causes rickets, osteomalacia, osteoporosis, and osteopenia.

When compensated, acidosis is mild with few signs/symptoms but when uncompensated, it can be severe and the signs/symptoms are multisystem. Subcategory E87.2 primarily represents lactic and metabolic acidosis, either of which can be acute or chronic.

> **Documentation Tip**
>
> **Code assignment cannot be based on ancillary test results, therapies, or clinical criteria alone. A diagnosis and its clinical significance must be supported by physician or other qualified healthcare professional documentation. When it is unclear or there is contradictory information, query the physician or other qualified healthcare professional for clarification.**

Lactic acidosis is a form of metabolic acidosis characterized by excess lactic acid, either from overproduction of lactate or decreased metabolism of lactate, or both. Along with acidemia, it includes a lactate level > 5 mEq/L. There are two types:

- Type A: due to tissue hypoperfusion and hypoxia (including localized skeletal muscle):
  - acute pulmonary edema
  - carbon monoxide poisoning
  - cardiopulmonary arrest
  - hypothermic shivering
  - massive rhabdomyolysis
  - sepsis
  - severe anemia
  - severe seizure
  - severe strenuous muscle activity
  - shock
- Type B: due to other condition not involving hypoperfusion and hypoxia:
  - diabetes mellitus
  - hypoglycemia
  - uremia
  - liver disease
  - infections
  - malignancy
  - total parenteral nutritional (TPN) therapy
  - inborn errors of metabolism
  - drugs/alcohol ingestion or poisoning
  - toxins
  - D-lactic acidosis from short bowel syndrome with colonic overgrowth of Lactobacilli

Metabolic acidosis is due to increased acid production, acid ingestion, decreased acid excretion by the kidneys or GI/Renal bicarbonate loss (HCO_3< 24 mEq/L). There are several types:

- Diabetic acidosis or diabetic ketoacidosis (DKA): this is excluded from subcategory E87.2- and found in category EØ8–E11, E13 with ketoacidosis
- Ketoacidosis: alcoholism, starvation

- Hyperchloremic acidosis is from excessive loss of sodium bicarbonate
  - severe diarrhea
  - colostomy or ileostomy or high stomal output due to short small bowel remnant
- Lactic acidosis: see previous entry above
- Kidney disease with impaired renal tubular function, as seen in distal or proximal renal tubular acidosis (N25.89) or underlying disease (i.e., hypoaldosteronism)
- Maintenance dialysis: result of both chronic renal failure (CRF) and dialysis
- Severe dehydration

Documentation Tip

Complications of care: The condition must be more than a routinely expected condition or event. The documentation must support that the condition is clinically significant with an indication that it is a complication by demonstrating:

- **A cause-and-effect relationship between the care or procedure and the condition**
- **That the condition resulted in altering the course of a procedure or surgery**

The term "complication" does not have to be explicitly documented.

Respiratory acidosis is due to a decrease in alveolar ventilation (hypoventilation) or a decrease in respiratory rate, or both. It results in increased blood carbon dioxide concentration (hypercapnia) and acidosis and usually hypoxia when hypoventilation is present.

Coding Tip

Respiratory acidosis described as acute or chronic has been reclassified to the respiratory chapter under code J96.Ø2 Acute respiratory failure with hypercapnia, or J96.12 Chronic respiratory failure with hypercapnia, respectively. If the respiratory acidosis is not further specified in the documentation, code E87.29 Other acidosis, may be assigned when the condition is not considered integral to the disease process. See the section titled "Respiratory Failure" in this manual for further information on coding and documentation requirements for respiratory failure.

Excluded

Metabolic acidosis with/complicated by respiratory acidosis, see E87.4.

Respiratory acidosis with/complicated by metabolic alkalosis/acidosis, see E87.4.

Newborn acidosis, see P84; late metabolic acidosis of newborn, see P74.Ø; metabolic acidemia in newborn, see category P19.

Diabetic acidosis or ketoacidosis, see category EØ8–E11, E13 with ketoacidosis.

Treatment is directed toward the underlying disease and correction of acidemia and associated metabolic or electrolyte imbalances.

Acidosis is reported in addition to the code for the underlying disease or condition. The exception to this is when acidosis is integral to the disease process, and then it is not assigned (i.e., sepsis, shock, respiratory failure, COPD, emphysema, asthma).

Coding Tip

Adverse effect: Nature of adverse drug effect: code for (adverse condition) followed by the code from T36–T5Ø with fifth or sixth character 5 to identify the drug.

Poisoning: Identify drug/chemical by the code from T36–T5Ø with fifth or sixth character of intent followed by a code for nature of adverse drug effect (manifestation).

Coding/Reporting Criteria	Clinical Criteria	
1. Physical Evaluation *(routine/expected in italics)*	• Symptoms depend on underlying disease or condition • Some symptoms can be seen in all types • Metabolic: – rapid, deep breathing (Kussmaul respirations) – hyperventilation – dyspnea – palpitations – chest pain – headache – nausea and/or vomiting – abdominal pain – diarrhea – muscle weakness – bone pain – tinnitus – visual disturbances – heart failure – confusion – lethargy – cranial nerve palsy – retinal edema – shock (severe) – death (severe)	• Respiratory – shortness of breath – anxiety – tremor – myoclonic jerks – asterixis – sleepiness – lethargy – stupor (CO_2 narcosis) – confusion – easy fatigue – papilledema • Severe acidemia (pH< 7.20) – Kussmaul respirations – lethargy – stupor – coma – seizures – ventricular tachycardia – decreased response to epinephrine – hypotension
2. Clinical Evaluation *(routine/expected in italics)*	• Testing for underlying condition can determine which tests are performed • *Arterial blood gas (ABG) analysis* • Serum electrolytes (basic metabolic panel) • Anion gap calculated • Delta gap calculated (HCO_3 equivalent) • Winter's formula for calculating compensatory changes	• Urine pH • Ketone level • Serum lactate level • Salicylate levels • Iron levels • Respiratory acidosis • Lactate acidosis: – pH < 7.36 – lactate level > 4-5 mEq/L
3. Diagnostic Px *(routine/expected in italics)*	• Chest x-ray • Imaging (kidneys, ureter, bladder) • Pulmonary function test	• Electrocardiology • Continuous pulse oximetry
4. Therapeutic Tx *(routine/expected in italics)*	• Correction of primary, underlying condition • Hemodynamic and/or respiratory support	• Use of sodium bicarbonate: small amounts are supported for very severe acidemia to maintain pH >7.20 • Alkalinizing agent
5. Increased Nursing Care and/or Monitoring	• Iatrogenic cause of underlying condition occurs postprocedure • Underlying cause/condition occurs during admission • D-Lactate acidosis: IV fluids, oral antibiotics, restriction of carbohydrates	• Thiamine therapy for total parenteral nutrition (TPN) induced lactic acidosis • Dialysis • Bronchodilator drugs • Oxygen • Noninvasive positive-pressure ventilation
6. Extends LOS	• Iatrogenic cause of underlying condition postprocedure	• Underlying cause/condition occurs during admission and delays discharge

Acidosis-Related Lab Value	Normal Arterial Range	Normal Venous Range
pH	7.35-7.45	7.31-7.41
pCO2	35-45 mmHg	41-51 mmHg
pO2	75-100 mmHg	30-40 mmHg
HCO3	22-26 mmol/L	23-29 mmol/L
O2 saturation	95-100%	60-80% (mixed venous)
Normal blood lactate	<2 mmol/L	<2mmol/L

Diagnoses

Condition	Documentation Example	ICD-10-CM Corresponding Codes
Routine/Expected/ Integral/Inherent/ Incidental*(italics only)*	1. *IP Progress Note: COPD with compensated respiratory acidosis.*	1. *Do not assign E87.29 when stated as "compensated respiratory acidosis" with COPD.*
Principal Diagnosis	1. IP Admit Note: ESRD patient admitted due to acute metabolic acidosis with maintenance dialysis.	1. Report E87.21 Acute metabolic acidosis, followed by N18.6 End-stage renal disease, and Z99.2 Dependence on renal dialysis.
Comorbidity	1. IP Discharge Summary: Acute renal failure with acute metabolic acidosis, dehydration, and urinary tract infection; acute renal failure and dehydration treated with IV hydration; urinary tract infection treated with IV antibiotics; metabolic acidosis monitored and corrected with treatment and resolution of the acute renal failure.	1. Report N17.9 Acute kidney failure, unspecified, followed by E86.Ø Dehydration; N39.Ø Urinary tract infection, site not specified; and E87.21 Acute metabolic acidosis.
Complication of Care	1. IP Progress Note: Patient developed hyperchloremic acidosis due to rapid isotonic saline infusion.	1. Report E87.2Ø Acidosis, unspecified; T8Ø.89XA Other complications following infusion, transfusion and therapeutic injection, initial encounter.
Poisoning or Adverse Effect of Medication/ Chemical	1. IP Progress Note: Acute lactic acidosis due to TPN. 2. IP Admit Note: Admitted with coma and Kussmaul respirations due to ethylene glycol poisoning suicide attempt, level 20 mg/dL by ED labs with metabolic acidosis 7.1; intubated for airway protection; IV crystalloids 250 mL/h started and Antizol IV loading dose given in ED.	1. Report E87.21 Acute metabolic acidosis, followed by T5Ø.3X5A Adverse effect of electrolyte, caloric and water-balance agents, initial encounter. 2. Report T52. 3X2A Toxic effect of glycols, intentional self-harm, initial encounter followed by R4Ø.2Ø Unspecified coma and E87.2Ø Acidosis, unspecified.

Additional References:

AHA CC: 4Q, 2022, p. 13-14; 3Q, 2020, p. 30

Acute Kidney Injury

N17.0	**Acute kidney failure with tubular necrosis**	MCC
N17.1	**Acute kidney failure with acute cortical necrosis**	MCC
N17.2	**Acute kidney failure with medullary necrosis**	MCC
N17.8	**Other acute kidney failure**	CC
N17.9	**Acute Kidney Failure, unspecified**	CC
N99.0	**Postprocedural (acute) (chronic) kidney failure**	

Associated terminology: acute kidney injury (nontraumatic); acute kidney failure, unspecified; acute post-op kidney failure; acute post-op kidney injury

Discussion

Nontraumatic acute kidney injury or impairment (AKI), also referred to as acute kidney or renal failure, is the rapid loss of kidney function within 48 hours in either pre-existing normal renal function or with pre-existing renal disease (acute on chronic). It is a syndrome of progressive kidney injury/impairment starting with RISK as an increase in absolute serum creatinine (SCr) of either ≥ 0.3 mg/dl (or a percentage increase of ≥ 50 percent or 1.5 fold from baseline) or a reduction in urine output and increases in designated stages of injury, failure and with outcomes of LOSS, and end-stage kidney disease (ESKD) or end-stage renal disease (ESRD). These stages were given the acronym RIFLE by the Acute Dialysis Quality Initiative to develop a uniformly accepted definition of AKI. Acute kidney injury is considered reversible until it progresses to the outcome of complete loss of renal function or ESRD. Treatment depends on both the underlying cause and the severity or stage of AKI.

At the present time, ICD-10-CM makes no distinction between the stages of AKI as identified by the RIFLE Classification system. AKI is classified to N17.9 Acute kidney failure, unspecified. When using the RIFLE Classification system for staging of severity, acute kidney failure represents stage III.

The Acute Kidney Injury Network (AKIN) also developed standardized clinical indicators to help diagnose AKI. The criteria involve the timing and amount of reduction in kidney function.

RIFLE Criteria (Risk, Injury, Failure, Loss, and End-stage kidney disease)

Class	GFR (Glomerular Filtration Rate)	Urine Output
Risk	↑ SCr × 1.5 or ↓ GFR >25%	<0.5 mL/kg/h × 6 h
Injury	↑ SCr × 2 or ↓ GFR >50%	<0.5 mL/kg/h × 12 h
Failure	↑ SCr × 3 or ↓ GFR >75% or if baseline SCr ≥4 mg/dL ↑ SCr >0.5 mg/dL	<0.3 mL/kg/h × 24 h or anuria × 12 h
Loss of kidney function	Complete loss of kidney function > 4 weeks	
ESRD	Complete loss of kidney function > 3 months	

AKIN Criteria (Acute Kidney Injury Network)

Stage	Serum Creatinine	Urine Output
Stage 1	↑ SCr of 0.3 mg/dL or 150% to 200% of baseline (1.5- to 2.0-fold)	<0.5 mL/kg/h × 6 h
Stage 2	↑SCr to >200%-300% of baseline (>2- to 3-fold)	<0.5 mL/kg/h × 12 h
Stage 3	↑ SCr to >300%of baseline (>3-fold) OR SCr 4.0 mg/dL with an acute rise of at least 0.5 mg/dL	<0.3 mL/kg/h × 24 h or anuria × 12 h

In 2012, a modified definition was proposed by the Kidney Disease: Improving Global Outcomes (KDIGO) AKI Workgroup, which reconciled the differences between the RIFLE and AKIN criteria. The KDIGO definition and staging system is the most current and preferred definition. KDIGO met in 2019 and discussed new advances and information for AKI definition and staging practices. At this time, however, the 2012 guidelines remain, although they may be revisited in the future.

Although these criteria cannot be used for code assignment without physician verification, presence of the criteria in the documentation ensures the appropriateness of reporting a code for AKI.

KDIGO Criteria (Kidney Disease Improving Global Outcomes)

Stage	Serum Creatinine	Urine Output
Stage 1	↑ SCr 1.5–1.9 times baseline OR ≥ 0.3 mg/dL increase	<0.5 mL/kg/h × 6 h
Stage 2	↑ SCr 2–2.9 times baseline	<0.5 mL/kg/h × 12 h
Stage 3	↑ SCr 3 times baseline OR ↑ SCr to ≥4 mg/dL OR initiation of renal replacement therapy (RRP)	<0.3 mL/kg/h × 24 h or anuria × 12 h

When acute kidney injury (AKI) is documented, if the clinical indicators for acute kidney failure are not met, clinical validators may query the provider if AKI represents "acute kidney insufficiency" (N28.9) as this is the early stage of renal impairment before it evolves into renal failure. Blood urea nitrogen (BUN) and serum creatinine values may be mildly elevated and other clinical symptoms may or may not be present or minimal. RIFLE/AKIN stages I and II represent acute kidney insufficiency, which are milder forms of impairment that do not meet clinical indicators for acute kidney failure.

If AKI is documented and the serum creatinine levels are less than 0.3 mg/L or lasts less than 24 hours, and returns to baseline with no to minor treatment, clinical validators may query for the clinical significance and note the inconsistency with clinical indicators for AKI. If not indicative of acute kidney insufficiency or acute kidney failure, the physician should be queried if the rise in creatinine represents azotemia (R79.89) or if it is integral to another condition, (i.e., hemoconcentration due to dehydration) with minimal rise in BUN/Cr ratio.

Documentation Tip

When documentation and serum creatine levels do not match, query the provider for clarification of the diagnosis.

Linking acute kidney injury to any type of nephropathy does not alter reporting N17.9 for documented AKI. Acute kidney injury/failure can occur in the presence of end-stage renal disease when caused by another condition; in such cases, both AKI/AKF and ESRD are reported.

The etiology of AKI should be documented and the link made to the underlying pathology; depending on the underlying condition, the category N17 code may be further defined. For example, if documented as acute kidney injury, meaning acute kidney failure, and is further specified as "with tubular, acute cortical or medullary necrosis," code N17.Ø, N17.1, or N17.2, respectively, would be reported.

Excluded

Posttraumatic renal failure, see T79.5-.

Traumatic kidney injury, see S37.Ø-.

The etiologies of acute kidney injury or failure are classified into three categories – pre-renal, intrinsic renal, and post-renal:

- Pre-renal: diminished blood flow to the kidneys or volume loss; oliguria
  - severe dehydration
  - shock
  - embolism
  - cardiac failure
  - hepatic failure
  - sepsis
  - excessive diuresis
  - hemorrhage
  - tense ascites
  - peritonitis
  - pancreatitis
  - burns
  - myocardial infarction
  - antihypertensive meds, NSAIDS, cyclosporine, tacrolimus, ACE inhibitors
  - anesthetics
  - renal artery obstruction/renal vein thrombosis

	

- Intrinsic/renal: diseases and disorders of the kidneys
  - acute tubular necrosis
  - SLE/glomerulonephritis
  - Sickle cell disease
  - nephrotoxins: IV iodinated radiologic contrast agents
  - renal ischemia
  - acute pyelonephritis
  - acute poststreptococcal glomerulonephritis
  - Wegener's granulomatosis
  - Goodpasture syndrome
  - acute tubulointerstitial nephritis as drug reaction
  - acute vascular nephropathy: vasculitis, malignant hypertension, systemic sclerosis
  - atheroembolism
  - infiltrative diseases: lymphoma, sarcoidosis, leukemia
- Post-renal: bilateral obstruction of urinary outflow; anuria
  - ureteral calculi
  - blood clot
  - neoplasm
  - BPH
  - urethral stricture
  - congenital defects
  - retroperitoneal fibrosis
  - ureteral trauma or surgical ureteral injury
  - phimosis
  - obstructed indwelling urinary catheter
  - anticholinergic meds
- Some of the associated conditions of AKI (acute kidney injury) are:
  - cardiac arrhythmia
  - hyperkalemia
  - acidemia
  - metabolic acidosis
  - hypernatremia
  - encephalopathy

When evaluating clinical indicators, it must be noted that when using AKIN criteria, serum creatinine (SCr) levels must represent an elevation (from baseline or seen between two creatinine levels within 48 hours) and not merely a "jump" and that this calculation is based on levels obtained after adequate fluid resuscitation, when possible. RIFLE criteria do not use these parameters. Stage is determined by whichever of the two criteria, serum creatinine (SCr) or urinary output (UO), is higher and only after meeting the criteria for AKI.

Documentation Tip

When a patient admitted with possible AKI is suspected of chronic kidney disease (CKD) with daily creatinine labs and baseline is unknown, Kidney Disease Improving Quality Outcomes (KDIGO) recommends that the lowest creatinine level reached during hospitalization be considered baseline to determine if AKI has occurred using the "1.5 times baseline" criterion. KDIGO also allows the provider to presume that the increase may have occurred within seven days. Therefore, it is appropriate to query the provider for CKD stage.

Documentation Tip

Code assignment cannot be based on ancillary test results, therapies, or clinical criteria alone. A diagnosis and its clinical significance must be supported by physician or other qualified healthcare professional documentation. When it is unclear or there is contradictory information, query the physician or other qualified healthcare professional for clarification.

Coding/Reporting Criteria	Clinical Criteria	
1. Physical Evaluation *(routine/expected in italics)*	• *Asymptomatic* • Symptoms of underlying condition • *Insufficiency*: s/s may be absent to minimal • Anorexia • Nausea/vomiting • Decreased urine output • Asterixis • Hyperreflexia • Weakness • Peripheral edema/fluid retention • Orthostasis	• Myoclonic jerks • Seizures • Confusion • Fluid overload • Uremic pericarditis – chest pain – pericardial friction rub – pericardial tamponade • Pulmonary edema – dyspnea – crackles on auscultation • Coma
2. Clinical Evaluation *(routine/expected in italics)*	• *Serum creatinine with "jump" or < 0.3 mg/L, short-term; indicating hemoconcentration of clinical dehydration* • Serum creatinine (SCr): – KDIGO - Increase of SCr by ≥0.3 mg/dl (≥26.4 µmol/L) within 48 hrs or increase 1.5–1.9 times from baseline (Stage I) - Increase of SCr by ≥0.3 mg/dl (≥26.4 µmol/L) within 48 hrs or increase 2.0–2.9 times from baseline (Stage II) - Increase of SCr ≥3.0 times from baseline or SCr ≥4.0 mg/dl (≥354 µmol/L) or treatment with RRT or in patients <18 years, decrease in estimated GFR to <35 ml/min per 1.73 m2 (Stage III) • Urine output (UO): – KDIGO - I. UO < 0.5 ml/kg/hr for 6–12 hours - II. UO < 0.5 ml/kg/hr for ≥ 12 hours - III. UO < 0.3 ml/kg/hr for ≥ 24 hours (oliguria) or anuria for ≥ 12 hours	• Serum BUN/Cr ratio > 20/1 • FENa < 1 (Fractional excretion of sodium) (< 1 prerenal; > 3 ATN) • GFR • Urinary sediment, protein, blood, casts • Urine: specific gravity > 1.018, osmolarity (> 500) • CBC • Electrolytes • Urine Na concentration > 20 • Postvoid residual bladder volume (postrenal cause suspected) • Peripheral smear • Fractional excretion of sodium and urea • Biomarkers (future)
3. Diagnostic Px *(routine/expected in italics)*	• Urine output < 500 mL/day • Kidney biopsy • EKG • Renal scan	• Ultrasound of kidney • KUB • IV pyelogram • Renal arteriography
4. Therapeutic Tx *(routine/expected in italics)*	• Oral hydration • IV hydration	• Dialysis
5. Increased Nursing Care and/or Monitoring	• Develops AKI postadmit	
6. Extends LOS	• AKI delays discharge	• Discharge delayed due to postprocedure AKI

Renal-Related Lab Value	Normal Range
GFR	90 – 120 ml/min
Serum Cr	0.5 – 1.1 mg/dL (females) 0.6 – 1.2 mg/dL (males)
BUN	5 – 20 mg/dL
Albumin	3.5 – 5.5 g/dL
Calcium	8.5 – 10.5 mg/dL
Phosphorus	2.5 – 4.5 mg/dL
Potassium	3.5 – 5.2 mEq/L
Sodium	135 - 145 mEq/L

Condition	Documentation Example	ICD-10-CM Corresponding Codes
Routine/Expected/ Integral/Inherent/ Incidental *(italics only)*	1. *IP Admit Note: Admitted due to persistent vomiting x two days; requires workup; mild dehydration with mild AKI; BUN/Cr is 30/1.3 with baseline creatinine 0.9, push fluid intake.* **(Query clinical significance of BUN/creatinine increase and if AKI represents acute kidney failure, acute kidney insufficiency, azotemia or hemoconcentration of dehydration.)**	*NA*
Principal Diagnosis	1. IP Discharge Summary: AKI due to bladder neck obstruction associated with BPH. Treated with dialysis.	1. Principal diagnosis is that condition established after study to be chiefly responsible for occasioning the admission of the patient to the hospital for care.
Comorbidity	1. IP Discharge Summary: Final diagnosis: AKI due to SLE nephritis. 2. IP Admit Note: Admit due to AKI, decompensated HF from noncompliance in ESRD by missing dialysis appointment, perform dialysis today.	1. Linking acute kidney injury to any type of nephropathy does not alter reporting N17.9 for documented AKI. 2. When two or more diagnoses equally meet the definition of principal diagnosis, any one of the diagnoses may be sequenced first.
Complication of Care	1. IP Discharge Summary: Discharge was delayed due to post on-pump CABG induced AKI with stage 4 chronic kidney disease. 2. IP Admit Note: Admit due to AKI from renal artery thrombosis, s/p kidney transplant (affecting the function of the transplanted organ).	1. Report by sequencing postprocedure (acute) (chronic) kidney failure N99.Ø before an additional code for type of kidney disease. 2. Report complication resulting from surgery or other medical care. Sequence complication code first followed by additional code to specify nature of complication if not included in complication code. For complications in T8Ø–T88 range, follow with a code for the specific complication.
Poisoning or Adverse Effect of Medication/ Chemical	1. IP Progress Note: AKI due to contrast dye following IV pyelogram (adverse effect)	1. Report result of adverse effect: AKI (N17.9), N14.11 for contrast induced nephropathy, followed by the adverse effect code from categories T36–T5Ø.

Additional References

AHA CC: 3Q, 2021, p. 10; 3Q, 2020, p. 22

Acute Kidney Injury Network (AKIN) and Risk, Injury, Failure, Loss of kidney function, and End-stage kidney disease (RIFLE): https://www.ncbi.nlm.nih.gov/pmc/articles/PMC5094385/

Kidney Disease Improving Quality Outcomes (KDIGO): www.kdigo.org

Diagnoses

Acute Myocardial Infarction

I21.Ø-	**ST elevation (STEMI) myocardial infarction of anterior wall (left main coronary artery, left anterior descending, other)**	MCC HCC
I21.1-	**ST elevation (STEMI) myocardial infarction of inferior wall (right coronary artery, other)**	MCC HCC
I21.2-	**ST elevation (STEMI) myocardial infarction of other sites (left circumflex coronary artery, other)**	MCC HCC
I21.3	**ST elevation (STEMI) myocardial infarction of unspecified site**	MCC HCC
I21.4	**Non-ST elevation (NSTEMI) myocardial infarction**	MCC HCC
I21.9	**Acute myocardial infarction, unspecified**	MCC HCC
I21.A-	**Other type of myocardial infarction (type 2, 3, 4 and 5)**	MCC HCC
I21.B	**Myocardial infarction with coronary microvascular dysfunction**	MCC HCC
I22-	**Subsequent ST elevation (STEMI) and non-ST elevation (NSTEMI) myocardial infarction**	MCC HCC
I25.2	**Old myocardial infarction**	
I5A	**Non-ischemic myocardial injury (non-traumatic)**	CC

Associated terminology: cardiac infarction, coronary artery embolism/occlusion/rupture/ thrombosis, ST segment elevation myocardial infarction (STEMI), non-ST segment elevation myocardial infarction (NSTEMI), acute Q wave infarction, acute transmural infarction, non-Q wave myocardial infarction, acute subendocardial infarction, type 2 due to demand ischemia, myocardial infarction with coronary microvascular disease, myocardial infarction with nonobstructive coronary arteries (MINOCA) with microvascular disease, non-ischemic myocardial infarction (non-traumatic)

Discussion

An acute myocardial infarction (AMI) occurs when the blood supply to the cardiac muscle is diminished or limited. The decreased blood supply leads to ischemia, which progresses to an oxygen shortage and irreversible damage and/or death to the cardiac muscle tissue. This damage and death of tissue is considered the infarction. An infarction may be further specified by the area of the cardiac muscle that is damaged, such as the following:

- Anterior wall
- Inferior wall
- Lateral wall
- Posterior wall
- Septal

The clinical condition of an acute myocardial infarction in ICD-10-CM is mainly divided into two subcategories: ST elevation and non-ST elevation. This distinction is made based on ECG changes. The ST segment of an ECG tracing relates to ventricle systolic depolarization. When cardiac muscle is damaged, the electrical properties change, thus changing the ST segment of the ECG. It is important to note that acute myocardial infarction is not the most common cause of ST elevation in patients presenting with chest pain. Therefore, other clinical factors must be present and correlate with a diagnosis of STEMI.

In addition to the ECG changes, further information may classify the AMI based on pathology. In cases where the ECG tracings show ST elevation and Q waves, this indicates a transmural infarction and is usually a result of complete loss of blood supply involving a major coronary artery. Transmural infarctions usually extend through the entire affected cardiac muscle. Where there is an ST depression on an ECG tracing, this may indicate a subendocardial infarction, which involves a small area of the left ventricle, ventricular septum, or papillary muscles that is especially predisposed to ischemia.

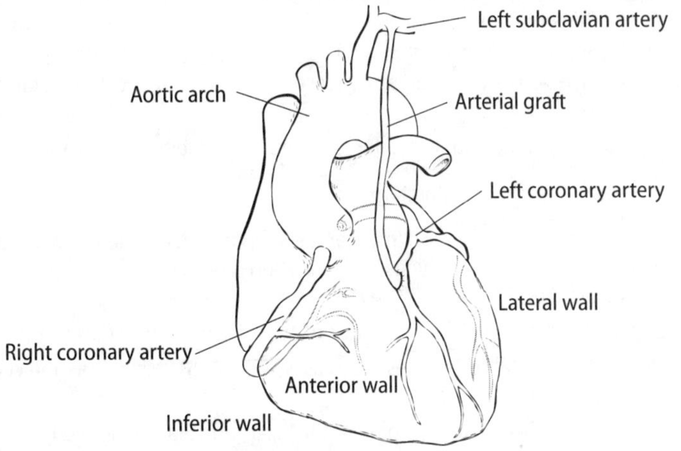

Documentation Tip

When reviewing charts for diagnosed or possible AMI:

- **Clarify whether documentation of demand ischemia is actually referring to a type 2 myocardial infarction. If type 2 MI is present, obtain specification of underlying cause, which is sequenced before the type 2 MI code.**
- **Review documentation for acute MI when acute coronary syndrome or unstable angina is diagnosed.**
- **For best practice, documentation of type 1 STEMI should identify the specific site of the left or right coronary artery.**
- **Documentation of cardiac or myocardial injury does not equate to an acute MI. Although ICD-10-CM categorizes "myocardial injury" as either myocardial (acute) (chronic) (nonischemic) (nontraumatic) or traumatic, with the instruction to "see Injury, heart," the new fourth universal definition of cardiac injury is a troponin elevation only without the other symptoms or criteria for an acute MI. In any case, neither traumatic cardiac injury nor non-MI troponin elevation secondary to a nonischemic cause (i.e., nonischemic myocardial injury) is reported with acute myocardial infarction codes. If an AMI is suspected, appropriate documentation must be obtained.**

Coding Tip

Code I21.B Myocardial infarction with coronary microvascular dysfunction also reports myocardial infarction with coronary microvascular disease and myocardial infarction with nonobstructive coronary arteries (MINOCA) with microvascular disease. Coronary microvascular dysfunction (CMD) is defined as small vessel disease that affects the walls and inner lining of microscopic coronary artery blood vessels; plaque is absent, but inner wall damage can cause spasms and decreased blood flow.

AMI not specified as STEMI or NSTEMI:

- Nonsubendocardial and transmural: report as type 1 STEMI by site or unspecified site (I21.0-, I21.1-, I21.2-, I21.3).
- Subendocardial and nontransmural: report as type 1 NSTEMI (I21.4).
- If an AMI is documented as nontransmural or subendocardial, but the site is provided, it is still coded as a subendocardial type 1 NSTEMI (I21.4).
- Code I21.3 ST elevation (STEMI) myocardial infarction, unspecified site, is assigned when the myocardial site of the type 1 infarction is not specified.
- Acute myocardial infarctions specified by site (except for subendocardial and non-transmural), but not specified as STEMI or non-STEMI, should be coded to acute MI type 1 STEMI by site.
- Code I21.9 Acute myocardial infarction, unspecified, is the default for unspecified acute myocardial infarction or unspecified type.

The etiology of an acute myocardial infarction is classified into five main types:

- **Type 1:** Spontaneous due to occlusion (i.e., atherosclerosis, plaque, etc.)
- **Type 2:** Ischemia due to increased oxygen demand or decreased oxygen supply (i.e., spasm, embolism, arrhythmias, etc.)
- **Type 3:** Unexpected cardiac death/cardiac arrest
- **Type 4:** Associated with coronary angioplasty
  - 4a: Percutaneous cardiac intervention
  - 4b: Stent thrombosis (identified during angiography or autopsy)
  - 4c: Myocardial infarction due to restenosis ≥50 percent after an initially successful percutaneous coronary intervention (PCI)
- **Type 5:** Associated with procedures on the heart itself (not stent) such as coronary artery bypass graft (CABG).

Other types of myocardial infarction:

- Type 2 myocardial infarction (myocardial infarction due to demand ischemia or secondary to ischemic imbalance), is assigned to code I21.A1 Myocardial infarction type 2. A code for the underlying cause of the imbalance is sequenced ***before*** the type 2 MI code (I21.A1).
- Do not assign code I24.8 Other forms of acute ischemic heart disease, for the demand ischemia if MI is documented.
- When a type 2 AMI code is described as NSTEMI or STEMI, only assign code I21.A1. Codes I21.01–I21.4 should only be assigned for type 1 AMIs.
- Acute myocardial infarctions type 3, 4a, 4b, 4c, and 5 are assigned to code I21.A9 Other myocardial infarction type.
- Myocardial infarction with coronary microvascular disease or myocardial infarction with nonobstructive coronary arteries (MINOCA) with microvascular disease is assigned to code I21.B Myocardial infarction with coronary microvascular dysfunction.
- The "Code also" and "Code first" notes should be followed related to complications, and for coding of postprocedural myocardial infarctions during or following cardiac surgery.

Coding Tip

Guideline I.C.9.e.1: "If a type 1 NSTEMI evolves to STEMI, assign the STEMI code. If a type 1 STEMI converts to NSTEMI due to thrombolytic therapy, it is still coded as STEMI."

When a myocardial infarction occurs without chest pain or any other symptoms, this is coined a "silent" MI. It is estimated that at least a quarter of myocardial infarctions are silent. Usually a silent MI is diagnosed using blood enzymes (troponins and CK-MB [creatine kinase]) or on autopsy, but many times it goes undiagnosed until revealed later on an electrocardiogram. When a myocardial infarction is found on ECG and the physician discusses its clinical significance and the patient is having no symptoms, code I25.2 Old myocardial infarction, is reported. This type of infarction is more prevalent in the elderly, diabetics, and heart transplant recipients.

Certain factors predispose people to having an acute myocardial infarction. Many of these factors are able to be modified and/or removed from a patient's daily activity or habits, thereby making infarctions preventable in many situations. Those risk factors that have an ICD-10-CM code should be reported. Some of the more avoidable risk factors are:

- Alcohol
- Obesity
- Oral contraceptive pills
- Sedentary lifestyle
- Tobacco smoking including secondhand smoke

Less avoidable but able to be controlled or maintained with proper medical advice and treatment:

- Coronary artery disease (CAD), atherosclerosis, or arteriosclerosis
- Diabetes mellitus
- Dyslipidemia/hyperlipidemia/hypercholesterolemia
- Hypertension or high blood pressure

Unchangeable risk factors:

- Age
- Air pollution exposure
- Family history of ischemic heart disease
- Gender (males are more at risk)
- Psychosocial factors (socioeconomic factors)

The World Health Organization (WHO) released guidelines that streamline the diagnosis of an acute myocardial infarction. Originally published in 1979, a revision emphasizing the importance of cardiac biomarkers in the formula was released in 2000. In 2018, the Joint Task Force of The European Society of Cardiology (ESC), American College of Cardiology Foundation (ACCF), The American Heart Association (AHA), and the World Heart Federation (WHF) redefined the universal definition of the diagnosis of an MI. This definition states that the term myocardial infarction is used when there is clinical evidence of acute myocardial ischemia and includes detection of a rise and/or fall of cardiac troponin (cTn) with at least one value above the 99th percentile and with at least one of the following:

- Symptoms of acute myocardial ischemia
- New ischemic electrocardiographic (ECG) changes
- Development of pathological Q waves
- Imaging evidence of new loss of viable myocardium or new regional wall motion abnormality in a pattern consistent with an ischemic etiology
- Identification of a coronary thrombus by angiography including intracoronary imaging or by autopsy (not for type 2 MI)
- Type 2 adds evidence of an imbalance between myocardial oxygen supply and demand

Coding Tip

When a subsequent type 1 acute MI occurs within 28 days of a prior type 1 or unspecified acute MI, the category I22 code must always be accompanied by a category I21 code with sequencing dependent upon the circumstances of the admission.

Do not assign code I22 for subsequent myocardial infarctions other than type 1 or unspecified. For subsequent type 2 AMI, assign only code I21.A1. For subsequent type 4 or type 5 AMI, assign only code I21.A9. If a subsequent myocardial infarction of one type (e.g., type 2) occurs within 28 days of an MI of a different type (e.g., type 1, NSTEMI) assign the appropriate codes from category I21 to identify each type. Do not use codes from I22.

Coding Tip

Complications of an AMI may occur immediately after the infarction to months or years later. If a complication arises in the 28 days after the infarction, a code from category I23 Certain current complications following ST elevation (STEMI) and non-ST elevation (NSTEMI) myocardial infarction (within the 28 day period), should be assigned in conjunction with a code from category I21 Acute myocardial infarction, or I22 Subsequent ST elevation (STEMI) and non-ST elevation (NSTEMI) myocardial infarction. Sequencing is dependent on the circumstances of the admission.

Coding/Reporting Criteria	Clinical Criteria	
1. Physical Evaluation *(routine/expected in italics)*	• *Asymptomatic* • Chest pain/angina • Shortness of breath (SOB) • Nausea • Vomiting • Palpitations • Diaphoresis • Anxiety	• Generalized weakness • Heartburn/indigestion • Left arm, lower jaw, neck, right arm, epigastric or back pain • Fatigue • Levine's sign • Lightheadedness • Loss of consciousness
2. Clinical Evaluation *(routine/expected in italics)*	• Laboratory tests – CK-MB – Troponin	
3. Diagnostic Px *(routine/expected in italics)*	• *ECG evidence only, asymptomatic* • ECG • Echocardiography • Cardiac MRI	• MIBI (methoxyisobutylisonitrile) scan (Technetium [Tc99m] sestamibi) • Cardiac catheterization with angiography
4. Therapeutic Tx *(routine/expected italics)*	• Percutaneous coronary intervention (PCI)/Cardiac catheterization • Coronary artery bypass (CABG) • Oxygen • Aspirin	• Sublingual nitroglycerin • Reperfusion therapy • Thrombolysis • Platelet inhibitor
5. Increased Nursing Care and/or Monitoring	• Occurred after admission	
6. Extends LOS	• AMI delays discharge	

Condition	Documentation Example	ICD-10-CM Corresponding Codes
Routine/Expected/ Integral/Inherent/ Incidental *(italics only)*	1. *Discharge Summary: Incidental finding of MI of indeterminate age on ECG, no symptoms.*	1. *Incidental findings are not reported without physician documentation of clinical significance. If the documentation is unclear, the provider or other qualified healthcare professional should be queried for clarification. If the physician documents this as clinically significant, report I25.2 Old myocardial infarction.*
Principal Diagnosis	1. History and Physical: Patient with known history of coronary artery disease (CAD) presents with unstable angina and diaphoresis; ST elevations on ECG; aspirin, sublingual nitroglycerine and beta blocker given in ED; admit for STEMI of the anterior wall. 2. Patient admitted with type 2 MI due to persistent atrial fibrillation.	1. Report I21.Ø9 ST elevation (STEMI) myocardial infarction involving other coronary artery of anterior wall, followed by I25.11Ø Atherosclerotic heart disease of native coronary artery with unstable angina pectoris. 2. According to guideline I.C.9.e.5 and the coding instruction at I21.A1, report I48.19 Other persistent atrial fibrillation, followed by the code I21.A1 Myocardial infarction type 2.
Comorbidity	1. History and Physical: Admitted for severe HF four days after being discharged for an AMI against medical advice. **(Query type of heart failure, systolic, diastolic or combined; query type and site of AMI.)**	1. Report I5Ø.9 Heart failure, unspecified, followed by I21.9 Acute myocardial infarction, unspecified.
Complication of Care	1. Discharge Summary: Acute inferior myocardial infarction due to coronary stent thrombosis. 2. Operative Note: Admitted for cardiac catheterization for refractory angina complicated intraoperatively by AMI of left descending artery due to the procedure.	1. Report T82.867A Thrombosis due to cardiac prosthetic devices, implants and grafts, initial encounter, followed by I21.A9 Other myocardial infarction type. AMI due to stent thrombosis is considered a type 4b MI regardless of whether the site is documented. 2. Report I2Ø.2 Refractory angina pectoris, followed by I97.79Ø Other intraoperative cardiac functional disturbances during cardiac surgery, and I21.A9 Other myocardial infarction type. AMI due to percutaneous cardiac intervention is considered a type 4a MI regardless of whether the site is documented.
Poisoning or Adverse Effect of Medication/ Chemical	1. ED: Cocaine-induced AMI, type 3, recreational use, patient DOA.	1. Report T4Ø.5X1A Poisoning by cocaine, accidental (unintentional), initial encounter, followed by I21.A9 Other myocardial infarction type.

Additional References

AHA CC: 1Q, 2024, p. 28; 4Q, 2023, p. 25; 2Q, 2023, p. 29; 4Q, 2022, p. 61, 66; 4Q, 2021, p. 14; 3Q, 2021, p. 6; 3Q, 2020, p. 32; 2Q, 2019, p. 6, 32; 4Q, 2018, p. 6, 57; 3Q, 2018, p. 5; 4Q, 2017, p. 12; 2Q, 2017, p. 11; 1Q, 2017, p. 44, 45; 4Q, 2016, p. 26, 60, 140; 2Q, 2015, p. 16

https://www.acc.org/latest-in-cardiology/articles/2018/08/24/14/26/fourth-universal-definition-of-mi-released-esc-2018

Acute Pulmonary Edema, Noncardiogenic

J68.1	**Pulmonary edema due to chemicals, gases, fumes and vapors**	MCC HCC
J7Ø.Ø	**Acute pulmonary manifestations due to radiation**	CC
J7Ø.8	**Respiratory conditions due to other specified external agents**	
J7Ø.9	**Respiratory conditions due to unspecified external agent**	
J8Ø	**Acute respiratory distress syndrome**	MCC HCC
J81.Ø	**Acute pulmonary edema**	MCC HCC
J95.84	**Transfusion-related acute lung injury (TRALI)**	CC
T7Ø.29XA	**Other effects of high altitude, initial encounter**	
T75.1XXA	**Unspecified effects of drowning and nonfatal submersion, initial encounter**	CC HAC

Associated terminology: acute pulmonary edema due to fluid overload, acute edema of lung, chemical pulmonary edema, radiation pneumonitis with acute pulmonary edema, near drowning with acute pulmonary edema, effects of high altitude with pulmonary edema (HAPE), acute respiratory distress syndrome (ARDS), adult hyaline membrane disease

Discussion

Acute pulmonary edema develops suddenly due to direct injury to the lung or injury mediated by high pressures within the pulmonary circulation; it can become life threatening. It is a buildup of fluid and protein in the alveoli caused by the fluid suddenly shifting from the pulmonary blood vessels into the lung. This leads to decreased oxygen transfer, hypoxemia, and respiratory distress.

There are conditions in which acute pulmonary edema (J81.Ø) is integral and not assigned as an additional code (i.e., ARDS, transfusion-related acute lung injury [TRALI]) and codes from categories J6Ø–J7Ø Lung diseases due to external agents.

Conditions in which acute (noncardiogenic) pulmonary edema would be assigned as an additional code include kidney disease with acute pulmonary edema, acute pulmonary edema as a postoperative complication, smoke inhalation and lung infection, sepsis or certain viral infections, and neurogenic pulmonary edema.

As an adverse effect of medication, acute pulmonary edema would be sequenced first; as a manifestation of drug overdose or poisoning it would be sequenced after a code from categories T36–T5Ø Poisoning by, adverse effects of, and underdosing of drugs, medicaments and biological substances, identifying the drug.

Coding and Documentation Tip

Acute pulmonary edema is also frequently documented as flash pulmonary edema. Assign code J81.Ø Acute pulmonary edema, for flash pulmonary edema.

When due to inhalation of gases, fumes, or vapors, the code for pulmonary edema (J68.1) should follow a code from categories T51–T65 Toxic effects of substances nonmedicinal as to source.

Acute pulmonary edema due to (near) drowning indexes to T75.1 Unspecified effects of drowning and nonfatal submersion. But special attention should be paid to the Excludes 1 note stating "specified effects of drowning-code to effects." Additionally, note that category J81 Pulmonary edema does not have an Excludes1 note for subcategory T75.1. Verify the accuracy of the alphabetic index-selected code with the tabular list, including following all notes. If it is understood that acute pulmonary edema is integral to T75.1 and, therefore, not considered an effect, then report T75.1 *without* J81.Ø for acute pulmonary edema due to near drowning.

Documentation Tip

Acute respiratory distress (RØ6.ØØ) and acute respiratory distress syndrome (ARDS) (J8Ø) are reported with two different codes. Accurate documentation is vital for proper code assignment and may affect treatment. ARDS generally occurs in critically ill patients and is often associated with sepsis and shock.

Coding/Reporting Criteria	Clinical Criteria
1. Physical Evaluation *(routine/expected in italics)*	• End-inspiratory crackles on auscultation • Shortness of breath on exertion/severe respiratory distress/dyspnea • Sudden respiratory distress after sleep • Difficulty breathing when prone • Coughing • Bubbly, wheezing or gasping sound when breathing • Severe acute pulmonary edema: – labored and rapid breathing – frothy, bloody fluid containing pus in sputum – fast pulse – possible cardiac dysrhythmia – cold, clammy, sweaty, and bluish skin – severe drop in blood pressure with thready pulse • Headache • Distended neck veins; raised jugular venous pressure • Can lead to ARDS • Can lead to cardiac arrest
2. Clinical Evaluation *(routine/expected in italics)*	• ABGs — usually show hypoxia and PCO_2 can be variable • CBC • Metabolic profile
3. Diagnostic Px *(routine/expected in italics)*	• Chest x-ray: patchy alveolar infiltrates; air space opacification; air bronchograms; lung white out with centrally positioned trachea • Pulmonary artery catheterization (Swan-Ganz): wedge pressure < 18 mmHg usually indicates noncardiogenic edema; to r/o ARDS • Pulmonary function tests
4. Therapeutic Tx *(routine/expected in italics)*	• Treatment is focused on both pulmonary edema and underlying cause • Upright position • Oxygen • Vent • Drug therapy: diuresis; nesiritide when resistant to standard-of-care therapies • Dialysis • IV nitrates • HBO: smoke inhalation • Prevention: High altitude: dexamethasone, sildenafil, Diamox, acetazolamide • Bronchodilators
5. Increased Nursing Care and/or Monitoring	• Acute pulmonary edema postadmit as an adverse effect of medication
6. Extends LOS	• Postoperative acute pulmonary edema

Condition	Documentation Example	ICD-10-CM Corresponding Codes
Routine/Expected/ Integral/Inherent/ Incidental *(italics only)*	*NA*	*NA*
Principal Diagnosis	1. IP Admit Note: Patient with morbid obesity, obstructive sleep apnea, admitted with acute noncardiogenic pulmonary edema with fluid overload due to dietary and medication noncompliance, intentional, due to financial hardship. 2. IP Discharge Summary: Smoke Inhalation with acute pulmonary edema.	1. Report J81.Ø Acute pulmonary edema, followed by E87.79 Other fluid overload; E66.Ø1 Morbid (severe) obesity due to excess calories; G47.33 Obstructive sleep apnea (adult) (pediatric); Z91.11Ø Patient's noncompliance with dietary regimen due to financial hardship; Z91.12Ø Patient's intentional underdosing of medication regimen due to financial hardship. 2. Report code J7Ø.5 Respiratory conditions due to smoke inhalation only, as the pulmonary edema is integral to the smoke inhalation.
Comorbidity	1. IP Admit Note: End-stage renal patient admitted with acute kidney failure, fluid overload and pulmonary congestion due to dialysis noncompliance. **(Query: If the pulmonary congestion can be further specified as acute or chronic; Query: Is the pulmonary congestion an indication of pulmonary edema, pneumonia, HF, other (specify) or unknown.)**	1. Report N17.9 Acute kidney failure, unspecified, followed by N18.6 End-stage renal disease; Z99.2 Dependence on renal dialysis; E87.79 Other fluid overload; RØ9.89 Other specified symptoms and signs involving the circulatory and respiratory systems; Z91.15 Patient's noncompliance with renal dialysis; if the query response is acute pulmonary edema, replace RØ9.89 with J81.Ø Acute pulmonary edema.
Complication of Care	1. IP Progress Note: Post extubation from surgery, patient experienced laryngospasm and was monitored, within two hours patient began coughing with respiratory distress; workup revealed acute negative pressure pulmonary edema related to extubation.	1. Report J95.89 Other postprocedural complications and disorders of respiratory system, not elsewhere classified, followed by J81.Ø Acute pulmonary edema.
Poisoning or Adverse Effect of Medication/ Chemical	1. IP Admit Note: A 60-year-old female patient took her HydroDIURIL for hypertension as prescribed, but within 15 minutes she experienced dyspnea and nausea/vomiting. Workup showed acute pulmonary edema, noncardiogenic, due to med. 2. IP Discharge Summary: Narcotic overdose, undetermined intent, with acute pulmonary edema, noncardiogenic.	1. Report J81.Ø Acute pulmonary edema, followed by T5Ø.2X5A Adverse effect of carbonic-anhydrase inhibitors, benzothiadiazides and other diuretics, initial encounter) and I10 Essential (primary) hypertension. 2. Report T4Ø.6Ø4A Poisoning by unspecified narcotics, undetermined, initial encounter, followed by J81.Ø Acute pulmonary edema.

Additional References

AHA CC: 1Q, 2023, p. 25; 4Q, 2020, p. 96; 3Q, 2020, p. 27; 1Q, 2017, p. 26

Anesthesia and Analgesia, June 1999: http://journals.lww.com/anesthesia-analgesia/Pages/issuelist.aspx

The Annals of Pharmacotherapy, 2016, archives: http://aop.sagepub.com

AIDS

B2Ø Human immunodeficiency virus [HIV] disease CC HCC

Associated terminology: AIDS, AIDS-related complex (ARC), HIV with AIDS defining illness

Diagnoses

Discussion

Acquired immunodeficiency syndrome (AIDS) is the final stage of human immunodeficiency virus (HIV) infection, stage 4 by World Health Organization (WHO) criteria (2007) and stage 3 by Centers for Disease Control and Prevention (CDC) (2008) criteria or clinical categories B or C (CDC). HIV is a retrovirus that destroys the immune system, disabling the body's ability to fight infections and causing some lymphomas and other malignancies. Clinically, AIDS is confirmed HIV infection with a CD4 count less than 200μL *or* confirmed HIV infection with certain opportunistic conditions known as "AIDS defining," as identified by the CDC.

Transmission is through contact with infected body fluids of blood, semen, vaginal secretions, breast milk, wounds, or skin and mucosal lesions. Contact is made by sexual intercourse, sharing needles, childbirth, breastfeeding, or medical procedures/situations that expose patient or employee to contamination. Testing of donated blood decreases the possibility of viral transmission through transfusion. However, risk is still present due to incorrect reporting of risk factors by donors, as well as blood donation during the "eclipse" period, an acute initial infection period of 10 to 15 days from contact during which the virus is undetectable by testing. Conditions that affect transmission are open wounds, mucosal inflammation, gonorrhea, chlamydia, trichomoniasis, chancroid, herpes, and syphilis.

There is no recognized cure for AIDS, although many medical breakthroughs have been made. Treatment consists of controlling the disease using combinations of five classes of antiretroviral drugs to block its reproduction. The intent of highly active antiretroviral therapy (HAART) is to reduce the plasma HIV RNA levels and to restore the CD4 count. This immune restoration, even when small, may improve outcomes by lessening opportunistic infections, other complications, and cancers. Sometimes after beginning HAART, patients experience serious reactions known as immune reconstitution inflammatory syndrome (IRIS) or immune recovery syndrome (D89.3 Immune reconstitution syndrome). This immune reaction to subclinical infections or antigens post-treatment can range from self-limiting conditions and those that respond to treatment with brief regimens of corticosteroids to fatal if due to cryptococcal meningitis.

Coding and Documentation Tip

Code B2Ø Human immunodeficiency virus [HIV] disease, may be reported only when provider documentation and/or the alphabetic index supports the coding of this condition, including cases for which:

- **AIDS or HIV disease is documented**
- **Treatment is being rendered for a documented HIV-related illness**
- **The patient is documented as having a condition(s) resulting from the patient's HIV status**
- **The patient is documented as having a history of HIV disease, HIV-related illness, or AIDS, and is maintained on antiretroviral medications**

Presence of a condition from CDC's AIDS-Defining Conditions or from MS-DRG MDC 25 alone is not sufficient to code B2Ø Human immunodeficiency virus [HIV] disease, without documentation from the provider that the patient has AIDS or an HIV-related illness.

A prior diagnosis of an AIDS defining condition is assigned as B2Ø. Once meeting AIDS criteria, the patient will always be assigned as B2Ø on every subsequent admission/encounter, allowing that it is documented within that record.

AIDS will be sequenced as the principal diagnosis when it is the reason for the admission/encounter or an AIDS-related condition is responsible for the admission/encounter.

AIDS will be sequenced as comorbidity or as an additional diagnosis when the reason for the encounter/admission is for a non-related condition and the patient has a confirmed diagnosis of AIDS.

AIDS can be a complication due to a misadventure or due to medical care.

Documentation Tip

Ensure that the patient's HIV status is clearly documented. Examine the record carefully, as terms such as "HIV positive," "known HIV," or "HIV test positive" refer to the patients' asymptomatic human immunodeficiency virus (HIV) status (code Z21) and do not mean the patient has AIDS.

Coding Tip

CDC's AIDS-defining conditions that classify HIV+ as AIDS (must have laboratory-confirmed HIV infection): Appendix A: http://www.cdc.gov/mmwr/preview/mmwrhtml/rr5710a2.htm

- **Bacterial infections, multiple or recurrent (in children <13 years)**
- **Candidiasis of esophagus, bronchi, trachea, or lungs**
- **Cervical cancer, invasive among adults and adolescents ≥ 13 years**
- **Coccidioidomycosis, disseminated or extrapulmonary**
- **Cryptococcosis, extrapulmonary**
- **Cryptosporidiosis, chronic intestinal (>1 month's duration)**
- **Cytomegalovirus disease (other than liver, spleen, or nodes), onset at age >1 month**
- **Cytomegalovirus retinitis (with loss of vision)**
- **Encephalopathy, HIV related**
- **Herpes simplex: chronic ulcers (>1 month's duration) or bronchitis, pneumonitis, or esophagitis (onset at age >1 month)**
- **Histoplasmosis, disseminated or extrapulmonary**
- **Isosporiasis, chronic intestinal (>1 month's duration)**
- **Kaposi sarcoma**
- **Lymphoid interstitial pneumonia or pulmonary lymphoid hyperplasia complex in children <13 years**
- **Lymphoma, Burkitt (or equivalent term), immunoblastic (or equivalent term), or primary of brain**
- ***Mycobacterium avium* complex or *Mycobacterium kansasii*, disseminated or extrapulmonary**
- ***Mycobacterium tuberculosis* of any site, pulmonary (Only among adults and adolescents aged ≥13 years), disseminated, or extrapulmonary**
- ***Mycobacterium*, other species or unidentified species, disseminated or extrapulmonary**
- ***Pneumocystis jiroveci* pneumonia (PJP) (formerly: *P. carinii* pneumonia [PCP])**
- **Pneumonia, recurrent (Only among adults and adolescents aged ≥ 13 years)**
- **Progressive multifocal leukoencephalopathy (PML), a demyelinating disease due to JC virus (human polyomavirus formerly known as papovavirus)**
- ***Salmonella* septicemia, recurrent**
- **Toxoplasmosis of brain, onset at age >1 month**
- **Wasting syndrome attributed to HIV (involuntary loss of 10% of body weight, chronic diarrhea, chronic weakness and fever)**

Symptoms and signs of AIDS include HIV infection, the associated conditions including complications of treatment and AIDS defining conditions. The list of the CDC's AIDS-defining conditions can be seen in the table above. The Centers for Medicare and Medicaid Services' Major Diagnostic Category (MDC) 25 also includes a list of diagnostic ICD-10-CM codes representing major HIV-related diagnoses. *The Merck Manual* and the AIDS Education and Training Centers (AETC) National Resource Center were consulted to compile the following list of associated conditions and complications. Please note that this list is not all inclusive:

- Adverse effects of antiretroviral medications: patient should be screened for anemia, pancreatitis, hepatitis, glucose intolerance, hyperlipidemia
- Anemia of chronic disease and/or due to treatment; autoimmune hemolytic anemia
- Anorexia
- Bacillary angiomatosis
- Cachexia (with temporal wasting)
- Hairy leukoplakia of the tongue
- HIV associated nephropathy (HIV AN)
- Hypersensitivity reaction to medications
- Immune reconstitution inflammatory syndrome (IRIS) or immune recovery syndrome
- Leukopenia
- Neurological complications
- Osteonecrosis
- Osteopenia
- Osteoporosis
- Pancytopenia
- Redistribution of fat/lipodystrophy (adverse effect of meds)
- Thrombocytopenia
- Thrush

Diagnoses

Coding Tip

Code assignment cannot be based on ancillary test results, therapies, or clinical criteria alone. A diagnosis and its clinical significance must be supported by physician or other qualified healthcare professional documentation. When it is unclear or there is contradictory information, query the physician or other qualified healthcare professional for clarification.

Coding/Reporting Criteria	Clinical Criteria	
1. Physical Evaluation *(routine/expected in italics)*	• AIDS-defining conditions • Associated conditions (i.e., anemia of chronic disease) • Blurred and distorted vision • Chronic diarrhea • Cough and shortness of breath • Headaches • Lymphadenopathy	• Persistent, unexplained fatigue • Persistent white spots or unusual lesions on tongue/mouth • Shaking chills or fever > 100 F (38 C) for several weeks • Skin rashes • Soaking night sweats • Weight loss
2. Clinical Evaluation *(routine/expected in italics)*	• Positive result from reactive enzyme immunoassay (EIA) test with confirmation by a positive result from a supplemental HIV antibody test (Western Blot or indirect immunofluorescence assay test) **or** • Positive result of a detectable quantity from any of the following: – HIV nucleic detection test (PCR) for HIV RNA – HIV p24 antigen test, including neutralization assay – HIV isolation (viral culture) – bDNA • *Baseline CD4+T lymphocyte cell count less than 200 µl (<200 cells/mm3 or CD4%<14%) (*AIDS diagnosis still stands when treatment results in rise in CD4 count above 200 µl) • CSF analysis: evaluation of associated conditions or some AIDS defining conditions • ELISA: enzyme-linked immunosorbent assay • *HIV+ that is symptomatic, meaning the patient currently or has been in the past, diagnosed with an AIDS-defining condition ("with" or "due to")(*AIDS-defining condition supersedes CD4 count) • HIV+ with pulmonary tuberculosis	• HIV+ with two occurrences of bacterial pneumonia within a 12-month period (x2/1 yr) • HIV+ woman with invasive cervical cancer • Immunochromatography with confirmation test • Immunoconcentration with confirmation test • Laboratory-confirmed evidence of HIV infection • Nucleic acid amplification assays to determine HIV RNA level (viral load) • Particle agglutination with confirmation test • Positive Coombs test: HIV-associated autoimmune hemolytic anemia • Screening: suggested routinely to adults and teens, pregnant women regardless of risk. For high risk, testing every six to 12 months • Western Blot (supplemental) • When CD4 count and CD4 percentage for severity stage is mixed, default to the more severe stage • When laboratory confirmation is not available: the provider's or other qualified healthcare professional's diagnostic statement that the patient is HIV+ based on lab criteria results that are described and documented in the medical record and has an AIDS defining illness or baseline CD4 count <200 is sufficient.
3. Diagnostic Px *(routine/expected in italics)*	• Bone marrow aspiration/biopsy: evaluation of associated cytopenias or some AIDS-defining conditions • CT/MRI: evaluation of associated conditions or AIDS-defining conditions	• Lumbar puncture: evaluation of AIDS-associated conditions
4. Therapeutic Tx *(routine/expected in italics)*	• Antiretroviral treatment: (HAART) combination (of) drugs recommended. For current list, see http://www.fda.gov • Erythropoietin therapy—first-line treatment of anemia • Medications for anorexia • Mytesi for treatment of antiretroviral treatment induced diarrhea	• Pain medications • Pre-exposure Prophylaxis Treatment (PrEP) • Secondary (postacute infection) prophylaxis for specified AIDS-defining conditions • Transfusions to treat associated conditions—limit to situations requiring immediate effect (i.e., correction of low hemoglobin levels)
5. Increased Nursing Care and/or Monitoring	• AIDS-related condition	• Complication(s) due to AIDS condition(s)
6. Extends LOS	• AIDS-related condition exacerbation post admit • Complication(s) due to AIDS condition(s)	• Transfer to palliative care

HIV-Related Lab Value	Normal Range
CD4 cell count	500 – 1200 cells/mm3
CD4 percentage	25 – 65%
Hgb	11.9 – 14.8 g/dL (females) 13.6 – 16.9 g/dL (males)
Hct (%)	35 – 43 (females) 40 – 50 (males)
Platelets	153 – 361 x10^3/microL (females) 152 – 324 x10^3/microL (males)
WBCs	3.8 – 10.3 x10^3/microL

Condition	Documentation Example	ICD-10-CM Corresponding Codes
Routine/Expected/ Integral/Inherent/ Incidental *(italics only)*	*NA*	*NA*
Principal Diagnosis	Admitted for/with: 1. w/u: s/s due to AIDS 2. AIDS-defining condition 3. AIDS-related condition with known AIDS dx 4. AIDS-related condition with confirmed HIV+ status 5. Hemolytic-uremic syndrome related to AIDS 6, Sepsis due to AIDS-related infection 7. Palliative care for AIDS	1. Report B2Ø AIDS. 2. Report B2Ø AIDS, followed by code for AIDS-defining condition. 3. Report B2Ø AIDS, followed by code for AIDS-related condition. 4. Report B2Ø AIDS, followed by code for AIDS-related condition. 5. Report D59.31 Infection-associated hemolytic-uremic syndrome, followed by B2Ø AIDS. 6. Report B2Ø AIDS, followed by sepsis and codes for all reported AIDS-related conditions. 7. Report B2Ø AIDS, followed by Z51.5 when admitted or transferred for palliative care, comfort care, end-of-life care.
Comorbidity	1. Admitted for open reduction with internal fixation (ORIF) open ankle fracture from fall; history of HIV disease, will continue current antiretroviral regimen. 2. Admitted for unrelated condition with HIV+ status and history/physical documents criteria for AIDS. **(Query regarding patient with HIV+ status and criteria for AIDS-defining condition(s), to confirm AIDS.)**	1. Report unrelated condition as principal diagnosis when an AIDS patient is admitted for a condition unrelated to AIDS or its complications. Code B2Ø can be reported when a patient with a documented history of HIV disease is being managed with antiretroviral medications. 2. Same as above.
Complication of Care	1. Admitted due to newly diagnosed AIDS as a result of contaminated transfusion as child.	1. Report T8Ø.29XA Infection following other infusion, transfusion and therapeutic injection, initial encounter, followed by B2Ø Human immunodeficiency virus [HIV] disease and Y64.Ø Contaminated medical or biological substance, transfused or infused.
Poisoning or Adverse Effect of Medication/ Chemical	1. Adverse effect of an antiviral drug 2–4. Poisoning by an antiviral drug All initial encounters	1. Adverse reaction to antiviral med: adverse condition + T37.5X5A Adverse effect of antiviral drugs. 2. Poisoning by antiviral med: T37.5X1A Poisoning by antiviral drugs, accidental (unintentional) + manifestation. 3. Poisoning by antiviral med: T37.5X2A Poisoning by antiviral drugs, intentional self-harm + manifestation. 4. Poisoning by antiviral med: T37.5X4A Poisoning by antiviral drugs, undetermined + manifestation.

Condition	Documentation Example	ICD-10-CM Corresponding Codes
Obstetrics	1. Admitted for planned C-section for post-term, patient HIV+.	1. Report reason for admission for cesarean O48.Ø Post-term pregnancy, followed by O98.72 Human immunodeficiency virus [HIV] disease complicating childbirth, followed by codes for HIV.
History of Exposure to HIV leading to AIDS	1. Status AIDS due to medical care/exposure	1. B2Ø followed by: W46.1XX[D,S] Contact with contaminated hypodermic needle [subsequent encounter, sequela] **or** Y64.Ø Contaminated medical or biological substance, transfused or infused **or** Y62.3 Failure of sterile precautions during injection or immunization **or** Y64.8 Contaminated medical or biological substance administered by other means
High-Risk Sexual Behavior	1. HIV risk due to patient's lifestyle/sexual behavior	1. Report Z72.51 High risk heterosexual behavior; Z72.52 High risk homosexual behavior; Z72.53 High risk bisexual behavior; or Z72.89 Other problems related to lifestyle.

Additional References

AHA CC: 4Q, 2022, p. 79; 1Q, 2022, p. 36; 4Q, 2021, p. 81; 1Q, 2021, p. 52; 2Q, 2020, p. 3; 1Q, 2019, p. 8

AIDS Education and Training Centers National Resource Center: https://aidsetc.org/

CDC: http://www.cdc.gov/mmwr/preview/mmwrhtml/rr5710a2.htm

Aspiration Pneumonia/Pneumonitis/Bronchitis

J69.Ø	**Pneumonitis due to inhalation of food and vomit**	MCC HCC
J69.1	**Pneumonitis due to inhalation of oils and essences**	MCC HCC
J69.8	**Pneumonitis due to inhalation of other solids and liquids**	MCC HCC
J95.4	**Chemical pneumonitis due to anesthesia**	CC
J95.89	**Other postprocedural complications and disorders of respiratory system, not elsewhere classified**	CC
O29.Ø1[1,2,3,9]	**Aspiration pneumonitis due to anesthesia during pregnancy, [first, second, third, unspecified] trimester**	
O74.Ø	**Aspiration pneumonitis due to anesthesia during labor and delivery**	
O89.Ø1	**Aspiration pneumonitis due to anesthesia during the puerperium**	

Associated terminology: aspiration (with): pneumonia/pneumonitis/bronchitis; postprocedural aspiration pneumonia; acid pulmonary syndrome; Mendelson's syndrome; postop aspiration pneumonia due to anesthesia; Mendelson's syndrome during labor/delivery, during pregnancy, during the puerperium

Diagnoses

Discussion

Note: Bacterial or viral pneumonia is due to aspiration of bacteria or viral organisms; this discussion focuses on primary aspiration pneumonia, aspiration pneumonitis and aspiration bronchitis that are a result of an aspiration event of substances noninfectious in origin.

Aspiration pneumonia, aspiration pneumonitis or aspiration bronchitis is an inflammation of the lungs and airways caused by inhalation of foreign substances of oropharyngeal or gastric secretion/contents or exogenous irritants/liquids/foreign body into the bronchial tree or lungs. A chemical pneumonitis (with or without pneumonia) develops due to the acidity of the aspirate, which is also known as acid pulmonary syndrome or Mendelson's syndrome. Microorganisms (bacterial, viral, anaerobic oral flora, colonization, hospital acquired, community acquired) may also be aspirated during or after the episode and contribute to the inflammation as a superimposed bacterial or viral pneumonia. Noninfectious aspirates include, but are not limited to: vomitus, food, saliva, nasal secretions, gastric contents (acid/peptic/solid particulate matter), barium, water (near drowning), mineral/vegetable oil (laxative oils), activated charcoal (in the treatment of overdose), pill fragments, blood, and foreign objects.

Aspiration of small amounts of saliva or stomach contents with microorganisms is not uncommon and does not cause disease in a healthy individual. Protective mucociliary and macrophagic activity maintains lower respiratory tract sterility and prevents mucus accumulation in the lungs. Aspiration becomes pathological based on the condition of the individual, volume of aspirated material, and nature of the aspirated substance. Presentation of a pathological process is acute, developing within a few to several hours of an aspiration event. The site of a pulmonary infiltrate or consolidation is related to the position of the patient during the event. These positions and related anatomic sites may include:

- Right middle and lower lobes (most common locations)
- The right middle and lower lobes are the most common location
- Standing: bilateral basal segments of lower lobes
- Left lateral decubitus lie: left lobe
- Prone: right upper lobe
- Supine: posterior segments upper lobes and apical segments lower lobes

Mendelson's syndrome (pneumonitis) or acid pulmonary syndrome will have the radiological appearance similar to pulmonary edema. When a superimposed bacterial pneumonia develops, the causative organism can be dependent on the setting in which the event occurs, by the anacrobic oropharyngeal colonizers present, or by use of antacids, such as proton pump Inhibitors (PPIs) or H2-receptor antagonists. Presence of a superimposed bacterial or viral pneumonia is coded as an additional diagnosis; if a specified organism is confirmed by physician documentation and supported by clinical evidence then a specific pneumonia code can be assigned. Aspiration pneumonia will recur due to predisposing conditions, especially if these conditions are not treated or managed. Hypoxemia is not integral to pneumonia; when hypoxemia is documented and meets additional diagnosis criteria, it can be coded in addition to the pneumonia.

Documentation Tip

Review all labs and treatments for signs of superimposed bacterial/viral pneumonia and clarify whether both aspiration pneumonia and infectious pneumonia are present. Each condition is coded separately.

Coding Tip

The following list of codes capture chemical pneumonitis (aspiration pneumonia due to chemical fumes or vapors/gases, toxic materials, respiratory effects of toxic materials, or smoke inhalation). These would be listed as a secondary diagnosis following a code from categories T51-T65 to identify the substance.

J68.Ø	**Bronchitis and pneumonitis due to chemicals, gases, fumes and vapors**
J69.1	**Pneumonitis due to inhalation of oils and essences**
J7Ø.5	**Respiratory conditions due to smoke inhalation**
J7Ø.8	**Respiratory conditions due to other specified external agents**
J7Ø.9	**Respiratory conditions due to unspecified external agent**

Fetal aspiration pneumonia/pneumonitis is located in category P24 Neonatal aspiration.

Predisposing conditions that place an individual at high risk for an aspiration episode can be categorized as:

- Esophageal/incompetent swallowing mechanism:
  - dysphagia: oropharyngeal dysphagia occurs frequently in the elderly
  - esophageal strictures, stenosis, obstruction
  - esophageal neoplasm
  - gastroesophageal reflux or esophagitis
  - achalasia
  - impaired pharyngeal reflex or gag reflex, airway defense
  - feeding/mastication disorder
- Physical state/positional:
  - vomiting
  - recumbency, bed confinement
  - deconditioning or debility
  - critical illness
  - pregnancy
  - severe COPD
- Altered consciousness/impaired airway maintenance:
  - alcohol intoxication or overdose; alcoholism
  - drug intoxication or overdose
  - seizure
  - cerebrovascular accident (stroke), acute or by history
  - head trauma, traumatic brain injury (TBI)
  - anesthesia/oversedation
  - near drowning
  - coma, comatose state
- Neurological disorders:
  - multiple sclerosis
  - dementia
  - Parkinson's
  - myasthenia gravis
  - quadriplegia
  - hypoxic ischemic encephalopathy (HIE)
- Presence of or procedure involving mechanical device:
  - nasogastric tube or intubation
  - endotracheal tube or intubation
  - tracheostomy
  - enteral feeding

Documentation Tip

When aspiration is documented, do not assume bronchitis or pneumonia as the site. Aspiration can occur anywhere along the respiratory tract and will be reported from category T17 Foreign body in respiratory tract, with the specified site when the aspiration is not causing bronchitis or pneumonia. Always review documentation, including radiology reports, to locate the site of aspiration. If it is unclear, query the site and nature of the aspiration, including if it is causing asphyxiation.

Documentation Tip

Code assignment cannot be based on ancillary test results, therapies, or clinical criteria alone. A diagnosis and its clinical significance must be supported by physician or other qualified healthcare professional documentation. When it is unclear or there is contradictory information, query the physician or other qualified healthcare professional for clarification.

Coding/Reporting Criteria	Clinical Criteria	
1. Physical Evaluation *(routine/expected in italics)*	• Shortness of breath • Difficulty breathing • Chest pain • Rigors • Respiratory distress • Coughing (with pink/frothy sputum) • Bronchospasm • Cyanosis (possible)	• Audible wheezing • Decreased breath sounds/wet/gurgling breaths/crackling • Dullness to percussion over consolidated areas • Rales • Pleural friction rub • Altered mental status
2. Clinical Evaluation *(routine/expected in italics)*	• Fever: ≥ 37.7°C • Hyperthermia: ≥ 40°C or hypothermia: ≤ 35°C • Hypotension: SBP <90 • Tachycardia/heart rate above 100 bpm • Tachypnea/respiratory rate above 25 • ABG analysis: – pH<7.35 – PO_2 < 60 or Sat < 90 – hypoxemia – respiratory alkalosis – normal to low partial pressure of carbon dioxide – pH of aspirated fluid <2.5, greater chance of chemical/acid pneumonitis • Lab: Na < 130; BUN >30 • CBC with differential: elevated WBC, increased neutrophils, anemia, thrombocytosis indicates anaerobic bacterial infection	• Basic metabolic panel • Aspiration: Large volume > 0.3mL/kg of body wt (20-25 mL in adults) • Sputum gram stain: to identify bacteria in conjunction with sputum cultures and chart documentation • Microscopy: to identify bacteria • Culture: to identify bacteria • Pulse oximetry • C-reactive protein (CRP): high levels may indicate bacterial pneumonia • Procalcitonin level-rise • Plasma soluble triggering receptor expressed on myeloid cells 1 (sTREM-1) elevation
3. Diagnostic Px *(routine/expected in italics)*	• Chest x-ray: infiltrate/consolidation; volume loss in any lobar area suggests obstruction; chemical pneumonitis appearance similar to pulmonary edema • Dehydration can obscure visibility of infiltrate on x-ray • When no infiltrate is seen with a diagnosis of pneumonia, query to confirm (suspected, not ruled out)	• Protective specimen brushing/catheter: suspected obstructing neoplasm or to retrieve foreign body • Bronchoscopy: suspected foreign body or food aspiration • Bronchoalveolar lavage • Tracheal aspirate • Swallowing evaluation • CT scan
4. Therapeutic Tx *(routine/expected in italics)*	• Antibiotics/antimicrobials: – if failure to resolve within 48 hours or with secondary bacterial/fungal infection – not recommended for uncomplicated chemical pneumonitis • IV fluids/electrolyte replacement • Bronchodilators/nebulizers • Tracheal suctioning	• Oxygen supplementation • Endotracheal intubation • Ventilation • Speech therapy training for swallowing/feeding strategies • Nasogastric feeding tube insertion • Enteral feeding • Gastrostomy or jejunostomy
5. Increased Nursing Care and/or Monitoring	• Aspiration precautions protocol • Cardiac monitoring • Pulse oximetry	• Consults • Repeat radiology
6. Extends LOS	• Discharge delayed due to postop aspiration pneumonia	

Diagnoses

Condition	Documentation Example	ICD-10-CM Corresponding Codes
Routine/Expected/ Integral/Inherent/ Incidental *(italics only)*	*NA*	*NA*
Principal Diagnosis	1. IP Admit Note: Patient aspirated (no other info; clinical data does not support pneumonia). **(Query location/nature of aspiration.)** 2. Aspiration pneumonia due to near drowning with acute respiratory failure. 3. Aspiration pneumonitis with SIRS. 4. Acute respiratory failure due to aspiration pneumonia.	1. Aspiration can occur anywhere along the respiratory tract; when the site is not stated, query (do not assume pneumonia); when causing asphyxia, index as foreign body, site of respiratory tract, causing asphyxia 2. Sequencing of aspiration pneumonia, acute respiratory failure and near drowning will be guided by OCG: I.C.10.b.1-3 and II.C. 3. Sequencing of aspiration pneumonitis and SIRS will follow OCG: I.C.18.g as aspiration pneumonitis or pneumonia is of non-infectious origin. 4. Sequencing of aspiration pneumonia and acute respiratory failure will be guided by OCG: I.C.10.b.1-3 and II.C.
Comorbidity	1. IP Progress Note: Patient aspirated (no other info; clinical data does not support pneumonia). **(Query the location and nature of the aspiration.)**	1. Aspiration can occur anywhere along the respiratory tract; when the site is not stated, query (do not assume pneumonia); when causing asphyxia, index as foreign body, site of respiratory tract, causing asphyxia.
Complication of Care	1. IP Progress Note: Patient with post CABG aspiration pneumonia due to procedure (not anesthesia). 2. Aspiration pneumonitis due to displaced enteral feeding (feeding tube) (post admit).	1. Report J95.89 Other postprocedural complications and disorders of respiratory system, not elsewhere classified, and a code from category J69 Pneumonitis due to solids and liquids. Both codes are required to identify the complication and the nature of the complication. 2. Report T85.528A Displacement of other gastrointestinal prosthetic devices, implants and grafts, initial encounter; J69.Ø Pneumonitis due to inhalation of food and vomit; and Y73.1 Therapeutic (nonsurgical) and rehabilitative gastroenterology and urology devices associated with adverse incidents.
Poisoning or Adverse Effect of Medication/ Chemical	1. Vomitus aspiration pneumonia due to nonprescription oxycodone use with alcohol intoxication with acute respiratory failure with hypoxia. 2. Mendelson's syndrome postop due to anesthesia (nonobstetric). 3. IP Progress Note: Suspect patient aspirated at time of delivery resulting in aspiration pneumonia (with identified clinical consequences/treatment).	1. Report T4Ø.2X1A Poisoning by other opioids, accidental (unintentional), initial encounter); T51.ØX1A Toxic effect of ethanol, accidental (unintentional), initial encounter; J69.Ø Pneumonitis due to inhalation of food and vomit; J96.Ø1 Acute respiratory failure with hypoxia. 2. Report J95.4 Chemical pneumonitis due to anesthesia, and use additional code from category T41 Poisoning by, adverse effect of and underdosing of anesthetics and therapeutic gases, with fifth or sixth character 5 (adverse effect) to identify drug. 3. Report O74.Ø Aspiration pneumonitis due to anesthesia during labor and delivery. An additional code is not required since the complication code identifies the nature of the complication.

Additional References

AHA CC: 2Q, 2019, p. 6, 31; 1Q, 2017, p. 24

Atelectasis

J95.89 **Other postprocedural complications and disorders of respiratory system, not elsewhere classified** CC

J98.11 **Atelectasis** CC

Associated terminology: atelectasis, postop atelectasis

Diagnoses

Discussion

Atelectasis is an incomplete expansion of lung segments that may result in partial or complete lung collapse. It occurs to some degree in many patients undergoing upper abdominal or thoracic surgery. Prognosis depends on prompt removal of any airway obstruction, relief of hypoxia, and re-expansion of the collapsed lung. Risk factors include, but are not limited to, anesthesia, mechanical ventilation, prolonged immobility, prolonged bedrest with minimal position changes, underlying lung diseases, or any condition that inhibits full lung expansion or lends to shallow or painful deep breathing.

Atelectasis is an expected condition within the first 48 hours postoperatively after a patient has undergone a general anesthetic with moderately high oxygen concentrations. It is often an incidental x-ray/physical finding that is self-limiting. Atelectasis will usually resolve spontaneously without treatment. The condition may be visible on x-ray for up to four to five days, though without increased temperature or need for treatment in an otherwise ambulatory patient, it is not considered a comorbidity or complication. This includes atelectasis seen on x-ray after a line placement in the absence of other clinical symptoms.

Atelectasis is reportable when it is associated with other clinically significant findings, such as fever or need for work-up and treatment (i.e., non-routine x-ray, urinalysis, blood culture, respiratory therapy, extended length of stay). (It must be documented as the definitive diagnosis for the symptom(s) that prompted the workup).

Excluded

Newborn (primary) atelectasis, see category P28.

Tuberculous atelectasis (current disease) (A15)

Documentation Tip

To ensure that documentation supports assignment of atelectasis as an additional diagnosis, clarify whether it was a complication of a procedure and/or report all significant symptoms. Any diagnostic or therapeutic workup should be discussed as well as whether the condition required an extended hospital stay.

Coding/Reporting Criteria	Clinical Criteria
1. Physical Evaluation *(routine/expected in italics)*	• *Chest pain*—not routine if w/u prompted • Coarse lung sound and/or decreased lung sound • Cough • *Dyspnea*—not routine if w/u prompted • *Shortness* of breath—not routine if w/u prompted • Splinting • Transudate pleural effusion **Note:** Early postoperative fever and atelectasis are not positively correlated.
2. Clinical Evaluation *(routine/expected in italics)*	• Tachycardia • Temp > 102 prompting workup (blood culture/UA) • WBC > 15 & Bands > 7% • WBC > 18
3. Diagnostic Px *(routine/expected in italics)*	• Bronchoscopy—not routine • *Chest x-ray: atelectasis—incidental finding/routine p/o (not prompted by workup)* • Repeat x-ray due to symptoms • Repeat x-ray to monitor progression/resolution

Diagnoses

Coding/Reporting Criteria	Clinical Criteria
4. Therapeutic Tx *(routine/expected in italics)*	• Bronchoscopy/removal of obstruction (mucus plug)—not routine • Early mobilization/ambulation • Encourage coughing, deep breathing • Glucocorticoid treatment • *Incentive spirometry (IS) routine order* • Incentive spirometry (IS) treatment performed • Intermittent positive pressure breathing (ventilation) (IPPB), continuous positive airway pressure (CPAP), or positive end expiratory pressure (ventilation) (PEEP)—not routine • Nasogastric suction when caused by abdominal distention due to intraluminal air • Paracentesis when due to tense ascites • Physical therapy • Prophylactic: – analgesics to facilitate deep breathing – antibiotics for associated infection • Upright positioning • Use of nebulized bronchodilators/aerosols of water/saline to liquefy/remove secretions—not routine
5. Increased Nursing Care and/or Monitoring	• Increase incentive spirometry • Placed on IPPB/CPAP/PEEP
6. Extends LOS	• Discharge delayed

Condition	Documentation Example	ICD-10-CM Corresponding Codes
Routine/Expected/ Integral/Inherent/ Incidental *(italics only)*	1. *Progress Note: Expected/incidental atelectasis not requiring treatment. Discharge Summary: Routine/incidental atelectasis.*	*NA - no code reported.*
Principal Diagnosis	NA	NA
Comorbidity	1. Progress Note: Fever (or other symptom) (workup) due to atelectasis. 2. Progress Note: Continue IS for atelectasis; day two progress note: repeat chest x-ray to evaluate atelectasis; discharge summary: atelectasis required evaluation/treatment. 3. IP Admit Note: Acute exacerbation bronchiectasis with massive atelectasis.	1. Report J98.11 Atelectasis; R5Ø.81 Fever presenting with conditions classified elsewhere. 2. Report J98.11 Atelectasis. 3. Report J47.1 Bronchiectasis with (acute) exacerbation; J98.11 Atelectasis.
Complication of Care	1. Progress Note: Atelectasis due to surgery, increase incentive spirometry (IS)/ use intermittent positive pressure breathing (ventilation) (IPPB)/continuous positive airway pressure (CPAP)/positive end expiratory pressure (ventilation)(PEEP). 2. Progress Note: Bronchoscopy to evaluate postsurgical atelectasis. Progress Note: Atelectasis due to surgery. 3. Progress Note: Postpone/hold dc due to atelectasis due to surgery. 4. Discharge Summary: Postoperative course was complicated by atelectasis due to surgery.	1. Report J95.89 Other postprocedural complications and disorders of respiratory system, not elsewhere classified; J98.11 Atelectasis. 2. Same as #1. 3. Same as #1. 4. Same as #1.
Poisoning or Adverse Effect of Medication/ Chemical	NA	NA

Bacteremia as a Principal Diagnosis

R78.81 Bacteremia CC

Z03.89 Encounter for observation for other suspected diseases and conditions ruled out

Associated terminology: bacteremia due to contaminant, bacteremia ruled out, bacteremia with sepsis

Excluded

R78.81 Bacteremia

Excludes 1: sepsis—code to specified infection

Discussion

Bacteremia is not an infection but an abnormal laboratory blood culture finding that indicates viable bacteria in the blood in the absence of two or more signs of sepsis. It does not represent a disease process. It occurs when an infection at another body site or normal flora seeds the bloodstream with a bacterial organism. Opportunistic paths for bacterial blood infiltration include dental procedures, foreign bodies, iatrogenic complications, IV drug use, localized infections, surgical procedures, and traumatic injuries.

Bacteremia can be transient and nonpathological. Prior to some procedures, prophylactic antibiotics are administered because there is an expectation of transient bacteremia. Transient bacteremia may cause fever but is otherwise usually asymptomatic. Procedures that facilitate transient bacteremia are often associated with mucous membrane trauma, such as cystoscopy, dental surgery, drainage, and sigmoidoscopy.

Intermittent bacteremia, a more common form, indicates that microorganisms enter the blood at various times. This type of bacteremia can be seen especially with extravascular infections. Examples of extravascular infections include pneumonia, osteomyelitis, and meningitis. Other infections produce continuous bacteremia in which microorganisms are always in the blood. Examples include intravascular infections such as endocarditis, suppurative thrombophlebitis, and infected aneurysm.

A fever can present when an immune response to the bacteria is sustained, or if the immune system is weakened or colonization occurs. To report bacteremia, it must be identified as clinically significant by the physician or other qualified healthcare professional.

Bacteria can spread to other sites, causing secondary site infections and complications of iatrogenic devices, such as prosthetic heart valves, without progressing to the state of sepsis. When this occurs, assign a code for the type of infection, followed by the bacteremia and the specified organism when it is identified by physician documentation.

Coding Tip

- **Fungemia is a fungal organism in the bloodstream.**
- **Viremia is a viral organism in the bloodstream.**
- **Septicemia is sepsis due to unspecified organism, see A41.9 Sepsis, unspecified organism.**

If the organism level becomes pathological and symptomatic and elicits a severe immune system response, it is now sepsis (septicemia). Bacteremia is not reported when documented with sepsis.

A single set of blood cultures consists of two bottles of growth medium, one for aerobes and one for anaerobes, in which 10 to 20 ml of blood drawn from the patient is introduced. Two to three sets are adequate to evaluate for infection.

Documentation Tip

Code assignment cannot be based on laboratory findings or clinical criteria alone. A diagnosis and its clinical significance must be supported by physician or other qualified healthcare professional documentation. When it is unclear or there is contradictory information, query the physician or other qualified healthcare professional for clarification.

Contamination of the blood culture can produce false results; therefore, it should be repeated at intervals and at different access sites to determine if the results are accurate. When results are due to contamination, bacteremia is not assigned. Common contaminants that produce a positive blood culture include:

- Coag negative *Staphylococcus* (gram positive cocci)
- *Corynebacterium* (gram positive rods)
- *Propionibacterium acnes* (anaerobic gram positive rods)
- *Bacillus* species (anaerobic gram positive rods)

Even though these are common contaminants, it is important to rule out true infection in the following settings that involve prosthetic devices, immunosuppressed patients or when multiple blood cultures from different sets are positive.

The following organisms are typically not skin contaminants and would warrant further workup:

- *Streptococcal* species
- *Staphylococcus aureus*
- *Enterococcus*
- *Candida*
- *Pseudomonas* and other gram negative rods

Empiric antibiotic treatment is given after blood cultures are obtained. If the patient received antibiotics prior to culture or is on maintenance antibiotics, culture results may be affected or not performed.

As a chapter 18 code, bacteremia should rarely be assigned as principal diagnosis on an inpatient admission. Review the record for a more definitive diagnosis or an uncertain diagnosis at discharge. If it is the only sign or symptom that warranted admission and at discharge it is stated only as "bacteremia" without a stated underlying cause, then it would meet OCG: II.A as principal diagnosis.

Bacteremia is integral to sepsis/septicemia and, therefore, is not assigned when sepsis/septicemia is the final diagnosis. It is not integral to other infections and can be assigned as an additional code when it meets criteria. As a manifestation of a complication, it is assigned to provide further information on the nature of the complication.

Documentation Tip

If bacteremia is ruled out due to contaminant, the principal diagnosis is ZØ3.89 Encounter for observation for other suspected diseases and conditions ruled out. Bacteremia (R78.91) is very rarely warranted for assignment as an inpatient principal diagnosis. Principal diagnosis would be the infection (not the contaminant) or infectious source (e.g., infected prosthetic), sepsis if present, or code ZØ3.89 if all other conditions are ruled out. Query to clarify if no condition is identified.

Coding/Reporting Criteria	Clinical Criteria	
1. Physical Evaluation *(routine/expected in italics)*	• *Asymptomatic* • Fever	
2. Clinical Evaluation *(routine/expected in italics)*	• *Blood culture—routine, pre-op* • Blood culture—when symptomatic or for workup to evaluate infection site(s) • Urinalysis	• CSF culture • Sputum culture • Gram stain • Antibiotic sensitivity/susceptibility test
3. Diagnostic Px *(routine/expected in italics)*	• Workup to evaluate infection site(s) • Echocardiography (cardiac valve vegetation) • Spinal tap	• CT • MRI • Gallium scan
4. Therapeutic Tx *(routine/expected in italics)*	• *Prophylactic antibiotics* • Empiric antibiotics	• Antibiotic regimen specific to organism • Antibiotics, wide spectrum
5. Increased Nursing Care and/or Monitoring	• Patient bacteremic, monitor for symptoms	
6. Extends LOS	• Delay discharge for workup of bacteremia etiology	

Condition	Documentation Example	ICD-10-CM Corresponding Codes
Routine/Expected/ Integral/Inherent/ Incidental *(italics only)*	1. *Antibiotic prophylaxis prior to procedure.* 2. *Transient bacteremia post-transrectal prostrate biopsy.*	1. *No code assigned.* 2. *No code assigned.*
Principal Diagnosis	1. Admit to IP: Bacteremia with blood culture 2/2 bottles positive, symptoms persists. **(Query if bacteremia, 2/2 bottles positive, symptomatic, indicates a serious infectious process; query for etiology/source of bacteremia.)** 2. Admit to IP: IV drug abuser with fever, workup shows. *Staphylococcus aureus* bacteremia and echocardiogram reveals tricuspid valve vegetation; final diagnosis is infective right sided endocarditis with *S. aureus* bacteremia due to IV drug abuse. **(Query if there is additional evidence that a more severe systemic infectious process is present [i.e., sepsis].)**	1. Symptomatic bacteremia is worked-up which indicates a serious infection, a query is necessary. 2. Sequence first underlying localized infection, I33.Ø Acute and subacute infective endocarditis, followed by R78.81 Bacteremia, and B95.61 Methicillin susceptible Staphylococcus aureus infection as the cause of diseases classified elsewhere. If sepsis/septicemia is ruled in, sequence sepsis as principal diagnosis and do not assign a code for bacteremia. An exception to sepsis sequencing would be in the case of complications.
Comorbidity	1. Postadmit: Fever, workup, blood culture positive, start antibiotics for bacteremia. 2. Urinary tract infection with *Escherichia coli* bacteremia. 3. Left arm laceration with cellulitis and with bacteremia.	1. When bacteremia is symptomatic with fever, assign R5Ø.9 Fever, unspecified, and R78.81 Bacteremia. 2. When bacteremia is present with a localized infection (UTI), sequence first underlying localized infection N39.Ø Urinary tract infection, site not specified, followed by R78.81 Bacteremia, in addition to the code for specified organism B96.2Ø Unspecified Escherichia coli [E. coli], as the cause of diseases classified elsewhere. 3. When bacteremia is present with traumatic wound infection, either the wound (S41.119A Laceration without foreign body of left upper arm, initial encounter) or the localized infection, cellulitis (LØ3.114A Cellulitis of left upper limb) may be sequenced first depending on circumstances of the admission, followed by R78.81 Bacteremia, in addition to the code for specified organism when identified by physician documentation.
Complication of Care	1. PICC line with bacteremia 2. Bacteremia with AV fistula	1. Bacteremia as a complication due to or resulting from device, implant, or graft, assign first the complication code followed by a code for the specific complication and manifestation. Report T8Ø.211A Bloodstream infection due to central venous catheter, initial encounter, followed by R78.81 Bacteremia, in addition to the code for specified organism. 2. T82.7XXA Infection and inflammatory reaction due to other cardiac and vascular devices, implants and grafts, initial encounter, followed by R78.81 Bacteremia, in addition to the code for specified organism.
Poisoning or Adverse Effect of Medication/ Chemical	NA	NA

Diagnoses

Cerebral Edema

G93.6	**Cerebral edema**	MCC HCC
SØ6.1XØA	**Traumatic cerebral edema without loss of consciousness, initial encounter**	MCC HCC
SØ6.1X[1,2,3,4]A	**Traumatic cerebral edema with loss of consciousness of [3Ø min or less, 31 min to 59 min, 1 hour to 5 hours 59 min, 6 hours to 24 hours], initial encounter**	MCC HAC HCC
SØ6.1X5A	**Traumatic cerebral edema with loss of consciousness greater than 24 hours with return to pre-existing conscious level, initial encounter**	MCC HAC HCC
SØ6.1X6A	**Traumatic cerebral edema with loss of consciousness greater than hours without return to pre-existing conscious level with patient 24 surviving, initial encounter**	MCC HAC HCC
SØ6.1X7A	**Traumatic cerebral edema with loss of consciousness of any duration with death due to brain injury prior to regaining consciousness, initial encounter**	MCC HAC
SØ6.1X8A	**Traumatic cerebral edema with loss of consciousness of any duration with death due to other cause prior to regaining consciousness, initial encounter**	MCC HAC
SØ6.1XAA	**Traumatic cerebral edema with loss of consciousness status unknown, initial encounter**	MCC HAC HCC
SØ6.1X9A	**Traumatic cerebral edema with loss of consciousness of unspecified duration, initial encounter**	MCC HAC HCC

Associated terminology: cerebral edema; traumatic cerebral edema

Excluded

- **Cerebral edema due to birth injury (with anoxia/hypoxia), see P11.Ø.**
- **Cerebral edema, newborn (anoxia, hypoxia), see P52.4.**

Discussion

Cerebral (brain) edema is the excess collection of fluid in the brain. It may result in brain swelling, which leads to elevated intracranial pressure (ICP) and compression. This displaces or herniates the brain tissue from one area to another with "a mass effect/midline shift." Its clinical significance ranges from none/low to being an independent risk factor for mortality. Causes of cerebral edema are varied and include cerebral infarction/hemorrhage/ischemia, trauma, neoplasm, infection, toxicity, and metabolic disorders affecting the nervous system.

The clinical significance of the cerebral edema must be documented; it is the determining factor for reporting. If the edema is clinically insignificant (i.e., expected [postsurgery]), small, asymptomatic and resolves spontaneously without treatment, without further workup or monitoring, then it will not be reported. If it is symptomatic, requires workup, monitoring, treatment or causing further complications (neurological symptoms, herniation), it can be reported as long as the link is made to the clinical criteria and its significance stated. When reportable, cerebral edema, as a manifestation of the underlying condition or as a concurrent condition to traumatic brain injury, is a reflection of the condition having a higher severity of illness and risk of mortality than if the cerebral edema was inconsequential. When the clinical significance is unclear or there is contradictory information or incomplete documentation, query the physician or other qualified healthcare professional.

Documentation Tip

Ensure that any connection between cerebral swelling or cerebral edema and a traumatic brain injury are clearly documented.

Although there is distinction among the types of cerebral edema, one type can lead to another and there is overlap between them. Key factors affecting cerebral fluid exchange include cellular metabolism function, blood-brain barrier (BBB), CSF-brain barrier, and osmolality. Compromised integrity of any of these mechanisms may lead to cerebral edema.

Types of cerebral edema:

- Vasogenic
  - BBB breakdown: plasma constituents (intravascular proteins and fluid) enter brain
  - extracellular space swelling, eventual intracellular swelling
  - evolves over hours to days: begins six to eight hours after ischemic onset with maximum peak two to four days after onset
  - considered irreversible and damaging
  - trauma (traumatic brain injury [TBI]) (shaken infant syndrome)
  - brain neoplasm:(stasis edema at compression site due to stasis in venous drainage areas)
  - infection: subdural empyema, encephalitis, toxoplasmosis, meningitis
  - focal inflammation
  - cerebral ischemia/hemorrhage/infarction: combination of vasogenic and cytotoxic
  - hypertensive encephalopathy; hydrostatic due to malignant hypertension
  - altitude sickness (high altitude cerebral edema [HACE]); high altitude induced hypoxic effects of the BBB
- Cytotoxic
  - BBB undisturbed: cellular metabolism dysfunction causes cellular retention of sodium and water
  - intracellular swelling
  - evolves over minutes to two to three hours
  - can be reversible
  - intoxications of drugs/chemicals
  - trauma (TBI) (shaken infant syndrome)
  - Reye's syndrome
  - severe hypothermia
  - early ischemia, cerebral infarction/hemorrhage, encephalopathy, hypoxia
  - cardiac arrest
  - pseudotumor cerebri
- Interstitial
  - CSF-brain barrier rupture: spread of CSF after it penetrates brain; since it is CSF, there is almost no protein in the fluid
  - extracellular spread of CSF
  - obstructive hydrocephalus
- Osmotic
  - due to plasma dilution by excess water intake causing the brain osmolality to exceed the serum osmolality; creates an abnormal pressure gradient that allows water to enter the brain
  - extracellular swelling
  - water intoxication
    hyponatremia
  - syndrome of inappropriate secretion of antidiuretic hormone (SIADH)
  - hemodialysis
  - hyperosmolar hyperglycemic state

Coding and Documentation Tip

When traumatic cerebral edema is noted, look for signs, symptoms, and/or documentation of cranial cerebrospinal fluid (CSF) leak. Cerebrospinal fluid discharging from the nose or the ear can be caused by a fracture of the frontal bone with tearing of the dura mater and arachnoid. It is characterized by watery drainage usually from only one side of the nose or one ear, headache, vision changes, and hearing loss. Traumatic cranial cerebrospinal fluid leak is captured with code G96.Ø8 Other cranial cerebrospinal fluid leak. Query provider if clinical indicators are present but CSF leak is not documented.

Coding Tip

Hospital-acquired condition (HAC): CMS does not allow a code to increase MS-DRG reimbursement by acting as a CC or MCC with a present on admission (POA) value of N or U. The case will be paid as though these conditions were not reported.

Coding/Reporting Criteria	Clinical Criteria	
1. Physical Evaluation *(routine/expected in italics)*	• *Asymptomatic* • Headache • Neck pain or stiffness • Nausea and/or vomiting • Dizziness • Irregular breathing • Vision loss or changes • Memory loss • Difficulty walking, ataxia • Disorientation • Difficulty speaking • Papilledema • Stupor • Seizures • Loss of consciousness • Hyperperfusion syndrome with cerebral edema (postsurgery)	• Pseudohypoxic brain swelling (PHBS) postsurgery due to suction drainage • Tumor lysis syndrome with cerebral edema as adverse effect of antineoplastic chemotherapy • Shaken infant (baby) syndrome: varies from mild to severe • Extreme irritability • Vomiting • Poor eating • Difficulty staying awake, lethargy • Tremors • Pale or bluish skin • Seizures • Paralysis • Loss of consciousness • Coma
2. Clinical Evaluation *(routine/expected in italics)*	• Toxicology • Blood tests • Fever	• Lactic acidosis • Blood glucose for hyperglycemia
3. Diagnostic Px *(routine/expected in italics)*	• *Postsurgery edema peaks between 48 and 60 hours following surgery* • Intracerebral hemorrhage/ischemic stroke: develops between four to 14 days • ICP and CPP: – maintain ICP < 20 mmHg – maintain CPP (cerebral perfusion pressure) at 60–70 mmHg • CT scan head: may be negative for first 24–36 hrs – hypodense or hypointense lesion with concomitant parenchymal hypoattenuation	• MRI brain: usually positive within three to four hours – T1 weighted = hypodense or hypointense lesion – T2 weighted = hyperintense (CSF) • Intracranial pressure monitoring via ICP catheter • ICP subdural bolt/screw for immediate ICP monitoring • Epidural sensor to monitor ICP • Ophthalmological exam • EEG • Neurological exam
4. Therapeutic Tx *(routine/expected in italics)*	• Administration of mannitol (osmotic agent) with or without DMSO or sodium added • Monitored administration of glycerol/sorbitol • Surgical excision of neoplasm when it is the etiology • Shunting for obstructive hydrocephalus • Administration of diuretics • Barbiturates to lower ICP • Surgical decompression of the brain or skull by craniectomy	• Raise the head of the bed 30° to assist in reducing ICP • Insertion of (EVD) ventricular catheter (ventriculostomy) for CSF drainage • Oxygen therapy • Corticosteroids • Glucocorticoid steroid: dexamethasone • Anticonvulsive meds • Hyperventilation therapy • IV fluids
5. Increased Nursing Care and/or Monitoring	• Progression of cerebral edema with mass effect/midline shift	
6. Extends LOS	• Hyperperfusion syndrome with cerebral edema • Cerebral edema during the postop period, complication of surgery	

Condition	Documentation Example	ICD-10-CM Corresponding Codes
Routine/Expected/ Integral/Inherent/ Incidental *(italics only)*	1. *Progress Note: Postglioblastoma excision with trace cerebral edema adjacent to surgical bed on postop imaging, progressing well.*	1. *No code assigned for cerebral edema.*
Principal Diagnosis	1. IP Discharge Summary: Closed frontal skull fracture, TBI with moderate cerebral edema and loss of consciousness (LOC) eight hours, cerebral edema treated with mannitol, resolved by day five.	1. Sequence the most serious injury as determined by the provider and the focus of treatment as principal diagnosis, noting that codes from subcategory SØ6.1X Traumatic cerebral edema, are combo codes that include both the cerebral edema and duration of LOC.
Comorbidity	1. Admit to IP: Shaken infant syndrome with cerebral edema. 2. IP: consultant report states cerebral edema increased causing herniation, treat with dimethyl sulfoxide (DMSO)/mannitol; the discharge summary does not mention the cerebral edema. **(Query the physician of the clinical significance of the cerebral edema with herniation treated by DMSO/mannitol as noted by the consult.)** 3. IP Progress note: After intrathecal methotrexate completed, patient experienced seizure; workup revealed cerebral edema: final diagnosis: Intracranial tumor lysis syndrome with cerebral edema causing seizure due to intrathecal methotrexate.	1. Report and sequence T74.4XXA Shaken infant syndrome, initial encounter, as principal diagnosis followed by any associated current injuries, including SØ6.1XØA Traumatic cerebral edema without loss of consciousness, initial encounter. 2. *If the query response is that it is not integral to the cause nor included in a combo code and its clinical significance is documented code G93.6 Cerebral edema, is reported as an additional diagnosis.* 3. Report intracranial tumor lysis syndrome with cerebral edema due to intrathecal methotrexate. Sequence E88.3 Tumor lysis syndrome, as principal diagnosis, followed by T45.1X5A Adverse effect of antineoplastic and immunosuppressive drugs, initial encounter, and G93.6 Cerebral edema, with an additional code for the neoplasm as appropriate.
Complication of Care	1. IP admit: Carotid endarterectomy five days ago, admitted due to seizure, workup revealed cerebral edema ipsilateral to surgery site. Final diagnosis: hyperperfusion syndrome with cerebral edema and seizure due to surgery.	1. Report hyperperfusion syndrome G97.82 Other postprocedural complications and disorders of nervous system, followed by G93.6 Cerebral edema, to identify the nature of the complication and R56.9 Unspecified convulsions.
Poisoning or Adverse Effect of Medication/ Chemical	NA	NA

Additional References

AHA CC: 3Q, 2022, p. 9, 10

CMS: Hospital Acquired Conditions (HAC) List
https://www.cms.gov/medicare/medicare-fee-for-service-payment/hospitalacqcond/icd10_hacs

Cerebrovascular Accident

G97.3[1,2]	**Intraoperative hemorrhage and hematoma of a nervous system organ or structure complicating a [nervous system, other] procedure**	CC
G97.5[1,2]	**Postprocedural hemorrhage of a nervous system organ or structure following a [nervous system, other] procedure**	CC
G97.6 [1,2]	**Postprocedural hematoma of a nervous system organ or structure following a [nervous system, other] procedure**	CC
I6Ø-	**Nontraumatic subarachnoid hemorrhage**	MCC HCC
I61-	**Nontraumatic intracerebral hemorrhage**	MCC HCC
I62.Ø[Ø,1,2,3]	**Nontraumatic [unspecified, acute, subacute, chronic] subdural hemorrhage**	MCC HCC
I62.1	**Nontraumatic extradural hemorrhage**	MCC HCC
I62.9	**Nontraumatic intracranial hemorrhage, unspecified**	CC HCC
I63-	**Cerebral infarction**	MCC HCC
I97.5[1,2]	**Accidental puncture and laceration of a circulatory system organ or structure during a [circulatory system, other] procedure**	CC
I97.81[Ø,1]	**Intraoperative cerebrovascular infarction during [cardiac, other] surgery**	CC
I97.82[Ø,1]	**Postprocedural cerebrovascular infarction during [cardiac, other] surgery**	CC
T45.695A	**Adverse effect of other fibrinolysis-affecting drugs, initial encounter**	
Z92.82	**Status post administration of tPA (rtPA) in a different facility within the last 24 hours prior to admission to current facility**	

Associated terminology: cerebrovascular accident with infarct; hemorrhagic CVA; cerebral hemorrhage/hematoma due to procedure; cerebral Infarct due to procedure; (prolonged) reversible ischemic neurological deficits; aborted CVA; cerebral hemorrhage due to tissue plasminogen activator (tPA)

Coding Tip

For category I63 Cerebral Infarction, use additional code, if known, to indicate National Institutes of Health Stroke Scale (NIHSS) score (R29.7-) The NIHSS scale is a tool used to evaluate neurological status based on clinical assessment of the effect of the CVA on the following neurological functions:

- **Levels of consciousness**
- **Language**
- **Neglect**
- **Visual-field loss**
- **Extraocular movement**
- **Motor strength**
- **Ataxia**
- **Dysarthria**
- **Sensory loss**

These NIHSS scale codes are reported as secondary codes following the acute CVA code and use scores from 0-42. NIHSS documentation may be taken from other clinicians that are not the patient's provider; however, the stroke diagnosis must be documented by the provider. Although multiple stroke scale scores may be captured, at the minimum, the initial score should be reported.

Discussion

Cerebrovascular accident (CVA) or stroke is a common term for a group of disorders that are classified as either ischemic (thrombosis/embolism/occlusion) or hemorrhagic that cause focal disruption of blood flow of the intracerebral or precerebral arteries with resulting neurological deficits and brain tissue damage. Symptom onset is sudden or abrupt, lasting longer than one hour and is related to the region of the brain involved and the type of CVA, ischemic or hemorrhagic. Evolving/in evolution means that the deficits are developing slowly, over 24–48 hours. Imaging should reveal an infarct or hemorrhage, usually within the first 48 hours. Associated conditions or complications, such as coma or encephalopathy, which are not integral or inherent to CVA infarct/hemorrhage, should be coded as additional diagnoses when present on admission or develop during the encounter.

It is important to note that MS-DRG assignment is affected by the administration of tissue plasminogen activator (tPA) by the facility billing for the encounter. A thorough review of the record is essential in determining if it was administered by the transferring hospital (Z92.82) or given in the receiving hospital.

Coding Tip

Impending CVA: There is no index listing for impending or threatened CVA. If it occurs, code as confirmed diagnosis per official coding guidelines. If it does not occur, assign the signs/symptoms or underlying condition in lieu of the code for CVA.

(P)RIND: (prolonged) reversible ischemic neurological deficit is a cerebral infarct that lasts between 24 and 72 hours. Per the ICD-10-CM index, code I63.9 should be reported for this condition.

Ischemic: blocked artery; associated with cerebral infarct; hemorrhagic conversion can occur: When hemorrhagic conversion occurs, report a code from category I63 Cerebral infarction, and an additional code for the hemorrhage (categories I6Ø–I62).

Documentation Checklist

- **Physician IP admit order: by admitting physician**
- **Medical necessity statement: need for IP admission**
- **History: medical history, family history relevant to encounter**
- **Onset: time of symptoms onset**
- **Identify: symptoms, associated conditions**
- **Duration: how long symptoms lasted**
- **Identify: type of stroke (thrombosis, embolism, other occlusion/stenosis, hemorrhagic; site of hemorrhage/infarct, including laterality; cause of hemorrhage (aneurysm, AVM, conversion, treatment)**
- **Treatment: stroke, associated conditions**
- **Neurology consult**
- **tPA administration: ED, outside hospital record, ICU, radiology**
- **Imaging results: infarct or hemorrhagic; is hemorrhage due to conversion or therapy**
- **Swallow test: identify presence and level of dysphagia**
- **Evaluation/therapy: PT/OT, speech, nutrition**
- **Medication: stroke treatment, treatment of associated conditions**
- **Discharge summary: provider confirms all relevant diagnoses, procedures, diagnostic testing results and consultant information and states discharge disposition, if known**
- **Discharge disposition: must be documented and correct Medicare code selected**

Types of CVA:

- Cerebral Infarct is focal brain necrosis.
- Thrombus: blood clot that forms inside a cerebral artery and blocks blood flow (atheromas, hypercoagulopathy disorders, atherosclerosis/atherothrombosis).
- Embolism: blood clot that originates outside the cerebral/precerebral arteries, dislodges from site of origin and travels to the brain, plugging a cerebral vessel and blocking blood flow (atrial fibrillation, vegetative endocarditis, prosthetic heart valve, fat emboli from long bone fracture, air embolism, post cardiac catheterization embolism).
- Occlusion or obstruction, nonatherothrombotic (lacunar infarct): occlusion usually caused by lipohyalinosis (degeneration of the middle layer of small, deep cortical arteries) and walls of artery are replaced by lipids and collagen (hypertension, diabetes, atherosclerosis of small vessels).
- Vasospasm: occlusion from vasospasm (migraine, cocaine or amphetamine use)

- Venous sinus thrombosis, nonpyrogenic: thrombosis of dural venous sinuses (postop, hypercoagulopathy, oral contraception).
- Watershed infarct (cortical or subcortical/internal): occurs at the border between cerebral vascular territories (prolonged systemic hypotension) (carotid stenosis) (any condition that causes significant hypotension).
- Hemorrhagic: a defective artery ruptures; occlusion not present:
  - Intracerebral: hemorrhage within the brain and ventricles (hypertension, amyloid cerebral angiopathy [cortical cerebral microbleeding], cocaine use, neoplasm, vasculitis, anticoagulation therapy)
  - Subarachnoid: hemorrhage occurs in the space between the brain and the skull; causes chemical meningitis; secondary vasospasm may cause TIA or infarct (ruptured cerebral aneurysm/ arteriovenous malformation (AVM), anticoagulation therapy, bleeding disorder, idiopathic).

Coding Tip

- **Occlusion/stenosis of cerebral/precerebral artery without infarction, see categories I65 Occlusion and stenosis of precerebral arteries, not resulting in cerebral infarction, and I66 Occlusion and stenosis of cerebral arteries, not resulting in cerebral infarction.**
- **Venous sinus thrombosis, septic, see code GØ8 Intracranial and intraspinal phlebitis and thrombophlebitis.**
- **Traumatic venous sinus thrombosis, see category SØ6 Intracranial injury.**
- **Cerebral infarction associated to traumatic brain injury, see category SØ6 Intracranial injury.**

Common neurological deficits with CVA/hemorrhage:

- Some neurological deficits will be reported as they are not inherent; report even when resolved by discharge or develop post admit and/or meet criteria as an additional diagnosis. Review the alphabetic index entry for the neurological deficit in order to determine if it is included in I63.
  - paralysis/paresis (hemiplegia) (monoplegia) (quadriplegia) (embolic/thrombotic; current episode)
  - paresthesia
  - dysphagia
  - dysphasia
  - ataxia; ataxic gait; acute ataxia
  - apraxia
  - dysarthria
  - homonymous hemianopia
  - aphasia
  - third cranial nerve pals
  - cognitive deficits
  - pseudobulbar affect
  - neurological/sensory/hemispatial neglect
  - facial droop/weakness
  - fluency disorder
  - locked-in state/other paralytic syndromes
  - seizure
  - visual defects/disturbance

Documentation Tip

When documentation and clinical criteria do not match, query the provider for clarification of the diagnosis.

Documentation Tip

Code assignment cannot be based on ancillary test results, therapies, or clinical criteria alone. A diagnosis and its clinical significance must be supported by physician or other qualified healthcare professional documentation. When it is unclear or there is contradictory information, query the physician or other qualified healthcare professional for clarification.

Documentation Tip

Complications of care: The condition must be more than a routinely expected condition or event. The documentation must support that the condition is clinically significant with an indication that it is a complication, by demonstrating:

- **A cause-and-effect relationship between the care or procedure and the condition**
- **That the condition resulted in altering the course of a procedure or surgery**

The term "complication" does not have to be explicitly documented.

Coding/Reporting Criteria	Clinical Criteria	
1. Physical Evaluation *(routine/expected in italics)*	• Symptoms with abrupt onset, vary and some reflect infarct or hemorrhage and origin (cerebral/precerebral) and area of brain involved • Infarct: neurological deficits will affect contralateral side of infarct hemispheric site • Symptoms last > 1 hour for infarct/hemorrhage and infarct/hemorrhage on imaging; if < 1 hour/transient, suspect TIA w/o infarct/hemorrhage on imaging • Confusion • Weakness/paresis • Hemiplegia/quadriplegia • Hemisensory loss • Gaze preference • Neurological neglect • Facial droop • Photophobia • Stiff neck/pain/chemical meningitis • Papilloedema • Monocular/binocular blindness • Blurred vision or visual field defects: homonymous hemianopia • Eye movement abnormalities (diplopia or nystagmus)	• Anisocoria • Hyperglycemia • Dysphagia • Dysarthria or difficulty understanding speech • Vertigo • Ataxia • Aphasia • Headache (worst headache of my life, thunderclap) • Nausea/vomiting • Syncope • New onset seizure • Acute neurological deficit • Altered loss of consciousness • Cytotoxic cerebral edema: causes deterioration during the first 48–72 hours after onset • Hydrocephalus • Increased intracranial pressure • Encephalopathy • Coma/obtunded (GCS ≤ 8) • Hypertension (systolic BP > 220 mm Hg) • Fever (indication of neurological deterioration) • Brain herniation/compression/midline shift • Decorticate/decerebrate posturing
2. Clinical Evaluation *(routine/expected in italics)*	• CBC • Platelet count • Prothrombin time test (PT)/partial thromboplastin time test (PTT) • Fasting blood glucose	• Lipid profile • Homocysteine • Erythrocyte sedimentation rate (ESR) • Other tests as warranted for specific dx workup
3. Diagnostic Px *(routine/expected in italics)*	• Neurological exam/consult • CT: after 24 hours ischemic infarct visible; initial neuroimaging • Diffusion weighted MRI: follow-up to CT, esp. when initial CT is negative • gradient echo MRI • Angiography	• Carotid duplex ultrasonography • ECG • Swallow study for dysphagia • Lumbar puncture for SAH • transesophageal echocardiography to evaluate cardiac etiology

Coding/Reporting Criteria	Clinical Criteria
4. Therapeutic Tx *(routine/expected in italics)*	• Treatment depends on the type (ischemic or hemorrhagic) • IV nicardipine; labetalol • Nimodipine to prevent vasospasm • Aspirin • Tissue plasminogen activator (tPA) administration (review ED record, transferring hospital records, ICU record, or radiology report): within 3 (or 4.5 hours with certain criteria) of onset • Anticoagulation for thrombosis • Antiplatelet therapy • Reversal of anticoagulation for hemorrhage: – FFP – vitamin K – platelet transfusions • Treat hypertension: – mean arterial pressure (MAP) > 130 mmHg – systolic BP > 185 mm Hg • Ventricular drain • Surgical evacuation of cerebellar hematomas > 3 cm • Stents with or without percutaneous angioplasty (PTA)/tPA: intracerebral or precerebral artery: atherosclerotic stenosis • Angioplasty • Coiling embolization of aneurysm/arteriovenous malformation (AVM) (ruptured): endovascular • Pipeline embolization device (PED) for aneurysm repair • Clipping of aneurysm/AVM (ruptured) • Mechanical thrombectomy/embolectomy: Merci Retrieval System®, with or without tPA • Endarterectomy • BrainsGate Ischemic Stroke System (ISS): sphenopalatine ganglion implantable neurostimulator; up to 24 hours of onset • Supportive measures • Treatment of complications: – airway support (intubation) – oxygen – mechanical ventilation – physical therapy/occupational therapy – speech therapy – feeding therapy/restrictions/gastrostomy – insertion of intracranial bolt for ICP monitor – CoolGard; intravascular cooling system • Medications to control blood pressure, edema, glucose, fever, seizures
5. Increased Nursing Care and/or Monitoring	• Cerebral infarct/hemorrhage develops post-admit
6. Extends LOS	• Cerebral infarct/hemorrhage due to complication of care

Condition	Documentation Example	ICD-10-CM Corresponding Codes
Routine/Expected/ Integral/Inherent/ Incidental *(italics only)*	*NA*	*NA*
Principal Diagnosis	1. IP Discharge Summary: A 70-year-old male admitted for right cortical intracerebral hemorrhage due to known amyloid cerebral angiopathy. 2. IP Discharge Summary: 80-year-old female admitted with embolic left middle cerebral artery infarct from rheumatic mitral stenosis, hemorrhagic intraventricular conversion on day two.	1. Report I61.1 Nontraumatic intracerebral hemorrhage in hemisphere, cortical; E85.4 Organ-limited amyloidosis; I68.Ø Cerebral amyloid angiopathy. 2. Report I63.412 Cerebral infarction due to embolism of left middle cerebral artery; I61.5 Nontraumatic intracerebral hemorrhage, intraventricular; IØ5.Ø Rheumatic mitral stenosis.
Comorbidity	1. IP Progress Note: A 92-year-old male admitted yesterday with aspiration pneumonia, acute hypoxic respiratory failure and massive right intracerebral infarct due to right carotid arteriosclerotic stenosis; intubated with mechanical vent on admit; patient expired. 2. A 78-year-old female admitted for right hemispheric CVA with resultant left-sided (nondominant) weakness.	1. Report J96.Ø1 Acute respiratory failure with hypoxia; J69.Ø Pneumonitis due to inhalation of food and vomit; I63.231 Cerebral infarction due to unspecified occlusion or stenosis of right carotid arteries. 2. In addition to the CVA code, code G81.94 Hemiplegia, unspecified affecting left nondominant side, is appropriate for the left-sided weakness. When weakness on one side is clearly documented as associated with the CVA, it is considered synonymous with hemiplegia/hemiparesis.

Condition	Documentation Example	ICD-10-CM Corresponding Codes
Complication of Care	1. IP Progress note: A 65-year-old patient exhibited dysarthria and encephalopathy while in the ICU post CABG; workup revealed embolic infarct right posterior cerebral artery. **(Query if the infarct is related to the surgery as a complication or unrelated and due to another specified condition.)**	1. Add an additional code when the complication of care code does not identify the specific nature of the complication or if an additional code provides additional information. For example, if documentation upholds a connection supporting the complication of/due to surgery, report I97.82Ø Postprocedural cerebrovascular infarction during cardiac surgery; I63.432 Cerebral infarction due to embolism of left posterior cerebral artery; R47.1 Dysarthria and anarthria; G93.49 Other encephalopathy.
Poisoning or Adverse Effect of Medication/ Chemical	1. IP Progress Note: A 30-year-old male admitted after taking extra doses of valium then becoming intoxicated with alcohol, stated as accidental without intent to harm self, workup revealed internal watershed infarction. 2. IP Discharge Summary: A 78-year-old male on Coumadin due to chronic atrial fibrillation, admitted due to left hemispheric subcortical intracerebral hemorrhage secondary to Coumadin coagulopathy, med taken as prescribed; reverse anticoagulation with vitamin K, transfuse FFP and monitor.	1. Report T42.4X1A Poisoning by benzodiazepines, accidental (unintentional), initial encounter; T51.ØX1A Toxic effect of ethanol, accidental (unintentional), initial encounter; F1Ø.92Ø Alcohol use, unspecified with intoxication, uncomplicated; I63.519 Cerebral infarction due to unspecified occlusion or stenosis of unspecified middle cerebral artery. • Poisoning: Identify drug/chemical by the code from T36–T5Ø with fifth or sixth character of intent followed by a code for nature of adverse drug effect (manifestation). 2. Report I61.Ø Nontraumatic intracerebral hemorrhage in hemisphere, subcortical; T45.515A Adverse effect of anticoagulants; initial encounter; I48.2Ø Chronic atrial fibrillation, unspecified; Z79.Ø1 Long term (current) use of anticoagulants. • Adverse effect: Nature of adverse drug effect: code for (adverse condition) followed by the code from T36–T5Ø with fifth or sixth character 5 to identify the drug.

Additional References:

AHA CC: 2Q, 2024, p. 25; 1Q, 2024, p. 26; 4Q, 2023, p. 42; 3Q, 2022, p. 9; 1Q, 2022, p. 25; 3Q, 2020, p. 24, 28; 2Q, 2020, p. 29; 2Q, 2019, p. 24; 2Q, 2017, p. 9; 4Q, 2016, p. 26

Chest Pain as Principal Diagnosis

RØ7.1	**Chest pain on breathing**
RØ7.2	**Precordial pain**
RØ7.81	**Pleurodynia**
RØ7.82	**Intercostal pain**
RØ7.89	**Other chest pain**
RØ7.9	**Chest pain, unspecified**

Associated terminology: chest pain of undetermined etiology; pleuritic chest pain; noncardiac chest pain; atypical chest pain; musculoskeletal chest pain; painful respiration; anterior (chest) wall pain; central chest pain

Diagnoses

Discussion

Chest pain requires medical evaluation as the etiology can range from critical to benign, but cannot be determined without a workup. A workup begins with a thorough history, noting the location, duration, character, and quality of chest pain, the precipitating events as well as triggers, and what relieves the pain. Associated symptoms and risk factors also aid in the direction of the investigation. Sometimes the clinical evaluation can determine the etiology of the chest pain, and along with trial of treatment, the suspected cause can be determined. Other times, the chest pain will be of unknown origin.

When chest pain is determined to be due to two or more contrasting or comparative diagnoses, all of the contrasting comparative diagnoses would be reported, with any of the contrasting or comparative diagnoses sequenced as principal diagnosis.

If the symptom of chest pain is integral to a diagnosis, it is not reported as a secondary code. If chest pain is not integral but a manifestation of the diagnosis, the symptom chest pain is reported as an additional diagnosis for an inpatient encounter (i.e., chest pain due to anxiety is assigned a code from category F41 Other anxiety disorders, followed by the code from category RØ7 Pain in throat and chest).

Documentation Tip

When the final diagnosis is chest pain with no further clarification as to the cause, but the workup or therapy suggests a possible definitive diagnosis, query if a definitive diagnosis was suspected, possible, probable, or if symptoms and treatment were consistent with a specified diagnosis.

Documentation Tip

Code assignment cannot be based on ancillary test results, therapies, or clinical criteria alone. A diagnosis and its clinical significance must be supported by physician or other qualified healthcare professional documentation. When it is unclear or there is contradictory information, query the physician or other qualified healthcare professional for clarification.

Observation status may be used for initial risk stratification assessment beyond ED time. For inpatient admission, document all comorbidities and factors that support inpatient admission.

Coding Tip

- **Adverse effect: Nature of adverse drug effect: code for (adverse condition) followed by the code from T36–T5Ø with fifth or sixth character 5 to identify the drug.**
- **Poisoning: Identify drug or chemical by the code from T36–T5Ø with fifth or sixth character of intent followed by a code for nature of the toxic drug effect (manifestation).**

Potential causes of chest pain:

- Myocardial infarction/angina/coronary disease
- Musculoskeletal: costochondritis (Tietze's syndrome), bruised or broken ribs, fibromyalgia
- Pleurisy/pleuritis/myocarditis
- Atelectasis
- Pneumothorax
- Shingles
- Pneumonia or chronic obstructive pulmonary disease (COPD) exacerbation
- Pulmonary embolus
- Pulmonary hypertension
- Panic attack, psychological stress, ventricular irritability (neurasthenia)
- Aortic dissection
- Reflux esophagitis/gastroesophageal reflux disease/dysphagia/esophageal rupture/gastric/duodenal ulcer/colitis
- Acute chest syndrome of sickle-cell disease
  Note: Some diagnoses in ICD-10-CM are combination codes that identify both the primary condition and an associated manifestation. This is true for sickle-cell disease with acute chest syndrome, which can be found in category D57 Sickle-cell disorders.
- Referred abdominal pain from gallbladder, pancreas

Coding Tip

To preempt possible denial by external audit: diagnoses made within the record but not listed or included in the discharge summary, query the provider for concordance and inclusion into discharge summary. (Note: CMS reinforces that omission by the provider of a consultant's diagnosis in the discharge summary or discharge note is not a conflict in documentation and, therefore, the consultant's diagnosis may be reported. However, denials of the consultant's diagnosis may be attempted by external auditors.)

Coding/Reporting Criteria	Clinical Criteria	
1. Physical Evaluation *(routine/expected in italics)*	• Symptoms or signs will be related to cause • Vital signs: – blood pressure – pulse rate – respiratory rate – temperature • Oxygen saturation • Rash: suggests shingles • Carotid bruit or heart murmur: suggests cardiac issue	• Chest palpation: suggests musculoskeletal issue • Abnormal breath sounds: suggests lung issue • Friction rubs: suggests lung or pleural issue • Abnormal heart sounds: suggests pericardial issues • Jugular venous distention: suggests pericardial, cardiac issue • Abdominal palpation: for masses or GI pain • Extremity pulses
2. Clinical Evaluation *(routine/expected in italics)*	• Workup is based on suspected cause based on presentation and history and physical • Troponin/creatine phosphokinase (CPK)s: rule out cardiac • Erythrocyte sedimentation rate: rule out myocarditis	• C-reactive protein: rule out myocarditis • Serum lipase: rule out pancreas • WBC: rule out infection • Arterial blood gas (ABG): rule out lung disorder • D-dimer
3. Diagnostic Px *(routine/expected in italics)*	• Workup is based on suspected cause based on presentation and history and physical • Chest x-ray • Serial ECGs • CT chest; CT abdomen • Transesophageal echocardiogram (TEE) • Echocardiology • Esophagoscopy with contrast: esophageal rupture • Esophagoscopy/esophagogastroduodenoscopy/colonoscopy/ileoscopy; with or without biopsy; *H. pylori*: rule out GI source • Motility studies	• Ultrasound: rule out gallbladder • Barium swallow: rule out esophageal motility disorder • Pulse oximetry • Cardiac angiogram; with or without ergonovine provocation test: rule out coronary disease/spasm • Ventilation-perfusion scan: rule out lung or embolism • Pulmonary angiogram or peripheral arteriogram: rule out embolism, deep vein thrombosis • Stress test: rule out cardiac disorder • Cardiac cath
4. Therapeutic Tx *(routine/expected in italics)*	• Treatment can be empirical, or based on suspected condition • Pain meds • Cardiovascular meds: aspirin, beta blockers, nitroglycerin • GI meds: acid blockers, antacids • Ice or warm compress for musculoskeletal pain • Anti-inflammatory meds • Thoracentesis: pleurisy/effusion	• Chest tube: pneumothorax • Oxygen therapy • Antiviral meds: shingles • Antibiotics: infection • Anticoagulation: embolism or thrombosis • Thrombolytic therapy: embolism or thrombosis • Angioplasty • Pericardiocentesis • Platelet inhibitor during cardiac catheterization
5. Increased Nursing Care and/or Monitoring	• Monitor efficacy of treatment plan	
6. Extends LOS	• NA	

Condition	Documentation Example	ICD-10-CM Corresponding Codes
Routine/Expected/ Integral/Inherent/ Incidental *(italics only)*	*NA*	*NA*
Principal Diagnosis	1. IP Discharge Summary: Admitted due to chest pain after minor motor vehicle accident with seat belt in place; unsure if chest hit steering wheel; cardiac contusion and thoracic dissection ruled out; chest wall contusion versus anxiety reaction.	1. Report RØ7.9 Chest pain, unspecified, followed by S2Ø.219A Contusion of unspecified front wall of thorax, initial encounter, and F41.1 Generalized anxiety disorder.
Comorbidity	1. IP Discharge Note: Admitted with precordial chest pain, suspected cardiac neurasthenia.	1. Report F45.8 Other somatoform disorders, followed by RØ7.2 Precordial pain.
Complication of Care	NA	NA
Poisoning or Adverse Effect of Medication/ Chemical	1. IP Admit Note: Admitted due to chest pain induced by cocaine toxicity.	1. Report T4Ø.5X1A Poisoning by cocaine, accidental (unintentional), initial encounter, followed by RØ7.9 Chest pain, unspecified.

Chronic Obstructive Pulmonary Disease (COPD) Exacerbation with Asthma/Bronchitis

J44.1 **Chronic obstructive pulmonary disease with (acute) exacerbation** CC HCC

Associated terminology: decompensated COPD; emphysema with chronic bronchitis with acute exacerbation; asthma with COPD exacerbation; chronic obstructive asthma with exacerbation; acute exacerbation of COPD (AECOPD)

Coding Tip

Category J44 Other chronic obstructive pulmonary disease, includes both chronic asthma and bronchitis.

Discussion

An acute exacerbation of chronic obstructive pulmonary disease (COPD) is a short and rapid onset of an increase in severity of symptoms of dyspnea, cough frequency, sputum quality/quantity, sputum purulence and in severe cases may include a failure to respond to the usual therapy. Exacerbations are most often triggered by infection with bronchitis or pneumonia. Less often, pollution, heart failure, pneumothorax, pulmonary embolism, aspiration, and inhalation exposure, among other environmental factors are the cause. Decompensation is the worsening or acute exacerbation of a chronic condition; therefore, documentation of decompensated COPD is interpreted to mean acute on chronic exacerbation. Also note, the term "acute" does not need to be stated in order to assign J44.1 as it is a nonessential modifier.

Hypoxia may be present and documented as due to the COPD. Since it is not inherent to COPD, it is coded separately. If it occurs without respiratory failure, code RØ9.Ø2 from chapter 18 would be added. If respiratory failure is documented, a combination code from category J96-, chapter 10, which includes both the type of respiratory failure and the hypoxia, would be appropriate.

Acute bronchitis is not equivalent to acute exacerbation; it is a separate condition. The tabular Excludes 2 note under J44.1 indicates that COPD with acute bronchitis (J44.Ø Chronic obstructive pulmonary disease with acute lower respiratory infection) is not included in J44.1, and when appropriate, both conditions may be reported together.

When asthma with COPD exacerbation is documented, code both J44.1 and the specified type of asthma from category J45 per the tabular instructional note under category J44 Other chronic obstructive pulmonary disease.

Documentation Tip

When emphysema with COPD is documented, it is reported with emphysema (J43.9) since emphysema is a more specific form of COPD. However, a code from category J44 Other chronic obstructive pulmonary disease, is assigned for chronic emphysematous bronchitis. A review of the includes and excludes notes under categories J43, J44, and J45 will assist with whether a query is needed to clarify the condition.

Medical necessity for inpatient admission status for exacerbation of COPD has been an audit issue. Facilities may want to initiate protocols for observation and inpatient criteria for COPD exacerbation. Physician admit orders must detail the clinical indicators that denote exacerbation and the therapies tried and failed, clinical judgment, and decision-making in order to support the condition and admission type. Some suggested criteria for hospitalization are:

- High-risk comorbidities: chronic respiratory failure, pneumonia, cardiac arrhythmia, heart failure/cor pulmonale (right heart failure), diabetes, renal failure, liver failure
- Failure of initial or outpatient therapies/failure to respond to controlled oxygen therapy or bronchodilators
- Increase in symptoms (quantify/comparison)
- Negative impact on activities of daily living requirements: sleep interruption, inability to eat
- Worsening hypoxemia or hypercapnia/quantify
- Inadequate home/residence support
- History of respiratory failure
- Aspiration risk/gastroesophageal reflux disease (GERD)
- Uncorrected moderate to severe acute hypoxemia

- Acute or severe respiratory acidosis/after O_2 therapy
- New arrhythmias
- Progressive respiratory fatigue, need for intubation
- Central nervous system depression, change in mental status/after O_2 therapy
- Advanced age

Another audit issue is the reporting of acute and/or chronic respiratory failure with COPD exacerbation. Some of the signs or symptoms of acute and chronic respiratory failure are the same for COPD and its acute exacerbation. Many, but not all, COPD patients have chronic respiratory failure. They may require supplemental home oxygen therapy for the first time after an exacerbation episode, but note that the need for supplemental oxygen should be reassessed 60 to 90 days after discharge as the patient may improve and no longer require supplemental oxygen. COPD can cause both hypoxemic and hypercapnic respiratory failure. Hypoxemic, also known as type I, is characterized by a drop in blood oxygenation. Hypercapnic, otherwise known as type II respiratory failure, can be determined by a rise in arterial CO_2 levels. In chronic respiratory failure, the patient's blood pH is normal (7.35–7.45) or slightly decreased; if pCO_2 remains well over 55 or CO_2 is 35 or above, along with other clinical indicators, a query for chronic respiratory failure may be indicated.

Global Initiative for Chronic Obstructive Lung Disease (GOLD) staging criteria is a set of clinical data established to classify COPD patients by measuring the level of pulmonary obstruction via pulmonary function tests (PFT). The GOLD staging criteria indicate GOLD IV is very severe COPD and the forced expiratory volume in 1 second (FEV1) predicted is less than 50 or chronic respiratory failure symptoms are present (usually meaning requires long-term supplemental oxygen). A query based on the GOLD criteria may assist in identifying chronic respiratory failure with COPD.

With respiratory acidosis pH less than 7.30 or worsening of respiratory symptoms, a 10–15 mm drop in PO_2 and/or significant increase in PCO_2 together with a decrease in pH, suspect acute respiratory failure. A decrease of 10 percent from baseline oxygenation may indicate acute respiratory failure in COPD. Again, with supporting clinical indicators, a query would be appropriate for acute respiratory failure in conjunction with COPD.

Documentation Tip

Medical necessity for inpatient admission for COPD exacerbation and reporting of respiratory failure due to COPD exacerbation are frequent targets of audits. Ensure adequate criteria is reported to support these conditions with thorough documentation of items such as comorbidities, increase of severe symptoms, pulmonary function tests (PFTs), prior failed treatments, and current treatment.

Coding/Reporting Criteria	Clinical Criteria	
1. Physical Evaluation *(routine/expected in italics)*	• Acute increase in symptoms beyond normal variations: – cough: increase in frequency and severity – sputum production: increase in volume and/or changes in quality, quantity, color, or purulence – worsening or resting dyspnea – decreased breath sounds – lethargy or somnolence: due to retention of CO_2 – diaphoresis – tachycardia; heart rate > 120 beats/min – anxiety – cyanosis – increased work of breathing	• Wheezing • Tripod positioning of the arms against the legs/exam table • Constitutional symptoms • Mild tachypnea; respiratory rate > 35 breaths/min • Pursed lip breathing • Use of accessory muscles • Increased respiratory phase of breathing •
2. Clinical Evaluation *(routine/expected in italics)*	• Arterial blood gas (ABG): to quantify hypoxemia and hypercapnia (severe exacerbations) • Sputum: yellow/green indicates neutrophils and suggests bacterial colonization/infection • Sputum culture: suspected infection	• Gram stain • Electrolytes • Renal function • Basic metabolic panel
3. Diagnostic Px *(routine/expected in italics)*	• Chest x-ray: stable/unchanged chest x-ray; hyperinflation; with emphysema/bullae • Pulmonary function tests: decrease in pulmonary function	• Pulse oximetry: low O_2 saturation • Electrocardiogram

Coding/Reporting Criteria	Clinical Criteria
4. Therapeutic Tx *(routine/expected in italics)*	• Treatment of both COPD exacerbation and cause • Antibiotic: moderate or severe exacerbation; purulent sputum • Bronchodilator: short acting B-agonist and anticholinergic: MDI or nebulizer • Corticosteroid dose and duration: 30–40 mg for 7–14 days for moderate to severe exacerbations • Adequate oxygenation (hypoxemic) (90–94%) and PaO_2 of 60–70 mmHg • Venturi mask: titrating FiO_2 • NPPV: moderate to severe exacerbations; contraindications are severely impaired consciousness, inability to clear secretions or protect airway, high aspiration risk • Vent/intubation • Anticoagulation based on mobility • Maintain nutrition • Tracheostomy • Pulmonary rehab
5. Increased Nursing Care and/or Monitoring	• Need for intubation/mechanical ventilation
6. Extends LOS	• Need for tracheostomy

Condition	Documentation Example	ICD-10-CM Corresponding Codes
Routine/Expected/ Integral/Inherent/ Incidental *(italics only)*	*NA*	*NA*
Principal Diagnosis	1. IP Admit Note: After failed outpatient treatment and increase in severity of symptoms, admit to IP for control of COPD decompensated with chronic respiratory failure on long-term home oxygen.	1. Report J44.1 Chronic obstructive pulmonary disease with (acute) exacerbation; J96.1Ø Chronic respiratory failure, unspecified whether with hypoxia or hypercapnia; Z99.81 Dependence on supplemental oxygen.
Comorbidity	1. IP Discharge Summary: Admitted for *Haemophilus influenzae* pneumonia with moderate exacerbation of COPD; pneumonia treated with IV antibiotics, COPD exacerbation treated with oxygen and nebulizers.	1. Assign both codes J44.Ø Chronic obstructive pulmonary disease with acute lower respiratory infection, and J44.1 Chronic obstructive pulmonary disease with (acute) exacerbation. Since the focus and intensity of the treatment is the pneumonia, and the prescribed treatment of the COPD exacerbation could have been treated as an outpatient if the pneumonia had not been present, sequence code J14 Pneumonia due to Hemophilus influenzae first, followed by J44.Ø and J44.1 for the COPD with acute lower respiratory tract infection and exacerbation. The "code also to identify the infection," instructional note at code J44.Ø indicates that a code should also be assigned to capture the specific type of infection. Sequencing of the pneumonia and COPD codes are governed by the Section II, "Selection of Principal Diagnosis," guidelines. In this case it was the pneumonia that was "chiefly responsible for occasioning the admission."
Complication of Care	1. Postoperative Note: Exacerbation of COPD due to lung resection in <24 hours prior.	1. Report J95.89 Other postprocedural complications and disorders of respiratory system, not elsewhere classified; J44.1 Chronic obstructive pulmonary disease with (acute) exacerbation.
Poisoning or Adverse Effect of medication/ Chemical	1. IP Admit Note: Acute exacerbation of COPD due to use of ammonia bathroom cleaner aerosol spray while cleaning the home bathroom.	1. Report T54.3X1A Toxic effect of corrosive alkalis and alkali-like substances, accidental (unintentional), initial encounter, followed by J68.3 Other acute and subacute respiratory conditions due to chemicals, gases, fumes and vapors, and J44.1 Chronic obstructive pulmonary disease with (acute) exacerbation.

Additional References

AHA CC: 2Q, 2024, p. 3-5; 1Q, 2019, p. 34, 35; 4Q, 2017, p. 96-98; 1Q, 2017, p. 26; 3Q, 2016, p. 15-16; 1Q, 2016, p. 35

Global Initiative for Chronic Obstructive Lung Disease: https://goldcopd.org/

MLN, *Medicare Quarterly Provider Compliance Newsletter*, July 2011, January 2012

Coagulopathy

R79.1	**Abnormal coagulation profile**	
T45.51[1,3,4]A	**Poisoning by anticoagulants, [accidental (unintentional), assault, undetermined], initial encounter**	
T45.512A	**Poisoning by anticoagulants, intentional self-harm, initial encounter**	HCC
T45.515A	**Adverse effect of anticoagulants, initial encounter**	

Associated terminology: coagulopathy due to anticoagulant; elevated PT/PTT/INR due to anticoagulant

Note: This clinical review is limited to coagulopathy related to anticoagulant use.

Discussion

Anticoagulant medication prevents blood from clotting by interfering with vitamin K levels or decreasing production of clotting proteins. An elevated or prolonged prothrombin time test (PT)/partial thromboplastin time test (PTT)/international normalized ratio test (INR) level is an expected outcome of anticoagulant therapy. This becomes problematic when these levels rise even further and result in adverse effects or indicate potential for adverse effects. The most common adverse effect of anticoagulant therapy is bleeding. Excessive anticoagulation can occur due to many variables (diet, other medications, noncompliance) and makes routine INR testing valuable. Coagulopathy is an intersection of elevated INR level, age, comorbid conditions and hemorrhage. Coagulopathy due to anticoagulant therapy is categorized as an abnormal coagulation profile (elevated PT/PTT/INR), and in coding may be considered an "adverse effect" or a "poisoning."

Note: Although many codes representing bleeding conditions are signs/symptoms that fall into chapter 18, they will be assigned as principal diagnosis when they identify the nature of an adverse effect and are the reason for admission.

Coagulopathy due to anticoagulant therapy is not located in categories D65–D69 Coagulation defects, purpura and other hemorrhagic conditions. Most of this category represents coagulopathy directly related to a disease process that causes deficient or missing naturally occurring coagulation factors or (intrinsic) circulating anticoagulants in the bloodstream. However code D68.32 Hemorrhagic disorder due to extrinsic circulating anticoagulants, which includes drug-induced hemorrhagic disorder, can be additionally reported for bleeding such as hematuria, hemoptysis, hematochezia, etc. associated with an anticoagulation therapy drug. Code sequencing is dependent on the circumstances of the admission.

Documentation Tip

Complications of care: The condition must be more than a routinely expected condition or event. The documentation must support that the condition is clinically significant with an indication that it is a complication, by demonstrating:

- **A cause-and-effect relationship between the care or procedure and the condition**
- **That the condition resulted in altering the course of a procedure or surgery**

The term "complication" does not have to be explicitly documented.

Elevated/Prolonged PT/PTT/ Supratherapeutic INR

An elevated or prolonged PT/PTT/INR is an expected result of anticoagulant use. These elevated levels place the patient at an increased risk for bleeding and a common side effect associated with the therapy is when the levels rise beyond therapeutic levels. The code R79.1 Abnormal coagulation profile, is reported to denote the elevated PT/PTT/INR or supratherapeutic INR when it is documented and no specific side effect is documented. When the elevated PT/PTT/INR due to therapeutic anticoagulation therapy is excessive, needs treatment, increases care/monitoring, or extends LOS, this is considered an adverse effect and is reported with code R79.1, followed by T45.515A Adverse effect of anticoagulants, initial encounter.

Documentation Tip

Code assignment cannot be based on ancillary test results, therapies, or clinical criteria alone. A diagnosis and its clinical significance must be supported by physician or other qualified healthcare professional documentation. When it is unclear or there is contradictory information, query the physician or other qualified healthcare professional for clarification.

Adverse Effect

When the anticoagulant therapy is correctly prescribed and properly administered, but the patient experiences an adverse effect, report a code for the nature of the adverse effect (manifestation) followed by T45.515A to identify the anticoagulant drug. Anticoagulant intoxication due to accumulative effect resulting in an adverse effect is also considered an adverse effect and not a poisoning.

Coding Tip

Some of the complications of care codes include the external cause or the external cause and intent. The code includes the nature of the complication in addition to the type of procedure that caused the complication and in some cases, the intent. When it includes the external cause or intent, no additional external cause code from category Y62–Y84 is necessary. When the external cause or intent is not included in the complication of care code, report all chapter 20 codes needed to completely describe the circumstances as appropriate for the type of encounter.

Examples: nature of adverse effect due to anticoagulant coagulopathy (not all inclusive)	T45.515A and D68.32: sequenced after code(s) for the nature of the adverse effects
Bleeding gums	KØ6.8
Blood in stool/melena	K92.1
Epistaxis	RØ4.Ø
Excessive bleed from AV fistula	T82.838A
Excessive bleed from Foley	T83.83XA
Excessive bleed from PICC	T82.838A
Gastritis with bleeding	K29- with a fifth character of 1
GI bleed of undetermined, unspecified site	K92.2
Gross hematuria	R31.Ø
Hemoperitoneum (nontraumatic) (spontaneous)	K66.1
Hemoptysis	RØ4.2
Hemorrhage of anus and rectum	K62.5
HIT (heparin induced thrombocytopenia)	D75.82-
Joint hemarthrosis	M25.Ø-
Muscle (Psoas) hematoma	M79.81
Retroperitoneal hematoma/hemorrhage	K66.1
Spontaneous ecchymoses	R23.3
Subdural hematoma (spontaneous) (nontraumatic)	I62.Ø-
Warfarin-induced skin necrosis (gangrene)	I96

Poisoning

When an error is made in administration of the anticoagulant medication, whether by the care provider or the patient, a poisoning code is reported. Examples of an error are:

- Error in prescription (dosage)
- Error in administration (e.g., wrong route)
- Overdose resulting in toxicity
- Nonprescribed drug taken with correctly prescribes/properly administered drug resulting in toxicity/reaction
- Reaction resulting from the interaction of drug and alcohol

Report T45.51[1, 2, 3, 4]A and sequence before the code(s) for any manifestations. The sixth character identifies the intent.

Documentation Tip

The symbols ↑ and ↓ do not indicate a diagnosis. Query the provider as to the meaning and if it represents a diagnosis, a sign of abnormal results, a condition, or an indication of a change over past results. Request that the information be fully stated, including the clinical significance.

Admission to Reverse or Discontinue Anticoagulation Therapy Prior to Procedure

When a patient is admitted prior to a planned procedure to stop, reverse, or adjust anticoagulation prior to the procedure, the principal diagnosis will be the reason for the procedure, followed by Z51.81 Encounter for therapeutic drug monitoring and Z79.Ø1 Long term (current) use of anticoagulants, and the condition that is under treatment/prophylaxis by the drug. This is the case even if the procedure would have been routinely performed as an outpatient.

Coding Tip

The seventh character extensions A, D, S affect the analysis of complications and quality of care and reimbursement.

Coding/Reporting Criteria	Clinical Criteria
1. Physical Evaluation *(routine/expected in italics)*	• *Asymptomatic* • Symptoms vary depending on the nature/site of the hemorrhagic condition • Hemorrhage, bleeding, hematoma, ecchymosis (bruising) • Heparin-induced thrombocytopenia (HIT) – arterial/venous thrombosis: cerebral vascular accident (CVA), pulmonary embolism (PE), myocardial infarction (MI), deep vein thrombosis (DVT)
2. Clinical Evaluation *(routine/expected in italics)*	• *PT/PTT/INR elevated therapeutically to the therapeutic level, not causing adverse reaction* • PT/PTT elevated beyond therapeutic levels – PTT: 1.5 to 2.5 x that of the reference range • INR: therapeutic range on anticoagulant 2.0–3.5 depending on diagnosis/reason for drug – INR > 4.0 risk factor for hemorrhage – overcoagulation: INR 5–9 • Anti-Xa test for low molecular weight heparin (LMWH) • HIT – serotonin release assay (SRA)—positive – heparin-induced platelet aggregation assay (HIPA)—positive – H-PF4 ELIZA solid phase immunoassay-positive – particle gel immunoassay – platelet count-decreased • CBC
3. Diagnostic Px *(routine/expected in italics)*	• CT scan if internal bleed is suspected • Vascular imaging for HIT sequela • Ultrasound
4. Therapeutic Tx *(routine/expected in italics)*	• Discontinue or withhold and decrease dose • Vitamin K • Transfusion: – coagulation factors – fresh frozen plasma (FFP) – prothrombin complex concentrate (PCC) • Overheparinization causing bleeding: – protamine sulfate • Therapy to control hemorrhage (e.g., nasal packing) • Therapy to drain hemorrhage (e.g., Psoas muscle drainage) • HIT: discontinue and avoid heparin products – start alternative anticoagulant drug
5. Increased Nursing Care and/or Monitoring	• Continued treatment of hemorrhagic condition or monitoring INR and drug levels
6. Extends LOS	• Post procedure monitoring after anticoagulant restart, discharge after therapeutic INR level obtained

Condition	Documentation Example	ICD-10-CM Corresponding Codes
Routine/Expected/ Integral/Inherent/ Incidental *(italics only)*	1. *IP Progress Note: ↑ INR therapeutic on warfarin for bioprosthetic mitral valve replacement.*	1. *Report Z79.01 Long term (current) use of anticoagulants, and Z95.3 Presence of xenogenic heart valve as additional diagnoses.* *It is not necessary to query the meaning of the up arrow as it would not be coded since it is at a therapeutic level.*
Principal Diagnosis	1. IP Progress Note: Admitted due to Coumadin toxicity. (**Query if the reaction or nature of the toxicity; query if the drug was correctly prescribed/administered when not stated or unclear.**)	1. When the reaction or nature of drug toxicity is not documented, a query is needed to define toxicity as either an adverse effect or as a poisoning and to identify the reaction/manifestation.
Comorbidity	1. IP Progress Note: Post-admit, elevated INR became symptomatic with warfarin-induced melena; workup revealed chronic gastritis with bleeding; chronic atrial fibrillation stable with adjusted warfarin dose.	1. Report K29.51 Unspecified chronic gastritis with bleeding; T45.515A Adverse effect of anticoagulants, initial encounter; D68.32 Hemorrhagic disorder due to extrinsic circulating anticoagulants; I48.2Ø Chronic atrial fibrillation, unspecified; Z79.Ø1 Long term (current) use of anticoagulants. • When elevated PT/PTT/INR is further specified as producing a reaction/manifestation, do not report R79.1 Abnormal coagulation profile.
Complication of Care	NA	NA
Poisoning or Adverse Effect of Medication/ Chemical	1. IP Admit Note: Admit due to HIT-induced acute right thigh DVT s/p right knee total arthroplasty on heparin prophylaxis. 2. IP Discharge Summary: Coumadin overdose due to elderly patient accidently taking additional doses, resulting in epistaxis; treated with nasal packing and oral vitamin K.	1. Report D75.829 Heparin induced thrombocytopenia (HIT); T45.515A Adverse effect of anticoagulants, initial encounter; I82.4Y1 Acute embolism and thrombosis of unspecified deep veins of right proximal lower extremity; Z96.651 Presence of right artificial knee joint; Z79.Ø1 Long term (current) use of anticoagulants. 2. Report T45.511A Poisoning by anticoagulants, accidental (unintentional), initial encounter; RØ4.Ø Epistaxis; D68.32 Hemorrhagic disorder due to extrinsic circulating anticoagulants; Z79.Ø1 Long term (current) use of anticoagulants.

Additional References

AHA CC: 1Q, 2021, p. 4; 1Q, 2016, p. 14; 2Q, 2013, p. 34

Journal of AHIMA, November/December 2005, "Classification of Coagulopathy," pp. 72–74

COVID-19

UØ7.1	**COVID-19**	MCC
A41.89	**Other specified sepsis**	MCC HCC
D89.83[1,2,9]	**Cytokine release syndrome [grade 1, grade 2, grade unspecified]**	
D89.83[3,4,5]	**Cytokine release syndrome [grade 3, grade 4, grade 5]**	CC
JØ6.9	**Acute upper respiratory infection, unspecified**	
J12.82	**Pneumonia due to coronavirus disease**	MCC
J2Ø.8	**Acute bronchitis due to other specified organisms**	
J22	**Unspecified acute lower respiratory infection**	
J4Ø	**Bronchitis, not specified as acute or chronic**	
J8Ø	**Acute respiratory distress syndrome**	MCC HCC
J96.Ø-	**Acute respiratory failure**	MCC HCC
J98.8	**Other specified respiratory disorders**	
M35.81	**Multisystem inflammatory syndrome**	CC HCC
UØ9.9	**Post COVID-19 condition, unspecified**	
ZØ1.84	**Encounter for antibody response examination**	
ZØ3.818	**Encounter for observation for suspected exposure to other biological agents ruled out**	
Z11.52	**Encounter for screening for COVID-19**	
Z2Ø.822	**Contact with and (suspected) exposure to COVID-19**	

Associated terminology: COVID-19, coronavirus 19, novel coronavirus (nCoV), severe acute respiratory syndrome-related coronavirus 2 (SARS-CoV-2), with or without acute upper or lower respiratory infection, with pneumonia, with acute respiratory failure with or unspecified whether with hypoxia or hypercapnia, with ARDS; test for COVID-19 antibodies, screening test for COVID-19 exposure; cytokine storm, cytokine release syndrome (CRS)

Discussion

COVID-19 is considered a zoonotic disease (passes from animals to humans) that was first identified in an outbreak of respiratory illness cases in Wuhan City, Hubei Province, China. It was initially reported to the World Health Organization (WHO) on December 31, 2019, and by January 30, 2020, the WHO declared the COVID-19 outbreak a global health emergency. On March 11, 2020, the first time since the H1N1 influenza outbreak of 2009, the WHO declared COVID-19 a global pandemic.

Although individuals of all ages can contract COVID-19 and severe disease, serious complications are more prevalent in ages 60 and older and those with chronic medical conditions. The mortality rate is higher in those age 70 or higher with or without chronic medical conditions. Data in the United States has indicated higher incidence of COVID-19 with higher hospitalization rate and death in ethnic minorities.

Symptoms of COVID-19 generally appear within four to five days of exposure, although they may take as long as 14 days post exposure to appear. Although COVID-19 is widely known to be respiratory in nature, it also accesses various body cells by attaching to ACE2 enzymes (membrane proteins on the cellular surface) found mainly in heart, intestinal, kidney, and lung cells. ACE2 serves as the entry point into cells for this coronavirus, where after binding to the ACE2 enzyme, it injects its viral RNA into the cell. Viral RNA takes over cellular activity, instructing cells to replicate and release the virus.

Alveoli walls thicken with debris, preventing exchange of O_2 and CO_2, and lesions develop in the lungs, ranging in size from grape to grapefruit. The following respiratory conditions have been frequently associated with COVID-19.

Viral pneumonia: Pneumonia is a serious infection/inflammation of one or both of the lungs in which the alveoli (air sacs) fill with pus or liquid rather than oxygen, making it difficult to breathe and difficult for oxygen to pass into the bloodstream. COVID 19 pneumonia typically affects bilateral lungs.

Symptoms include fever, cough, shortness of breath, fatigue, altered mentation, elevated WBCs, possible left shift, tachycardia, tachypnea, dullness to percussion, and diaphoresis. Treatments include supplemental O_2, IV antibiotics, antipyretics, cough medication (antitussants), hydration, breathing treatments, and pulmonary and infectious disease consults.

- Coding: For pneumonia confirmed as due to COVID-19, assign code UØ7.1 COVID-19, as the primary or first-listed diagnosis and J12.82 Pneumonia due to coronavirus disease.
- Documentation: Provider should clearly state the causative organism (when known) and that the specific organism caused the pneumonia (i.e., "viral pneumonia due to confirmed COVID-19 disease"). Unclear documentation such as "infiltrate on CXR" or "infectious lung process" cannot be reported as pneumonia. Query to clarify.

Diagnoses

Acute bronchitis: Inflammation of the mucous membrane within the bronchi, inducing symptoms such as cough that is dry or with thickened mucus, shortness of breath, fatigue, post-nasal drip, and bronchospasm. Treatments include NSAIDs, analgesics, and cough suppressants. Bronchospasms are sudden constrictions in muscle of the bronchiole walls, which can impede breathing. They are treated with inhaled, short-acting beta2-agonists, such as Ventolin or Proventil (albuterol) to help open airways.

- Coding: If acute bronchitis occurs due to COVID-19, sequence UØ7.1 COVID-19, followed by J2Ø.8 Acute bronchitis due to other specified organisms.
- Documentation: Specify bronchitis as acute or chronic and link to (due to) COVID-19 when applicable. Document any other conditions present, such as chronic obstructive pulmonary disease (COPD) and asthma, with further specificity for both diagnoses.

Acute respiratory distress syndrome (ARDS): ARDS, a sudden failure of the respiratory system, has been notable in severe COVID-19 cases. In ARDS, the alveoli become inflamed and engorged with fluid, resulting in flooding and collapse of the alveolar space. As a result, pulmonary gas exchange is compromised, and the patient becomes hypoxic. ARDS usually occurs only in critically ill patients. Symptoms of ARDS include dyspnea, tachypnea, hypoxemia, left atrial hypertension, pulmonary hypertension, and cyanosis. Diagnosis can be confirmed by identifying abnormalities on chest x-ray. The condition is also defined by the P/F ratio (the partial pressure of oxygen in the patient's arterial blood to the fraction of oxygen in the inspired air). Most definitions state that ARDS can be diagnosed when the P/F ratio is <300 mm Hg. Prognosis varies, depending on the underlying etiologies and health status of the patient at the time of the critical illness. Treatment requires intensive care management with ventilatory and hemodynamic support and adjuvant drug therapies. ARDS is also called shock lung.

- Coding: For ARDS due to COVID-19, assign codes UØ7.1 COVID-19, and J8Ø Acute respiratory distress syndrome.
- Documentation: The term "respiratory distress" is not enough to code ARDS. If the clinical condition indicates ARDS, a query is needed to clarify whether that is indeed the case.
- Documentation: When acute respiratory failure documented as related to COVID-19 progresses to acute respiratory distress syndrome (ARDS), assign only codes U07.1 COVID-19, and J80 Acute respiratory distress syndrome, as ARDS is a severe life-threatening form of respiratory failure that should be reported to the highest level of specificity. This is supported by the Excludes 1 note at category J96 Respiratory failure, not elsewhere classified, where code J80 Acute respiratory distress syndrome, is listed, indicating that only code J80 should be reported when both conditions are documented in the medical record.

Acute respiratory failure: Respiratory failure occurs when there is an inadequate gas exchange of O_2 intake and CO_2 elimination in the lungs, which results in the inability to maintain arterial oxygen and/or carbon dioxide levels within their normal ranges. This imbalance leads to hypoxemia, with or without hypercapnia. It is life-threatening and always due to another condition.

Hypoxemic respiratory failure is diagnosed in patients without chronic lung disease when there is falling pulse oximetry from 92 percent saturation or initial pulse oximetry below 80 percent saturation on room air. Severe respiratory failure is diagnosed when arterial blood gas shows PaO_2 of <60 mmHg (<8 kPa) on room air.

Hypercapnic respiratory failure is diagnosed in patients without chronic lung disease when there is hypoxia and acute elevation of arterial $PaCO_2$ >45 to 50 mmHg (>6.0 to 6.7 kPa) and associated acidosis (pH <7.35).

Acute respiratory failure develops over minutes to hours as evidenced by a pH of less than 7.30 (acidemia). Chronic respiratory failure develops over days or longer, which allows for renal compensation with an increase in bicarbonate concentration with only a slight decrease in pH level. Treatment is directed towards both the respiratory failure and the underlying cause, when identified.

Clinical indicators include dyspnea or tachypnea (RR >20), cyanosis (bluing of fingers, toes, around lips), tripod position or leaning forward, increased work of breathing and use of accessory muscles, hypotension and changes in mentation—confusion or altered level of consciousness (LOC). Treatment often requires monitored ICU status with frequent arterial blood gases (ABGs) checks and O_2 saturation monitoring and supplemental O_2, including continuous positive airway pressure (CPAP), bilevel positive airway pressure (BIPAP), or mechanical ventilation. (See "Respiratory Failure" in this publication for more details)

- Coding: For acute respiratory failure due to COVID-19, sequence first UØ7.1 COVID-19, followed by J96.Ø- Acute respiratory failure (with appropriate specificity).
- Documentation: Respiratory failure—Specify acuity: acute, chronic, acute-on-chronic and mechanism such as hypoxic, hypercapnic, or combination of both. If the respiratory failure is chronic, consider if the patient is dependent on home O_2. Look for ABGs, pulmonary function tests (PFTs), and P/F ratio to support a diagnosis of acute respiratory failure.

Documentation Tip

If the patient is exhibiting signs and symptoms of respiratory *failure* but the documentation reflects only insufficiency or distress, it is appropriate to query for clarification to move the documentation away from these otherwise nonspecific terms. Insufficiency and distress are reported with codes RØ6.89 and RØ6.Ø3, which classify unspecified abnormalities of breathing, in Major Diagnostic Category (MDC) chapter 18 for Signs, Symptoms, and Abnormal Clinical and Lab Findings. Respiratory distress refers to difficulty breathing that may be due to conditions such as asthma, aspiration, heart disease, etc. Respiratory distress is not associated with a respiratory system inability to supply adequate oxygen and/or eliminate carbon dioxide to maintain metabolism.

Coding and Documentation Tip

Since the principal diagnosis for COVID-19 with sepsis depends on the circumstance of admission, it is imperative to clarify whether the sepsis was present on admission (POA) and necessitated the admission in order to use A41.89 Other specified sepsis, as the principal diagnosis. If sepsis clearly developed over the course of the admission and COVID-19 was POA, code first UØ7.1 COVID-19.

Coding Tip

When a patient who previously had COVID-19 and is without residual symptoms or conditions is seen for a follow-up exam and the COVID-19 test is negative, assign codes ZØ9 Encounter for follow-up examination after completed treatment for conditions other than malignant neoplasm, and Z86.16, Personal history of COVID-19.

Note: Cytokine release syndrome (CRS) is a nonrespiratory condition worth noting as it has been prevalent in COVID-19 cases. The syndrome is an overreaction of the immune system—the body floods itself with cytokines, which are proteins created and released from immune cells. The proteins mediate and regulate immunity, inflammation, and hematopoiesis. The condition vasodilates the blood vessels, which can lead to hypotension and shock even when the patient has sufficient fluids. The vessels, in their state of vasodilation, do not pump blood efficiently, leading to hypoxemic states throughout the body and potential organ failure. CRS also activates the release of cytokines during hemophagocytic lymphohistiocytosis, a condition whereby the body makes too many activated immune cells, specifically macrophages and lymphocytes. In cases of too much inflammation, the immune cells destroy each other instead of attacking infected and damaged cells in the body. Microscopic evidence shows these cells "eating" other cells (hemophagocytic). Clinical indicators include fevers, rash, enlarged liver/spleen/lymph nodes, anemia, low platelets and WBCs, jaundice, hepatitis and liver failure, respiratory issues, seizures, and altered mentation. The patient may also present with disseminated intravascular coagulation (DIC), and multiorgan failure. Treatments include chemotherapy, immunotherapy, steroids, and antivirals.

- Coding: As noted in the coding instructions at subcategory D89.83- Cytokine release syndrome, code first the underlying cause, such as COVID-19 or complication of transplanted organ.
- Documentation: The condition may also be called cytokine storm. Documentation should link to COVID-19, when applicable.

Coding and Documentation Tip

Multisystem inflammatory syndrome (MIS) is a serious condition that can affect children and adults with a current or previous COVID-19 infection. This rare condition can produce elevated inflammatory markers and damage to the heart and other vital organs. If COVID-19 is currently active, code UØ7.1 COVID-19, is listed as the principal diagnosis, followed by M35.81 Multisystem inflammatory syndrome, as secondary for the MIS. If the MIS is a residual of a past COVID-19 infection, code first the M35.81, followed by UØ9.9 Post COVID-19 condition, unspecified as secondary. Query the provider if documentation is not clear whether the COVID-19 infection is active or resolved (history) and/or the provider does not establish a clear link between the MIS and COVID-19 infection.

Coding and Documentation Tip

Code UØ9.9 Post COVID-19, unspecified, is to be used when documentation references persistent or new symptoms or sequela related to a previous COVID-19 infection. Codes for the new or persistent symptoms or conditions should be coded first with UØ9.9 coded as secondary.

Common persistent symptoms or sequela often associated with post COVID-19 (not exhaustive):

- **Fatigue**
- **Cough**
- **Hypoxia**
- **Chest pain**
- **Joint pain**
- **Muscle pain**
- **Numbness**
- **Fever**
- **Headache**
- **Dizziness**
- **Rash**
- **Loss of smell (anosmia)**
- **Loss of taste (parosmia)**
- **Mood changes**

A patient may experience residual, or sequela, conditions related to a past COVID infection *and* develop symptoms or conditions related to a current or active COVID infection. Codes UØ7.1 and UØ9.9 can be reported together in this instance. Codes for any symptoms or conditions related to the active infection and/or the post COVID infection may also be assigned.

Coding/Reporting Criteria	Clinical Criteria	
1. Physical Evaluation *(routine/expected in italics)*	• Fever or chills • Dyspnea/shortness of breath • Cough • Tachycardia • Tachypnea: increased breathing rate • Altered mentation • Loss of taste and/or smell	• Muscle or joint aches • Headache • Sore throat • Congestion or runny nose • Nausea, vomiting • Diarrhea • Fatigue
2. Clinical Evaluation *(routine/expected in italics)*	• Lymphopenia • Neutrophilia • Elevated serum alanine aminotransferase and aspartate aminotransferase levels • Elevated lactate dehydrogenase • High ferritin/CRP • Elevated D-dimer • High plasma levels of Inflammatory markers • Lung tissue inflammation usually from bacterial or viral source	• Bilateral air-space consolidation • Bilateral, peripheral ground glass opacities • Mild thrombocytopenia • Prolonged prothrombin time • CBC diff (esp. total lymphocyte count) • CPK creatine kinase • Positive blood culture • Monitor ferritin/CRP (first 2 wks of hospitalization) • PT/PTT/fibrinogen
3. Diagnostic Px *(routine/expected in italics)*	• Chest x-ray • Viral (nucleic acid or antigen) test for COVID-19 • Sputum culture • Chest CT	• EKG • Pulmonary function test • LDH (repeat daily if elevated) • Troponin (repeat q2-3d if elevated)

Coding/Reporting Criteria	Clinical Criteria	
4. Therapeutic Tx *(routine/expected in italics)*	• Frequent ABG checks and O_2 saturation monitoring • Supplemental O_2, including CPAP, BIPAP, or mechanical ventilation • Antipyretics • Cough medication (antitussants) • Hydration • Management of underlying condition(s) • Antimicrobials in setting of superimposed infection • Remdesivir (RDV) for patients who require supplemental oxygen but who are not on high-flow oxygen, noninvasive ventilation, mechanical ventilation, or ECMO (BI).	• Prophylactic anticoagulation with low-molecular-weight heparin (LMWH) in the absence of any contraindications • For cytokine storm—anakinra, baricitinib, siltuximab, tocilizumab • Dexamethasone for use in patients who require supplemental O_2 only • For AKI—continuous (or intermittent) renal replacement therapy (CRRT)
5. Increased Nursing Care and/or Monitoring	• Monitored ICU bed	• Isolation precautions
6. Extends LOS	• Discharge delayed due to mechanical ventilation	• Discharge delayed due to physical rehabilitation (transfer to rehab unit)

Condition	Documentation Example	ICD-10-CM Corresponding Codes
Routine/Expected/ Integral/Inherent/ Incidental *(italics only)*	1. *IP Discharge Summary: High fever, cough, and shortness of breath, suspect COVID-19.* (Query for COVID-19 test results)	1. *For positive test code only UØ7.1 COVID-19. Other symptoms integral.* If negative or no results, code only symptoms RØ5.9 Cough, unspecified. RØ6.Ø2 Shortness of breath, R5Ø.9 Fever
Principal Diagnosis	1. IP Admit Note: Patient with acute bronchitis. Tests positive for COVID-19. 2. Patient admitted with sepsis. Tests positive for COVID-19. 3. Patient readmitted with pneumothorax d/t previous hx of COVID-19	1. Code first UØ7.1 COVID-19, followed by J2Ø.8 Acute bronchitis due to other specified organisms. 2. Code first A41.89 Other specified sepsis, followed by UØ7.1 COVID-19. Pdx depends on circumstances of admission 3. J93.83 Other pneumothorax, is principal dx, followed by UØ9.9 Post COVID-19 condition, unspecified.
Comorbidity	1. Throughout stay, COVID-19 patient treated for signs, symptoms of ARDS. Discharge Summary: Acute respiratory distress. (Query for acute respiratory distress syndrome [ARDS])	1. Code UØ7.1 COVID-19, with J8Ø Acute respiratory distress syndrome, which is an MCC if query agrees. Acute respiratory distress (RØ3.Ø3) is a symptom of COVID-19 and is not reported separately.
Complication of Care	NA	NA
Poisoning or Adverse Effect of Medication/ Chemical	NA	NA

Additional References

AHA: Frequently Asked Questions Regarding ICD-10-CM/PCS Coding for COVID-19, revised May 9, 2023 (codingclinicadvisor.com)

AHA CC: 2Q, 2022, p. 28; 4Q, 2021, p. 31; 1Q, 2021, p. 25, 31; 4Q, 2020, p. 12; 3Q, 2020, p. 13-14; 2Q, 2020, p. 3; 1Q, 2020, p. 34, 40

CDC: https://www.cdc.gov/covid/index.html
https://www.cdc.gov/mis/index.html

Deep Vein Thrombosis of Upper and Lower Extremities

I82.4-	**Acute embolism and thrombosis of deep veins of lower extremity**	CC HAC HCC
I82.5-	**Chronic embolism and thrombosis of deep veins of lower extremity**	CC HCC
I82.62-	**Acute embolism and thrombosis of deep veins of upper extremity**	CC HCC
I82.72-	**Chronic embolism and thrombosis of deep veins of upper extremity**	CC HCC
I82.A-	**Embolism and thrombosis of axillary vein**	CC HCC
I82.B-	**Embolism and thrombosis of subclavian vein**	CC HCC
I82.C-	**Embolism and thrombosis of internal jugular vein**	CC HCC
I82.8-	**Embolism and thrombosis of other specified veins**	CC
I82.9-	**Embolism and thrombosis of unspecified vein**	CC
I97.89	**Other postprocedural complications and disorders of the circulatory system, not elsewhere classified**	CC
T82.868A	**Thrombosis due to vascular prosthetic devices, implants and grafts, initial encounter**	CC
Z86.718	**Personal history of other venous thrombosis and embolism**	

Associated terminology: deep vein thrombosis; DVT not otherwise specified; acute DVT; chronic DVT

Discussion

Deep vein thrombosis (DVT) is a condition in which thrombus or a blood clot develops and originates within a deep vein. The deep blood vessels are those that lie within and below muscles. These occur most commonly in the veins of the lower extremity, but may occur in the upper extremity as well. A complication of a DVT is embolism or thromboembolism in which the thrombus dislodges and occludes a distant blood vessel; the most common is pulmonary embolism due to leg DVT. This complication is reported using a code from category I26 Pulmonary embolism, or code I27.82 Chronic pulmonary embolism.

DVT is not limited to a certain group of people and can be found in a patient of any race, gender, or health status. Common risk factors for a DVT are:

- Venous injury from fracture, muscle injury, or surgery
- Thoracic outlet syndrome (TOS)
- Slow blood flow from prolonged immobility
- Increased estrogen
- Chronic illnesses, including but not limited to:
  - heart disease
  - lung disease
  - cancer and cancer treatment
  - irritable bowel syndrome, Crohn's disease, or ulcerative colitis
- Personal or family history of DVT or pulmonary embolism (PE)
- Obesity
- Over 40 years of age
- Presence of a central venous catheter (CVC)
- Genetic clotting disorders

Documentation Tip

Complications of care: The condition must be more than a routinely expected condition or event. The documentation must support that the condition is clinically significant with an indication that it is a complication, by demonstrating:

- **A cause-and-effect relationship between the care or procedure and the condition**
- **That the condition resulted in altering the course of a procedure or surgery**

The term "complication" does not have to be explicitly documented.

Another common issue is postphlebitic syndrome, in which the veins have been damaged by the blood clot, creating resistance and decreasing blood flow. This may happen fairly quickly to years after the initial DVT occurs. Common symptoms are leg edema with pain and skin discoloration. Wearing compression stockings and/or taking aspirin or diuretics treat the symptoms of the syndrome. This condition is reported using a code from subcategory I87.Ø Postthrombotic syndrome.

Another finding that is extremely common with DVT is thrombophlebitis, which is the inflammation of the lining of a vein. A thrombus can develop without causing inflammation in the blood vessel. Therefore, the phlebitis is not integral to a DVT and a code from category I8Ø Phlebitis and thrombophlebitis, should be reported as an additional diagnosis when both DVT and thrombophlebitis are present at the same site. An exception would be with subcategories I82.4, I82.5, I82.81 per the Excludes 1 note at category I8Ø that indicates these codes may not be reported together. It is important that both codes are reported when both conditions are present for those subcategories that allow both codes.

Coding Tip

Some of the complications of care codes include the external cause or the external cause and intent. The code includes the nature of the complication in addition to the type of procedure that caused the complication and in some cases, the intent. When it includes the external cause or intent, no additional external cause code from category Y62–Y84 is necessary. When the external cause or intent is not included in the complication of care code, report all chapter 20 codes needed to completely describe the circumstances as appropriate for the type of encounter.

When a physician documents "history of DVT" and the patient is currently maintained on an anticoagulant such as heparin, warfarin, or Coumadin, and there is no further indication of the status of the DVT, the physician should be queried to establish whether the anticoagulant is being given prophylactically to prevent recurrence or as a treatment for chronic DVT. If the reason is prophylaxis, the appropriate code to report would be Z86.718 Personal history of other venous thrombosis and embolism. If chronic, select a code from subcategory I82.5.

Chronic DVTs (clots that are one month to several months old) can harden and develop intravascular scarring, causing occlusive symptoms such as chronic leg swelling, skin discoloration, ulceration, cellulitis, or other complications.

When DVT is due to vascular prosthetic devices, implants, and grafts, report the complication code and the code identifying the specified site.

Documentation Tip

Since only *acute* DVT is considered a hospital acquired condition, it is important that documentation clearly indicates whether a DVT was chronic and present on admission or occurred during the inpatient encounter.

It is important to note that the term acute is a nonessential modifier for DVT and, therefore, is not needed in order to report a code from subcategory I82.4. In fact, if not further specified, the default code selection for DVT is acute rather than chronic. There is also no defined time frame established to distinguish when a DVT is chronic; only the physician's clinical training and judgment make that determination.

Recurrent DVT indicates the condition has occurred more than once. Recurrent DVT would be reported with the default "acute" unless the provider documents the recurrent DVT is chronic, as there is no specific code for "recurrent DVT."

Documentation Tip

If documented, acute and chronic embolism and thrombosis of the lower extremities can be further specified by anatomic site: femoral, iliac, popliteal, tibial, peroneal, and calf muscular veins. Although an unspecified vein option is available, specificity is always preferred.

Coding/Reporting Criteria	Clinical Criteria	
1. Physical Evaluation *(routine/expected in italics)*	• *Swelling of affected extremity* • Pain in extremity	• Redness of the skin
2. Clinical Evaluation *(routine/expected in italics)F*	• D Dimer blood test • Activated protein C resistance • Antithrombin III levels	• Antiphospholipid antibodies • Lupus anticoagulant • Protein C and S levels
3. Diagnostic Px *(routine/expected in italics)*	• Duplex ultrasound • Venography	• MRI • CT scan
4. Therapeutic Tx *(routine/expected in italics)*	• *Increased mobilization* • *Compression stockings* • *Lower leg exercises*	• Anticoagulants • Thrombectomy • Vena cava (Greenfield) filter insertion
5. Increased Nursing Care and/or Monitoring	• DVT occurs post admit	
6. Extends LOS	• Discharge delayed due to DVT	

Diagnoses

Condition	Documentation Example	ICD-10-CM Corresponding Codes
Routine/Expected/ Integral/Inherent/ Incidental *(italics only)*	1. *Patient on Coumadin for DVT prophylaxis.*	1. *Report Z86.718 Personal history of other venous thrombosis and embolism, followed by Z79.01 Long term (current) use of anticoagulants.*
Principal Diagnosis	1. Discharge Summary: A 65-year-old male was admitted for DVT and thrombophlebitis of right popliteal vein; treated with thrombectomy.	1. Report I82.431 Acute embolism and thrombosis of right popliteal vein.
Comorbidity	1. Discharge Summary: Final Diagnosis: Massive acute pulmonary embolism due to chronic DVT **(Query the site of DVT.)**	1. Report I26.99 Other pulmonary embolism without acute cor pulmonale, followed by I82.4Ø9 Acute embolism and thrombosis of unspecified deep veins of unspecified lower extremity.
Complication of Care	1. Discharge Summary: The patient was admitted for a DVT of the right brachial vein due to the presence of a CVC.	1. Report T82.868A Thrombosis of vascular prosthetic devices, implants and grafts, initial encounter, followed by I82.621 Acute embolism and thrombosis of deep veins of right upper extremity.
Poisoning or Adverse Effect of Medication/ Chemical	1. History and Physical: Recurrent, chronic DVT of left tibial vein due to patient noncompliance with warfarin regimen because he could not afford the prescription.	1. Report I82.542 Chronic embolism and thrombosis of left tibial vein, followed by T45.516A Underdosing of anticoagulants, initial encounter, and Z91.12Ø Patient's intentional underdosing of medication regimen due to financial hardship.

Additional References

AHA CC: 3Q, 2023, p. 12; 2Q, 2023, p. 8; 2Q, 2020, p. 20; 4Q, 2019, p. 8

CDC: http://www.cdc.gov

CMS: Hospital Acquired Conditions (HAC) List
https://www.cms.gov/medicare/medicare-fee-for-service-payment/hospitalacqcond/icd10_hacs

Dehydration as Principal Diagnosis

E86.Ø	**Dehydration**	
E87.Ø	**Hyperosmolality and hypernatremia**	CC
E87.1	**Hypo-osmolality and hyponatremia**	CC

Associated terminology: dehydration; dehydration with hypernatremia; dehydration with hyponatremia; cachexia due to dehydration

Discussion

Dehydration is a state of water and/or sodium imbalance due to the amount of total water or sodium loss being greater than the amount taken in. It is usually due to an associated condition, such as diarrhea, vomiting, diabetes, neoplasm, etc. The severity is measured by the percentage of body weight reduction due to fluid loss:

- Mild: 1–2 percent loss of body weight
  - typically does not need medical intervention; treat by increasing fluid intake enhanced with sodium/electrolytes
- Moderate: 3–5 percent loss of body weight
  - requires medical treatment; IV fluids/electrolyte/carbohydrate replacement
- Severe: > 5 percent loss of body weight; 7–9 percent loss of body weight is critical; > 10 percent loss of body weight (high risk of mortality)
  - requires hospitalization; IV fluids, electrolyte, or carbohydrate replacement

When sequencing dehydration and its cause, consider whether either condition could have been treated on an outpatient basis or if the treatment was consistent with outpatient therapy. If both were treated equally with therapy that requires inpatient admission, then review coding guidelines and coding guidance for sequencing.

Coding Tip

Principal diagnosis is that condition established after study to be chiefly responsible for occasioning the admission of the patient to the hospital for care.

Coding Tip

When the admission/encounter is for management of dehydration due to malignancy and only the dehydration is being treated (intravenous rehydration), the dehydration is sequenced first, followed by the code(s) for the malignancy.

Before reporting dehydration, dehydration with hypernatremia, or dehydration with hyponatremia, ensure the clinical criteria support the diagnostic statement. If there are discrepancies, query the physician for clarification. Also, physician documentation should include all comorbidities, especially those that influence the condition and treatment of dehydration.

Reporting dehydration *with* hypernatremia or hyponatremia requires two codes: E86.Ø *and* either E87.Ø or E87.1.

Coding Tip

When two or more diagnoses equally meet the definition of principal diagnosis, any one of the diagnoses may be sequenced first.

Documentation Tip

Code assignment cannot be based on ancillary test results, therapies, or clinical criteria alone. A diagnosis and its clinical significance must be supported by physician or other qualified healthcare provider documentation and clinical criteria. When it is unclear or there is contradictory information, query the physician or other qualified healthcare provider for clarification.

Documentation Tip

The symbols ↑ and ↓ do not indicate a diagnosis. Query the provider as to the meaning and if it represents a diagnosis, a sign of abnormal results, a condition, or an indication of a change over past results. Request that the information be fully stated, including the clinical significance.

Coding/Reporting Criteria	Clinical Criteria	
1. Physical Evaluation *(routine/expected in italics)*	• Elderly patients may exhibit some signs/symptoms due to age or other factors • Headache/head rush • Diminished skin turgor (degree of elasticity) • Dry mucous membranes • Tachycardia • Tachypnea • Orthostatic hypotension • Decreased urine output • Patient complains of thirst • Urine concentration showing as progressively yellow color to amber • Lack of tears • Sweating may stop (check armpit/groin)	• Muscle cramps • Nausea/vomiting • Heart palpitations • Lightheadedness • Skin: cool/clammy/dry/flushed • Constipation • Severe: – oliguria – weakness – confusion – seizure – organ failure/kidney failure – shock – coma – cerebral edema
2. Clinical Evaluation *(routine/expected in italics)*	• Serum electrolytes • BUN/creatinine: elevated • Plasma osmolality	• Urine chemistries/urine specific gravity • CBC • Blood chemistry
3. Diagnostic Px *(routine/expected in italics)*	• Work up for underlying cause • Mental status evaluation	• Vital signs • Temperature (rectal): to evaluate for fever
4. Therapeutic Tx *(routine/expected in italics)*	• Treatment of underlying cause and complications • Administration: sodium • Fluid resuscitation: oral (clear fluids) or IV • Clear fluids: – water – clear broths – popsicles – Jello – other replacements fluids that may contain electrolytes	
5. Increased Nursing Care and/or Monitoring	• Monitor fluid intake/output	
6. Extends LOS	• Fluid overload due to overhydration	

Condition	Documentation Example	ICD-10-CM Corresponding Codes
Routine/Expected/ Integral/Inherent/ Incidental *(italics only)*	*NA*	*NA*
Principal Diagnosis	1. IP Admit Note: Frail 82-year-old female with moderate dehydration due to gastroenteritis; admit for IV hydration and continue po Imodium.	1. Report E86.Ø Dehydration, followed by K52.9 Noninfective gastroenteritis and colitis, unspecified.
Comorbidity	1. IP Discharge Summary: UTI with dehydration with hyponatremia; treated with IV antibiotics and IV hydration.	1. Report N39.Ø Urinary tract infection, site not specified, E86.Ø Dehydration, and E87.1 Hypo-osmolality and hyponatremia
Complication of Care	NA	NA
Poisoning or Adverse Effect of Medication/ Chemical	NA	NA

Additional References

AHA CC: 2Q, 2019, p. 7; 1Q, 2019, p. 12; 1Q, 2014, p. 7

Diagnoses

Diabetic Ketoacidosis

EØ8.1Ø	**Diabetes mellitus due to underlying condition with ketoacidosis without coma**	MCC HAC HCC
EØ8.11	**Diabetes mellitus due to underlying condition with ketoacidosis with coma**	MCC HAC HCC
EØ9.1Ø	**Drug or chemical induced diabetes mellitus with ketoacidosis without coma**	MCC HAC
EØ9.11	**Drug or chemical induced diabetes mellitus with ketoacidosis with coma**	MCC HAC
E1Ø.1Ø	**Type 1 diabetes mellitus with ketoacidosis without coma**	MCC HAC HCC
E1Ø.11	**Type 1 diabetes mellitus with ketoacidosis with coma**	MCC HAC HCC
E11.1Ø	**Type 2 diabetes mellitus with ketoacidosis without coma**	MCC HAC HCC
E11.11	**Type 2 diabetes mellitus with ketoacidosis with coma**	MCC HAC HCC
E13.1Ø	**Other specified diabetes mellitus with ketoacidosis without coma**	MCC HAC HCC
E13.11	**Other specified diabetes mellitus with ketoacidosis with coma**	MCC HAC HCC

Associated terminology: diabetic ketoacidosis, DKA

Discussion

Diabetic ketoacidosis (DKA) is a potentially life-threatening complication of diabetes mellitus characterized by hyperglycemia, the production of ketone bodies, and systemic acidosis, due to a shortage of insulin in which the body switches to burning fatty acids and producing acidic ketone bodies.

Common causes of DKA include insulin noncompliance, missed or inadequate insulin dosage, or an acute infection such as sepsis, urinary tract infection or pneumonia. DKA may be complicated by changes in mental status/consciousness that can vary from somnolence to lethargy, stupor and coma.

DKA most typically occurs in patients with type 1 diabetes. It can also be found, although less commonly, in patients with type 2 diabetes under conditions of extreme stress, such as severe infection, trauma, myocardial or cerebral infarction, and, less frequently, as the initial presentation of a disorder called ketosis-prone type 2 diabetes.

Coding Tip

Although ketosis-prone type 2 diabetes is a variant form of type 2 diabetes, in ICD-10-CM "ketosis-prone" is an inclusion term under type 1 diabetes and is, therefore, reported with a code from category E1Ø Type 1 diabetes mellitus.

Patients with type 2 diabetes more frequently develop hyperosmolar hyperglycemic states (HHS), which can be confused with DKA. However, ketone levels are low or absent in patients with HHS, pH is greater than 7.3 and serum bicarbonate is greater than 15 mEq/L. HHS presents with impaired mental status, severe hyperglycemia (plasma glucose >600 mg/dl) and elevated serum osmolality (>320 mOsm/kg).

Other causes of high anion gap metabolic acidosis, such as those mentioned in the differential diagnoses below, must be ruled out.

Differential diagnoses include:

- Gastroenteritis
- High anion gap metabolic acidosis:
  - advanced chronic renal failure
  - alcoholic ketoacidosis
  - lactic acidosis
  - rhabdomyolysis
  - salicylate poisoning
- Hyperosmolar hyperglycemic state
- Myocardial infarction
- Pancreatitis
- Renal tubular acidosis
- Starvation ketosis

The diagnosis of DKA is based on an elevated serum glucose level greater than 250 mg/dL, an elevated serum ketone level, a pH less than 7.3, and a serum bicarbonate level less than 15 mEq/L.

Arterial blood gas measurement to determine pH is performed. In some cases where arterial blood gases are not available, venous pH level is an option if the patient is hemodynamically stable.

The severity of DKA is determined by the arterial pH, bicarbonate level, anion gap, and mental status of the patient. Generally, mild DKA is classified by a pH level of 7.25–7.3, serum bicarbonate level between 15–18 mEq/L, and anion gap greater than 10; moderate DKA has a pH between 7.0–7.24, serum bicarbonate level of 10 to less than 15 mEq/L; and severe DKA has a pH less than 7.0 and bicarbonate less than 10 mEq/L.[17]. In moderate or severe DKA the anion gap is greater than 12.

Treatment of DKA involves identification and treatment of the precipitating condition(s), correction of hyperglycemia, dehydration, and any electrolyte imbalances. Hyperglycemia is treated with regular insulin by IV infusion, except in mild episodes. Fluid status, cardiac status, urine output, blood pressure, and electrolyte levels are monitored. DKA is resolved when the serum glucose level is less than 200 mg/dL, pH is greater than 7.3, and the bicarbonate level is 18 mEq/L or higher.

Cerebral edema is the most severe complication of DKA, but other complications can include hyperkalemia, hypoglycemia, acute renal failure, shock, rhabdomyolysis, and thrombosis.

Goals for prevention include patient education regarding the signs and symptoms of DKA, adjusting insulin therapy, frequency of self-monitoring of blood glucose levels, checking urine ketone levels with a dipstick test if the glucose level is greater than 240 mg/dL, as well as nutrition management during periods of acute illness. Patients with an insulin pump should be familiar with their pump settings, and have backup insulin available in case of pump failure.

Coding Tip

Diabetes with ketoacidosis is inherently uncontrolled diabetes, and includes hyperglycemia. There is no default ICD-10-CM code for "uncontrolled diabetes." In ICD-10-CM, uncontrolled diabetes is classified by the type of diabetes and the presence of hyperglycemia or hypoglycemia. It is, therefore, not necessary to report an additional code for diabetes with hyperglycemia or a separate code for hyperglycemia in patients with diabetic ketoacidosis.

Coding Tip

If there are other diabetic complications besides ketoacidosis, any combination of diabetes codes can be assigned together, unless one diabetic condition is inherent in another. Take care to be consistent in coding the type of diabetes. It would not be appropriate to report one diabetic complication as type 1, and another as type 2, for example.

Coding Tip

DKA in a patient with gestational diabetes, with no evidence or history of pre-existing diabetes mellitus, is reported with code O24.419 Gestational diabetes mellitus in pregnancy, unspecified control, and E87.2 Acidosis.

Diagnoses

Documentation Tip

Type 1 diabetes may be documented as juvenile onset, ketosis-prone, idiopathic, brittle, due to autoimmune process, due to immune mediated pancreatic islet beta-cell destruction.

Type 2 diabetes may be documented as due to insulin secretory defect, insulin resistant, insulin use, if any.

Drug or chemical induced diabetes should have documentation of the causal drug or chemical, and insulin use, if any.

Diabetes due to an underlying condition should include documentation of the underlying condition, such as Cushing syndrome, cystic fibrosis, malignant neoplasm, malnutrition, pancreatitis and other diseases of pancreas, and insulin use, if any.

Diabetes due to other specified causes can include diabetes due to genetic defects of beta-cell function, genetic defects in insulin action, postpancreatectomy or postprocedural diabetes, or diabetes documented as secondary without a specified cause.

Coding/Reporting Criteria	Clinical Criteria	
1. Physical Evaluation *(routine/expected in italics)*	• Thirst or dry mouth • Polyuria • Polydipsia • Polyphagia • Weakness • Nausea and/or vomiting • Abdominal pain • Difficulty breathing/shortness of breath • Confusion or loss of consciousness (coma)	• Signs of dehydration – dry mucus membranes – decreased skin turgor – tachycardia – hypotension • Acetone smelling breath (fruity odor) • Hyperglycemia • Ketonuria/ketonemia • Acidosis • Hypothermia (even with infection)
2. Clinical Evaluation *(routine/expected in italics)*	• Testing for precipitating condition can determine which tests are performed • Arterial blood gas or venous pH level • Serum electrolytes (potassium, sodium, chloride, magnesium, calcium, phosphorus) • Amylase and lipase levels • Plasma glucose levels • Anion gap calculated (Na+(mEq/L) – [Cl-(mEq/L) + HCO3-(mEq/L)]) • Serum bicarbonate	• Urinalysis with pH and ketones • Serum ketone levels • Blood urea nitrogen (BUN) and creatinine • Beta-hydroxybutyrate (predominant ketone in DKA) • Serum osmolality • Glasgow coma scale • Complete blood count with differential • Hemoglobin A1c level
3. Diagnostic Px *(routine/expected in italics)*	• Chest x-ray • Head CT or MRI scanning • Electrocardiography • Continuous pulse oximetry	• Telemetry • Bacterial cultures of urine, blood, sputum, or other sites of suspected infection
4. Therapeutic Tx *(routine/expected in italics)*	• Correction of precipitating or underlying condition • Hemodynamic and/or respiratory support • Use of sodium bicarbonate: small amounts are supported for very severe acidemia (pH less than 6.9) to maintain pH >7.2	• IV insulin • IV fluids, oral antibiotics • Electrolyte replacement
5. Increased Nursing Care and/or Monitoring	• Increased monitoring of fluids, glucose level, insulin, potassium levels and treat accordingly • Iatrogenic cause of underlying condition occurs postprocedure	• Underlying cause/condition occurs during admission
6. Extends LOS	• Iatrogenic cause of underlying condition postprocedure	• Underlying cause/condition occurs during admission and delays discharge

Condition	Documentation Example	ICD-10-CM Corresponding Codes
Routine/Expected/ Integral/Inherent/ Incidental *(italics only)*	*NA*	*NA*
Principal Diagnosis	1. IP History and Physical: 12 y/o boy with no PMH presents with two-week hx of shortness of breath, polyuria, polydipsia and nocturia. He then developed headache, dizziness, agitation and altered level of consciousness. Glasgow coma scale (GCS) of 13/15 on admit, normal tone and reflexes. IP Discharge Summary: 12 y/o boy with no family history of diabetes was admitted in a state of ketoacidosis with a mild altered level of consciousness but no coma. He was diagnosed with initial presentation of diabetic ketoacidosis due to uncontrolled type 1 diabetes. The patient and his parents received education regarding management of type 1 diabetes and insulin administration.	1. Report E1Ø.1Ø Type 1 diabetes mellitus with ketoacidosis without coma
Comorbidity	1. IP Discharge Summary: 88 y/o male admitted in septic shock due to underlying E.coli sepsis of undetermined infectious source. Patient is a type 2 diabetic, usually well controlled on oral hypoglycemics, but developed ketoacidosis without coma due to the systemic insult.	1. Report code A41.51, Sepsis due to Escherichia coli [E. coli]), followed by R65.21, Severe sepsis with septic shock; E11.1Ø Type 2 diabetes mellitus with ketoacidosis without coma; and Z79.84 Long term (current) use of oral hypoglycemic drugs
Complication of Care	1. IP Admit Note: 40 y/o female admitted with type 1 diabetes with ketoacidosis and coma. IP Progress Note: Glucose 400 mg/dL. Insulin pump malfunctioned, failed to administer insulin dose. IP Discharge Summary: 40 y/o female with type 1 diabetes diagnosed at age 14, admitted with ketoacidosis and coma due to inadequate dosage of insulin from pump failure. Patient received IV insulin and DKA resolved, with patient returning to previous level of consciousness.	1. Report T85.614A Breakdown (mechanical) of insulin pump, initial encounter as principal diagnosis, followed by T38.3X6A Underdosing of insulin and oral hypoglycemic (antidiabetic) drugs, initial encounter, and E1Ø.11 Type 1 diabetes mellitus with ketoacidosis with coma
Poisoning or Adverse Effect of Medication/ Chemical	1. IP Discharge Summary Note: Final dx: 30 y/o male admitted with steroid induced diabetes mellitus presenting as diabetic ketoacidosis, without significant loss of awareness. Patient was taking methylprednisolone as prescribed for acute exacerbation of Crohn's disease.	1. Report EØ9.1Ø Drug or chemical induced diabetes mellitus with ketoacidosis without coma, followed by T38.ØX5A Adverse effect of glucocorticoids and synthetic analogues, initial encounter; K5Ø.9Ø Crohn's disease, unspecified, without complications; and Z79.52 Long term (current) use of systemic steroids

Additional References

AHA CC: 3Q, 2020, p. 30; 4Q, 2017, p. 6; 2Q, 2016, p. 10; 3Q, 2013, p. 20

American Diabetes Association www.diabetes.org

CMS: Hospital Acquired Conditions (HAC) List
https://www.cms.gov/medicare/medicare-fee-for-service-payment/hospitalacqcond/icd10_hacs

Diagnoses

Diagnoses

Empyema, Pleural or Pyothorax

J86.Ø	**Pyothorax with fistula**	MCC HCC
J86.9	**Pyothorax without fistula**	MCC HCC
J95.88	**Other intraoperative complications of respiratory system, not elsewhere classified**	CC
J95.89	**Other postprocedural complications and disorders of respiratory system, not elsewhere classified**	CC
S27.6[3,9]XA	**[Laceration, Other injury] of pleura, initial encounter**	CC
S27.6[3,9]XD	**[Laceration, Other injury] of pleura, subsequent encounter**	
S27.6[3,9]XS	**[Laceration, Other injury] of pleura, sequela**	

Associated terminology: empyema; infective loculated pleural effusion; pleural abscess; chest abscess; purulent pleuritis

Discussion

Empyema, also called pyothorax, is infected pleural fluid or pus that develops due to infection, aspiration, injury, or penetrating trauma with secondary infection from the lungs, pleura, thorax, or adjacent/distal sites that seed through hematologic extension. It is a complicated parapneumonic pleural exudate effusion with infection or abscess. When free-flowing they are large, more than half the hemithorax. Collections trapped in the pleural cavity by adhesions, fissure, or fibrin septa are noted on imaging as loculations or loculated pleural effusion (due to infection). Loculations that are fibrinopurulent are also empyema. Pleural effusion with loculations that are not infected or fibrin only are not considered to be an empyema.

When the infection extends beyond the thoracic cavity and into the chest wall it is known as empyema necessitatis. In this rare complication, an additional code would be assigned to represent the soft tissue infection.

A lung abscess can be reported separately when present with a pleural empyema as they are separate anatomical site abscesses. Long-term sequelae of empyema are bronchopleural fistula formation and scarring of the pleural membranes, which restricts lung expansion. Empyema can recur, itself being a sequela of previous trauma or surgery.

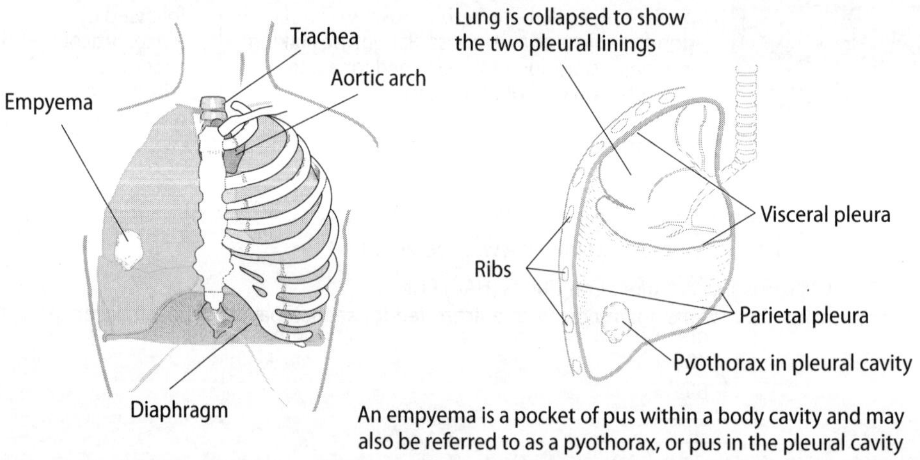

An empyema is a pocket of pus within a body cavity and may also be referred to as a pyothorax, or pus in the pleural cavity

Coding Tip

Principal diagnosis is that condition established after study to be chiefly responsible for occasioning the admission of the patient to the hospital for care.

Note: When due to trauma, either blunt or penetrating, bronchoalveolar lavage (BAL) or sputum cultures will seldom have any correlation to empyema culture indicating that the etiology is not a pneumonic process but due to the trauma.

Surgical procedures most commonly associated with empyema are thoracentesis, tube insertion, lung surgery, or as an extended infection from abdominal surgery.

> **Documentation Tip**
>
> **Complications of care: The condition must be more than a routinely expected condition or event. The documentation must support that the condition is clinically significant with an indication that it is a complication, by demonstrating:**
>
> - **A cause-and-effect relationship between the care or procedure and the condition**
> - **That the condition resulted in altering the course of a procedure or surgery**
>
> **The term "complication" does not have to be explicitly documented.**

> **Documentation Tip**
>
> **Code assignment cannot be based on ancillary test results, therapies, or clinical criteria alone. A diagnosis and its clinical significance must be supported by physician or other qualified healthcare professional documentation. When it is unclear or there is contradictory information, query the physician or other qualified healthcare professional for clarification.**

> **Coding Tip**
>
> **The seventh character extensions A, D, S affect the analysis of complications and quality of care and reimbursement.**

Coding/Reporting Criteria	Clinical Criteria	
1. Physical Evaluation *(routine/expected in italics)*	• Pleuritic chest pain (inflammation of the parietal pleura) • Cough • Fever and chills (persist > 48 hours after initiation of antibiotic treatment) • *Rales or crackles* • Bronchial breathing, breath sounds, or egophony • Malaise • Shortness of breath	• Excessive sweating, especially at night • Pleural friction rub • Weight loss • Decreased or absent breath sounds • Dullness to percussion • Decreased tactile fremitus (vibration felt while the patient is speaking with hand held against the chest) • Tracheal deviation away from a large effusion
2. Clinical Evaluation *(routine/expected in italics)*	• Pleural fluid aspiration with pleural fluid analysis (simple effusion is sterile; complicated has organisms and cellular debris) • Cytology • Sputum culture • Leukocytosis • Positive Gram stain or culture of pleural fluid • Pleural fluid pH < 7.20 with normal peripheral blood pH; indication of empyema with nonpurulent, culture-negative fluid • Lactic acid dehydrogenase (LDH) > 1000 U/L and glucose < 40 mg/dL or a pH < 7.00 and a glucose < 40 mg/dL • Blood cell count and differential: WBC > 50,000 cells/μL	• Exudative: ≥ 1 of the following marked with: – fluid LDH ≥ 2/3 upper limit of normal for serum LDH (or > 0.6) – pleural fluid: serum total protein ratio ≥ 0.5 – pleural fluid: serum LDH ratio ≥ 0.6 – fluid total protein ≥ 3 g/dL – fluid cholesterol ≥ 43 mg/dL or ≥ 60 mg/dL – pleural fluid: serum cholesterol ratio ≥ 0.3 – serum protein-pleural fluid protein ≤ 3.1 g/dL – cloudy appearance – specific gravity > 1.020 • Macroscopic presence of pus

Diagnoses

Coding/Reporting Criteria	Clinical Criteria	
3. Diagnostic Px *(routine/expected in italics)*	• Chest x-ray: appears as white area on posteroanterior position. Lateral decubitus x-rays are more sensitive • Blunted posterior costophrenic angles lateral upright on chest x-ray by 75mL of fluid; blunting of lateral angle by ~175 mL to 500 mL • Large effusions may cause mediastinal shift • Effusions > 4 – may cause complete opacification of hemithorax and mediastinal shift to the contralateral side • Ultrasound • CT: Gas bubbles in pleural spec without recent thoracentesis	• Loculated effusions: fluid trapped by pleural adhesions/pulmonary fissures, typical of empyema/pyothorax • Bronchoscopy • Mediastinoscopy • Pleural biopsy • Thoracoscopy • Immediate pleural effusion injection into blood culture bottles for aerobic/anaerobic after aspiration • Polymerase chain reaction (PCR) or antigen detection
4. Therapeutic Tx *(routine/expected in italics)*	• Thoracentesis: pleural fluid ≥ 10 mm thickness, > 1 cm on decubitus x-ray, or new, or uncertain etiology; in heart failure when chest pain, fever or when diuresis fails, or effusions ≥ 3 days • Prompt chest tube drainage • IV then oral antibiotics/antifungals for bacterial/fungal etiologies • Pain medication • Intercostal drain • Pleurodesis, surgical or chemical	• Pleurectomy • Fibrinolysis with both fibrinolytic and mucolytic of fibrin loculations • Saline injection for breaking up fibrin loculations • Pleuroperitoneal shunt • Decortication • Oxygen therapy • Video-assisted thoracoscopy (VATS) or open drainage • Thoracoplasty
5. Increased Nursing Care and/or Monitoring	• Monitoring of chest tube output	
6. Extends LOS	• Signs of severe sepsis (SIRS due to infection) develop post admit	

Condition	Documentation Example	ICD-10-CM Corresponding Codes
Routine/Expected/ Integral/Inherent/ Incidental *(italics only)*	*NA*	*NA*
Principal Diagnosis	1. Discharge Summary: Empyema due to aspiration pneumonia from vomiting with superimposed bacterial pneumonia; treated with VATs drainage, IV antibiotics.	1. Report J86.9 Pyothorax without fistula, followed by J69.Ø Pneumonitis due to inhalation of food and vomit; and J15.9 Unspecified bacterial pneumonia.
Comorbidity	1. Progress Note: Admitted with severe sepsis with shock due to empyema with *Pseudomonas* pneumonia; thoracentesis analysis confirms *Pseudomonas* as did sputum and blood culture 2/2 bottles.	1. Report A41.52 Sepsis due to Pseudomonas, followed by R65.21 Severe sepsis with septic shock; J86.9 Pyothorax without fistula; and J15.1 Pneumonia due to Pseudomonas.
Complication of Care	1. Discharge Summary: MRSA empyema with bronchopleural fistula due to previous pneumonectomy; initial drainage was by closed tube followed by open thoracostomy.	1. Report J95.89 Other postprocedural complications and disorders of respiratory system, not elsewhere classified, followed by J86.Ø Pyothorax with fistula; B95.62 Methicillin resistant Staphylococcus aureus infection as the cause of diseases classified elsewhere; and Z9Ø.2 Acquired absence of lung [part of].
Poisoning or Adverse Effect of Medication/ Chemical	NA	NA

Encephalopathy

G92.8	**Other toxic encephalopathy**	MCC
G92.9	**Unspecified toxic encephalopathy**	MCC
G93.40	**Encephalopathy, unspecified**	CC
G93.41	**Metabolic encephalopathy**	MCC
G93.49	**Other encephalopathy**	CC

Associated terminology: toxic, metabolic, or toxic-metabolic encephalopathy; encephalopathy of unknown etiology

Note: This clinical review is limited to toxic, metabolic, other, and unspecified encephalopathy. Hepatic encephalopathy (K76.82) is reviewed under the section Hepatic Encephalopathy/Hepatic Coma in this publication.

Discussion

Encephalopathy is a general term indicating a syndrome of diffuse brain dysfunction which alters brain function or structure. It is a complication of a primary condition or disease, organic or inorganic, and it can be permanent or reversible. The symptom that is integral to encephalopathy is altered mental status. When associated conditions are present, such as myoclonus, dementia, coma, etc. they will be reported as additional diagnoses.

The type or cause of encephalopathy should be identified and the alphabetic index lists many codes to be reported for specific causes, such as septic, metabolic, drug induced, traumatic (postconcussional), hypertensive, etc. Encephalopathy due to infection, tumor, cerebral infarction, cerebral ischemia will usually be identified as metabolic; toxic encephalopathy is identified with drugs, poisonings, chemical substances. Toxic-metabolic encephalopathy (G92.8) can be found in organ failure or intoxication.

Encephalopathy due to a postictal state due to seizure/epilepsy will not be reported separately as the encephalopathy is integral to the postictal state.

When encephalopathy is documented and the etiology is not identified or clear, query the cause based on the record. When a cause cannot be identified, then G93.40 Encephalopathy, unspecified, will be reported. When a type of encephalopathy is identified or specified, but does not fit into any of the classifications listed in the alphabetic index, G93.49 Other encephalopathy, Encephalopathy NEC, would be reported (e.g., due to inflammation, such as encephalitis, noninfectious).

Documentation Tip

If the type of encephalopathy is not documented, review the medical record for results of blood tests, spinal fluid examination, imaging studies, and EEG to formulate a query for the underlying cause.

Sequencing will depend on the index, guidelines, and other coding instructions.

EEG findings are nonspecific in differentiating between etiologies, but provide a demonstrable measure of severity, prognosis, and efficacy of treatment. There are four grades of encephalopathy:

- Grade I: altered mental status, altered mood, impaired concentration and psychomotor function, rousable
- Grade II: drowsy, inappropriate behavior, able to talk
- Grade III: very drowsy, disoriented, agitated, aggressive
- Grade IV: coma, may respond to painful stimuli

Coding Tip

- **Adverse effect: Nature of adverse drug effect: code for (adverse condition) followed by the code from T36–T50 with fifth or sixth character 5 to identify the drug.**
- **Poisoning: Identify drug/chemical by the code from T36–T50 with fifth or sixth character of intent followed by a code for nature of adverse drug effect (manifestation).**

Coding/Reporting Criteria	Clinical Criteria
1. Physical Evaluation *(routine/expected in italics)*	• Altered mental status: only s/s or manifestation integral to encephalopathy • When these manifestations are present, they may be reported as an additional diagnosis, unless otherwise indicated by the index and tabular notes or other guideline: – loss of cognitive function – subtle personality changes – inability to concentrate – lethargy – depressed consciousness – myoclonus – asterixis – nystagmus – tremor – seizure – Cheyne-Stokes respirations – apneic respirations – progressive loss of memory – dementia – muscle atrophy – weakness – loss of ability to swallow – loss of ability to speak – ataxia – brain swelling – brain herniation – coma
2. Clinical Evaluation *(routine/expected in italics)*	• Evaluation of underlying cause • Blood tests/CBC • Spinal fluid analysis • Blood pressure • Metabolic tests • Drug and toxin levels • Blood/body fluid analysis for infection workup • Creatinine
3. Diagnostic Px *(routine/expected in italics)*	• Evaluation of underlying cause • Lumbar puncture • Imaging studies • EEG
4. Therapeutic Tx *(routine/expected in italics)*	• Varies depending on etiology/type and severity • Oxygen • IV fluids • Oral lactulose: hepatic • Antibiotics • Dialysis: uremic • Glucose: diabetic hypoglycemia • Removal blood glucose: diabetic hyperglycemia • Medications to control hyper- or hypotension
5. Increased Nursing Care and/or Monitoring	• Prevention teaching: importance of diet, medication, dialysis compliance
6. Extends LOS	• Encephalopathy postadmit or postoperative

Condition	Documentation Example	ICD-10-CM Corresponding Codes
Routine/Expected/ Integral/Inherent/ Incidental *(italics only)*	*NA*	*NA*
Principal Diagnosis	1. IP Discharge Summary: An 85-year-old female with acute encephalopathy, unknown cause, second presentation after change in mental status, ataxic gait with stumbling incident, no serious trauma, soft restraints x24 hours due to agitation with combative behavior, patient is a fall risk, workup nonspecific, monitored; recommendations for placement discussed with family.	1. Report G93.40 Encephalopathy unspecified, followed by R26.0 Ataxic gait; R45.1 Agitation; Z91.81 At risk for falling; Z78.1 Physical restraint status.
Comorbidity	1. IP Discharge Summary: Urinary tract infection due to *E. coli*, severe dehydration, encephalopathy; UTI treated with IV antibiotics and dehydration resolved with IV fluids **(Query if the encephalopathy was related to either of or both conditions of UTI or dehydration.)**	1. Report N39.0 Urinary tract infection, site not specified, followed by B96.20 Unspecified Escherichia coli [E. coli] as the cause of diseases classified elsewhere; E86.0 Dehydration, unspecified; G93.40 Encephalopathy, unspecified. • If the query response links the encephalopathy to either condition, then G93.41 Metabolic encephalopathy, would be reported.
Complication of Care	1. IP Progress Note: Encephalopathy post- coronary artery bypass graft (CABG) encephalopathy, multifactorial, monitor and treat symptomatically.	1. Report G97.82 Other postprocedural complication and disorder of nervous system, followed by G93.49 Other specified encephalopathy.
Poisoning or Adverse Effect of Medication/ Chemical	1. ED order to transfer to IP: A 19-year-old male with encephalopathy with stupor, seizure, and vomiting due to alcohol overdose, blood alcohol 410, engaged in beer chugging contest with friends in yard at home of neighbor.	1. Report T51.0X1A Toxic effect of ethanol, accidental (unintentional), initial encounter), followed by G92.8 Other toxic encephalopathy, for toxic encephalopathy due to drugs; R40.1 Stupor; R56.9 Seizure; R11.10 Vomiting; and Y90.2 Blood alcohol level of 40–59 mg/100 ml.

Additional References

AHA CC: 2Q, 2024, p. 14; 2Q, 2021, p. 3; 1Q, 2021, p. 13; 4Q, 2018, p. 16; 2Q, 2018, p. 22, 24; 2Q, 2017, p. 8, 9; 3Q, 2016, p. 42; 3Q, 2015, p 21

Diagnoses

Fracture, Pathological

M48.4-	**Fatigue fracture of vertebra, initial encounter**
M48.5-	**Collapsed vertebra, not elsewhere classified, initial encounter**
M8Ø.Ø-	**Age-related osteoporosis with current pathological fracture**
M8Ø.8-	**Other osteoporosis with current pathological fracture**
M84.3-	**Stress fracture**
M84.4-	**Pathological fracture, not elsewhere classified**
M84.5-	**Pathological fracture in neoplastic disease**
M84.6-	**Pathological fracture in other disease**
M96.6-	**Fracture of bone following insertion of orthopedic implant, joint prosthesis, or bone plate**
M96.A-	**Fracture of ribs, sternum and thorax associated with compression of the chest and cardiopulmonary resuscitation**
M97.-	**Periprosthetic fracture around the internal prosthetic joint**

Associated terminology: chronic fracture; fatigue fracture; fragility fracture; stress fracture; stress fracture NOS; March fracture; stress reaction; osteoporotic fracture; non-traumatic fracture; periprosthetic fracture

Note: CC and HCC designation for the codes listed above is dependent on the specific seventh character assigned and, in some instances, the specific anatomical site. Refer to an approved coding manual or the CMS website to determine which codes are CCs or HCCs.

Discussion

Fractures, partial or complete breaks of the bone, occur from underlying pathology, such as cancer or osteoporosis, or from trauma due to external force against the bone. Pathologic fractures are covered in Chapter 13: Diseases of the Musculoskeletal System and Connective Tissue (M00–M99). Traumatic fractures are covered in Chapter 19: Injury, Poisoning, and Certain Other Consequences of External Causes (S00–T88).

Pathological fractures occur at sites weakened by pre-existing disease. These fractures differentiate from traumatic fractures by the magnitude of the trauma or stress causing the fracture. Minor trauma or stress can cause a pathological fracture in bones diseased by disseminated bone disorders, inflammatory bone diseases, metabolic bone disease, neoplasms, Paget's disease, or any other condition that compromises bone strength and integrity. Despite common references in the medical field that pathological fractures are specifically related to neoplastic disease, the ICD-10-CM code set encompasses multiple potential chronic and pathological etiologies beyond cancer. Pathologic fractures are also referred to as chronic fractures due to the chronic nature of the underlying disease processes. It must be noted that only a provider can determine that a sustained fracture is out of proportion to the level of trauma leading to the fracture; documentation must support appropriate code selection.

Coding Tip

Stress or fatigue fractures, reported under subcategory M48.4 are different from pathological fractures in that stress fractures are caused by repetitive overuse, such as in sports, strenuous exercise, or from heavy physical labor.

Osteoporosis, the cause of many pathologic fractures, is characterized by decreased osteoblastic formation of matrix combined with increased osteoclastic resorption of bone. This leads to a marked decrease in bone mass. The condition is systemic, affecting all bones of the musculoskeletal system. Osteoporosis often presents with osteopenia, a decrease in bone mineralization. Signs and symptoms of osteoporosis include chronic and intermittent back pain (due to vertebral microfractures), skeletal remodeling such as dorsal kyphosis, or loss of height. Bone scans and radiographs determine the extent and severity of osteoporosis and osteopenia and may reveal new or historical evidence of pathological fractures.

Category M80 includes osteoporosis with current "fragility fracture," a traumatic fracture in a patient with osteoporosis due to a minor fall or trauma, in which the causal event would not normally cause fracture in healthy bone. ICD-10-CM combination codes in category M80 classify the combination of osteoporosis and pathological fracture and facilitate reporting of certain specific types of osteoporosis, anatomic site of fracture, and laterality.

Coding Tip

Pathological fracture due to a neoplasm, when the focus of care is on the fracture, is coded by sequencing the fracture code first (subcategory M84.5 Pathological fracture in neoplastic disease), followed by the code for the neoplasm. If the focus of treatment is the neoplasm, the neoplasm code should be sequenced first, followed by a code from subcategory M84.5 for the pathological fracture.

Diagnoses

Periprosthetic fractures occur around or near an implanted prosthetic joint. Despite their proximity to a prosthesis, these fractures are not complications of the prosthesis, but rather they are due to trauma or disease and are coded from category M97. If known, first code the specific type and cause of fracture, if it is traumatic or pathological. These fractures occur specifically around prostheses of the hips, knees, elbows, and shoulders, as well as those of the smaller digital joints.

To fully code any fracture (pathological or traumatic), the medical record must include the following:

- Anatomic site
- Laterality
- Type (i.e., open, closed, pathologic, stress/fatigue, displaced/nondisplaced)
- Pattern (i.e., comminuted, oblique, spiral)
- Encounter type (initial, subsequent, sequela)
- Status at time of subsequent encounters (i.e., routine/delayed healing, malunion, nonunion)

Coding/Reporting Criteria	Clinical Criteria	
1. Physical Evaluation *(routine/expected in italics)*	• Fracture from minor trauma or stress • Presence of neoplastic disease, osteoporosis, infection • Pain/swelling/discomfort at fracture site • Bruising at fracture site • Numbness or tingling	• Fracture at joint prosthesis site • Decreased mobility and range of motion at site • Muscle weakness • Fever or chills in the setting of osteomyelitis/infection
2. Clinical Evaluation *(routine/expected in italics)*	• Evaluation of underlying cause	
3. Diagnostic Px *(routine/expected in italics)*	• Imaging studies; pathological fractures often have a transverse pattern • MRI/CT scan/nuclear bone scan • Bone density test	• Calcium level • CBC • Electrolytes • C-reactive protein: assess for inflammation
4. Therapeutic Tx *(routine/expected in italics)*	• Internal/external fixation • Limited motion • Analgesic medication • Treatment of underlying cause	• Physical/occupational therapy • Vitamin D and calcium replacement • Use of supportive devices (cane, walker)
5. Increased Nursing Care and/or Monitoring	• Bedside assist with activities of daily living (ADLs)	• Pain management
6. Extends LOS	• Underlying cause may require diagnosis/management	• Surgical intervention with recovery

Condition	Documentation Example	ICD-10-CM Corresponding Codes
Routine/Expected/ Integral/Inherent/ Incidental *(italics only)*	*NA*	*NA*
Principal Diagnosis	1. IP Discharge Summary: 90-year-old female with osteoporosis fell from bed at assisted living and sustained a right ulnar fracture. Provider states fracture was due to advanced-age osteoporosis. 2. IP Discharge Summary: 56-year-old male status post left shoulder replacement presents with periprosthetic fracture after walking into a door frame and having immediate pain. Physician note indicates that after study, the patient was determined to have a pathological fracture of the left shoulder.	1. Report M80.031A Age-related osteoporosis with current pathological fracture, right forearm, initial encounter and W06.XXXA Fall from bed, initial encounter, as the external cause. 2. Report M84.412A Pathological fracture, left shoulder, initial encounter and M97.32XA Periprosthetic fracture around internal prosthetic left shoulder joint, initial encounter.
Comorbidity	1. Progress Note: A 72-year-old female admitted for multiple myeloma treatment complained of left ankle pain after walking to the bathroom. She was diagnosed with left ankle pathological fracture from neoplastic disease.	1. Report C90.00 Multiple myeloma not having achieved remission, followed by M84.572A Pathological fracture in neoplastic disease, left ankle.
Complication of Care	1. History and Physical: 68-year-old male admitted after surgery for management of right femoral fracture sustained after implantation of bone plate.	1. Report M96.661 Fracture of femur following insertion of orthopedic implant, joint prosthesis, or bone plate, right leg.
Poisoning or Adverse Effect of Medication/ Chemical	NA	NA

Additional References:

AHA CC: 4Q, 2023, p. 33; 4Q, 2020, p. 32; 2Q, 2018, p. 12

Gastrointestinal Hemorrhage

I85.[Ø,1]1	**[Esophageal, secondary esophageal] varices with bleeding**	MCC HCC
K13.79	**Other lesions of oral mucosa**	
K2Ø.[8,9]1	**Esophagitis [other, unspecified] with bleeding**	MCC
K21.Ø1	**Gastro-esophageal reflux disease with esophagitis, with bleeding**	MCC
K22.11	**Ulcer of esophagus with bleeding**	MCC
K22.6	**Gastro-esophageal laceration-hemorrhage syndrome**	MCC
K22.8-	**Other specified diseases of esophagus**	
K25.[Ø,4]	**[Acute, chronic or unspecified] gastric ulcer with hemorrhage**	MCC
K25.[2,6]	**[Acute, chronic or unspecified] gastric ulcer with both hemorrhage and perforation**	MCC HCC
K26.[Ø,4]	**[Acute, chronic or unspecified] duodenal ulcer with hemorrhage**	MCC
K26.[2,6]	**[Acute, chronic or unspecified] duodenal ulcer with both hemorrhage and perforation**	MCC HCC
K27.[Ø,4]	**[Acute, chronic or unspecified] peptic ulcer, site unspecified with hemorrhage**	MCC
K27.[2,6]	**[Acute, chronic or unspecified] peptic ulcer, site unspecified with both hemorrhage and perforation**	MCC HCC
K28.[Ø,4]	**[Acute, chronic or unspecified] gastrojejunal ulcer with hemorrhage**	MCC
K28.[2,6]	**[Acute, chronic or unspecified] gastrojejunal ulcer with both hemorrhage and perforation**	MCC HCC
K29.[Ø,2,3,4,5,6,7]1	**[Acute, alcoholic, chronic superficial, chronic atrophic, unspecified chronic, other, unspecified] gastritis with bleeding**	MCC
K29.[8,9]1	**[Duodenitis, unspecified gastroduodenitis] with bleeding**	MCC
K31.811	**Angiodysplasia of stomach and duodenum with bleeding**	MCC
K31.82	**Dieulafoy lesion (hemorrhagic) of stomach and duodenum**	MCC
K5Ø.[Ø,1,8,9]11	**Crohn's disease of [small intestine, large intestine, both small and large intestine, unspecified] with rectal bleeding**	CC HCC
K51.[Ø,2,3]11	**Ulcerative [pancolitis, proctitis, rectosigmoiditis] with rectal bleeding**	CC HCC
K51.[5,8,9]11	**[Left-sided, other, unspecified] ulcerative colitis with rectal bleeding**	CC HCC
K51.411	**Inflammatory polyps of colon with rectal bleeding**	CC HCC
K55.21	**Angiodysplasia of colon with hemorrhage**	MCC
K55.9	**Vascular disorder of intestine, unspecified**	CC
K57.[Ø,2,4,8]1	**Diverticulitis of [small intestine, large intestine, both small and large intestine, intestine part unspecified] with perforation and abscess with bleeding**	MCC

Diagnoses

Diagnoses

K57.1[1,3]	**[Diverticulosis, Diverticulitis] of small intestine without perforation or abscess with bleeding**	MCC
K57.3[1,3]	**[Diverticulosis, Diverticulitis] of large intestine without perforation or abscess with bleeding**	MCC
K57.5[1,3]	**[Diverticulosis, Diverticulitis] of both small and large intestine without perforation or abscess with bleeding**	MCC
K57.9[1,3]	**[Diverticulosis, Diverticulitis] of intestine, part unspecified, without perforation or abscess with bleeding**	MCC
K62.5	**Hemorrhage of anus and rectum**	CC
K63.81	**Dieulafoy lesion of intestine**	MCC
K91.6[1,2]	**Intraoperative hemorrhage and hematoma of a digestive system organ or structure complicating a [digestive system, other] procedure**	CC
K91.84[Ø,1]	**Postprocedural hemorrhage and hematoma of a digestive system organ or structure following a [digestive system, other] procedure**	CC
K92.Ø	**Hematemesis**	CC
K92.1	**Melena**	CC
K92.2	**Gastrointestinal hemorrhage, unspecified**	CC
K94.[Ø,1,2,3]1	**[Colostomy, enterostomy, gastrostomy, esophagostomy] hemorrhage**	CC HCC

Associated terminology: gastrointestinal hemorrhage, unspecified; esophageal hemorrhage; anal/rectal hemorrhage; hematemesis, vomiting blood; melena; hematochezia; heme+stool; occult blood in feces; GI hemorrhage intraop/postop; esophageal varices with bleeding; esophagitis with bleeding; ulcer of esophagus with bleeding; gastroesophageal laceration-hemorrhage syndrome; gastric ulcer with hemorrhage; duodenal ulcer with hemorrhage; peptic ulcer with hemorrhage; gastrojejunal ulcer with hemorrhage; gastritis with bleeding; duodenitis with bleeding; angiodysplasia with bleeding; hemorrhagic Dieulafoy lesion; Crohn's disease with rectal bleeding; ulcerative colitis with rectal bleeding; colitis with rectal bleeding; ischemic colitis; diverticulitis with bleeding; diverticulosis with bleeding; stomal hemorrhage

Discussion

The site of gastrointestinal (GI) bleeding or hemorrhage can originate anywhere along the GI tract, from the mouth to the anus. When blood is overt and able to be seen without aid, it is referred to as "gross." Occult blood is viewed by microscopic exam or by a laboratory test. An upper GI origin manifests by mouth and esophageal bleeding, hematemesis, or occult positive stool, or melena from the small bowel. A lower GI origin is demonstrated by melena, occult positive stool, and hematochezia.

Complications of GI bleeding are anemia, angina/myocardial infarction due to coronary hypoperfusion, aspiration and shock. Decision for encounter type will be made based on the clinical scenario: whether the bleed is acute or chronic, brisk/massive or minimal/intermittent, patient is high risk or low risk, age, and comorbidities (heart failure, ischemic heart disease, etc.). The terms used to indicate GI bleeding and their definitions are as follows:

- Hematemesis: vomiting red blood indicates acute bleed, whereas vomitus described as coffee-ground emesis is bleeding that has slowed or stopped.
- Hematochezia: gross bright-colored blood passed from the anus, usually in or with stools.
- Melena: black, tarry stool due to dark colored blood which may continue to be seen a few days after bleeding has actually ended. Foods and medications can cause black stools also so it must be determined if the symptom is due to blood or not. Physicians sometimes document black, tarry stool as "melanotic" but this term is incorrect. Melanotic refers to containing melanin, the dark skin pigment present in moles and melanoma. The correct term is "melenic" stool or "melena." Melena or melenic stools indicate an "upper" gastrointestinal tract bleed or source of

hemorrhage because the tarry appearance is caused by exposure to digestive juices only present in the stomach and upper small intestine.

- Occult blood in stool: laboratory testing with positive results that indicate the presence of blood.

With significant blood loss, the initial focus of treatment will be blood volume restoration. The associated complications will be treated concurrently. Evaluation for the site and cause and control of hemorrhage as indicated. When GI bleeding and an associated complication or an underlying condition are present on admission, sequencing will be determined by the circumstances of admission and the focus of diagnostic workup and treatment, the clinical significance of each, including resource utilization considerations.

***Example*:**

POA: 68-year-old male, melena x 2 weeks, fatigue, h/o gastric ulcer

Workup: lab work for anemia; EGD for source

Results: Hb 9.0; gastric ulcer, chronic with evidence of recent bleed

Diagnosis, clinical significance: Acute on chronic blood loss anemia requiring transfusion; chronic gastric ulcer with stigmata of recent bleeding requiring IV Protonix

Sequencing: chronic gastric ulcer with bleeding, acute on chronic blood loss anemia

Rationale: The workup by EGD focused on evaluation for a source was more intensive than obtaining blood for lab; therefore, the workup was not equal.

When diagnostic workup reveals a confirmed source of bleed, assign the specified condition as "with bleeding" or "hemorrhagic" and do not assign an additional code for the bleeding. If the condition does not have these selections as subterms for the condition, review the alphabetic index main term for a nonessential modifier indicating hemorrhage/hemorrhagic. The qualifiers "acute,""chronic," or "acute on chronic" should be included in the diagnostic statement.

***Examples*: (Alphabetic Index)**

Ischemic colitis K55.9 incudes "hemorrhagic" because it is a subterm of the main term Colitis which includes "hemorrhagic" as a nonessential modifier.

Dieulafoy lesion of intestine K63.81 includes the nonessential modifier "hemorrhagic" in the main term Dieulafoy lesion. It is also important to note the hemorrhage is integral to a Dieulafoy lesion.

Gastritis includes the subterm "with bleeding" and subterms for acute and chronic, "with bleeding."

Excluded

- **Newborn gastrointestinal hemorrhage, see code P54.3.**
- **Gastrointestinal hemorrhage due to trauma, see category S36.**

A condition that does not have inclusion terms for hemorrhage or bleeding and hemorrhage/bleeding is not integral to the diagnosis, a code for hemorrhage is assigned as an additional diagnosis in order to show the symptomatic manifestation.

Documentation Tip

When documentation and clinical criteria do not match, query the provider for clarification of the diagnosis.

Code assignment cannot be based on ancillary test results, therapies, or clinical criteria alone. A diagnosis and its clinical significance must be supported by physician or other qualified healthcare professional documentation. When it is unclear or there is contradictory information, query the physician or other qualified healthcare professional for clarification.

If, upon evaluation, one or more conditions are found that could potentially be the cause of the GI hemorrhage, query the provider to identify if the single finding or which, if any, in the case of multiple findings is the source, if the link is not clearly stated. Include in the query if the condition is acute, chronic, or acute on chronic. If the provider states that a condition found could not have caused the bleed (due to extent of bleed, or insignificance of the finding, etc.) or is incidental and unrelated, code the hemorrhage/bleeding separately when they are not linked. In order to assign a code that includes hemorrhage/bleeding, the hemorrhage/bleeding must be either contemporaneous with the encounter, signs or stigmata of bleed, or linked in the documentation, even if the hemorrhage/bleeding was not actively demonstrated on exam or during the encounter.

Coding Tip

The classification presumes a causal relationship between two conditions linked by the terms "with bleeding" or "with hemorrhage," under the main term in the alphabetic index or tabular list. These conditions should be coded as related even in the absence of provider documentation explicitly linking them, unless the provider documents a different etiology of bleeding or clearly states the conditions are unrelated. (Guideline I.A.15)

GI Anatomical Site	Measurement (approximate)	
Esophagus-cervical	C6–T1, 15–18 cm from incisors	
Esophagus-thoracic	T1–T4 upper, 18–23 cm from incisors; T4–T8 mid, 24–32 cm from incisors; T8–T10 lower, 32–38 cm from incisors (including abdominal) 32–40 cm from incisors	
Esophagus-abdominal (below diaphragm) (LES/CE junction)	T10–T11, 38–40 cm from incisors	
Esophagus upper 1/3	Proximal, C6–T3, 15–23.3 cm from incisors (approx. upper thoracic)	
Esophagus middle 1/3	Middle, T3–T8, 23.3–31.6 cm from incisors (approx. mid thoracic)	
Esophagus lower 1/3	Distal, T8–T11, 31.6–40 cm from incisors (lower thoracic/abdominal)	
Stomach	Portion that connects to duodenum	At junction of esophagus and cardia of stomach; relaxing opens to allow food to enter stomach, closure prevents reflux
	Z line	Squamocolumnar epithelium where esophageal tissue meets gastric tissue
	GEJ	Where esophagus meets the cardia of the stomach
	Cardia	Most proximal portion of stomach that surrounds the orifice
	Fundus	Area to left and above the orifice
	Body	Central portion
	Lesser curvature	Medial side
	Greater curvature	Lateral side
Pylorus	Pyloric antrum	Distal portion
	Pyloric canal	Segment between stomach and pylorus
	Pylorus	Portion anterior to sphincter, connects stomach to duodenum
Pyloric sphincter	Allows food to pass from stomach to duodenum	
Duodenum (joined to stomach by pyloric sphincter) (includes bulb = 5 cm)	25 cm long	
Jejunum	200 cm long	
Ileum (joins cecum at ileocecal valve)	300 cm long	
Anus (dentate line: divides upper 2/3 and lower 1/3 of the anal canal)	0–4 cm (from anal verge)	
Rectum	4–16 cm (from anal verge)	
Rectosigmoid	15–17 cm (from anal verge)	
Sigmoid (left colon)	17–57 cm (from anal verge)	
Descending (left colon)	57–82 cm (from anal verge)	
Splenic flexure (left colon)	82 cm (from anal verge)	
Transverse (left half: left colon)(right half: right colon)	82–132 cm (from anal verge)	
Hepatic flexure (right colon)	132 cm (from anal verge)	
Ascending (right colon)	132–147 cm (from anal verge)	
Cecum (right colon)	150 cm (from anal verge)	

Documentation Tip

Complications of care: The condition must be more than a routinely expected condition or event. The documentation must support that the condition is clinically significant with an indication that it is a complication, by demonstrating:

- **A cause-and-effect relationship between the care or procedure and the condition**
- **That the condition resulted in altering the course of a procedure or surgery**

The term "complication" does not have to be explicitly documented.

Coding/Reporting Criteria	Clinical Criteria	
1. Physical Evaluation *(routine/expected in italics)*	• *Expected bleed at biopsy/polypectomy site* • Epigastric/abdominal pain • Vomiting • Orthostatic changes • Tachycardia (HR > 100) • Syncope • Weakness • Diaphoresis • Fatigue • Pallor	• Chest pain/angina • Dizziness • Melena • Hematemesis • Hematochezia • Coffee-ground emesis • Hemodynamic instability • Weight loss • Shock
2. Clinical Evaluation *(routine/expected in italics)*	• Guaiac/fecal occult blood test/hemoccult positive stool • CBC • Coagulation profile (prothrombin time test (PT)/partial thromboplastin time test (PTT)/platelet count) • Hematocrit/hemoglobin (every six hrs in severe bleeding)	• Bun/cr • Lytes • Alanine aminotransferase (ALT)/aspartate aminotransferase ratio (AST) • Type/screen packed red blood cells (PRBC) • Hypovolemia
3. Diagnostic Px *(routine/expected in italics)*	• Workup based on suspected source • Digital rectal exam/exam under anesthesia • Barium contrast upper GI series with small bowel follow-through: not for acute bleeding • Barium swallow • Barium enema • Enteroclysis • Push enteroscopy (double balloon enteroscopy) • Technetium-99m-tagged red blood cell scan	• Meckel's scan • X-ray • Angiography • Arteriography-brisk bleeding • Endoscopy • Capsule endoscopy • EKG • Pulse oximetry
4. Therapeutic Tx *(routine/expected in italics)*	• *Endo/hemoclip application/coagulation during scope for routine hemostasis*] • Endo/hemoclip for hemostasis of non-routine bleeding due to other condition • Endotracheal intubation to prevent aspiration: with inadequate gag reflex, unconsciousness • IV hydration/NS • Nasogastric aspiration/suction • Gastric lavage/ice lavage • Transfusion	• Oxygen for respiratory distress/chest pain • H2 antagonist/blocker • Embolectomy, revascularization, resection • Coagulation, vasopressin injection, sclerotherapy, embolization, oversewing, polypectomy • Iron therapy: anemia • Transjugular intrahepatic portosystemic shunt (TIPS)
5. Increased Nursing Care and/or Monitoring	• Rebleed post treatment	
6. Extends LOS	• Postop hemorrhage	

Condition	Documentation Example	ICD-10-CM Corresponding Codes
Routine/Expected/ Integral/Inherent/ Incidental *(italics only)*	1. *OP Report: After polypectomy, oozing and endoclip placed at site for hemostasis.*	*NA*
Principal Diagnosis	1. Discharge Note: Admitted with melena for one week and syncopal episode; patient with history of peptic gastric ulcers and currently on Coumadin prophylaxis for atrial fibrillation. Workup by upper endoscopy revealed minimal superficial chronic gastritis, healed gastric ulcers; discharged stable; scheduled outpatient colonoscopy for further workup. **(Query: Based on patient history and workup findings and need for further investigation, determine if an etiology of the melena found: minimal superficial chronic gastritis with bleed, melena as an adverse effect of Coumadin, other/specify, or undetermined/unknown etiology.)**	1. Report K92.1 Melena, followed by R55 Syncope and collapse; I48.91 Unspecified atrial fibrillation, Z87.11 Personal history of peptic ulcer disease; K29.3Ø Chronic superficial gastritis without bleeding; Z79.Ø1 Long term (current) use of anticoagulants. • If the query response identifies a definitive etiology, report the definitive etiology.
Comorbidity	NA	NA
Complication of Care	1. IP Discharge Summary: Aortoduodenal fistula related to post AAA graft repair six months ago; presented with melena, developed hematemesis in ED; workup found aortoduodenal fistula at suture line of graft.	1. Report T81.83XA Persistent postprocedural fistula, initial encounter, followed by I77.2 Rupture of artery; K91.841 Postprocedural hemorrhage and hematoma of a digestive system organ or structure following other procedure. • Intra- or postprocedural complication of specified body system category K91 and category T81 Complications of procedures, NEC, may be reported together when appropriate following the Excludes 2 note under category T81. • Additional codes may be assigned with complications of care codes if they identify the nature of the complication and the complication code does not fully describe the complication.
Poisoning or Adverse Effect of Medication/ Chemical	1. Discharge Note: Hematemesis due to Coumadin therapy supratherapeutic levels; history of deep vein thrombosis of lower right leg with Coumadin prophylaxis; medication regimen adjusted.	1. Report K92.Ø Hematemesis, followed by T45.515A Adverse effect of anticoagulants, initial encounter; Z79.Ø1 Long-term (current) use of anticoagulants; Z86.718 Personal history of other venous thrombosis and embolism.

Additional References

AHA CC: 3Q, 2023, p. 10; 1Q, 2023, p. 16, 20; 4Q, 2021, p. 15; 1Q, 2021, p. 11; 1Q, 2020, p. 16, 19; 1Q, 2019, p. 21; 3Q, 2018, p. 21, 22; 3Q, 2017, p. 27; 1Q, 2016, p. 15

MLN Medicare Quarterly Provider Compliance Newsletter, July 2011

SEER Training Modules, National Cancer Institute

Heart Failure (non-rheumatic)

I11.Ø	**Hypertensive heart disease with heart failure**	HCC
I13.Ø	**Hypertensive heart and chronic kidney disease with heart failure and stage 1 through stage 4 chronic kidney disease, or unspecified chronic kidney disease**	CC HCC
I13.2	**Hypertensive heart and chronic kidney disease with heart failure and with stage 5 chronic kidney disease, or end stage renal disease**	CC HCC
I5Ø.1	**Left ventricular failure, unspecified**	CC HCC
I5Ø.[2,3,4]Ø	**Unspecified [systolic, diastolic, combined systolic and diastolic] (congestive) heart failure**	CC HCC
I5Ø.[2,3,4]1	**Acute [systolic, diastolic, combined systolic and diastolic] (congestive) heart failure**	MCC HCC
I5Ø.[2,3,4]2	**Chronic [systolic, diastolic, combined systolic and diastolic] (congestive) heart failure**	CC HCC
I5Ø.[2,3,4]3	**Acute on chronic [systolic, diastolic, combined systolic and diastolic] (congestive) heart failure**	MCC HCC
I5Ø.81[1,2,3]	**[Acute, chronic, acute on chronic] right heart failure**	HCC
I5Ø.814	**Right heart failure due to left heart failure**	HCC
I5Ø.82	**Biventricular heart failure**	HCC
I5Ø.83	**High output heart failure**	HCC
I5Ø.84	**End stage heart failure**	HCC
I5Ø.9	**Heart failure, unspecified**	HCC

Associated terminology: hypertensive heart failure with or without chronic kidney disease; congestive heart failure (CHF); diastolic failure; systolic failure; heart failure; combined heart failure; left sided heart failure; right sided heart failure secondary to left; biventricular heart failure; cardiac asthma; stage D heart failure

Discussion

Heart failure is a condition in which the heart over time is no longer is able to pump sufficient blood to keep up with the body. Right sided heart failure occurs when the heart is unable to pump enough blood to the lungs. Left sided heart failure is when the heart cannot pump the oxygenated blood to the rest of the body. Left sided heart failure can be further subdivided into two additional categories:

- Diastolic: The left ventricle does not relax; therefore, the chamber does not fill with blood appropriately.
- Systolic: The left ventricle no longer has the ability to contract hard enough to push the blood into circulation.

Both right and left heart failure cause edema and jugular vein distention (JVD). Left heart failure may also cause shortness of breath (SOB), malaise, and fatigue. As the heart grows weaker, symptoms progress. Fluid buildup (edema) causes weight gain, frequent urination, and a cough indicative of pulmonary edema (worse lying supine). Fluid buildup in tissues is considered congestive heart failure or CHF.

If it is documented that a patient has heart failure (congestive or not) and systolic and/or diastolic dysfunction, the heart failure is assumed to be related in nature. A direct link or exact verbiage stating systolic or diastolic heart failure is unnecessary in these cases as the assumption allows the coder to report the more specific diagnosis code in this scenario. However, if the dysfunction is mentioned in absence of heart failure, do not assume the presence of heart failure. The physician should be queried for documentation of heart failure if clinical criteria are met or a code for the dysfunction, I51.89 Other ill-defined heart diseases, is reported rather than a code from category I5Ø Heart failure.

Documentation Tip

Results of an echocardiogram will assist in differentiating between systolic and diastolic heart failure. Systolic shows a decreased ejection fraction while diastolic has normal or nearly normal ejection fraction. Ensure that this information is pulled into the documentation for appropriate coding.

Coding and Documentation Tip

According to information from the American College of Cardiology (ACC), documentation of heart failure with reduced ejection fraction (HFrEF) is synonymous with systolic heart failure and heart failure with preserved ejection fraction (HFpEF) equates to diastolic heart failure. This is reflected in inclusion notes in Subcategory I50.2 Systolic (congestive) heart failure, I50.3 Diastolic (congestive) heart failure, and I50.4 Combined systolic (congestive) and diastolic (congestive) heart failure.

According to *AHA Coding Clinic for ICD-10-CM,* third quarter 2020, page 32, documentation of heart failure with mid-range or mildly reduced ejection fraction (HFmrEF) is synonymous with systolic heart failure and documentation of heart failure with recovered ejection fraction (EF) is synonymous with diastolic heart failure.

The most common causes of heart failure are coronary artery disease (CAD), hypertension, and diabetes. Treating and controlling these diseases can prevent heart failure and improve patient outcomes in patients already diagnosed. Other causes are cardiomyopathy, endocarditis, heart valve disorders, cardiac arrhythmias, congenital defects, thyroid disorders, alcohol and illicit drug use, HIV, AIDS, and chemotherapy. Obstructive sleep apnea (OSA) is known to exacerbate heart failure by depriving the heart of oxygen and, thereby, increasing its workload.

Although heart failure is common in rheumatic heart disease and occasionally valve disorders and endocarditis may lead the coder to rheumatic heart failure, it is not correct to assume rheumatic heart failure unless the physician documents it as such. If there is a question as to whether the heart failure may be rheumatic in nature and this is not clearly defined in the documentation, a physician query should be drafted.

Although it is common in children with congenital cardiac defects, the focus of this section is on adult heart failure. Heart failure is more prevalent in certain adult demographics:

- Age 65 years or older
- African American
- Overweight/obese
- History of acute myocardial infarction
- Men

There are two commonly recognized classifications of heart failure patients. The New York Heart Association (NYHA) Functional Classification categorizes patients based on the severity of their symptoms or the risk of their lifestyle. The American Heart Association (AHA)/American College of Cardiology (ACC) staging system focuses on the progression of the disease from risk to severe. Either may be referenced, depending on the message the provider is trying to convey.

NYHA Heart Failure Classification

Class	Description
1 (Mild)	No limitation of physical activity—ordinary physical activity does not cause tiredness, heart palpitations, or shortness of breath
2 (Mild)	Slight limitation of physical activity—comfortable at rest, but ordinary physical activity results in tiredness, heart palpitations, or shortness of breath
3 (Moderate)	Marked or noticeable limitations of physical activity—comfortable at rest, but less than ordinary physical activity causes tiredness, heart palpitations, or shortness of breath
4 (Severe)	Severe limitation of physical activity—unable to carry out any physical activity without discomfort. Symptoms also present at rest. If any physical activity is undertaken, discomfort increases.

AHA/ACC Heart Failure Stages

Stage	Description
A	People at high risk for developing heart failure but who do not have heart failure or damage to the heart
B	People who have developed structural heart disease that is strongly associated with the development of heart failure (such as those with a history of heart attack, those with a low ejection fraction, valve disease with no symptoms) but without signs and symptoms of heart failure
C	Patients with known structural heart disease and current or prior symptoms. Most common symptoms include shortness of breath, fatigue, reduced ability to exercise
D	People who have advanced heart failure and severe symptoms difficult to manage with standard treatment (Patients with end-stage heart failure fall into this stage, and are characterized by advanced structural heart disease and pronounced symptoms of heart failure at rest or upon minimal physical exertion, despite maximal medical treatment.)

Coding Tip

Other types of heart failure:

- **Right heart failure, including right heart failure due to left heart failure, is included in subcategory I5Ø.81. Code I5Ø.814 Right heart failure due to left heart failure includes an instructional note to code also the type of left ventricular failure, if known (I5Ø.2–I5Ø.43).**
- **Patients with biventricular failure can have right heart disease due to one cause and left heart disease due to another, unlike most cardiomyopathies that have a single cause with right ventricular failure secondary to left ventricular failure (I5Ø.814). Report I5Ø.82 when there is a different disease causing heart failure in each ventricle.**
- **Biventricular heart failure, code I5Ø.82, also includes an instructional note to code also the type of left ventricular failure, if known (I5Ø.2–I5Ø.43).**
- **High output heart failure, code I5Ø.83, occurs when the high demand for blood exceeds the capacity of a normally functioning heart to meet the demand.**
- **End-stage heart failure, AHA/ACC classification stage D, code I5Ø.84, with an instructional note to code also type of heart failure as systolic or diastolic, if known.**

In ICD-10-CM, the acuity of heart failure is an important factor when selecting the appropriate code to represent the patient's illness. The stages and classifications above identify patients in the chronic stages of the disease but occasionally due to a variety of stressors, heart failure may worsen or exacerbate. In cases where the documentation only includes the verbiage "heart failure decompensation/exacerbation," it is correct to assign a code from category I5Ø with a fifth or sixth character of 3 representing acute on chronic. This is based on the definition of decompensation as discussed in the American Hospital Association's *Coding Clinic for ICD-10-CM*, second quarter 2013, page 33. Documented "history" of heart failure should be reported as "chronic" or in ICD-10-CM a code from category I5Ø with a fifth or sixth character of 2.

Another important factor to consider when selecting codes to report heart failure is whether or not the patient has any underlying conditions that may require an additional code or a combination code to identify the heart failure as a manifestation or related to another condition. This is most imperative when the heart failure is identified as being hypertensive in nature or linked to hypertension. In this case code I11.Ø Hypertensive heart disease with heart failure, is reported followed by a code from category I5Ø to identify the nature of the heart failure. If chronic kidney disease or end-stage renal disease is also present, a code from category I13 Hypertensive heart and chronic kidney disease, would be reported rather than I11.Ø.

Coding Tip

The hypertension classification presumes a causal relationship between hypertension and heart involvement and between hypertension and kidney involvement as these conditions are linked to the main term hypertension by the term "with" in the alphabetic index. These conditions should be coded as related even in the absence of provider documentation explicitly linking them, unless the documentation clearly states the conditions are unrelated. (Guideline I.C.9.a)

It should be noted that it is common for pleural effusions and pulmonary edema to be present with CHF. It is inappropriate to report an additional code for pulmonary edema of cardiogenic origin in addition to a code for CHF. However, dependent upon the documentation of clinical significance and evaluation and treatment of pleural effusion, a code for this condition may be reported as an additional diagnosis.

Coding/Reporting Criteria	Clinical Criteria	
1. Physical Evaluation *(routine/expected in italics)*	• Shortness of breath (on minimal exertion) • Fatigue • Swelling ankles, feet, legs • Ascites or swelling in the abdomen	• Pitting edema • Jugular venous distention (JVD) • Cough, worsens when supine
2. Clinical Evaluation *(routine/expected in italics)*	• Elevated BNP • I&Os	• Daily weights
3. Diagnostic Px *(routine/expected in italics)*	• LVEF under 40 • EKG—heart muscle thickening indicative of increased effort/weakness • CXR—cardiomegaly, pulmonary edema, pleural effusion • ECG	• Doppler ultrasound • Holter monitor • Stress test • Cardiac catheterization • Cardiac angiography • Cardiac MRI
4. Therapeutic Tx *(routine/expected in italics)*	• Low-salt diet • Restricted fluid intake • Pharmaceuticals: – diuretics – angiotensin-converting enzyme INH – aldosterone antagonists – angiotensin II receptor blockers (ARB) – beta blockers – digoxin – isosorbide dinitrate/hydralazine hydrochloride	• Autonomic implantable cardioverter defibrillator (AICD) • Cardiac resynchronization therapy (CRT) device • Left ventricular assist device • Dialysis for heart failure
5. Increased Nursing Care and/or Monitoring	• Monitoring IV medication	
6. Extends LOS	• Discharge delayed due to HF	

Condition	Documentation Example	ICD-10-CM Corresponding Codes
Routine/Expected/ Integral/Inherent/ Incidental *(italics only)*	*NA*	*NA*
Principal Diagnosis	1. History and Physical: Patient four days status postacute myocardial infarction (AMI) now admitted for chest pain and dyspnea secondary to HF. **(Query if acute, chronic or acute on chronic; query if systolic, diastolic or combined; query site of AMI.)**	1. Report I5Ø.9 Heart failure, unspecified, followed by I21.3 ST elevation (STEMI) myocardial infarction of unspecified site.
Comorbidity	1. History and Physical: Admitted for left total hip replacement for advanced degenerative joint disease (DJD), history of HF and systolic dysfunction on digoxin and Lasix.	1. Report M16.12 Unilateral primary osteoarthritis, left hip, followed by I5Ø.22 Chronic systolic heart failure.
Complication of Care	1. Progress Note: Increased shortness of breath and edema—HF exacerbation secondary to overhydration with normal saline due to IV line malfunction; known diastolic dysfunction; start Lasix.	1. Report T82.594A Other mechanical complication of infusion catheter, initial encounter, followed by I5Ø.33 Acute on chronic diastolic heart failure; and Y63.Ø Excessive amount of blood or other fluid given during transfusion or infusion.
Poisoning or Adverse Effect of Medication/ Chemical	1. Discharge Summary: Actos-induced HF, patient with diabetes type 2.	1. Report I5Ø.9 Heart failure, followed by T38.3X5A Adverse effect of insulin and oral hypoglycemic [antidiabetic] drugs; E11.9 Type 2 diabetes mellitus without complications and Z79.84 Long term (current) use of oral hypoglycemic drugs.

Additional References

AHA CC: 2Q, 2024, p. 9; 3Q, 2023, p. 14; 3Q, 2020, p. 32; 4Q, 2017, p. 15; 1Q, 2017, p. 45-47; 3Q, 2016, 46; 1Q, 2016, 10; 2Q, 2015, p. 15; 4Q, 2014, p. 21; 2Q, 2013, p. 33

American College of Cardiology: https://www.acc.org

American Heart Association: http://www.heart.org/

National Heart, Lung, and Blood Institute: http://www.nhlbi.nih.gov/

Hepatic Encephalopathy/Hepatic Coma

K70.40	**Alcoholic hepatic failure without coma**	HCC
K70.41	**Alcoholic hepatic failure with coma**	MCC HCC
K71.10	**Toxic liver disease with hepatic necrosis, without coma**	
K71.11	**Toxic liver disease with hepatic necrosis, with coma**	MCC
K72.00	**Acute and subacute hepatic failure without a coma**	MCC
K72.01	**Acute and subacute hepatic failure with coma**	MCC
K72.10	**Chronic hepatic failure without coma**	HCC
K72.11	**Chronic hepatic failure with coma**	MCC HCC
K72.90	**Hepatic failure, unspecified without coma**	HCC
K72.91	**Hepatic failure, unspecified with coma**	MCC HCC
K76.82	**Hepatic encephalopathy**	HCC
K91.82	**Postprocedural hepatic failure**	CC

Associated terminology: hepatic encephalopathy; hepatic coma

Note: This clinical review is limited to hepatic encephalopathy and hepatic failure (with and without coma). Toxic, metabolic, other, and unspecified encephalopathy is reviewed under the section Encephalopathy in this publication.

Discussion

Encephalopathy is a general term indicating a syndrome of diffuse brain dysfunction which alters brain function or structure. It is a complication of a primary condition or disease, organic or inorganic, and it can be permanent or reversible. The symptom integral to encephalopathy is altered mental status. The type or cause of encephalopathy should be identified and the alphabetic index consulted, which lists many codes for specific causes, such as septic, hepatic, metabolic, drug induced, traumatic (postconcussional), hypertensive, etc.

Hepatic encephalopathy occurs secondary to decreased liver function. The liver's main purpose is to filter toxins (such as ammonia) from the bloodstream, removing the toxins or rendering them harmless. When liver function is impaired, these toxic substances can build up, causing deterioration of the brain. Symptoms of hepatic encephalopathy can range from minimal changes in memory and coordination to amnesia and profound confusion. Lab findings include elevated ammonia levels. Treatment may include lactulose, a laxative that when used in higher doses reduces ammonia absorption from the colon.

Hepatic coma is the most severe and often terminal stage of hepatic encephalopathy. The presence of coma requires explicit physician documentation.

Coding and Documentation Tip

Determine whether Glasgow coma scale scores are evident in the medical record; the physician may use these to assess patients with hepatic coma.

According to the ICD-10-CM guidelines, Glasgow coma scale codes should be reported only in conjunction with traumatic brain injury codes. Although the reporting of Glasgow coma scale codes would not be appropriate in addition to hepatic coma codes, this guideline is not intended to restrict the use of the Glasgow coma scale in assessing these patients.

Coding Tip

Two codes should be reported for documented hepatic encephalopathy—code K76.82 and a code for the underlying liver disease described as "without coma." If hepatic coma is documented, only one code is reported, that for the underlying liver disease described as "with coma."

Coding/Reporting Criteria	Clinical Criteria	
1. Physical Evaluation *(routine/expected in italics)*	• Altered mental status: only s/s or manifestation integral to encephalopathy	• Glasgow coma scores available
2. Clinical Evaluation *(routine/expected in italics)*	• Evaluation of underlying cause • Ammonia level • Blood tests/CBC • Spinal fluid analysis • Blood pressure	• Metabolic tests • Drug and toxin levels • Blood/body fluid analysis for infection work-up • Creatinine • Serum electrolytes
3. Diagnostic Px *(routine/expected in italics)*	• Evaluation of underlying cause • Lumbar puncture	• Imaging studies • EEG
4. Therapeutic Tx *(routine/expected in italics)*	• Varies depending on etiology/type and severity • Oxygen • IV fluids • Oral lactulose: hepatic	• Antibiotics • Dialysis: Extracorporeal albumin dialysis (ECAD) • Medications to control hyper- or hypotension
5. Increased Nursing Care and/or Monitoring	• Prevention teaching; importance of diet, medication, dietary compliance	
6. Extends LOS	• Encephalopathy postadmit	

Condition	Documentation Example	ICD-10-CM Corresponding Codes
Routine/Expected/ Integral/Inherent/ Incidental *(italics only)*	*NA*	*NA*
Principal Diagnosis	1. IP Discharge Summary: An 85-year-old male with hepatocerebral intoxication, due to chronic liver failure presented with change in mental status; soft restraints x24 hours due to agitation with combative behavior; patient is a fall risk, work-up for mental status changes, monitored; treated with lactulose. **(Query physician for presence of hepatic coma.)**	1. Report K76.82 Hepatic encephalopathy; K72.1Ø Chronic hepatic failure without coma; Z91.81 At risk for falling, Z78.1 Physical restraint status. If query resulted in documentation of hepatic coma, report K72.11 Chronic hepatic failure with coma, followed by the Z codes.
Comorbidity	1. IP Discharge Summary: Admitted with urinary tract infection due to *E. coli*, severe dehydration. After admission developed mental status changes and was found to have hepatic encephalopathy due to acute hepatitis C. UTI treated with IV antibiotics and dehydration resolved with IV fluids. Hepatic encephalopathy improved with oral lactulose and antivirals given for acute hepatitis C. Follow up tests will be initiated.	1. Report N39.Ø Urinary tract infection, site not specified, followed by B96.2Ø Unspecified Escherichia coli [E. coli] as the cause of diseases classified elsewhere; E86.Ø Dehydration, unspecified; B17.1Ø Acute hepatitis C without hepatic coma; and K76.82 Hepatic encephalopathy.
Complication of Care	NA	NA
Poisoning or Adverse Effect of Medication/ Chemical	NA	NA

Additional References

AHA CC: 4Q, 2022, p. 27; 1Q, 2022, p. 52; 1Q, 2021, p. 13

Hypernatremia

E87.Ø **Hyperosmolality and hypernatremia** CC

Associated terminology: hypernatremia/hyperosmolality/hypertonic dehydration

Discussion

Hypernatremia is an elevated sodium level in the blood. This happens either as a loss of free water or a gain of sodium or a combination of both. Hyperosmolality or hypertonic refers to the increase of plasma osmolarity resulting in cellular dehydration and shrinkage.

Further classification of hypernatremia by extracellular fluid volume status and causes are:

- Hypovolemic: Decreased total body Na+ with relatively greater decrease in total body water (TBW)
  - excess water loss or inadequate water intake; most common
  - disability with inability to freely access water, debility, impaired thirst mechanism
  - severe diarrhea
  - severe vomiting
  - burns
  - excessive sweating
  - excess use of osmotic diuretics (glucose, Mannitol, urea) or loop diuretics, thiazide diuretics
  - nasogastric suctioning
  - intrinsic renal disease
- Euvolemic: near normal total body Na+ with decreased TBW
  - disability, chronic illness, impaired thirst mechanism
    hyperventilation or mechanical ventilation
  - excessive sweating (can occur before hypovolemic)
  - prolonged fever
  - ketoacidosis
  - diabetes insipidus
  - vasopressin malfunction
- Hypervolemic: increased Na+ with normal or increased TBW
  - hypertonic fluid administration with restricted free water intake: iatrogenic administration of hypertonic sodium bicarbonate solution or saline
  - TPN, lactulose
  - ingestion of sodium chloride (NaCl) tablets
  - sodium modeling in hemodialysis
  - ingestion of seawater
  - ingestion of excessive amount of sports drink
  - mineralocorticoid excess with restricted free water intake: adrenal tumor, congenital adrenal hyperplasia

Documentation Tip

Code assignment cannot be based on ancillary test results, therapies, or clinical criteria alone. A diagnosis and its clinical significance must be supported by physician or other qualified healthcare professional documentation. When it is unclear or there is contradictory information, query the physician or other qualified healthcare professional for clarification.

Infancy, advanced age, debilitation, long-term care residency, impaired mental status, brain injury status, and hospitalization are high-risk factors for developing hypernatremia. Identification of the underlying cause is important in management. The efficacy of treatment is influenced by the onset; acute hypernatremia, which develops in less than 24 hours should be corrected rapidly (< 24 hrs); chronic hypernatremia of unknown duration developing over a course of 48 hours should be corrected more slowly (> 24 hrs) due to the risk of cerebral edema during treatment. Treatment variables depend on whether the hypernatremia is acute or chronic, the classification, severity of the symptoms, the patient's weight (use in formulae) and the underlying cause.

Coding Tip

- **Diabetes insipidus is found in categories E23 Hypofunction and other disorders of the pituitary gland, or N25 Disorders resulting from impaired renal tubular function.**
- **Diabetes mellitus with hyperosmolarity is found in categories EØ8, EØ9, E11, E13.**
- **Hypernatremia in newborn is reported with P74.21 Hypernatremia of newborn.**

When both dehydration and hypernatremia are documented, query the provider if the relationship between the dehydration and hypernatremia can be linked or can be further specified.

Reporting dehydration with hypernatremia or hyponatremia requires two codes: E86.Ø and either E87.Ø or E87.1.

Documentation Tip

The ↑ and ↓ symbols do not indicate a diagnosis. Query the provider as to the meaning and if it represents a diagnosis. Request that the information be fully stated, including the clinical significance.

Coding/Reporting Criteria	Clinical Criteria	
1. Physical Evaluation *(routine/expected in italics)*	• *Asymptomatic* • Headache • Extreme thirst • Dry mucus membranes • Decreased skin turgor • Dizziness • Orthostatic blood pressure changes • Tachycardia (pulse > 90) • Nausea/vomiting • Weakness/fatigue	• Edema • Muscle spasm/tremors • Weight loss • Confusion • Lethargy • Oliguria • Obtundation • Seizure • Coma
2. Clinical Evaluation *(routine/expected in italics)*	• Serum sodium (Na+): > 145 mEq/L • Serial measurements of serum sodium to monitor/adjust treatment • Serum electrolytes • Glucose level • Urea (BUN) • Creatinine • Increased hemoglobin/hematocrit (H/H) after hydration	• Height/weight measurement: calculation of body fluid requirements; changes in daily weight indicate fluid loss or gain (1 lb Δ = 500 ml fluid volume Δ) • Measure intake/output • Urine/plasma osmolality • Urine electrolytes • 24-hour urine volume • Plasma arginine vasopressin level (if indicated)
3. Diagnostic Px *(routine/expected in italics)*	• Serial neurologic exams	
4. Therapeutic Tx *(routine/expected in italics)*	• *Untreated (chronic and asymptomatic)* • Diet therapy with oral fluid replacement: matching intake with output • Oral fluid rehydration therapy: fluid loss replaced liter for liter • Parenteral fluid replacement	• Diuretics • Vasopressin • IV fluid (H2O with dextrose/saline) with electrolytes: replacement for severe fluid loss • Dialysis (volume overload)
5. Increased Nursing Care and/or Monitoring	• Development of drug-induced hypernatremia, monitor Na+ levels; treated	
6. Extends LOS	• Discharge delayed due to hypernatremia due to (stated cause)	

Condition	Documentation Example	ICD-10-CM Corresponding Codes
Routine/Expected/ Integral/Inherent/ Incidental *(italics only)*	1. *Progress Note: Chronic hypernatremia, asymptomatic*	1. *No code assigned.*
Principal Diagnosis	1. IP: Admit due to lithium-induced hypernatremia, sodium level 162, patient compliant with regimen. 2. IP: Admit due to encephalopathy due to hypernatremic dehydration, begin IV rehydration.	1. Report E87.Ø Hyperosmolality and hypernatremia, followed by T43.595A Adverse effect of other antipsychotics and neuroleptics, initial encounter. 2. Report E87.Ø Hyperosmolality and hypernatremia, followed by E86.Ø Dehydration, and G93.41 Metabolic encephalopathy. The condition responsible for the admission will be sequenced as principal diagnosis, with consideration of the workup and the focus of treatment. The underlying cause of the encephalopathy is the hypernatremic dehydration and it is the focus of treatment.
Comorbidity	1. Progress Note: ↑Na, continue treatment **(Query the meaning of ↑Na and its clinical significance, noting it is under treatment and any associated lab values as documented by the provider.)** 2. IP Discharge Summary: Uncontrolled diabetes, type 1, with acute hyperglycemic hyperosmolar syndrome (HHS).	1. Codes cannot be assigned based on arrows as the only documentation. 2. Report E1Ø.69 Type 1 diabetes with other specified complication; followed by E1Ø.65 Type 1 diabetes mellitus with hyperglycemia; E87.Ø Hyperosmolality and hypernatremia.
Complication of Care	1. Progress Note: Hospital-acquired hypernatremia due to over-hydration with normal saline in a patient with increased water losses in setting of restricted free water intake and on prescribed diuretic. 2. Admit to OBV Note: Postdialysis fluid overload with hypernatremia due to error in sodium modeling dialysate.	1. Report T5Ø.3X1A Poisoning by electrolytic, caloric and water-balance agents, accidental (unintentional), initial encounter, followed by E87.Ø Hyperosmolality and hypernatremia. 2. Report T5Ø.3X1A Poisoning by electrolytic, caloric and water-balance agents, accidental (unintentional), initial encounter, followed by E87.Ø Hyperosmolality and hypernatremia.
Poisoning or Adverse Effect of Medication/ Chemical	NA	NA

Additional References

AHA CC: 1Q, 2022, p. 28; 1Q, 2014, p. 7

Diagnoses

Hyponatremia

E87.1 Hypo-osmolality and hyponatremia CC

Associated terminology: hyponatremia/hypo-osmolality/hypotonic dehydration

Diagnoses

Discussion

Hyponatremia is decreased sodium level in the blood. Serum osmolarity is low in true hyposmolar hyponatremia. It occurs from a loss of total body sodium or dilution of serum sodium due to excess water in plasma. The latter mechanism is the most common cause of hyponatremia. The lowered sodium level allows excess water to enter cells, causing them to swell.

Infancy, advanced age, debilitation, long-term care residency, impaired mental status, brain injury status, and hospitalization are high-risk factors for developing hyponatremia. Identification of the underlying cause is important in the management. The efficacy of treatment is influenced by the onset; acute hyponatremia has a rapid drop of sodium level < 48 hours. The results can cause critical physiologic effects. Acute hyponatremia that is severe should be corrected slowly, with increase in serum Na concentration not exceeding 10 mEq/L over the first 24 hours; chronic hyponatremia has a gradual drop of sodium level over several days (> 48 hours) or weeks. The results are usually moderate; can be asymptomatic. When it is symptomatic, it should be corrected slowly due to the risk of cerebral edema during treatment. Treatment variables depend on whether the hyponatremia is acute or chronic, the classification (fluid balance), and severity of the symptoms, the patients' weight (use in formulae) and the underlying cause.

Documentation Tip

Code assignment cannot be based on ancillary test results, therapies, or clinical criteria alone. A diagnosis and its clinical significance must be supported by physician or other qualified healthcare professional documentation. When it is unclear or there is contradictory information, query the physician or other qualified healthcare professional for clarification.

Further classification of hypotonic hyponatremia by extracellular fluid volume status and causes are:

- Hypovolemic: decreased total body Na+ to a greater extent than total body water (TBW) decrease (without presence of edema)
  - vomiting/diarrhea
  - excess sweating
  - burns
  - excessive blood loss
  - acute on chronic renal insufficiency
  - ascites
  - peritonitis
  - pancreatitis
  - rhabdomyolysis
  - small bowel obstruction
  - diuretics
  - TBI/ruptured brain aneurysm/intracranial surgery with cerebral salt wasting syndrome
  - exercise-induced (exertional) hyponatremia
  - Grand Canyon hiker's hyponatremia
- Euvolemic: Total body Na+ near normal with TBW increase (without presence of edema)
  - syndrome of inappropriate secretion of antidiuretic hormone (SIADH)
  - cortisol deficiency
  - hypothyroidism
  - psychogenic polydipsia
  - drugs
  - iatrogenic administration of hypotonic fluids
  - iatrogenic bowel prep
  - water intoxication (delusional hyponatremia): infants at high risk; fraternity hazing; over-hydration with ecstasy use
- Hypervolemia: total body Na+ increase with TBW increase to a greater extent (edema present)
  - congestive heart failure
  - cirrhosis
  - nephrotic syndrome/kidney failure
  - beer potomania
  - medication induced

There are several conditions that result in a low serum sodium level, but are not true hyponatremia:

- Redistribution or translocational hyponatremia: hypertonic: serum osmolarity is normal or elevated: dilution of serum sodium due to glucose causing water shift from the intracellular space to the extracellular space. It corrects as normoglycemia is re-established.
  - extreme hyperglycemia (hypovolemic)
  - administration of glycerol or mannitol
  - administration of radiocontrast agents in advanced renal disease
- Pseudohyponatremia: serum osmolarity is normal; serum is diluted with excessive proteins or lipids; a decrease in plasma water fraction
  - use of flame emission spectrophotometry or indirect potentiometry used to assay serum sodium levels
  - hypertriglyceridemia
  - hyperlipidemia
  - multiple myeloma with hyperproteinemia

Excluded

SIADH (syndrome of inappropriate secretion of antidiuretic hormone), see E22.2 Syndrome of inappropriate secretion of antidiuretic hormone.

When both dehydration and hyponatremia are documented, query the provider if the relationship between the dehydration and hyponatremia can be linked or be further specified.

Reporting dehydration with hypernatremia or hyponatremia requires two codes: E86.Ø and either E87.Ø or E87.1.

Documentation Tip

The ↑ and ↓ symbols do not indicate a diagnosis. Query the provider as to the meaning and if it represents a diagnosis, request that the information be fully stated, including the clinical significance.

Coding Tip

Hyponatremia in newborn is reported with P74.22 Hyponatremia of newborn.

Coding/Reporting Criteria	Clinical Criteria
1. Physical Evaluation *(routine/expected in italics)*	• *Asymptomatic* • Headache • Anorexia • Nausea/vomiting (peristalsis may be palpated or seen) • Lethargy • Fatigue • Restlessness/irritability • Muscle weakness, cramps, spasms • Fluid overload • Metabolic encephalopathy • Seizure • Cerebral edema • Intracranial pressure (ICP) • Tentorial brain herniation/compression • Obtundation • Coma • Noncardiogenic pulmonary edema • Respiratory arrest • Infant: – changes in mental status – low body temperature ≤ 97° – facial swelling/puffiness – seizure – with dehydration: fewer than 3 wet diapers in 24 hours • Hypovolemic – dry mucous membranes – tachycardia – poor skin turgor – orthostasis • Hypervolemia: – pulmonary rales/edema – S3 gallop – Jugular venous distention – peripheral edema – ascites • Severe acute: – fixed, unilateral, dilated pupil – decorticate/decerebrate posturing – acute, severe hypertension • Chronic: – status epilepticus – osmotic demyelination syndrome (cerebral pontine myelinolysis)

Diagnoses

Coding/Reporting Criteria	Clinical Criteria	
2. Clinical Evaluation *(routine/expected in italics)*	• Serum sodium (Na+): < 136 mEq/L (severe < 109-120 mEq/L) • Serum osmolarity: low in hyposmolar hyponatremia; normal in pseudohyponatremia; normal or elevated in hypertonic hyponatremia-hyperglycemic • Serial measurements of serum sodium to monitor/adjust treatment • Serum electrolytes • Glucose level • Urea • Creatinine	• Thyroid stimulating hormone (TSH)/free thyroxine levels • Height/weight measurement: calculation of body fluid requirements; changes in daily weight indicate fluid loss or gain (1 lb Δ = 500 ml fluid volume Δ) • Measure intake/output • Urine/plasma osmolality/sodium levels • Urine electrolytes • 24-hour urine volume • Plasma arginine vasopressin level (if indicated) • Adrenal function
3. Diagnostic Px *(routine/expected in italics)*	• Serial neurologic exams • Chest x-ray: underlying cause	• CT brain with neurological symptoms
4. Therapeutic Tx *(routine/expected in italics)*	• *Untreated (chronic and asymptomatic)* • Treatment of the underlying disorder • Diet induced: change in diet/habits • Infants: breast milk or formula that is not over-diluted; avoid straight water and electrolyte enriched pediatric drinks for routine hydration • Diet therapy with oral fluid restriction: small adjustments in mild cases • Oral fluid hydration therapy: restriction of free water • Place patient in an upright position • Diuretics • Vasopressin • ACE inhibitor in HF	• Chronic: 3% hypertonic saline – < 10–12 meg/L over 24 hours – < 18 mEq/L over 48 hours – 8 mEq/L for first 24 hours • Acute/severe: – hypertonic saline or vasopressin initially to increase Na by 1–2 mEq/L per hour until Na = 125 mEq/L or s/s diminish • IV fluid (H2O with saline) with electrolytes – hypovolemic; 0.9% saline – hypervolemic: fluid restriction; diuretic as indicated – euvolemic: treatment of cause • Adrenal gland insufficiency: hormone replacement • Dialysis (volume overload) • Intubation/vent
5. Increased Nursing Care and/or Monitoring	• Development of drug induced hyponatremia, monitor Na+ levels; treated	
6. Extends LOS	• Discharge delayed due to hyponatremia due to (stated cause)	

Condition	Documentation Example	ICD-10-CM Corresponding Codes
Routine/Expected/ Integral/Inherent/ Incidental *(italics only)*	1. *Progress Note: Chronic hyponatremia, asymptomatic, untreated.*	1. *No code assigned.*
Principal Diagnosis	1. IP: Admit due to encephalopathy secondary to hyponatremic dehydration, begin IV hydration NS. 2. IP: Admit due to psychogenic polydipsia induced hyponatremia with acute exacerbation of chronic paranoid schizophrenia; once hyponatremia is corrected, transfer to psych IP.	1. Report E87.1 Hypo-osmolality and hyponatremia, followed by E86.Ø Dehydration, and G93.41 Metabolic encephalopathy. The underlying cause of the encephalopathy is the hyponatremic dehydration and it is the focus of treatment. 2. Report E87.1 Hypo-osmolality and hyponatremia, followed by R63.1 Polydipsia. As a chapter 18 code, R63.1 would not be sequenced as principal diagnosis since the definitive diagnosis that warranted admission and treatment is E87.1.
Comorbidity	1. Progress Note: ↓Na, continue treatment. **(Query the meaning of ↓Na and its clinical significance, noting it is under treatment and any associated lab values as documented by the provider.)**	1. Codes cannot be assigned based on arrows as the only documentation.
Complication of Care	NA	NA
Poisoning or Adverse Effect of Medication/ Chemical	1. IP: Admit due to thiazide-induced hyponatremia, sodium level 130, patient compliant with regimen.	1. Report E87.1 Hypo-osmolality and hyponatremia, followed by T5Ø.2X5A Adverse effect of carbonic-anhydrase inhibitors, benzothiadiazides and other diuretics, initial encounter.

Additional References

AHA CC: 2Q, 2022, p. 10; 1Q, 2020, p. 5; 1Q, 2014, p. 7

Iatrogenic (Intraoperative) Puncture or Laceration (Tear) (Rent)

D78.1-	**Accidental puncture and laceration of the spleen during a procedure**	CC
E36.1-	**Accidental puncture or laceration of an endocrine system organ or structure during a procedure**	CC
G97.4-	**Accidental puncture or laceration of a nervous system organ or structure during a procedure**	CC
H59.2-	**Accidental puncture or laceration of eye and adnexa during a procedure**	CC
H95.3-	**Accidental puncture or laceration of ear and mastoid process during a procedure**	CC
I97.5-	**Accidental puncture or laceration of a circulatory system organ or structure during a procedure**	CC
J95.7-	**Accidental puncture or laceration of a respiratory system organ or structure during a procedure**	CC
K91.7-	**Accidental puncture or laceration of a digestive system organ or structure during a procedure**	CC
L76.1-	**Accidental puncture or laceration of skin and subcutaneous tissue during a procedure**	CC
M96.82-	**Accidental puncture or laceration of a musculoskeletal structure during a procedure**	CC
N99.7-	**Accidental puncture or laceration of a genitourinary system organ or structure during a procedure**	CC

Diagnoses

Associated terminology: durotomy; enterotomy during lysis of adhesions; intraoperative splenic tear; bladder tear by trocar during laparoscopic surgery; dural rent

Discussion

Intraoperative puncture, perforation, laceration, or tear of an organ should be reported when it is clinically significant, documented as a complication, or requires more than routine homeostasis or simple suture or glue repair. A full-thickness violation of an organ usually exhibits evidence of injury according to the organ site, such as exudate at site, bleeding, escape of contents, neurological deficits, or is described as injury to the organ. Minor tears described as incidental or serosal (without associated organ violation), small injury, or inadvertent tears are usually not clinically significant and may be considered inherent with the type of surgery. The exception is a dural tear to the dura mater of the brain, spinal cord, or spinal nerves. A dural tear is always considered clinically significant.

There may also be occasions in which a durotomy, bleeding, or serosal tear are not due to the procedure, but due to underlying conditions such as tissue friability, thinning of the dura, adhesions, or spinal osteophytes. A dural tear, when not a complication of surgery, is reported using ICD-10-CM code, G96.11 Dural tear. A nonsurgical serosal tear is not reported or is reported using only the code for the cause (i.e., adhesions).

Documentation Tip

Complications of care: The condition must be more than a routinely expected condition or event. The documentation must support that the condition is clinically significant with an indication that it is a complication, by demonstrating:

- **A cause-and-effect relationship between the care or procedure and the condition**
- **That the condition resulted in altering the course of a procedure or surgery**

The term "complication" does not have to be explicitly documented.

Hemorrhage or hematoma caused by an intraoperative puncture or laceration is included in some of the codes for puncture/laceration per the Excludes 1 note found under some of the intraoperative hemorrhage/hematoma subcategories; therefore, it is not appropriate to code the intraoperative bleed separately.

Intraoperative coronary artery dissection during cardiac catheterization or angioplasty without puncture or laceration is I97.88 Other intraoperative complication of the circulatory system, not elsewhere classified, reported in conjunction with I25.42 Coronary artery dissection when it is reported as clinically significant or as a complication.

Documentation Tip

If there is any question whether the puncture or laceration is clinically significant and a complication, query the provider or procedure physician.

Coding/Reporting Criteria	Clinical Criteria	
1. Physical Evaluation) *(routine/expected in italics)*	• *Incidental, asymptomatic: no clinical significance* • Clinical presentation is specific to organ injured • Clinically significant injury, intraoperative • Bleeding • Cerebral infarct	• Exudate • Escape of contents • Extravasation • Gas in Foley bag or hematuria
2. Clinical Evaluation *(routine/expected in italics)*	• Post-op monitoring • Specific to organ injured	• Urinalysis: hematuria • Hgb/Hct
3. Diagnostic Px *(routine/expected in italics)*	• Post-op monitoring • Specific to organ injured	• Imaging
4. Therapeutic Tx *(routine/expected in italics)*	• Specific to organ injured • *No treatment or simple suture/oversewn/hemostasis* • Suture: layered, complicated repair • Fibrin glue • Blood Patch • Dural graft; fat, muscle, allograft, Gortex • Supine "head on bed" ≥ 24 hours • Resection	• Stent • Excision • Bypass • Urinary catheter • Splenectomy • Occlusion • Mesh repair • Peritoneal toileting
5. Increased Nursing Care and/or Monitoring	• Monitor for cerebrospinal fluid leak after intraoperative spinal durotomy; 24 hour supine	
6. Extends LOS	• Discharge cancelled due to intracerebral hemorrhage due to cerebral artery puncture by Merci Retrieval System® thrombectomy catheter	

Condition	Documentation Example	ICD-10-CM Corresponding Codes
Routine/Expected/ Integral/Inherent/ Incidental *(italics only)*	1. *IP Operative Report: Incidental serosal rent during lysis of adhesions, oversewn.*	1. *No code assigned.*
Principal Diagnosis	1. IP Admit Note: Admitted from ambulatory surgery with intraoperative splenic laceration by trocar during attempted laparoscopic cholecystectomy; open splenorrhaphy.	1. Report D78.12 Accidental puncture and laceration of the spleen during other procedure.
Comorbidity	1. Tracheal laceration during intubation.	1. Report J95.71 Accidental puncture and laceration of a respiratory system organ or structure during a respiratory system procedure.
Complication of Care	1. IP Discharge Summary: Intraoperative bladder tear during open hysterectomy, confirmed as complication; repaired by urology.	1. Report N99.71 Accidental puncture and laceration of a genitourinary system organ or structure during a genitourinary system procedure.
Poisoning or Adverse Effect of Medication/ Chemical	NA	NA

Additional References

AHA CC: 1Q, 2024, p. 20;1Q, 2022, p. 22, 51; 2Q, 2021, p. 11; 2Q, 2019, p. 23-24, 33; 4Q, 2014, p. 24

Ileus

K31.5	**Obstruction of duodenum**	CC
K56.Ø	**Paralytic ileus**	CC HCC
K56.3	**Gallstone ileus**	CC HCC
K56.69[Ø,1,9]	**Other intestinal obstruction [partial, complete, unspecified]**	CC HCC
K56.7	**Ileus, unspecified**	CC HCC
K59.81	**Ogilvie syndrome**	
K59.89	**Other specified functional intestinal disorders**	
K91.3[Ø,1,2]	**Postprocedural intestinal obstruction [unspecified, partial, complete]**	CC
K91.89	**Other postprocedural complications and disorders of digestive system**	CC

Associated terminology: ileus; gallstone ileus; duodenal ileus; mechanical/obstructive ileus; neurogenic/paralytic ileus; pseudo-obstruction ileus; intraop/post-op intestinal obstruction; atony; Ogilvie syndrome

Discussion

Ileus (paralytic ileus, adynamic ileus) is a disruption of intestinal peristalsis that can lead to partial or complete non-mechanical blockage or obstruction of the small and/or large intestine. Handling the bowel during abdominal surgery/dissection can cause peristalsis to stop, making these patients at risk for experiencing ileus (surgery at other sites is not "due to surgery"). Another cause is the use of certain drugs, especially opioid analgesics either during an operation or in the postoperative phase, anticholinergic drugs, and certain chemotherapy drugs. When this occurs it is considered an adverse effect of the specified drug. Ileus from nonabdominal sites would be due to medication, not surgery. Severe electrolyte imbalance or a loss of nerve or blood supply to the intestine can also cause the loss of normal peristaltic function.

Ileus is a common condition occurring within the first 24 to 72 hours postoperatively, lasting usually only 48 to 72 hours. There will be a reduction or absence of bowel sounds. The patient is not allowed to eat or drink anything until intestinal function normalizes or returns. Fluids and electrolytes (such as sodium, chloride, and potassium) are given intravenously to restore balance.

Ileus is reportable when it is associated with significant findings, such as abdominal distention, nausea/vomiting, severe constipation, bowel obstruction, or requires further diagnostic or therapeutic work up, such as abdominal x-ray (as part of work up, not incidentally), CT scan, ultrasound, blood tests or colonoscopy, therapy by bed rest/bowel rest (no food PO), insertion of nasogastric or rectal tube for decompression, administration of drugs that promote intestinal motility (cisapride or vasopressin) or is linked to an extended hospital stay. (It must be documented as the definitive diagnosis for the symptoms that prompted the workup).

Coding Tip

Atony of colon, also called lazy colon or colon stasis, is a dysfunction of the colon caused by lack of muscle tone or strength within the colon and may result in chronic constipation. It is captured with code K59.89 Other specified functional intestinal disorders. Ogilvie syndrome mimics a mechanical obstruction in the colon but is caused by massive dilatation without a physical obstruction. Ogilvie syndrome is reported with code K59.81.

Documentation Tip

Complications of care: The condition must be more than a routinely expected condition or event. The documentation must support that the condition is clinically significant with an indication that it is a complication, by demonstrating:

- **A cause-and-effect relationship between the care or procedure and the condition**
- **That the condition resulted in altering the course of a procedure or surgery**

The term "complication" does not have to be explicitly documented.

Diagnoses

Coding/Reporting Criteria	Clinical Criteria	
1. Physical Evaluation *(routine/expected in italics)*	• *Reduced or absent bowel sounds* • Abdominal pain—not routine if w/u prompted • Nausea or vomiting—not routine if w/u prompted	• Abdominal distention—not routine if w/u prompted • Constipation (severe) and/or diarrhea—not routine if w/u prompted
2. Clinical Evaluation *(routine/expected in italics)*	• Temp > 102 prompting workup (blood culture/UA) • WBC > 18	• WBC > 15 & Bands > 7% • Electrolyte imbalance (severe)
3. Diagnostic Px *(routine/expected in italics)*	• *Abdominal x-ray: ileus (bulging loops of intestine)—incidental finding/routine p/o (not prompted by workup)* • CT scan—not routine if w/u prompted	• Ultrasound—not routine if w/u prompted • Repeat x-ray, CT, ultrasound due to symptoms • Colonoscopy—not routine • Blood tests
4. Therapeutic Tx *(routine/expected in italics)*	• *Bed rest/npo routine order* • Fluids and replacement of electrolytes (sodium, chloride, potassium) • Nasogastric tube inserted for decompression/feeding/aspiration • Rectal tube inserted for decompression	• Administration of drugs to promote peristalsis (prokinetic agents) • Supervised bed rest • IV nutrition/total parenteral nutrition (TPN) • IV crystalloid solutions • Aspiration, at intervals or siphon, via nasogastric tube
5. Increased Nursing Care and/or Monitoring	• Workup or treatment prompted by severity of symptoms or duration • Supervised bed rest	• IV nutrition/TPN • IV crystalloid solutions • Aspiration, at intervals or siphon, via nasogastric tube
6. Extends LOS	• Discharge delayed	

Condition	Documentation Example	ICD-10-CM Corresponding Codes
Routine/Expected/ Integral/Inherent/ Incidental *(italics only)*	1. *Progress Note: Expected/incidental ileus not requiring treatment.* 2. *Discharge Summary: Routine/incidental ileus.*	1. *No code assigned.* 2. *No code assigned.*
Principal Diagnosis	NA	NA
Comorbidity	1. Progress Note (1): (symptom) (workup) due to ileus. Progress Note (2): Decompression for ileus. Progress Note (3): Evaluate ileus. Discharge Summary: Ileus requiring evaluation/treatment (if due to med/anesthesia, state). **Query type of ileus.**	1. Report K56.7 Ileus, unspecified.
Complication of Care	1. Progress Note (1): (symptom) (workup) due to ileus from surgery. Progress Note (2): Decompression for ileus due to surgery. Progress Note (3): Evaluate ileus, surgical. Discharge Summary: Ileus due to surgery requiring evaluation/treatment (if due to med/anesthesia, state). **Query type of ileus further specified.**	1. Report K91.89 Other postprocedural complications and disorders of digestive system, with code K56.7 Ileus, unspecified. If due to anesthesia/medication, report as adverse effect of medicine and not surgical.
Poisoning or Adverse Effect of Medication/ Chemical	1. Progress Note: Adynamic ileus due to spinal anesthesia (or opioid).	1. Report K56.Ø Paralytic ileus followed by T41.3X5A Adverse effect of local anesthetics, initial encounter.

Additional References

AHA CC: 3Q, 2023, p. 11; 4Q, 2020, p. 29; 2Q, 2020, p. 22; 4Q, 2017, p. 16; 2Q, 2017, p. 12; 1Q, 2017, p. 40

Intraoperative or Postoperative Hemorrhage (not due to device, implant, or graft)

D78.Ø-	**Intraoperative hemorrhage and hematoma of the spleen complicating a procedure**	CC
D78.2-	**Postprocedural hemorrhage of the spleen following a procedure**	CC
E36.Ø-	**Intraoperative hemorrhage and hematoma of an endocrine system organ or structure complicating a procedure**	CC
E89.81-	**Postprocedural hemorrhage of an endocrine system organ or structure following a procedure**	CC
G97.3-	**Intraoperative hemorrhage and hematoma of a nervous system organ or structure complicating a procedure**	CC
G97.5-	**Postprocedural hemorrhage of a nervous system organ or structure following a procedure**	CC
H59.1-	**Intraoperative hemorrhage and hematoma of eye and adnexa complicating a procedure**	CC
H59.31-	**Postprocedural hemorrhage of eye and adnexa following an ophthalmic procedure**	CC
H59.32-	**Postprocedural hemorrhage of eye and adnexa following other procedure**	CC
H95.2-	**Intraoperative hemorrhage and hematoma of ear and mastoid process complicating a procedure**	CC
H95.4-	**Postprocedural hemorrhage of ear and mastoid process following a procedure**	CC
I97.4-	**Intraoperative hemorrhage and hematoma of a circulatory system organ or structure complicating a procedure**	CC
I97.61-	**Postprocedural hemorrhage of a circulatory system organ or structure following a circulatory procedure**	CC
I97.62Ø	**Postprocedural hemorrhage, of a circulatory system organ or structure following other procedure**	CC
J95.6-	**Intraoperative hemorrhage and hematoma of a respiratory system organ or structure complicating other procedure**	CC
J95.83-	**Postprocedural hemorrhage of a respiratory system organ or structure following a procedure**	CC
K91.6-	**Intraoperative hemorrhage and hematoma of a digestive system organ or structure complicating a procedure**	CC
K91.84-	**Postprocedural hemorrhage of a digestive system organ or structure following a procedure**	CC
L76.Ø-	**Intraoperative hemorrhage and hematoma of skin and subcutaneous tissue complicating a procedure**	CC
L76.2-	**Postprocedural hemorrhage of skin and subcutaneous tissue following a procedure**	CC
M96.81-	**Intraoperative hemorrhage and hematoma of a musculoskeletal structure complicating a procedure**	CC

Diagnoses

M96.83- **Postprocedural hemorrhage of a musculoskeletal structure following a procedure** CC

N99.6- **Intraoperative hemorrhage and hematoma of a genitourinary system organ or structure complicating a procedure** CC

N99.82- **Postprocedural hemorrhage of a genitourinary system organ or structure following a procedure** CC

Associated terminology: intraoperative hemorrhage complicating procedure; postprocedural/postoperative hemorrhage following procedure

Discussion

There is no all-inclusive definition of intraoperative or postoperative hemorrhage. Intraoperative hemorrhage as a complication is relative to patient characteristics, diagnosis, procedure/surgery being performed, treatment/control, volume of blood lost, and its clinical significance and physician judgment. Hemorrhage itself is not only a cause of morbidity and mortality by causing cardiac arrest, hypoxia, etc., but so are complications such as anemia and treatments such as transfusion, which can cause iron overload and other complications. Allowable blood loss can be calculated by formula with the variables of gender, weight, estimated blood volume, and initial and final hematocrit and their average.

Prevention, or at least mitigation of blood loss, starts prior to the surgery or procedure through a detailed history or physical, medical history, and medication history of the patient. It also includes operating room and procedure protocols that go into effect when and if intraoperative hemorrhaging begins.

The degree of hemorrhage is a consideration as well as the type of treatment. Bleeding considered incidental, minor, minimal, integral or expected, small amount, easily controlled, slight oozing, treated with manual pressure/compression at bedside, superficial, etc., usually are not clinically significant as a diagnosis or procedure and would not be reported. Query to have the medical significance clarified when there is a question as to the appropriateness of reporting.

Excluded

- **For obstetrics, see chapter 15.**
- **For birth injury, see chapter 16.**
- **Hemorrhage due to prosthetic devices, implants and grafts, see subcategories T82.83, T83.83, T84.83,T85.83.**

When the amount of intraoperative blood loss is expected, it is not considered a complication of surgery. But if the expected blood loss results in a complication of acute blood loss anemia requiring treatment, the anemia is medically significant. Intraoperative hemorrhage must be correctly identified as to the source: bleeding as a consequence of acute trauma or neoplasm would not be a complication of the surgery. The reporting of intraoperative/postoperative hemorrhage complicating or as a complication of procedure is determined by its clinical significance and the physician's documentation that it is a complication.

If patients refuse blood transfusion due to religious reasons, report the additional code Z53.1 Procedure and treatment not carried out because of patient's decision for reasons of belief and group pressure. Note the Excludes 1 notes under hemorrhage/hematoma codes: if hemorrhage or hematoma is due to a puncture or laceration, only the puncture or laceration code is reported.

Documentation Tip

When postoperative or intraoperative hemorrhage occurs, review medical record for labs and treatment indicating acute blood loss anemia and ensure it is documented if present.

Documentation Tip

Complications of care: The condition must be more than a routinely expected condition or event. The documentation must support that the condition is clinically significant with an indication that it is a complication, by demonstrating:

- **A cause-and-effect relationship between the care or procedure and the condition**
- **That the condition resulted in altering the course of a procedure or surgery**

The term "complication" does not have to be explicitly documented.

An ICD-10-PCS code should be assigned for any procedure performed to achieve hemostasis beyond what is considered integral to the original procedure. This would be captured using the root operation Control unless the procedure performed to control the postoperative bleeding is described by a more specific root operation such as Bypass, Detachment, Excision, Extraction, Reposition, Replacement, or Resection; see OCG: B3.7. For more information regarding the control of postoperative bleeding, see the section regarding "Control of Bleed, Postoperative" in this guide.

Documentation Tip

Code assignment cannot be based on ancillary test results, therapies, or clinical criteria alone. A diagnosis and its clinical significance must be supported by physician or other qualified healthcare professional documentation. When it is unclear or there is contradictory information, query the physician or other qualified healthcare professional for clarification.

Coding/Reporting Criteria	Clinical Criteria	
1. Physical Evaluation *(routine/expected in italics)*	• Adhesions: risk for intra-op tear/hemorrhage • Brisk or profuse bleeding • Arterial: pulsatile; spurts with every heartbeat; bright red; larger volume • Venous: steady flow or oozing; darker blood; lower volume	• Capillary: oozing • Bleeding from organ/system suggesting hemorrhage: hematuria, vaginal bleeding, increased output thoracostomy tube
2. Clinical Evaluation *(routine/expected in italics)*	• *Comparison of pre-op hemoglobin/hematocrit to post-op* • *Serial hemoglobin/hematocrit (H/H)* • Expected blood loss: specific to procedure and patient: – 10%–15% blood volume loss – joint replacements/neoplasm resections: 20%–30% blood volume loss – massive/critical/severe: > 25% patient's blood volume or requires emergency intervention • Allowable blood loss calculated • Hemorrhage grades: blood volume 7% adult/5 liter – class 1 minimal: blood volume loss ≤ 15%; ≤ 750ml; HR normal to mild increase; slightly anxious; capillary refill brisk (<2 sec), normal: pulse <100, BP, pH, respiratory rate 14–20, renal output ≥ 30 ml/hr – class 2 mild: blood volume loss 15%–30%; 750–1500 ml; Tachycardia > 100, diminished peripheral pulses, mild tachypnea 20–30, mildly anxious, confused, combative, cool extremities, mottling, delayed capillary refill, oliguria or 20–30 ml/hr, increased specific gravity; normal: BP and pH	– class 3 moderate: blood volume loss 30%–40%; 1500–2000 ml; significant tachycardia >120, thready peripheral pulses, hypotension, metabolic acidosis, moderate tachypnea 30–40, anxious, confused, lethargic, diminished pain response, cold extremities, mottling, pallor, prolonged capillary refill, oliguria 5-15 ml/hr, BUN increased – class 4 severe: blood volume loss ≥ 40%; ≥ 2000 ml; severe tachycardia ≥ 140, thready central pulses, significant hypotension, significant acidosis, severe tachypnea > 35, lethargic, coma, cold extremities, pallor, cyanosis, anuria/negligible • CBC
3. Diagnostic Px *(routine/expected in italics)*	• *Pulse dosimeter, intra-op*	• Duplex ultrasound to assess for pseudoaneurysm
4. Therapeutic Tx *(routine/expected in italics)*	• *Manual compression* • Pre-op treatment • Requires blood transfusion/PRBC, FFP/platelets • Iron supplement/Procrit • Fluid resuscitation • Cell saver blood salvage • Hemorrhage grades: – class 1: crystalloid – class 2: crystalloid – class 3: crystalloid + blood – class 4: crystalloid + blood	• Thrombin injection for pseudoaneurysm • Suture of site, blood vessel • Vasopressin injection • Coagulation • Resection, bypass, detachment, excision, extraction, reposition, replacement of organ/site of hemorrhage • Embolization
5. Increased Nursing Care and/or Monitoring	• Monitor hemoglobin/hematocrit (H/H) levels	
6. Extends LOS	• Cancel discharge due to post-op hemorrhage	• Procedure converted to open due to intraop bleed

Condition	Documentation Example	ICD-10-CM Corresponding Codes
Routine/Expected/ Integral/Inherent/ Incidental *(italics only)*	1. *IP Progress Note: Puncture site with minor oozing and small hematoma at right groin, controlled with manual pressure, continue to follow per protocol; usual hemoglobin/hematocrit (H/H) reporting.* **(Query if in question, query medical significance, if any, of small hematoma treated with manual compression; was it a complication due to procedure, expected outcome, incidental, etc.)**	1. *Reporting a complication code is based on documentation by the physician that it is a complication and related to surgery/procedure.*
Principal Diagnosis	1. IP Admit Note: Patient presents with hemothorax post needle decompression of tension pneumothorax three days ago in the ED; admit for drainage and monitoring.	1. Report J95.83Ø Postprocedural hemorrhage of a respiratory system organ or structure following a respiratory system procedure, followed by J94.2 Hemothorax.
Comorbidity	1. IP Discharge Summary: Patient admitted upon transfer from outside hospital for treatment of right groin pseudoaneurysm with brisk hemorrhage post left heart catheterization; treated by open suture of common femoral artery puncture site pseudoaneurysm, pressure and dressing.	1. Report I97.89 Other postprocedural complications and disorders of the circulatory system, not elsewhere classified, followed by I97.61Ø Postprocedural hemorrhage of a circulatory system organ or structure following a cardiac catheterization, and I72.4 Aneurysm of artery of lower extremity, other aneurysm of lower extremity (femoral artery).
Complication of Care	1. OP Report: Intraoperative complication: attempted robotic-assisted partial nephrectomy with hemorrhage of renal tissue necessitating conversion to open.	1. Report N99.61 Intraoperative hemorrhage and hematoma of a genitourinary system organ or structure complicating a genitourinary system procedure.
Poisoning or Adverse Effect of Medication/ Chemical	NA	NA

Additional References

AHA CC: 2Q, 2023, p. 28; 1Q, 2020, p. 19; 4Q, 2016, p. 99; 1Q, 2016, p. 15

Intravenous/Dialysis Line/Catheter Infections

T8Ø.211A	**Bloodstream infection due to central venous catheter, initial encounter**	CC HAC
T8Ø.212A	**Local infection due to central venous catheter, initial encounter**	CC HAC
T8Ø.218A	**Other infection due to central venous catheter, initial encounter**	CC HAC
T8Ø.219A	**Unspecified infection due to central venous catheter, initial encounter**	CC HAC
T82.7XXA	**Infection and inflammatory reaction due to other cardiac and vascular devices, implants and grafts, initial encounter**	CC HAC

Associated terminology: Tesio® catheter infection; central line infection; peripherally inserted central catheter (PICC) infection; bacteremia due to Hickman® catheter; cellulitis at central line insertion site; sepsis due to PORT-A-CATH®; peripheral venous catheter (PVC) thrombophlebitis

Diagnoses

Discussion

Central venous catheter (CVC) lines or central venous access devices (CVAD) are for long-term use. They may be inserted into the internal jugular vein of the neck, the subclavian vein in the upper chest under the clavicle, the femoral vein in the leg, groin, or the inferior vena cava and terminate at or near to the heart in one of the great vessels (the internal jugular vein, subclavian, brachiocephalic [innominate] or external/common iliac veins, femoral veins, aorta, the superior or inferior vena cava, pulmonary artery, or the right atrium and in neonates the umbilical artery or vein). CVC lines can have one, two, three, or more ports that connect to IV tubing, medications, or monitors. Nontunneled catheters are inserted percutaneously directly into a vein and are secured at the insertion site. Some are surgically tunneled under the skin, then into the vein to emerge at a distal exit site where they are secured. Procedures such as these are performed in the operating room or interventional radiology procedural suite.

Totally implanted venous access devices (TIVAD) are a type of vascular access device (VAD) with a port that is implanted in a pocket created in the subcutaneous tissue. VADs are used for blood sampling, medication administration, fluid administration, total parenteral nutrition (TPN), dialysis, transfusions, chemotherapy, cardiovascular, and fluid status monitoring.

Documentation Tip

Complications of care: The condition must be more than a routinely expected condition or event. The documentation must support that the condition is clinically significant with an indication that it is a complication, by demonstrating:

- **A cause-and-effect relationship between the care or procedure and the condition**
- **That the condition resulted in altering the course of a procedure or surgery**

The term "complication" does not have to be explicitly documented.

Chronic dialysis catheters have both an arterial and a venous port. They are tunneled catheters with cuffs that are placed using interventional radiology expertise.

Peripherally inserted central (venous) catheter (PICC) is a CVC with entry sites usually in the superficial veins of the arms, legs, feet or hands or head, such as basilic or cephalic vein and terminates in the subclavian, brachiocephalic (innominate) or iliac veins, the superior or inferior vena cava, or the right atrium. Since these are often inserted by nurses, it is important to review nursing documentation for capture of this procedure in the documentation.

Peripherally inserted venous access device catheters (PVC) or midline catheters are inserted into peripheral veins of the hand or forearm and terminate before the level of the axillary line. They are considered short peripheral intravenous catheters, usually less than three inches for PVC and three to eight inches for Midline. They perform the same functions as CVCs. One way to distinguish these from a CVC is where the line terminates: peripheral lines do not extend to near the heart nor do they enter central veins.

The acronym CLABSI stands for central line-associated (laboratory-confirmed) bloodstream infection. Code T8Ø.211A Bloodstream infection due to central venous catheter, initial encounter, represents CLABSI and is a designated hospital-acquired condition when the present on admission indicator is N or U, among other criteria, and is also one of the Agency for Healthcare Research and Quality's, patient safety indicators, #7 Central venous catheter-related blood stream infection rate. Sepsis, as a systemic infection, is categorized using this code. Bacteremia, although not defined as a classic infection, will also use this code assignment. It is important to note that the code for the specified infection is assigned as an additional code followed by a code identifying the organism, if not identified by the manifestation code.

Documentation Tip

Code assignment cannot be based on ancillary test results, therapies, or clinical criteria alone. A diagnosis and its clinical significance must be supported by physician or qualified healthcare professional documentation. When it is unclear or there is contradictory information, query the physician or qualified healthcare professional for clarification.

Coding Tip

When the catheter infection evolves to sepsis, assign first a code from subcategory T8Ø.2- Infections following infusion, transfusion and therapeutic injection, followed by the code for the infection (e.g., A41.9 Sepsis, unspecified organism or specific organism if known). If organ dysfunction occurs due to the sepsis, code also R65.2- Severe sepsis (with or without septic shock) and any codes for the organ dysfunction.

Coding Tip

The seventh character extensions A, D, S affect the analysis of complications and quality of care and reimbursement.

Local infections are specific to site, port, or reservoir and tunnel infections, such as cellulitis or abscess. This is reported using code T8Ø.212A Local infection due to central venous catheter, initial encounter, and is also a hospital-acquired condition when the present on admission indicator is N or U. It is important to note that the code for the specified infection or manifestation is assigned as an additional code followed by a code identifying the organism, if not identified by the manifestation code.

Code T8Ø.218A Other infection due to central venous catheter, initial encounter, represents other infections that are specified as due to the catheter, such as bacterial or infectious endocarditis, empyema, osteomyelitis, infectious (thrombo)phlebitis, or lymphangitis, etc. This code is HAC when the present on admission indicator is N or U. Assign a code the specified infection as an additional code.

Colonization of the catheter tip, without signs or symptoms of an infection, will be reported as carrier status of the organism, Z22 Carrier of infectious disease, category only, without a code from category T8Ø Complications following infusion, transfusion and therapeutic injection, or T82 Complications of cardiac and vascular prosthetic devices, implants, and grafts.

Note: "Suspected", "likely", "probable", "questionable", "rule out", "compatible with", and "consistent with" terms will not be reported as CLABSI when they do not have confirmed laboratory blood infections or are not included in the secondary site criteria.

Examples of CVCs/CVADs are:

- Cordis catheters
- Hickman® catheters
- BROVIAC® catheters
- GROSHONG® catheters
- Triple lumen catheters
- Double lumen catheters
- PICC
- Quinton™ catheter
- Umbilical venous catheter

Examples of TIVAD's are:

- PORT-A-CATH
- BardPort
- Infusaport
- Medi-Port
- P.A.S. Port® peripheral vascular access system

Coding Tip

Hospital-acquired condition (HAC): CMS does not allow a code to increase MS-DRG reimbursement by acting as a CC or MCC with a present on admission (POA) value of N or U. The case will be paid as though these conditions were not reported.

Coding/Reporting Criteria	Clinical Criteria	
1. Physical Evaluation *(routine/expected in italics)*	• Conditions not attributed to another source • Distal infection sites will have s/s related to the site (i.e., infective endocarditis, osteomyelitis, etc.) • Blood stream infection must be laboratory-confirmed for CLABSI • Fever > 38° • Chills • Hypotension • Nausea/vomiting	• Malaise • Localized site erythema/redness/warmth • Tachycardia • Thrombophlebitis (with signs of infection); palpable venous cord • Swelling at insertion site • Pain/tenderness at insertion site • Purulent discharge at insertion site
2. Clinical Evaluation *(routine/expected in italics)*	• Distal infection sites will require workup related to site • Elevated WBCs	• Culture catheter tip • Blood culture: one or more positive culture • CBC
3. Diagnostic Px *(routine/expected in italics)*	• Infection sites will require workup related to site	
4. Therapeutic Tx *(routine/expected in italics)*	• Remove CVC, VAD, PICC or peripheral line (with severe sepsis, hemodynamic instability, evidence of distal infection, suppurative thrombophlebitis, persistent bacteremia > 72 hours of antimicrobial therapy) or blood stream infection due to certain organisms	• Salvage: uncomplicated catheter related blood stream infection, not due to certain pathogens • Guidewire exchange, except for sepsis; if cath tip positive, new cath should have new site location • Antibiotics or antifungals • Thrombolytics with thrombophlebitis • Heat compress
5. Increased Nursing Care and/or Monitoring	• Infection postadmit	
6. Extends LOS	• Infection postadmit	

Condition	Documentation Example	ICD-10-CM Corresponding Codes
Routine/Expected/Integral/ Inherent/Incidental *(italics only)*	*NA*	*NA*
Principal Diagnosis	1. IP Discharge Summary: Admitted due to MRSA sepsis from hemodialysis catheter.	1. Report T82.7XXA Infection and inflammatory reaction due to other cardiac and vascular devices, implants and grafts, initial encounter, followed by A41.Ø2 Sepsis due to Methicillin resistant Staphylococcus aureus.
Comorbidity	1. Progress Note: *Staphylococcus epidermidis* right forearm cellulitis of PICC site.	1. Report T8Ø.212A Local infection due to central venous catheter, initial encounter, followed by LØ3.113 Cellulitis of right upper limb, and B95.7 Other staphylococcus as the cause of diseases classified elsewhere.
Complication of Care	1. IP Discharge Summary: Acute *Staphylococcus aureus* endocarditis due to Port-a-Cath with associated bacteremia.	1. Report T8Ø.218A Other infection due to central venous catheter, initial encounter, followed by I33.Ø Acute and subacute infective endocarditis; R78.81 Bacteremia; and A49.Ø1 Methicillin susceptible Staphylococcus aureus infection, unspecified site.
Poisoning or Adverse Effect of Medication/Chemical	NA	NA

Additional References

AHA CC: 1Q, 2019, p. 13-14; 4Q, 2018, p. 89; 1Q, 2015, p. 3

CDC Guidelines for the Prevention of Intravascular Catheter-Related Infections: https://www.cdc.gov/infectioncontrol/guidelines/BSI/index.html

Centers for Disease Control and Prevention (CDC) National Healthcare Safety Network (NHSN) Protocol

CMS: Hospital Acquired Conditions (HAC) List https://www.cms.gov/medicare/medicare-fee-for-service-payment/hospitalacqcond/icd10_hacs

Diagnoses

Diagnoses

Malnutrition

E40	**Kwashiorkor**	MCC
E41	**Nutritional marasmus**	MCC
E42	**Marasmic kwashiorkor**	MCC
E43	**Unspecified severe protein-calorie malnutrition**	MCC
E44.0	**Moderate protein-calorie malnutrition**	CC
E44.1	**Mild protein-calorie malnutrition**	CC
E46	**Unspecified protein-calorie malnutrition**	CC
K91.2	**Postsurgical malabsorption, not elsewhere classified**	CC
K94.23	**Gastrostomy malfunction**	CC HCC
Z68.1	**Body mass index [BMI] 19.9 or less, adult**	CC

Associated terminology: malnutrition, severe, moderate, mild; protein-calorie malnutrition; malnutrition following GI surgery; malnutrition due to gastrostomy mechanical complication

Discussion

Malnutrition, also known as undernutrition and protein-calorie malnutrition, is a nutritional insufficiency that is commonly due to inadequate dietary intake, a defect in the body's ability to absorb or use the food ingested, loss of nutrients, increase in nutritional needs or a disproportion of certain foods/nutrients. Associated risk factors for malnutrition include infancy/childhood, pregnancy/breastfeeding, old age, vegetarian diets, "fad" diets, use of certain pharmaceuticals, chronic disease, infection, alcohol/drug dependency, cerebrovascular accident with dysphagia, eating disorders, and obesity. This disease occurs in stages that develop over time, starting with low levels of nutrients within the blood and tissues, which then progressively change the intracellular structure and function. Once the cellular changes are drastic, clinical signs and symptoms appear. These signs and symptoms vary greatly and may affect multiple body systems as demonstrated in the table below.

Body System	Sign or Symptom
Generalized	Weight loss, fatigue, dizziness, ascites, lethargic, apathetic, cachexia
Oral	Swollen/bleeding gums, tooth decay, stomatitis, glossitis, parotic enlargement, mottled tooth enamel, delayed tooth eruption in children
Eye	Dry eyes, pale conjunctiva, periorbital edema
Musculoskeletal	Fragile bones, osteoporosis, muscle loss (especially in the buttocks and thighs), weakness
Neurological	Neurological slow reaction, dementia, memory loss, developmental delay, loss of knee and ankle reflexes
Cardiovascular	Tachycardia, bradycardia, hypotension, reduced cardiac output
Integumentary	Dry/cracked skin, poor wound healing, dull sparse brittle hair, hypopigmentation, alopecia, thin, soft nails, fissures or ridges in nails, pallor, petechiae
Hematological	Anemia
Electrolyte	Dehydration
Other systems	Renal impairment, decreased lung capacity, interstitial problems, stomach irregularities, abnormal menstrual cycles (female)

Protein calorie malnutrition is also classified by the extent it has progressed, from mild to severe. There are a variety of scoring methods to determine the severity. Mild nutrition is described as grade 1 and may have little, if any symptoms. Moderate malnutrition, also known as grade 2, involves further intracellular changes and, therefore, more intensified symptoms. In severe malnutrition, grade 3, the patient is clearly exhibiting symptoms. Severe malnutrition is further subdivided by the types of nutritional deficiency, such as kwashiorkor and marasmus. Marasmus is characterized by energy deficiency, peeling skin, and hair discoloration. It is caused by a lack of total nutrition in the diet. Kwashiorkor is a lack of protein in the diet and develops more physical and severe manifestations such as edema, distended abdomen, ulcerating dermatoses, hepatomegaly, marked hypoalbuminemia, anemia, lethargy, growth and development retardation, edema, changes in skin pigmentation, and hair loss or discoloration. Kwashiorkor is an extremely rare disorder in the United States and should, therefore, not be routinely reported. Marasmus is more common in the U.S. than kwashiorkor but usually only affects very young children.

Coding Tip

When a patient is admitted with malnutrition that progresses from one stage to another such as moderate present on admission (POA) and severe by discharge, report only the code that captures the highest level of severity.

The OIG Work Plan for Fiscal Year 2017 indicated that ongoing review was planned of Medicare payments made to hospitals for claims that include a diagnosis of kwashiorkor to determine whether the diagnosis is adequately supported by documentation in the medical record. A diagnosis of kwashiorkor on a claim substantially increases the hospitals' reimbursement from Medicare. Prior OIG reviews have identified inappropriate payments to hospitals for claims with a kwashiorkor diagnosis. For calendar years (CY) 2010 and 2011, Medicare paid hospitals $711 million for claims that included a diagnosis code for kwashiorkor. The OIG review of "Payments for Patients Diagnosed with Malnutrition" has been completed with a conclusion that kwashiorkor in the ICD-9 CM classification for malnutrition was inadequate. CMS concurred with recommendations that Medicare claims for kwashiorkor be reviewed and additional guidance be published.

The OIG updates its work plan website monthly to align with the work planning process and includes any new work plan items on the "Recently Added Items" page. Active items, including those underway or planned, are listed on the "Active Work Plan Items Page." Completed work plan items will be removed.

The OIG review of "Hospitals Billing for Severe Malnutrition on Medicare Claims" has been completed and is no longer included in the active work plan Items. The OIG determined after its review that providers were not complying with Medicare billing requirements when assigning the diagnosis codes for treating severe types of malnutrition on inpatient hospital claims.

The OIG in the cumulative report to CMS recommended that the agency review provider Medicare claims to ensure the diagnosis code for kwashiorkor is being used correctly by providers. This is because severe malnutrition—specifically codes E41 Nutritional marasmus, and E43 Unspecified severe protein-calorie malnutrition—are classified as MCCs, which can result in a higher payment. In written comments, CMS concurred with the recommendations and requested that the American Hospital Association publish additional coding guidance on the use of the kwashiorkor diagnosis code to address concerns that it was still being used incorrectly by some providers.

There are clinical guidelines that have been established to clinically validate mild to severe malnutrition. At least two of the following conditions should be present before considering reporting an ICD-10-CM code for undernutrition:

- Insufficient energy intake
- Weight loss
- Loss of muscle mass
- Loss of subcutaneous fat
- Localized/generalized fluid accumulation (edema)
- Diminished functional status (hand grip strength)

Note: In order to report kwashiorkor or marasmus, these conditions must be specifically documented and the more severe symptoms outlined earlier must be present in addition to those bulleted above.

Coding Tip

The code for kwashiorkor (E4Ø) is found in the Alphabetic Index under kwashiorkor and not under Malnutrition. Severe malnutrition with signs of kwashiorkor (and marasmus) (E42) is located under Malnutrition. Kwashiorkor (E4Ø) is very rare in the United States—this code should only be used in rare circumstances and only when specifically documented.

Documentation Tip

The use of the term kwashiorkor in the US should be carefully scrutinized for supporting clinical documentation with a query when it is in question.

Body mass index (BMI) should be assigned along with malnutrition codes. Body mass index for adults, subcategories Z68.1–Z68.4, covers persons age 20 years or older. Pediatric codes in subcategory Z58.5 is for persons age 2 to 19 years of age.

Documentation Tip

BMI can be reported based on documentation by clinicians, nurses, and dietitians who are not the patient's provider. However, the specific diagnosis of malnutrition and/or obesity must be based on physician or provider documentation.

The degree or severity of malnutrition (i.e., moderate, mild, severe) cannot be coded using documentation by dietician or other clinician. This information must be documented by the patient's provider (i.e., physician or other qualified healthcare practitioner legally accountable for establishing the patient's diagnosis).

Coding Tip

Documentation of emaciated or emaciation without documentation of malnutrition is not coded with a malnutrition code. Assign R64 Cachexia for emaciated, which is a descriptor referring to unusually thin or wasting.

Coding Tip

Wasting disease (syndrome) due to an underlying condition is reported with code E88.A. This code also represents cachexia due to an underlying condition. Wasting disease is seen in chronic illnesses, such as neoplastic disease and HIV. Code first the underlying condition when wasting disease is present. Code E88.A excludes the conditions of cachexia NOS (R64) and nutritional marasmus (E41).

Coding and Documentation Tip

The diagnosis of malnutrition cannot be reported based solely on clinical indicators. The provider must explicitly document the malnutrition. If clinical indicators are present with no diagnosis, query the provider.

Coding/Reporting Criteria	Clinical Criteria	
1. Physical Evaluation *(routine/expected in italics)*	• Weight loss (< 95% of normal body weight) • Loss of muscle mass • Loss of subcutaneous fat • Localized/generalized fluid accumulation (edema)	• Diminished functional status (hand grip strength) • Apathy • Weakness • Dizziness • BMI < 19.9
2. Clinical Evaluation *(routine/expected in italics)*	• Decreased albumin, prealbumin, total protein, total lymphocyte count, and/or A/G ratio	• Poor dietary intake with one of the following present: – tachyarrhythmia – renal dysfunction – dyspnea
3. Diagnostic Px *(routine/expected in italics)*	• Decreased mineralization in bone on radiological exam	• Swallow function study
4. Therapeutic Tx *(routine/expected in italics)*	• Total parenteral nutrition (TPN) • IV hydration with electrolytes • Caloric/nutrient supplements (Ensure) • Feeding tube	• Appetite stimulants • Gastrostomy placement • PICC placement
5. Increased Nursing Care and/or Monitoring	• IV nutrition • TPN	• IV hydration • Attention to gastrostomy
6. Extends LOS	• Discharge delayed due to malnutrition or procedure to evaluate or treat malnutrition	

Condition	Documentation Example	ICD-10-CM Corresponding Codes
Routine/Expected/ Integral/Inherent/ Incidental *(italics only)*	*NA*	*NA*
Principal Diagnosis	1. Progress Note: (symptom) (workup) due to/for (mild to severe) malnutrition. Orders: TPN, caloric supplements, gastrostomy placement Discharge Summary: Malnutrition requiring evaluation and treatment H&P: (mild to severe malnutrition); any signs/symptoms. **(Query mild, moderate, or severe.)**	1. Report appropriate code from E40–E46.
Comorbidity	1. Progress Note: (symptom) (work up) due to/for (mild to severe) malnutrition. Orders: TPN, caloric supplements Discharge Summary: (mild to severe) malnutrition requiring evaluation/treatment. **(Query mild, moderate, or severe.)**	1. Report appropriate code from E40–E46 Malnutrition.
Complication of Care	1. Admit Note: A 6-year-old patient admitted with severe malnutrition suspected secondary to caregiver neglect.	1. Report T76.02 Child neglect or abandonment, suspected, followed by E43 Unspecified severe protein-calorie malnutrition.
Poisoning or Adverse Effect of Medication/ Chemical	NA	NA

Additional References

AHA CC: 4Q, 2023, p. 14; 1Q, 2022, p. 13; 1Q, 2020, p. 4; 1Q, 2019, p. 26; 4Q, 2018, p. 77; 4Q, 2017, p. 108; 3Q, 2017, p. 24, 25; 1Q, 2017, p. 39

American Society for Parenteral and Enteral Nutrition (ASPEN) Malnutrition Criteria
https://www.nutritioncare.org/guidelines_and_clinical_resources/Malnutrition_Solution_Center/

Office of Inspector General Active Work Plan Items
https://oig.hhs.gov/reports-and-publications/workplan/active-item-table.asp

Diagnoses

Pleural Effusion

J9Ø	**Pleural effusion, not elsewhere classified**	CC
J91.Ø	**Malignant pleural effusion**	CC HCC
J91.8	**Pleural effusion in other conditions classified elsewhere**	CC
J94.Ø	**Chylous effusion**	CC
J95.88	**Other intraoperative complications of respiratory system, not elsewhere classified**	CC
J95.89	**Other postprocedural complications and disorders of respiratory system, not elsewhere classified**	CC

Associated terminology: malignant pleural effusion; influenza with pleural effusion; parapneumonic pleural effusion

Discussion

Pleural effusion is the abnormal collection of excess (greater than 20 mL) of pleural fluid, serous, blood, chyle or pus, between the two layers lining the pleural space of the lungs. When symptomatic, usually more than 300 mL of fluid is present, clinical signs are evident presenting as respiratory difficulties by limiting lung expansion during ventilation. Based on lab characteristics, pleural effusion can be classified one of two ways. As transudate, due to systemic conditions that alter the pleural pressure or permeability, or exudate, due to local conditions that cause inflammation, which affects permeability. Pleural effusions usually do not require workup or treatment when asymptomatic or with solely radiographic findings. It does, however, have clinical significance when symptomatic, requires workup, requires monitoring and/or treatment, and may be assigned as an additional code following the code for the etiology of the effusion when known.

Pleural effusion will be sequenced as a principal diagnosis when it is the reason for admission and no underlying condition is found.

The etiologies are many, but it is common to have pleural effusions for which a cause is not found, even after extensive workup.

Malignant pleural effusion, J91.Ø, stated as such, will be sequenced after the malignancy. When pleural effusion is present with a malignancy, but not confirmed or stated as "malignant," it will be reported as J9Ø Pleural effusion, not elsewhere classified. If a workup suggests or confirms it is a malignant pleural effusion related to the malignancy, query the provider for clarification between the clinical findings and diagnostic statement. It is important to note that malignant pleural effusion is not the same as pleural metastasis; malignant pleural effusion only indicates malignant cells in the pleural fluid. Fibrin loculations of pleural effusion can occur with malignancies.

Pleural effusion is integral to heart failure (HF) and, therefore, will typically not be reported. If the pleural effusion has demonstrated clinical significance by requiring monitoring or evaluation with additional x-rays or treatment by thoracentesis or chest tube, then it may be reported as a secondary diagnosis.

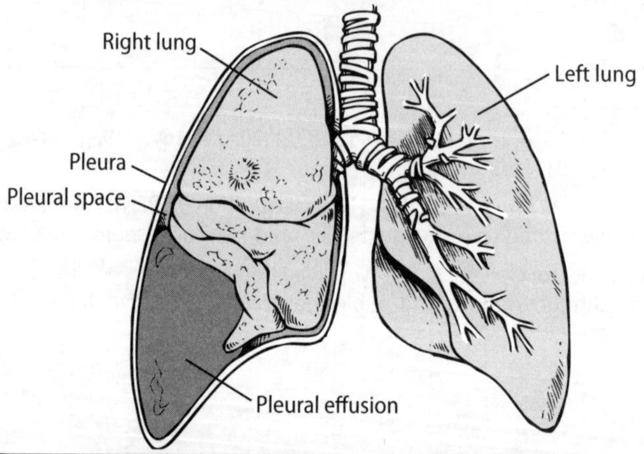

Excluded

- **Tuberculous pleural effusion, see code A15.6 Tuberculous pleurisy.**
- **Pleural effusion, tuberculosis, primary (progressive), see code A15.7 Primary respiratory tuberculosis.**
- **Pleural effusion, newborn, see code P28.89 Other specified respiratory conditions of newborn.**
- **Empyema (with or without fistula), see category J86 Pyothorax.**

Systemic lupus erythematosus (SLE) related pleural effusion will be reported as M32.13 Lung involvement in systemic lupus erythematosus, followed by J91.8 Pleural effusion in other conditions classified elsewhere, with documented clinical significance.

Documentation Tip

Complications of care: The condition must be more than a routinely expected condition or event. The documentation must support that the condition is clinically significant with an indication that it is a complication, by demonstrating:

- **A cause-and-effect relationship between the care or procedure and the condition**
- **That the condition resulted in altering the course of a procedure or surgery**

The term "complication" does not have to be explicitly documented.

Parapneumonic pleural effusion due to pneumonia will be reported by sequencing the pneumonia first, followed by J91.8 Pleural effusion in other conditions classified elsewhere, when it has documented clinical significance. If the associated pleural effusion is loculated, infected, or fibrinopurulent, query if this represents an empyema, represented by a code from the J86 Pyothorax, category, rather than pleural effusion.

Infected loculated pleural effusions are empyemas or pyothorax, see category J86 Pyothorax.

A chylous pleural effusion (J94.Ø) is effusion due to lymphatic fluid because of damage or obstruction to the thoracic duct or one of the main lymphatic vessels that drain it. Some causes of chylous effusion are chest trauma, complications of surgery, malignancy, and mediastinitis, among others.

Coding Tip

Principal diagnosis is that condition established after study to be chiefly responsible for occasioning the admission of the patient to the hospital for care.

The following are examples of the etiology of the two types of pleural effusion (not all inclusive):

- Transudate:
  - left ventricular failure (heart failure)
  - renal failure (hypoalbuminemia)
  - cirrhosis (liver failure) with ascites
  - hydronephrosis
  - constrictive pericarditis
  - atelectasis
  - peritoneal dialysis
- Exudate:
  - pneumonia (bacterial) (parapneumonic effusion)
  - neoplasm
  - pulmonary embolism
  - viral infection
  - postcoronary bypass surgery
  - insertion of central venous catheter (CVC) lines
  - systemic lupus erythematosus
  - sarcoidosis
  - pancreatitis
  - drugs
  - superior vena cava syndrome

Documentation Tip

Code assignment cannot be based on ancillary test results, therapies, or clinical criteria alone. A diagnosis and its clinical significance must be supported by physician or other qualified healthcare professional documentation. When it is unclear or there is contradictory information, query the physician or other qualified healthcare professional for clarification.

Coding/Reporting Criteria	Clinical Criteria	
1. Physical Evaluation *(routine/expected in italics)*	• *Asymptomatic* • Dyspnea • Pleuritic chest pain (inflammation of the parietal pleura) • Tactile fremitus (vibration felt while the patient is speaking with hand held against the chest) • Dullness to percussion over the fluid • Decreased breath sounds over the fluid • Decreased movement of the chest on the affected side	• Pleural friction rub • Bronchial breathing • Respiration rapid and shallow with large effusions • Tracheal deviation away from the effusion • Fever • Cough • Shortness of breath • Rales or crackles in lung base
2. Clinical Evaluation *(routine/expected in italics)*	• *Natriuretic peptide (NT-proBNP)* • Pleural fluid analysis • Fungal/gram stain • Culture	• Exudative: ≥ 1 of the following marked with – fluid lactic acid dehydrogenase (LDH) ≥ 2/3 upper limit of normal for serum LDH (or > 0.6) or > 200 IU – pleural fluid: serum total protein ratio ≥ 0.5 – pleural fluid: serum LDH ratio ≥ 0.6 – fluid total protein ≥ 3 g/dL – fluid cholesterol ≥ 43 mg/dL or ≥ 60 mg/dL – pleural fluid: serum cholesterol ratio ≥ 0.3 – serum protein-pleural fluid protein ≤ 3.1 g/dL – cloudy appearance – specific gravity > 1.020 • Cytology
3. Diagnostic Px *(routine/expected in italics)*	• *Chest x-ray: appears as white area on posteroanterior position* • Lateral decubitus x-rays are more sensitive when further workup or monitoring is needed • Blunted posterior costophrenic angles lateral upright on chest x-ray by 75mL of fluid; blunting of lateral angle by ~175 mL to 500 mL • Large effusions may cause mediastinal shift • Effusions > 4 – may cause complete opacification of hemithorax and mediastinal shift to the contralateral side	• Ultrasound • CT • Loculated effusions: fluid trapped by pleural adhesions or pulmonary fissures, typical of empyema or pyothorax • Bronchoscopy • Mediastinoscopy • Pleural biopsy • Thoracoscopy
4. Therapeutic Tx *(routine/expected in italics)*	• *Diuresis* • Thoracentesis: pleural fluid ≥ 10 mm thickness, > 1 cm on decubitus x-ray, or new, or uncertain etiology; in HF when chest pain, fever or when diuresis fails, or effusions ≥ 3 days • Anticoagulation for pulmonary embolism • Antibiotics for bacterial etiologies • Treatment for malignant pleural effusion	• Pain medication • Intercostal drain • Pleurodesis, surgical or chemical • Pleurectomy • Fibrinolysis of fibrin loculations • Saline injection for breaking up fibrin loculations • Lysis of loculation adhesions • Pleuroperitoneal shunt
5. Increased Nursing Care and/or Monitoring	• Increased monitoring of symptomatic pleural effusions	
6. Extends LOS	• Postsurgical pleural effusion	

Condition	Documentation Example	ICD-10-CM Corresponding Codes
Routine/Expected/ Integral/Inherent/ Incidental *(italics only)*	1. IP Discharge Summary: Acute decompensated HF with small pleural effusion on chest x-ray treated with diuretics. **(Query type of heart failure, systolic, diastolic, combined.)**	1. *Report I50.9 Heart failure, unspecified.*
Principal Diagnosis	1. IP Discharge Summary: First time large pleural effusion of undetermined etiology, thoracentesis analysis nonspecific; if it occurs again will plan pleural biopsy with thoracentesis.	1. Report J9Ø Pleural effusion, not elsewhere classified.
Comorbidity	1. IP Admit Note: Systemic lupus erythematosus (SLE) with symptomatic pleural effusion, schedule thoracentesis.	1. Report M32.13 Lung involvement in systemic lupus erythematosus, followed by J91.8 Pleural effusion in other conditions classified elsewhere.
Complication of Care	1. IP Discharge Summary: Patient admitted with large early pleural effusion related to coronary bypass surgery two weeks ago; thoracentesis performed for symptomatic relief.	1. Report J95.89 Other postprocedural complications and disorders of respiratory system, not elsewhere classified, followed by J9Ø Pleural effusion, not elsewhere classified.
Poisoning or Adverse Effect of Medication/ Chemical	1. Discharge Summary: Amiodarone-induced interstitial pneumonitis with large pleural effusion requiring thoracentesis.	1. Report J84.89 Other specified interstitial pulmonary diseases, followed by J9Ø Pleural effusion, and T46.2X5A Adverse effect of other antidysrhythmic drugs, initial encounter.

Diagnoses

Additional References

AHA CC: 2Q, 2024, p. 11; 3Q, 2022, p. 14; 2Q, 2015, p. 15

Poisoning and Toxic Effects of Illicit Drugs, Prescribed Drugs, Nonprescribed Drugs, Alcohol, Chemicals, and Other Substances

Diagnoses

T36-	**Poisoning by, adverse effect of and underdosing of systemic antibiotics**
T37-	**Poisoning by, adverse effect of and underdosing of other systemic anti-infectives and antiparasitics**
T38-	**Poisoning by, adverse effect of and underdosing of hormones and their synthetic substitutes and antagonists, not elsewhere classified**
T39-	**Poisoning by, adverse effect of and underdosing of nonopioid analgesics, antipyretics and antirheumatics**
T4Ø-	**Poisoning by, adverse effect of and underdosing of narcotics and psychodysleptics [hallucinogens]**
T41-	**Poisoning by, adverse effect of and underdosing of anesthetics and therapeutic gases**
T42-	**Poisoning by, adverse effect of and underdosing of antiepileptic, sedative-hypnotic and antiparkinsonism drugs**
T43-	**Poisoning by, adverse effect of and underdosing of psychotropic drugs, not elsewhere classified**
T44-	**Poisoning by, adverse effect of and underdosing of drugs primarily affecting the autonomic nervous system**
T45-	**Poisoning by, adverse effect of and underdosing of primarily systemic and hematological agents, not elsewhere classified**
T46-	**Poisoning by, adverse effect of and underdosing of agents primarily affecting the cardiovascular system**
T47-	**Poisoning by, adverse effect of and underdosing of agents primarily affecting the gastrointestinal system**
T48-	**Poisoning by, adverse effect of and underdosing of agents primarily acting on smooth and skeletal muscles and the respiratory system**
T49-	**Poisoning by, adverse effect of and underdosing of topical agents primarily affecting skin and mucous membrane and by ophthalmological, otorhinolaryngological and dental drugs**
T5Ø-	**Poisoning by, adverse effect of and underdosing of diuretics and other and unspecified drugs, medicaments and biological substances**
T51--T65-	**Toxic effects of substances chiefly nonmedicinal as to source**

Associated terminology: alcohol poisoning; drug overdose, toxicity of drug and alcohol; accidental overmedication; toxic interaction of prescribed medication with OTC medication; ecstasy overdose; huffing of Freon with toxicity; bath salts overdose; caffeine overdose with "sheets"

Note: Although the above-listed categories of codes include adverse effect and underdosing of drug, only the poisoning and toxic effects are discussed in this section. Only the codes in the categories above with a sixth character of 2, representing poisoning due to intentional self-harm, are considered HCCs.

Discussion

Drug poisoning, toxic effects of drugs, and the combining of drugs with nonmedicinal substances include errors in prescription/dosage, overdose, taking a nonprescribed drug with a correctly prescribed and properly administered drug, and interaction of drug and alcohol and abuse with intoxication of nonmedicinal substances.

Improper use of medication includes overdose or taking more than prescribed with resulting toxic effects, wrong substance given or taken in error, and wrong route of administration. When a nonprescribed drug is taken with a prescribed drug taken correctly and results in toxicity or other reaction from the interaction, this is reported as a poisoning. A reaction from the interaction of alcohol and any drug is also classified as a poisoning. Intoxication of an illicit drug with manifestations will be reported as a poisoning.

When reporting poisoning and toxic effects, the code from categories T36–T5Ø Poisoning by, adverse effects of and underdosing of drugs, medicaments and biological substances, and T51–T65 Toxic effects of substances chiefly nonmedicinal as to source, will be sequenced before the manifestations. Report a code for each drug or substance related to the poisoning. Code all manifestations documented, including coma, that are not integral to overdose or poisoning. Assign an additional code for drug dependence or abuse.

The intent of the overdose or toxicity should be documented. The intent will be identified by the fifth or sixth character as accidental, intentional, self-harm, assault, or undetermined. Undetermined intent is assigned when the documentation of the intent specifies that the intent cannot be determined. When the intent is unknown or unspecified, then it is coded as accidental by default.

When an overdose or toxicity is transferred to another hospital for transplant evaluation or procedure, if the toxicity is no longer present (i.e., its management is complete), and the sole reason for transfer is management of the organ failure or transplant evaluation, then report the organ failure as principal diagnosis for receiving hospital and the poisoning sequela code secondary (seventh character S). For example, end-stage kidney failure due to suicide attempt with acetaminophen overdose, report N18.6 End-stage renal disease, and T39.1X2S Poisoning by 4-aminophenol derivatives, intentional self-harm, sequela.

In the occasional unusual circumstance where multiple unknown drugs are suspected (for example, patient dies with no toxicology performed), a code from subcategory T5Ø.91- Poisoning by, adverse effect of and underdosing of multiple unspecified drugs, medicaments and biological substances, may be used.

Drug/Substance	ICD-10-CM Subcategory
Alcohol	T51.ØX
Crystal meth	T43.65
Ecstasy	T43.64
Ephedrine	T44.99
GHB	T43.8X
Ketamine	T41.29
2CB	T43.69
DXM	T48.3X
Caffeine	T43.61

Drug/Substance	ICD-10-CM Subcategory
Bath salts	T43.69
Dust Off	T53.5X
Spice	T4Ø.9Ø
K2	T4Ø.9Ø
Rohypnol	T42.4X
Crack cocaine	T4Ø.5X
Adderall	T43.62
Toluene solvent	T52.2X
Cannabis	T4Ø.711

Coding and Documentation Tip

A disorder of the respiratory or other systems that is documented as due to vaping is not captured in chapter 19, "Injury, Poisoning and Certain Other Consequences of External Causes." Chapter 22 contains codes for special purposes, provisional use, and emergency use. It currently holds codes for vaping-related disorder, COVID-19, and post-COVID-19 condition.

Respiratory illness or injury can be caused by harmful aerosolized substances and chemicals produced by electronic cigarettes, vapes, e-pipes, and other battery-powered vaping devices. Symptoms may include shortness of breath and fever, while some patients experience severe, sometimes fatal, lung damage.

Synonyms: e-cigarette and vaping product use-associated lung injury, EVALI

For patients admitted with conditions relating to vaping, such as acute respiratory failure, ARDS, or pneumonitis, code first UØ7.Ø Vaping related disorder, followed by any additional codes for manifestations. No additional code is needed for associated respiratory signs and symptoms such as cough or shortness of breath when a definitive diagnosis has been established. However, it is appropriate to code gastrointestinal symptoms such as diarrhea or abdominal pain separately.

Coding/Reporting Criteria	Clinical Criteria	
1. Physical Evaluation *(routine/expected in italics)*	• Symptoms vary depending on the substance and the amount taken • Delirium • Nausea/vomiting • Temperature: abnormal • Pulse rate: abnormal • Respiratory rate: abnormal • Blood pressure: abnormal • Sleepiness • Drowsiness • Confusion • Skin: cool/sweaty or warm/dry or bluish color • Dizziness • Lack of coordination/balance • Abdominal pain • Chest pain • Diarrhea • Disturbed vision	• Agitation • Abnormal pupil size • Nosebleed • Internal bleeding • Seizures • Tonic-clonic movements • Psychomotor retardation • Encephalopathy • Aspiration • Coma • Other organ effects: – respiratory failure – liver failure – kidney Failure – stroke – myocardial Infarction – cardiac arrest – ketamine associated ulcerative cystitis – anoxic brain damage
2. Clinical Evaluation *(routine/expected in italics)*	• Blood screen • Urine screen • Imbalance of pH: iron overdose	• Drug screen • Blood gases
3. Diagnostic Px *(routine/expected in italics)*	• Imaging: to evaluate manifestations	• ECG
4. Therapeutic Tx *(routine/expected in italics)*	• Gastric lavage • Activated charcoal • Narcan: IM or nasal spray • Intubation • Oxygen • Vent	• IV fluids • Dialysis • Antidote: Mucomyst (acetaminophen); Narcan (narcotics) • Chelation therapy: iron overdose
5. Increased Nursing Care and/or Monitoring	• Treatment of manifestations	
6. Extends LOS	• Drug overdose with acute kidney injury requiring dialysis	

Condition	Documentation Example	ICD-10-CM Corresponding Codes
Routine/Expected/ Integral/Inherent/ Incidental *(italics only)*	*NA*	*NA*
Principal Diagnosis	1. IP Discharge Summary: A 16-year-old male admitted with accidental "Spice" toxicity, intoxication with acute diffuse interstitial lung fibrosis, acute respiratory failure. When the pattern of substance use (dependence, abuse, or use) is not documented, query the physician for clarification.	1. Report T4Ø.711A Poisoning by cannabis, accidental (unintentional), initial encounter; J96.ØØ Acute respiratory failure, unspecified whether with hypoxia or hypercapnia; J68.3 Other acute and subacute respiratory conditions due to chemicals, gases, fumes and vapors. With no query or response, code F12.929 Cannabis use, unspecified with intoxication, unspecified.
Comorbidity	1. Progress Note: A 68-year-old female admitted with C3 displaced fracture w/o cord injury due to motor vehicle accident after taking prescribed Oxycontin with excessive alcohol, which caused transient LOC when driving.	1. Report S12.2ØØA Unspecified displaced fracture of third cervical vertebra, initial encounter for closed fracture, followed by T4Ø.2X1A Poisoning by other opioids, accidental (unintentional), initial encounter; T51.ØX1A Toxic effect of ethanol, accidental (unintentional), initial encounter; and R55 Syncope and collapse.
Complication of Care	1. IP History and Physical: Home health nurse mistakenly administered Risperdal to patient instead of Requip for Parkinson's; noticed increase in Parkinsonian tremors, with hypotension and bradycardia.	1. Report T43.591A Poisoning by other antipsychotics and neuroleptics, accidental unintentional, initial encounter, followed by I95.2 Hypotension due to drugs; RØØ.1 Bradycardia, unspecified; and G2Ø Parkinson's disease.
Poisoning or Adverse Effect of Medication/ Chemical	1. IP Discharge Summary: Suicide attempt by overdose of tricyclic antidepressant with seizure and sinus tachycardia.	1. Report T43.Ø12A Poisoning by tricyclic antidepressants, intentional self-harm, initial encounter, followed by R56.9 Unspecified convulsions; and RØØ.Ø Tachycardia, unspecified.

Additional References

AHA CC: 2Q, 2023, p. 10; 1Q, 2023, p. 39; 4Q, 2022, p. 23, 33, 45; 2Q, 2022, p. 10-11; 4Q, 2021, p. 30; 3Q, 2021, p. 8; 4Q, 2020, p. 40; 2Q, 2020, p. 24; 1Q, 2020, p. 8; 4Q, 2019, p. 17; 2Q, 2019, p. 24, 28; 1Q, 2019, p. 17, 20; 4Q, 2018, p. 30; 1Q, 2018, p. 4; 2Q, 2017, p.9; 1Q, 2017, p. 39-40; 4Q, 2016, p. 72; 2Q, 2016, p. 8; 1Q, 2016, p. 14-15; 1Q, 2015, p. 21; 4Q, 2014, p. 22; 4Q, 2013, p. 121; 2Q, 2013, p.34

Postoperative Anemia

D50.0	**Iron deficiency anemia secondary to blood loss (chronic)**	
D62	**Acute posthemorrhagic anemia**	CC
D64.9	**Anemia, unspecified**	

Associated terminology: anemia due to blood loss, postoperative/postprocedure, (acute) (posthemorrhagic); anemia, postoperative/postprocedure, not otherwise classified

Discussion

Anemia is a decrease in red blood cell volume, hemoglobin (Hgb or Hb) concentration, or hematocrit (Hct). Acute posthemorrhagic anemia develops several hours after acute blood loss. In order to determine when low hemoglobin/hematocrit (H/H) levels represent postoperative blood loss anemia, the pre-op baseline H/H level should be known or documentation should indicate relevant change. A 25 percent drop of hemoglobin from baseline is considered a safe allowable blood loss; therefore, a greater drop would be indicative of clinically significant blood loss anemia. Variables that influence the diagnosis of clinically significant anemia by H/H levels are age, sex, comorbidities, type of surgery, presence of dehydration or volume overload or hemodilution, repeated blood sampling, and hemorrhage volume.

Documentation Tip

When documentation and lab results or clinical criteria do not match, query the provider for clarification of the diagnosis.

It must be stressed:

- A diagnosis of anemia must be made by the provider in order to report the code.
- Lab values alone must not be used as a substitute for provider documentation to substantiate the code.
- Levels for H/H must be clinically indicative of anemia based on the clinical scenario.
- The anemia must be stated as being attributed to the surgery or other contributing factors (e.g., hemorrhagic condition that required the surgery), or both (code D62 includes acute posthemorrhagic, not necessarily just surgical blood loss).
- The surgery must involve hemorrhage, high estimated blood loss (EBL) or significant blood loss in order for anemia to be "due to surgery."
- A physician query must never be leading; it must identify all criteria, results and documentation on which it is based.

Many patients have preoperative low H/H levels or pre-op anemia. Patients at risk of anemia may decide to be treated preoperatively to lessen the consequences of surgery. Therefore, to determine if a diagnosis of anemia due to blood loss related to surgery is appropriate, many factors must be considered and documented. Whether transfusion is performed as treatment is not a deciding factor in whether the code should be assigned or not.

The code for anemia due to blood loss related to surgery, D62 Acute posthemorrhagic anemia, is not classified as a complication nor is it on the list of hospital acquired conditions (HAC). The code is a CC and, therefore, may impact MS-DRG assignment when reported as an additional diagnosis. Also, in order to report D62, the anemia must be stated as "due to blood loss." The term "acute" is a nonessential modifier in the alphabetic index for postoperative anemia due to blood loss; therefore, it is not absolutely necessary in the final diagnostic statement in order to assign D62. In contrast, posthemorrhagic must state "acute" in order to report D62. Anemia documented as due to surgery but not further specified is D64.9 and is neither a CC/MCC nor an HAC. In order to report either code as a consequence of surgery or procedure, the link must be made by the provider to the surgery/procedure as the cause of the anemia. If only the term "postoperative" is documented, it should be queried as to its meaning as either a link to the surgery or as a time frame.

Some factors to evaluate symptomatic or clinically significant blood loss anemia:

- Acute drop in hemoglobin to a level of 7–8 g/dL
- A greater than 25 percent drop of hemoglobin from baseline

- Levels lower than the lower limits of hemoglobin and hematocrit
  - women: Hb = 12.0 g/dL, Hct = 35%
  - men: Hb = 13.0 g/dL, Hct = 40%

If the amount of surgical blood loss is expected but the H/H level is consistent with anemia, and documentation states anemia and requires monitoring or extends length of stay (LOS), it can be reported with code D64.9 as the monitoring or extended LOS meeting the criteria as an additional diagnosis. Documentation should link to surgery, with the clinical significance indicated by requiring monitoring or extending LOS.

Documentation Tip

Code assignment cannot be based on ancillary test results, therapies, or clinical criteria alone. A diagnosis and its clinical significance must be supported by physician or other qualified healthcare professional documentation. When it is unclear or there is contradictory information, query the physician or other qualified healthcare professional for clarification.

According to the alphabetic index, documentation of low hemoglobin and low hematocrit can be reported with D64.9 Anemia, unspecified. Caution should be used if attempting to assign a diagnosis of anemia based solely on low H/H as these levels are relative. Query the provider if evidence of workup, monitoring, or treatment and clinical criteria/circumstances suggests a specific diagnosis along with its clinical significance.

Documentation Tip

The ↑, ↓ symbols do not indicate a diagnosis. Query the provider as to the meaning and if it represents a diagnosis, a sign of abnormal results, a condition or an indication of a change over past results, request that the information be fully stated, including the clinical significance.

Coding Tip

When both acute and chronic blood loss anemia are present, assign a code only for acute blood loss anemia.

Coding/Reporting Criteria	Clinical Criteria	
1. Physical Evaluation *(routine/expected in italics)*	• *Asymptomatic* • Paleness • Skin coldness • Faint/light headedness • Dizziness • Weakness • Sweating • Thirst	• Respirations > 20 • Weak pulse > 90 • Orthostatic hypotension • Diaphoresis • Shortness of breath • Chest pain • Shock
2. Clinical Evaluation *(routine/expected in italics)*	• *H/H levels due to expected blood loss without diagnosis of anemia not requiring monitoring* • Decreased hemoglobin concentration due to hypervolemia • H/H levels reflect effects of hemodilution • CBC	• Hemoglobin/hematocrit levels below baseline preprocedure – Hb < 8.0 g/dL (stable patient) Hb < 10.0 g/dL (decrease of 2+ g) (>65 year old, high risk) – Hct < 28 – or safe allowable blood loss: 25% of hemoglobin drop from baseline
3. Diagnostic Px *(routine/expected in italics)*	• If dramatic drop in H/H post-op, procedures may be performed to evaluate for acute hemorrhagic condition	

Coding/Reporting Criteria	Clinical Criteria	
4. Therapeutic Tx *(routine/expected in italics)*	• *No treatment* • IV fluids • Ferrous sulfate (iron), with or without erythropoietin • Ferrous gluconate • Transfusion: blood type and crossed – packed red blood cells (PRBC) – blood products (fresh frozen plasma [FFP]) • Blood volume loss – < 15%: not necessary unless pre-existing anemia – 15%–30%: treat with crystalloids/colloids in young/healthy patients or in pre-existing anemia/cardiopulmonary disease transfusion may be indicated – 30%–40%: requires rapid volume replacement; RBC transfusion probably needed – > 40%: life threatening; volume replacement with RBC transfusion required	• Hemoglobin concentration: – > 10 g/dL: transfusion rarely indicated – 6–10 g/dL: need for transfusion based on patient's risk of inadequate oxygenation from ongoing bleeding and/or high-risk factors. – < 6 g/dL: transfusion almost always indicated • Procedure to control postsurgical bleeding
5. Increased Nursing Care and/or Monitoring	Monitor anemia and treat per regimen	
6. Extends LOS	Discharge delayed due to surgical blood loss anemia	

Condition	Documentation Example	ICD-10-CM Corresponding Codes
Routine/Expected/ Integral/Inherent/ Incidental *(italics only)*	1. *IP Discharge Summary: A 35-year-old male, post left knee total arthroplasty, pre-op Hb 15.0 g/dL; -post-op Hb 11.95, asymptomatic*	1. *No code assigned.*
Principal Diagnosis	1. IP Admit Note: Patient readmitted due to symptomatic acute blood loss anemia posthysterectomy with intra-op bleed, which was controlled intra-op; treat with transfusion and monitor; patient had been discharged previously after refusing transfusion and insisting to be discharged on po iron medication.	1. Report D62 Acute posthemorrhagic anemia; Z90.710 Acquired absence of both cervix and uterus; Z91.19 Patient's noncompliance with other medical treatment and regimen.
Comorbidity	1. IP Consult: Post-op day two; anemia due to blood loss during CABG; transfuse. (This info is not included in the discharge summary.) **(Query the physician to include the information in the final diagnostic statement if they concur with the consultant's diagnosis.)** 2. IP Progress Note: Several notes indicate H/H levels postsurgery and po iron is given; review of the pre-op and post-op H/H levels suggest clinical criteria for anemia are met. **(Query: Due to the workup/monitoring, clinical criteria, clinical circumstances and treatment suggest a diagnosis with clinical significance to the encounter.)** 3. IP Progress Note: Anemia, post-op, transfuse. (Patient is s/p 360 spinal fusion.) **(Query if the clinical criteria and clinical circumstances suggest more specification; query if the type of anemia can be further specified.)**	1. Report D62 as an additional diagnosis. To preempt possible denial by external audit: diagnoses made within the record but not listed/included in the discharge summary, query the provider for concordance and inclusion into discharge summary. (Note: CMS reinforces that omission by provider of a consultants diagnosis is not a conflict, but denials may be attempted.) 2, 3. A query is appropriate when documentation describes workup, monitoring, clinical criteria, clinical circumstances, with or without treatment and is not linked to a specific condition, diagnosis or procedure but suggests clinical significance.
Complication of Care	NA	NA
Poisoning or Adverse Effect of Medication/ Chemical	NA	NA

Additional References

AHA CC: 1Q, 2023, p. 15-16; 3Q, 2019, p. 11, 17; 4Q, 2018, p. 88

Postoperative (Postprocedural) (Wound) Infection

J98.51	**Mediastinitis**	MCC HAC
O86.ØØ	**Infection of obstetric surgical wound, unspecified**	
O86.Ø1	**Infection of obstetric surgical wound, superficial incisional site**	
O86.Ø2	**Infection of obstetric surgical wound, deep incisional site**	
O86.Ø3	**Infection of obstetric surgical wound, organ and space site**	
O86.Ø4	**Sepsis following an obstetrical procedure**	MCC
O86.Ø9	**Infection of obstetric surgical wound, other surgical site**	
T81.4ØXA	**Infection following a procedure, unspecified, initial encounter**	CC HAC
T81.41XA	**Infection following a procedure, superficial incisional surgical site, initial encounter**	CC HAC
T81.42XA	**Infection following a procedure, deep incisional surgical site, initial encounter**	CC HAC
T81.43XA	**Infection following a procedure, organ and space surgical site, initial encounter**	CC HAC
T81.44XA	**Sepsis following a procedure, initial encounter**	CC HAC
T81.49XA	**Infection following a procedure, other surgical site, initial encounter**	CC HAC

Associated terminology: infection at surgical wound site; stitch abscess; mediastinitis as a complication of coronary artery bypass graft surgery

Discussion

Postoperative infections include surgical site infections (SSI), and systemic and distal site extensions due to surgery. Possible causes are poor preoperative preparation, wound contamination, poor antibiotic selection or coverage, and patient condition or comorbidities.

SSIs are classified by the tissue infected, either incisional or organ or space manipulated during an operation. SSIs of the incision can be described as either superficial, meaning involving skin and subcutaneous tissue, deep, which involves deep soft tissue, fascia, and muscle, or organ and space surgical site.

Documentation Tip

Complications of care: The condition must be more than a routinely expected condition or event. The documentation must support that the condition is clinically significant with an indication that it is a complication, by demonstrating:

- **A cause-and-effect relationship between the care or procedure and the condition**
- **That the condition resulted in altering the course of a procedure or surgery**

The term "complication" does not have to be explicitly documented.

When reporting a code from subcategory T81.4-, follow the tabular instruction note to use an additional code to identify the infection, which includes not only the organism B95-B97, but the specific manifestation, such as sepsis, peritonitis, epidural abscess, cellulitis, subphrenic abscess, etc. Identification of an organism must be based on provider documentation or confirmation and not on laboratory results only.

Coding Tip

For sepsis following a postprocedural wound (surgical site) infection, a code from T81.41 to T81.43 Infection following a procedure; T81.49 Infection following a procedure, other surgical site; or a code from O86.ØØ to O86.Ø3 Infection of obstetric surgical wound, or code O86.Ø9 Infection of obstetric surgical wound, other surgical site, that identifies the site of the infection should be sequenced first, if known. Assign an additional code for sepsis following a procedure (T81.44) or sepsis following an obstetrical procedure (O86.Ø4). Use an additional code to identify the infectious agent. If the patient has severe sepsis, the appropriate code from subcategory R65.2 should also be assigned with the additional code(s) for any acute organ dysfunction.

When an infection develops after surgery that involves insertion of an implanted device, prosthesis, or graft, and the infection is described as superficial, it may not be due to the implant. The correlation between the infection and the implant must be documented in order to assign a code from either category T81 Complications of procedures, not elsewhere classified, for a superficial wound infection or from categories T82–T85 Complications of prosthetic devices, implants and grafts, if the infection is due to and/or involving the implant.

Patient conditions that increase risk of infection that have an associated ICD-10-CM code should be reported, such as diabetes, long-term use of steroid medication, smoking, obesity, malnutrition, etc.

There is no time frame for postsurgical or postprocedure infections. Report the infection as a complication of surgery when identified as such, regardless of the remoteness of the procedure.

Coding Tip

Hospital-acquired condition (HAC): CMS does not allow a code to increase MS-DRG reimbursement by acting as a CC or MCC with a present on admission (POA) value of N or U. The case will be paid as though these conditions were not reported.

Coding Tip

Sepsis: *Suspected/presumptive/clinical/culture-negative:* Negative or inclusive blood cultures do not preclude a diagnosis of sepsis. The presence of one or more risk factors, the appropriate clinical presentation, and specific treatment in conjunction with physician confirmation validates the diagnosis. If the documentation is not clear, however, the physician should be queried.

Guideline I.C.1.d.1.i: "Negative or inconclusive blood cultures do not preclude a diagnosis of sepsis in patients with clinical evidence of the condition; however, the provider should be queried."

Coding/Reporting Criteria	Clinical Criteria	
1. Physical Evaluation *(routine/expected in italics)*	• Some symptoms will be specific to site • *Low-grade fever: 100 F first two days postsurgery* • Fever > 101 F lasting 48 or more hours post-op and/or with workup • Abnormal redness, warmth, or pain at surgical site • Abnormal drainage from wound	• Cellulitis or abscess at surgical wound site • Acute respiratory distress • Encephalopathy • Shock • Coma
2. Clinical Evaluation *(routine/expected in italics)*	• Workup due to symptoms: – cultures: blood, urine, wound, fluids • Leukocytosis	• Anemia or disseminated intravascular coagulation (DIC) • Hyperglycemia > 200 during first 48 hours following surgery as a reaction to infection
3. Diagnostic Px *(routine/expected in italics)*	• *Chest x-ray: routine follow up* • Chest x-ray: workup of symptoms	• Imaging: workup of symptoms • Re-opening of operative site or inspection
4. Therapeutic Tx *(routine/expected in italics)*	• *Antibiotics: prior to or ordered the day of surgery: prophylactic or empiric* • *Incentive spirometry: as routine post-op care* • *Patient mobilization: routine; as appropriate* • Begin/change in antibiotics to IV due to symptom(s) • Control of perioperative blood glucose levels • Use of perioperative supplemental oxygen	• Incision and drainage • Debridement • Excision • Resection • Bypass • Destruction • Drainage
5. Increased Nursing Care and/or Monitoring	• Post-op wet and dry dressings for debridement of wound infection	
6. Extends LOS	• Discharge cancelled due to sepsis due to subphrenic abscess	

Condition	Documentation Example	ICD-10-CM Corresponding Codes
Routine/Expected/ Integral/Inherent/ Incidental *(italics only)*	1. *IP Progress Note: Surgical incision site with erythema, watch for signs of infection.*	1. *No code assigned.*
Principal Diagnosis	1. IP Admit Note: Admitted due to subphrenic abscess related to laparoscopic cholecystectomy.	1. Report T81.43XA Infection following a procedure, organ and space surgical site, initial encounter for the subphrenic abscess which is in the organ space between the diaphragm, liver and spleen, followed by K65.1 Peritoneal abscess, and Z90.49 Acquired absence of other specified parts of digestive tract.
Comorbidity	1. IP Progress Note: Abdominal wall suture site with cellulitis and drainage; sutures removed; incision and drainage performed at bedside.	1. Report T81.41XA Infection following a procedure, superficial incisional surgical site, initial encounter followed by L03.311 Cellulitis of abdominal wall.
Complication of Care	1. IP Discharge Summary: Postlumbar discectomy one month ago, now with psoas muscle abscess at surgical site.	1. Report T81.42XA Infection following a procedure, deep incisional surgical site, initial encounter for the infection into the muscle followed by K68.12 Psoas muscle abscess.
Poisoning or Adverse Effect of Medication/ Chemical	NA	NA

Additional References

AHA CC: 1Q, 2024, p. 19; 2Q, 2020, p.32; 2Q, 2019, p. 39; 4Q, 2018, p. 33, 57; 4Q, 2016, p. 29; 1Q, 2014, p. 23

CMS: Hospital Acquired Conditions (HAC) List
https://www.cms.gov/medicare/medicare-fee-for-service-payment/hospitalacqcond/icd10_hacs

Diagnoses

Pressure Ulcer

L89- with a sixth character of Ø Pressure ulcer, unstageable HCC

L89- with a sixth character of 1 Pressure ulcer, stage 1

L89- with a sixth character of 2 Pressure ulcer, stage 2 HCC

L89- with a sixth character of 3 Pressure ulcer, stage 3 MCC HAC HCC

L89- with a sixth character of 4 Pressure ulcer, stage 4 MCC HAC HCC

L89- with a sixth character of 6 Pressure-induced deep tissue damage

L89- with a sixth character of 9 Pressure ulcer, unspecified stage

Associated terminology: pressure ulcer progressed to stage 3 to 4 by discharge; decubitus ulcer, unspecified stage; deep tissue wound, non-traumatic (meaning pressure ulcer); bed sore; plaster sore; pressure area; healing pressure ulcer; deep tissue injury

Discussion

Pressure ulcers, also known as decubitus ulcers, are areas of nontraumatic tissue wounds due to pressure alone or in conjunction with friction, shearing, or moisture. Areas most prone to formation of pressure ulcers are those in which promontory bone and external surfaces meet causing compression of the tissue over the bone, resulting in ischemia. Factors, such as age, poor vasculature, neuropathy, immobilization, poor nutrition, poor hygiene, sweating, and incontinence place patients at risk for developing these wounds.

Prevention is key; best practices include procedures and techniques used for at-risk patients. Risk factors that have an ICD-10-CM code should be reported. Treatment follows an integrated systemic approach from focused wound care to nutrition therapy.

Healing consists of granulation tissue filling the defect before re-epithelialization. Healing does not affect stage: it is described in terms of the original stage or depth. Documentation should include progress and efficacy of treatment by describing the characteristics of the wound (color, size, depth, amount of necrotic tissue, amount of exudate, tracking, undermining, odor, and presence of infection), and the site of the wound. It is important to note that an ulcer with an intact eschar is considered unstageable.

Nontraumatic deep tissue injury or ulcer is an area of discoloration, blister, or dark wound bed due to damaged underlying soft tissue. When this documentation is present and not further clarified, query the physician regarding the nature and cause of the wound, whether pressure, cancer, venous stasis, venous insufficiency, etc.

Pressure ulcer stages:

- Stage 1: Intact defined area of skin, persistent nonblanchable focal erythema or discoloration, as compared to adjacent tissue there are changes in temperature (warmer/cooler), tissue consistency (firmer/softer), sensory changes (pain/itching) or more tender, edema, induration; actual ulcer is not present but conditions favor its development
- Stage 2: Partial thickness tissue loss including epidermis or dermis or both, superficial ulcer (abrasion, blister, shallow [dry] crater)
- Stage 3: Full-thickness skin loss extending through and including subcutaneous tissue but not fascia, deep crater ulcer; depth varies by anatomical site
- Stage 4: Necrosis of full-thickness soft tissue loss down through to underlying muscle and including bone or cartilage
- Unstageable: Ulcer with intact eschar is unstageable; depth is obscured by slough and stage cannot be determined until removed; or deep tissue injury (nontraumatic)

Four Stages of Pressure Ulcer

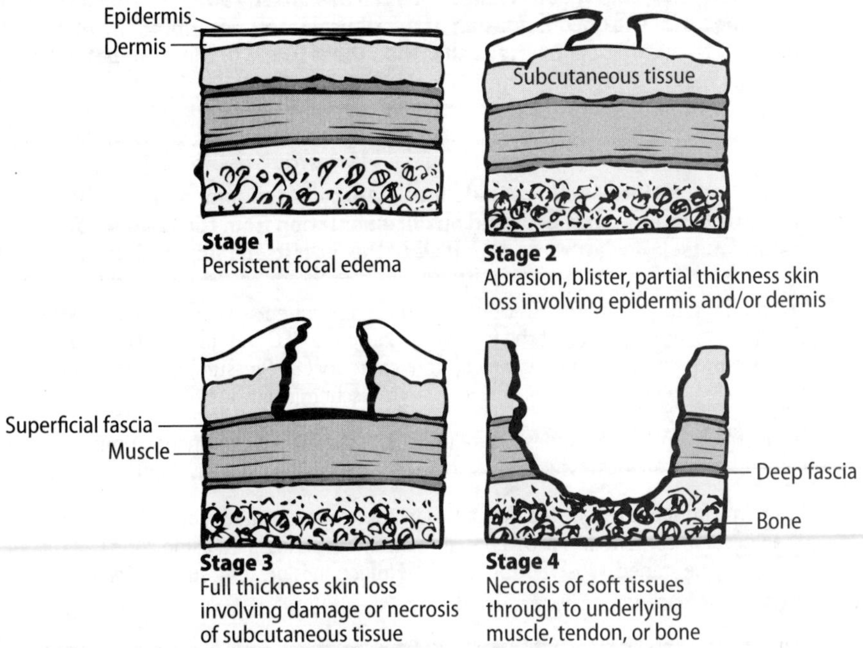

When pressure-induced deep tissue injury (DTPI) is documented, report the appropriate code from category L89 with specific site and sixth character 6. No stage is required for pressure-induced deep tissue damage or deep tissue pressure injury (DTPI) which is defined by the National Pressure Injury Advisory Panel (NPIAP) as "intact or non-intact skin with localized area of persistent non-blanchable deep red, maroon, purple discoloration or epidermal separation revealing a dark wound bed or blood filled blister. Pain and temperature change often precede skin color changes. Discoloration may appear differently in darkly pigmented skin. This condition results from intense and/or prolonged pressure and shear forces at the bone-muscle interface. The wound may evolve rapidly to reveal the actual extent of tissue injury, or may resolve without tissue loss."

Documentation Tip

It may be difficult to discern whether pressure ulcer (which needs a stage) or pressure-Induced tissue damage/injury is present (which needs no stage). A query may be necessary to clarify. Additionally, if tissue injury is documented, clarify whether it is a traumatic or nontraumatic (pressure) injury.

Pressure ulcers documented as healed are not reported. If an admission is for pressure ulcer treatment, which is found to be healed, assign a code from category Z09 Encounter for follow-up examination after completed treatment for conditions other than malignant neoplasm, with history code, Z87.2 Personal history of disease of the skin and subcutaneous tissue. If an ulcer is present on admission but healed at the time of discharge, assign the code for the site and stage of the pressure ulcer at the time of admission. If a patient has an unstageable pressure ulcer, but during the encounter a debridement procedure reveals the stage of the ulcer, assign only the code for the stage of the ulcer discovered after the debridement. If a patient is admitted with a pressure ulcer that evolves from one stage to another stage, two separate codes should be assigned: one code for the site and stage of the ulcer on admission and a second code for the same ulcer site and the highest stage reported during the stay. Facilities should have a written guide for coders on reporting or querying for pressure ulcer staging when vague documentation is present such as "stage 2 or 3" or "stage 3–4," defining if the facility policy is to query, report the lower stage, or report the higher stage.

Coding and Documentation Tip

Codes for unstageable pressure ulcer (L89.--Ø) should be based on the clinical documentation and should be used only for pressure ulcers whose stage cannot be clinically determined (e.g., the ulcer is covered by eschar or has been treated with a skin or muscle graft). These codes should not be confused with the codes for unspecified stage (L89.--9). When there is no documentation regarding the stage of the pressure ulcer, assign the appropriate code for unspecified stage (L89.-- 9). See guideline I.C.12.a.2.

Diagnoses

Coding Tip

Assignment of pressure ulcer stage code can be made by either the documentation of the stage, such as stage 1 or stage 2, or the documentation of the clinical terms describing the ulcer that are found in the alphabetic index. If terms are documented other than those found in the alphabetic index, then the provider should be queried for clarification.

Documentation Tip

According to Official Coding Guideline I.B.14, code assignment for pressure ulcer stage and depth of chronic non-pressure ulcer may be based on documentation from clinicians who are not the patient's provider (e.g., wound nurse). However, the diagnosis of the ulcer itself must be documented by the patient's provider.

When gangrene or gangrenous cellulitis is present, sequence a code from category I96 Gangrene, not elsewhere classified, to represent any of the following: gangrene NEC, gangrenous cellulitis, or skin/subcutaneous necrosis, before a code representing the pressure ulcer from category L89 Pressure ulcer. Note that gas gangrene is excluded from category I96, which represents only wet, dry, or ischemic gangrene.

The instruction of the Excludes 2 note under L89 indicates that skin infections in categories LØØ to LØ8 Infections of the skin and subcutaneous tissue, may also be reported when clinically confirmed (or suspected) and documented.

Note: Incontinence associated dermatitis in adults, also termed diaper dermatitis, can be confused with pressure ulcer. It can occur in conjunction with a pressure ulcer, but is classified using code L22 Diaper dermatitis, and the dermatitis should not be staged. When a superimposed infection is present, such as *Candida*, it should be reported as an additional code.

Documentation Tip

Hospital-acquired condition (HAC): CMS does not allow a code to increase MS-DRG reimbursement by acting as a CC or MCC with a present on admission (POA) value of N or U. The case will be paid as though these conditions were not reported. Therefore, it is important to identify in documentation whether the ulcer was actually present on admission. (POA – Y)

Documentation Tip

When the term Kennedy ulcer is used, it is necessary to obtain documentation of the stage of this pressure ulcer. Kennedy terminal ulcers occur in terminal patients and evolve quickly from multi-organ failure.

Coding/Reporting Criteria	Clinical Criteria	
1. Physical Evaluation *(routine/expected in italics)*	• Stage 1: Intact defined area of skin, persistent nonblanchable focal erythema or discoloration, as compared to adjacent tissue there are changes in temperature (warmer/cooler), tissue consistency(firmer/softer), sensory changes(pain/itching) or more tender, edema, induration; actual ulcer is not present but conditions favor its development • Stage 2: Partial thickness tissue loss including epidermis or dermis or both, superficial ulcer (abrasion, blister, shallow (dry) crater) • Stage 3: Full-thickness skin loss extending through and including subcutaneous tissue but not fascia, deep crater ulcer; depth varies by anatomical site	• Stage 4: Necrosis of full-thickness soft tissue loss down through to underlying muscle and including bone or cartilage • Unstageable: Ulcer with intact eschar is unstageable; depth is obscured by slough and stage cannot be determined until removed • Pressure-induced deep tissue injury/damage: Intact or nonintact skin with localized area of persistent nonblanchable deep red, maroon, purple discoloration or epidermal separation revealing a dark wound bed or blood filled blister often preceded by pain and temperature change.
2. Clinical Evaluation *(routine/expected in italics)*	• Wound culture: not routinely, as needed for superimposed infection	• Blood culture • Nutritional workup
3. Diagnostic Px *(routine/expected in italics)*	• Bone biopsy/culture, when possible, if osteomyelitis is suspected • MRI	

Coding/Reporting Criteria	Clinical Criteria	
4. Therapeutic Tx *(routine/expected in italics)*	• Pressure reduction or repositioning • Direct ulcer care or wound care • Pain management • Antibiotics or antifungals • Surgery: grafts • Debridements: mechanical and excisional	• Adjunctive therapy: negative-pressure therapy, topical recombinant growth factors, electrical stimulation therapy, therapeutic ultrasonography, electrical magnetic, heat, massage, and hyperbaric oxygen therapies • Nutrition therapy
5. Increased Nursing Care and/or Monitoring	• Continued wound care	
6. Extends LOS	• Pressure ulcer develops postadmit	

Diagnoses

Condition	Documentation Example	ICD-10-CM Corresponding Codes
Routine/Expected/ Integral/Inherent/ Incidental *(italics only)*	*NA*	*NA*
Principal Diagnosis	1. IP Discharge Summary: Infected stage 3 sacral pressure ulcer with methicillin susceptible *Staphylococcus aureus*	1. Report L89.153 Pressure ulcer of sacral region stage 3, followed by B95.61 Methicillin susceptible Staphylococcus aureus infection as the cause of diseases classified elsewhere.
Comorbidity	1. IP Admit Note: Admitted with stage 4 right heel decubitus ulcer with gangrene. 2. IP H&P: no documentation of pressure ulcer; DC summary 3 days later, stage 3 pressure ulcer of right ankle. Review chart to confirm whether pressure ulcer was present on admission. Nursing notes may provide this information. Query should be generated to provider to confirm whether pressure ulcer was actually present on admission and if so, if it was a stage 3 or evolved from another stage to stage 3.	1. Report I96 Gangrene, not elsewhere classified, followed by L89.614 Pressure ulcer of right heel stage 4. 2. Code L89.513 Pressure ulcer of right ankle, stage 3 is reported for the pressure ulcer with a POA of N for current documentation. If it was not POA, although a stage 3 ulcer is an MCC, no reimbursement will be made as it will be considered a hospital acquired condition. If query response indicated that the ulcer evolved, code both the admission stage and highest stage during stay. If it was amended to stage 3 on admission, use Y for POA indicator with code L89.513. If provider confirms the ulcer, notes from other clinicians may be used for staging.
Complication of Care	1. IP Admit Note: Admitted from personal care home with unstageable coccyx decubiti, debridement procedure performed revealing stage 2; physical neglect by staff with poor personal hygiene due to functional quadriplegia with severe dementia.	1. Report T74.Ø1XA Adult neglect or abandonment confirmed, initial encounter, followed by L89.152 Pressure ulcer of sacral region, stage 2; R53.2 Functional quadriplegia; and FØ3.CØ Unspecified dementia, severe, without behavioral disturbance, psychotic disturbance, mood disturbance, and anxiety.
Poisoning or Adverse Effect of Medication/ Chemical	NA	NA

Additional References

AHA CC: 2Q, 2022, p. 8; 3Q, 2021, p. 10; 1Q, 2021, p. 24; 4Q, 2019, p. 10, 52; 4Q, 2018, p. 57; 3Q, 2018, p. 3; 2Q, 2018, p. 21; 4Q, 2017, p. 109; 4Q, 2016, p. 118, 142

CMS: Hospital Acquired Conditions (HAC) List
https://www.cms.gov/medicare/medicare-fee-for-service-payment/hospitalacqcond/icd10_hacs

Pulmonary and Respiratory Insufficiency or Distress

J8Ø	**Acute respiratory distress syndrome**	MCC HCC
J95.1	**Acute pulmonary insufficiency following thoracic surgery**	MCC
J95.2	**Acute pulmonary insufficiency following nonthoracic surgery**	MCC
J95.3	**Chronic pulmonary insufficiency following surgery**	MCC
J98.4	**Other disorders of lung**	
RØ6.ØØ	**Dyspnea, unspecified**	
RØ6.Ø3	**Acute respiratory distress**	
RØ6.89	**Other abnormalities of breathing**	

Associated terminology: acute respiratory distress syndrome (ARDS); acute pulmonary insufficiency following surgery; pulmonary insufficiency following trauma; pulmonary insufficiency following shock; respiratory insufficiency; respiratory distress; adult respiratory distress

Discussion

Respiratory insufficiency and respiratory distress are chapter 18 codes for signs and symptoms. Respiratory insufficiency is reported using code RØ6.89 Other abnormalities of breathing, and respiratory distress is reported with RØ6.Ø3 Acute respiratory distress, which also includes respiratory distress not documented as "acute." This difficulty in breathing can be associated with underlying conditions, such as chronic obstructive pulmonary disease or asthma, and is not reportable as an integral sign or symptom of these conditions. Respiratory insufficiency or distress is also not reported when it is within limits of an expected outcome following surgery or certain procedures, including extubation. These signs or symptom codes will not be reported when they are related or integral to an established definitive diagnosis and when they are an expected outcome, or without clinical significance. These codes would be reported only when they are the sign or symptom for which a workup is performed or treatment rendered for, and no definitive diagnosis is established at discharge. Documentation of "postoperative respiratory insufficiency," meaning the patient is being routinely weaned for postsurgical extubation or is given routine incentive spirometry, will not be reported as it does not clinically meet criteria as a reportable diagnosis. Neither does it get reported as a complication as these are both expected and routine therapies for a postoperative patient.

Acute respiratory distress syndrome (ARDS) represents severe hypoxia with pulmonary edema due to acute lung injury (ALI) due to trauma or illness and is a clinically significant critical condition. ARDS includes pulmonary edema and acute hypoxemic respiratory failure. ARDS is a diagnosis of exclusion; workup should rule out other etiologies of the presentation.

Coding Tip

Acute respiratory distress, reported with code RØ6.Ø3 Acute respiratory distress, is distinctly separate from the more life-threatening condition referred to as acute respiratory distress syndrome (ARDS), reported with J8Ø. Hypoxemia, dyspnea, and fluid buildup associated with ARDS cause dangerously low levels of oxygen in the blood, threatening organ function, while respiratory distress (acute) is not associated with inadequate oxygen supply but refers only to breathing difficulty.

Documentation Tip

When the phrase respiratory distress is documented on the medical record of a critically ill patient or those with acute lung injury (ALI), review the chart for signs of severe hypoxia, and/or pulmonary edema, and clarify whether acute respiratory distress syndrome (ARDS) may be applicable.

Note: ICD-10-CM no longer classifies ARDS and acute respiratory failure following trauma and surgery in the same category. Also, acute respiratory failure due to trauma no longer has a separate code. Category J96 Respiratory failure, not elsewhere classified, has an Excludes 1 note for ARDS. Therefore when both acute respiratory failure and ARDS is documented, only code J8Ø Acute respiratory distress syndrome, is reported.

Coding Tip

Code J8Ø Acute respiratory distress syndrome, is assigned for acute respiratory failure that is present on admission but progresses to ARDS after admission. According to the Excludes 1 note under category J96, only code J8Ø should be assigned when both respiratory failure and ARDS are documented to capture the highest level of severity with a POA indicator of Y for code J8Ø, since the patient experienced worsening respiratory status, progressing to ARDS, a life-threatening form of respiratory failure.

Acute respiratory distress does not have an index entry for "impending" or "threatened." Therefore, when documented as such, follow official coding guideline I.B.11. If it occurs, the appropriate code is reported; if it does not occur, report the existing underlying condition.

Coding Tip

Guideline I.B.11 provides instruction for impending or threatened diagnosis as follows:

- **If it did occur, code as confirmed diagnosis.**
- **If it did not occur reference the Alphabetic Index to determine if the condition has a subentry for "impending" or "threatened" and also reference main term entries for impending and for threatened.**
- **If the subterms are listed, assign the given code.**
- **If the subterms are not listed, code the existing underlying condition(s) and not the condition described as impending or threatened.**

Excluded

Respiratory distress (syndrome) of newborn, see category P22.

Coding Tip

When acute respiratory distress syndrome (ARDS) occurs as a result of vaping, code first UØ7.Ø Vaping related disorder, followed by J8Ø Acute respiratory distress syndrome. When a patient is admitted with ARDS and COVID-19, UØ7.1 COVID-19, is the principal diagnosis, followed by J8Ø Acute respiratory distress syndrome.

Coding/Reporting Criteria	Clinical Criteria	
1. Physical Evaluation *(routine/expected in italics)*	• *Expected respiratory insufficiency postsurgery or postextubation* • Labored breathing • Dyspnea/shortness of breath • Tachypnea: increased breathing rate • Cyanosis • Grunting • Nose flaring • Retractions	• Sweating • Cool or clammy skin • Wheezing • Tachycardia • Peripheral vasoconstriction • Agitation • Confusion • Hypotension • Fatigue
2. Clinical Evaluation *(routine/expected in italics)*	• Arterial blood gas: fall in arterial oxygen pressure; increase of CO_2 pressure • Blood tests • Sputum cultures	• Hypoxemia: $PaO_2/FIO_2 \leq 300$ (ALI) or ≤ 200 (ARDS) • Absence of left atrial hypertension (PAOP ≤ 18 mmHg) or no clinical evidence of left atrial hypertension
3. Diagnostic Px *(routine/expected in italics)*	• Chest x-ray: diffuse bilateral infiltrates • CT scan • Bronchoscopy	• Pulmonary function test • Ventilation perfusion lung (V/Q) scan
4. Therapeutic Tx *(routine/expected in italics)*	• *Vent support for expected respiratory insufficiency postsurgery* • Positive end-expiratory pressure ventilation (PEEP) • Continuous positive airway pressure (CPAP), bilevel positive airway pressure (BiPAP)	• Intubation with mechanical ventilation • Supplemental oxygen • Spirometry: beyond routine • Bag-valve-mask ventilation • Treatment includes treatment of underlying cause
5. Increased Nursing Care and/or Monitoring	• Acute respiratory distress occurs post admission	
6. Extends LOS	• Postponed discharge due to acute respiratory distress postoperatively as a complication of care	

Condition	Documentation Example	ICD-10-CM Corresponding Codes
Routine/Expected/ Integral/Inherent/ Incidental *(italics only)*	1. *IP Progress Note: Post-extubation to determine respiratory insufficiency.* **(Query to determine if this represents a complication due to surgery, due to other condition or is it at an expected outcome postextubation.)**	1. *Query response will determine if it is a complication due to surgery, due to other condition or an expected outcome.*
Principal Diagnosis	1. IP Discharge Summary: Near drowning with ARDS from accidental fall into pool; requiring intubation/vent for 48 hours.	1. Report J8Ø Acute respiratory distress syndrome, followed by W16.Ø11A Fall into swimming pool striking water surface causing drowning and submersion, initial encounter.
Comorbidity	1. IP Progress Note: Acute respiratory distress due to right lung contusion in motor vehicle accident. 2. IP Progress Note: Dyspnea, due to impending pulmonary distress or exacerbation of chronic obstruction pulmonary disease (COPD); following note the next day states dyspnea resolved with bronchodilator, COPD stable.	1. Report code S27.321A Contusion of lung, unilateral, initial encounter, followed by RØ6.Ø3 Acute respiratory distress. 2. Report RØ6.ØØ Dyspnea, unspecified, followed by J44.9 Chronic obstruction pulmonary disease, unspecified.
Complication of Care	1. IP Progress Note: Acute pulmonary insufficiency as a result of nonthoracic surgery; place patient on CPAP and monitor.	1. Report J95.2 Acute pulmonary insufficiency following nonthoracic surgery.
Poisoning or Adverse Effect of Medication/ Chemical	NA	NA

Additional References

AHA CC: 2Q, 2024, p. 20; 2Q, 2021, p. 23; 1Q, 2021, p. 25; 4Q, 2020, p. 80, 96; 1Q, 2020, p. 34; 4Q, 2017, p. 23, 97; 1Q, 2017, p. 26

Respiratory Failure

J95.821	**Acute postprocedural respiratory failure**	MCC
J95.822	**Acute and chronic postprocedural respiratory failure**	MCC
J96.00	**Acute respiratory failure, unspecified whether with hypoxia or hypercapnia**	MCC HCC
J96.01	**Acute respiratory failure with hypoxia**	MCC HCC
J96.02	**Acute respiratory failure with hypercapnia**	MCC HCC
J96.10	**Chronic respiratory failure, unspecified whether with hypoxia or hypercapnia**	CC HCC
J96.11	**Chronic respiratory failure with hypoxia**	CC HCC
J96.12	**Chronic respiratory failure with hypercapnia**	CC HCC
J96.20	**Acute and chronic respiratory failure, unspecified whether with hypoxia or hypercapnia**	MCC HCC
J96.21	**Acute and chronic respiratory failure with hypoxia**	MCC HCC
J96.22	**Acute and chronic respiratory failure with hypercapnia**	MCC HCC
J96.90	**Respiratory failure, unspecified, unspecified whether with hypoxia or hypercapnia**	MCC HCC
J96.91	**Respiratory failure, unspecified with hypoxia**	MCC HCC
J96.92	**Respiratory failure, unspecified with hypercapnia**	MCC HCC

Associated terminology: respiratory failure; acute and/or chronic; with or unspecified hypoxia or hypercapnia; postprocedural

Discussion

Respiratory failure occurs when there is an inadequate gas exchange of O_2 intake and CO_2 elimination in the lungs, which results in the inability to maintain arterial oxygen and/or carbon dioxide levels within their normal ranges, leading to hypoxemia, with or without hypercapnia. It is life threatening and always due to another condition. Treatment is directed towards both the respiratory failure and the underlying cause, when identified. Acute respiratory failure develops over minutes to hours as evidenced by a pH less than 7.30 (acidemia). Chronic respiratory failure develops over days or longer, which allows for renal compensation with an increase in bicarbonate concentration with only a slight decrease in pH level.

Respiratory failure is assigned as principal diagnosis when it is determined to be the reason for admission or when the circumstances of the admission allow it to be sequenced before another acute condition according to official guidelines. It may also be sequenced first when it equally meets the definition of principal diagnosis as another acute condition and sequencing is optional. When it is the manifestation or nature of a drug adverse effect, it is sequenced before the code for the adverse effect of the drug.

Respiratory failure is a comorbidity/secondary diagnosis when it develops after admission or when a chapter-specific guideline takes precedence (e.g., obstetrics, poisoning, HIV, newborn/sepsis). For example, when it is a manifestation of a poisoning/overdose, then it is sequenced after the poisoning code. It may be sequenced as an additional code when it equally meets the definition of principal diagnosis as another acute condition and sequencing is optional.

Coding Tip

Code J80 Acute respiratory distress syndrome, is assigned for acute respiratory failure that is present on admission but progresses to ARDS after admission. According to the Excludes 1 note under category J96, only code J80 should be assigned when both respiratory failure and ARDS are documented to capture the highest level of severity with a POA indicator of Y for code J80, since the patient experienced worsening respiratory status, progressing to ARDS, a life-threatening form of respiratory failure.

Coding Tip

When acute respiratory failure occurs as a result of vaping, code first U07.0 Vaping related disorder, followed by a code in subcategory J96.0- Acute respiratory failure. When a patient is admitted with acute respiratory failure and COVID-19, U07.1 COVID-19, is the principal diagnosis, followed by the appropriate code from subcategory J96.0.

As a complication, respiratory failure is assigned when documented as "due to" or a "complication of" a procedure or surgery.

Long-term care hospital (LTCH) issue: when a patient is transferred to an LTCH for continued treatment of respiratory failure and it is not clear whether the respiratory failure is current, query if the patient is still in respiratory failure or if the treatment is for the underlying condition, and if it is current. If current, query also for acute/chronic and with or without hypercapnia. If the patient is admitted for vent weaning and respiratory failure is no longer a current diagnosis, assign Z99.11 Dependence on respirator [ventilator] status, for weaning.

The following are the different types of respiratory failure:

- Type I or hypoxic without hypercapnia (oxygenation failure)
  - most common form: usually acute, rarely chronic
  - airspace flooding
  - due to V/Q mismatch: parenchymal disease
  - due to shunting: right to left shunt, pulmonary embolism
  - due to interstitial lung disease: pneumonia, emphysema, pulmonary edema (cardio- and noncardiogenic)
  - PaO_2: low (< 60 mmHg)
  - $PaCO_2$: normal or low (< 50 mmHg)
- Type II or hypercapnic (ventilatory failure) (pump failure)
  - may be acute or chronic
  - due to increased airways resistance: chronic obstructive pulmonary disease (COPD), asthma, suffocation
  - due to reduced breathing effort: drug effects/overdose, morbid obesity, traumatic brain injury
  - due to decreased lung area: chronic bronchitis
  - due to neuromuscular disorder: cervical spinal cord injury, myasthenia gravis
  - Due to spinal/chest deformity: kyphoscoliosis, ankylosing spondylitis, flair chest
  - PaO_2: decreased (< 60 mmHg)
  - $PaCO_2$: increased (> 50 mmHg)
  - pH: decreased (chronic: pH level higher)
- Mixed respiratory failure is a combination of types I and II or acute on chronic
- Type III or peri- or postoperative
  - usually caused by atelectasis
  - treatment of atelectasis: incentive spirometry, adequate analgesia, upright positioning, early mobilization; due to abdominal distention: nasogastric suction, paracentesis
- Type IV or shock
  - hypoperfusion
  - due to acidosis, sepsis, acute hemorrhage, myocardial infarction (MI), shock

Documentation Tip

Code assignment cannot be based on ancillary test result, therapies, or clinical criteria alone. A diagnosis and its clinical significance must be supported by physician or other qualified healthcare professional documentation. When it is unclear or there is contradictory information, query the physician or other qualified healthcare professional for clarification.

Documentation Tip

Ongoing mechanical ventilation in a postsurgical or post-trauma scenario does not necessarily indicate acute respiratory failure. A patient may require ventilation for airway protection if they are unable to independently maintain an open airway. To appropriately report acute respiratory failure, the patient must meet clinical criteria. Clarify with the provider whether a diagnosis of acute respiratory failure is appropriate, or if the mechanical ventilation was meant for prevention of respiratory failure and/or maintenance of airway patency.

Coding/Reporting Criteria	Clinical Criteria	
1. Physical Evaluation *(routine/expected in italics)*	• Tachypnea (respirations > 20) • Tachycardia (pulse > 100) • Dyspnea • Wheezing • Headache • Impaired motor function • Altered mental status • Air hunger • Use of accessory muscles of respiration to breath • Cyanosis	• Shortness of breath • Crackles on auscultation • Restlessness • Confusion • Arrhythmia • Somnolence • Unconsciousness/coma/obtundation • Encephalopathy • Myoclonus/seizure in severe hypoxemia • Respiratory arrest

2. Clinical Evaluation
(routine/expected in italics)
	• Hypoxemia
	• Hypercapnia
	• Hypocapnia
	• Respiratory acidosis (pH < 7.30) (severe: pH < 7.20)
	• Pulse ox < 90%RA or < 95% on O_2
	• Respirations > 20
	• Arterial blood gasses (ABG):
	• No pre-existing lung disease
	  – PaO_2 < 60mmHg
	  – $PaCO_2$ > 50mm Hg
		• Pre-existing chronic lung disease
		  – pH<7.30 (acute)
		  – pH normal or >7.45 (chronic)
		  – degree of change in PO_2 < 60 or 10-15mm Hg below
		  – baseline
		  – degree of change in $PaCO_2$ > 50 or 10–15mm Hg above baseline
		• CBC

3. Diagnostic Px *(routine/expected in italics)*	• Chest x-ray • CT	• EKG • Pulmonary function test

4. Therapeutic Tx
(routine/expected in italics)
	• *Intubation for airway protection (with vent support) (due to neurological compromise) w/o dx of respiratory failure*
	• *Intubation/vent support continues postsurgery < 48 hours for routine post-op ventilation w/o dx of respiratory failure*
	• *Weaning from ventilation postoperatively with all organ systems stable/tolerating weaning (vent management)*
	• *Electively maintained on respiratory support (vent management)*
	• Re-intubation post-op/extubation (with vent support) due to respiratory failure
	• Ventilation extended post-op > 48 hours due to respiratory failure
	• Oxygen therapy/supplemental oxygen
		• Ventilation:
		  – nonmechanical: Positive end expiratory pressure (PEEP)
		  – mechanical:
		    - noninvasive (face mask/nasal mask): noninvasive positive pressure ventilation (NIPPV) assistance: continuous positive airway pressure (CPAP), bi-level positive airway pressure (BIPAP), inspiratory positive airway pressure (IPAP), expiratory positive airway pressure (EPAP)
		• Invasive performance: mechanical ventilation via ETT/tracheostomy: intermittent mandatory ventilation (IMV), continuous mandatory ventilation (CMV), synchronized intermittent mandatory ventilation (SIMV), noninvasive mechanical ventilation (NIMV), airway pressure release ventilation (APRV) Respiratory stimulants
		• Bronchoscopy
		• Aerosolized bronchodilators
		• Steroids
		• Pulmonary rehab
		• Physiotherapy
		• Treatment of underlying cause

5. Increased Nursing Care and/or Monitoring	• Re-intubation post-op/extubation (with vent support) due to respiratory failure • Ventilation extended post-op > 48 hours due to respiratory failure	• Requires high-flow oxygen post-op • Frequent arterial blood gas monitoring post-op
6. Extends LOS	• Re-intubation post-op/extubation (with vent support) due to respiratory failure • Ventilation extended post-op > 48 hours due to respiratory failure	• Discharge delayed due to respiratory failure • Admit/transfer to OBV due to respiratory failure

Condition	Documentation Example	ICD-10-CM Corresponding Codes
Routine/Expected/ Integral/Inherent/ Incidental *(italics only)*	1. *Progress Note: Weaning from ventilation postoperatively with all organ systems stable/tolerating weaning (vent management).* 2. *Progress Note: Electively maintained on respiratory support (vent management).* 3. *Progress Note: Vent management (< 48 hours postsurgery).* 4. *ED: Intubated/vent for airway protection due to stated condition (respiratory failure not documented).* 5. *ED: Acute respiratory failure with acute exacerbation of COPD. (The clinical criteria to support respiratory failure are not present.)* **(Query conflict between the diagnosis documented and the absence of clinical criteria to support dx.)**	1–5. No code assigned.
Principal Diagnosis	1. Admit Note: Impending/threatened acute respiratory failure (subsequently confirmed and supported by clinical criteria). Progress Note: Respiratory failure (dx made by other qualified healthcare professional and confirmed by physician). Discharge Summary: Respiratory failure (clinical criteria supports dx). 2. ED Respiratory failure (documented by ED physician but not documented by physician). **(Query to confirm.)** Admit Note: Near drowning with respiratory failure; Discharge Summary: Aspiration pneumonia with respiratory failure. **(Query with hypoxia or hypercapnia; query acute or chronic or acute on chronic; query underlying cause, when not stated; query conflict between dx and clinical criteria.)**	1. Report J96.ØØ Acute respiratory failure, unspecified whether with hypoxia or hypercapnia. Report codes for specified contributing diagnosis in addition to the respiratory failure if the physician confirms. 2. Report J96.9Ø Respiratory failure, unspecified, unspecified whether with hypoxia or hypercapnia; J69.8 Pneumonitis due to inhalation of other solids and liquids, and any external cause codes that are applicable.
Comorbidity	1. Progress Note: Acute on chronic respiratory failure due to AIDS. 2. Discharge Summary: Respiratory failure due to sepsis with septic shock. **(Query with hypoxia or hypercapnia; query acute or chronic or acute on chronic; query underlying cause if not stated; query conflict between dx and clinical criteria.)**	1. Report B2Ø Human immunodeficiency virus [HIV] disease, followed by J96.2Ø Acute and chronic respiratory failure, unspecified whether with hypoxia or hypercapnia. 2. Report A41.9 Sepsis, unspecified organism, followed by R65.21 Severe sepsis with septic shock; and J96.9Ø Respiratory failure, unspecified, unspecified whether with hypoxia or hypercapnia.
Complication of Care	1. Discharge Summary: Respiratory failure due to orthopedic reconstructive surgery. 2. Progress Note: Re-intubation due to Respiratory failure due to procedure 3. Progress Note: Remains intubated/vent post-op (> 48 hrs) due to respiratory failure. ***(*Query with hypoxia or hypercapnia; query acute or chronic or acute on chronic; query: underlying cause/reason for extended intubation (> 48 hours) or re-intubation or if stated as post-op; if not related to procedure or surgery, do not assign as complication due to procedure; query if conflict between dx and clinical criteria.)**	1, 2, 3. Report J95.821 Acute postprocedural respiratory failure, followed by a code for any specified contributing diagnosis (i.e., atelectasis, pulmonary edema, etc.).
Poisoning or Adverse Effect of Medication/ Chemical	1. ED Record: Acute respiratory failure due to alcohol poisoning. **(Query with hypoxia or hypercapnia; Query acute or chronic or acute on chronic.)**	1. Report T51.ØX1A Toxic effect of ethanol, accidental (unintentional), initial encounter, followed by J96.9Ø Respiratory failure, unspecified, unspecified whether with hypoxia or hypercapnia. When the intent is not specified, accidental is assumed. Undetermined intent is only used when the documentation specifies that the poisoning is literally undetermined, not lacking in documentation.

Additional References

AHA CC: 2Q, 2024, p. 11; 4Q, 2021, p. 101; 4Q, 2020, p. 96; 3Q, 2020, p. 9; 3Q, 2016, p. 8; 1Q, 2016, p. 38; 1Q, 2015, p. 3; 4Q, 2013, p. 121, 127

Sepsis

AØ2.1	**Salmonella sepsis**	MCC HCC
A22.7	**Anthrax sepsis**	MCC HCC
A24.1	**Acute and fulminating melioidosis**	CC
A26.7	**Erysipelothrix sepsis**	MCC HCC
A31.2	**Disseminated mycobacterium avium-intracellulare complex (DMAC) (MAC sepsis)**	CC HCC
A32.7	**Listerial sepsis**	MCC HCC
A4Ø.[Ø,1,3]	**Sepsis due to streptococcus, [streptococcus group A, streptococcus group B, Streptococcus pneumoniae]**	MCC HCC
A4Ø.[8,9]	**[Other, unspecified] streptococcal sepsis**	MCC HCC
A41.Ø-	**Sepsis due to Staphylococcus aureus (Methicillin susceptible Staphylococcus aureus, Methicillin resistant Staphylococcus aureus)**	MCC HCC
A41.[1,2]	**Sepsis due to [other specified, unspecified] staphylococcus**	MCC HCC
A41.3	**Sepsis due to Hemophilus influenzae**	MCC HCC
A41.4	**Sepsis due to anaerobes**	MCC HCC
A41.5-	**Gram-negative sepsis (unspecified, due to Escherichia coli [E. coli], due to Pseudomonas, due to Serratia, Acinetobacter baumannii, other Gram-negative sepsis)**	MCC HCC
A41.8-	**Other specified sepsis (Sepsis due to Enterococcus, Other specified sepsis)**	MCC HCC
A41.9	**Sepsis, unspecified organism**	MCC HCC
A42.7	**Actinomycotic sepsis**	MCC HCC
A54.86	**Gonococcal sepsis**	MCC HCC
BØØ.7	**Disseminated herpesviral disease**	MCC HCC
B37.7	**Candidal sepsis**	MCC HCC
O86.Ø4	**Sepsis following an obstetrical procedure**	MCC
R65.2Ø	**Severe sepsis without septic shock**	MCC HCC
R65.21	**Severe sepsis with septic shock**	MCC HCC
T81.12XA	**Postprocedural septic shock, initial encounter**	MCC
T81.44XA	**Sepsis following a procedure, initial encounter**	CC HAC

Associated terminology: sepsis, septicemia, severe sepsis, severe sepsis with septic shock, severe sepsis following procedure, postprocedural septic shock, sepsis with organ dysfunction, SIRS

Diagnoses

Discussion

Sepsis is a serious, potentially life-threatening complication of a localized infection caused by systemic or body-wide chemical response to the infectious agent, with the majority of sepsis cases being due to a bacterial infection. It can lead to shock, organ failure, and even death. Systemic inflammatory response syndrome (SIRS) is the body's inflammatory reaction in response to an assault by chemical, traumatic, or infectious stimuli. The first stage of the physiological response is directed at repair and protection; the second stage is homeostasis; if homeostasis is not achieved, during the third stage the system begins to self-destruct, which leads to end organ dysfunction.

A task force that comprises leading sepsis experts has published new recommendations regarding sepsis and septic shock definitions and criteria, which aid physicians in more quickly diagnosing at risk patients. The more recent definition of Sepis 3, the first change since 2001, emphasizes the 10 percent potential life-threatening mortality of sepsis based on organ dysfunction. Unlike the current ICD-10-CM codes, which offer both Sepsis (without organ dysfunction) and Severe Sepsis (with organ dysfunction), the Sepsis 3 definition "life threatening organ dysfunction caused by a dysregulated host response to infection" suggests that all sepsis is with organ dysfunction.

Clinical criteria for organ dysfunction are based on a Sequential Organ Failure Assessment (SOFA) or quickSOFA (qSOFA) score. The SOFA score is a table that measures respiratory, coagulation, liver, cardiovascular, central nervous system and renal functions, which assumes a baseline of 0 for no preexisting organ dysfunction. Sepsis, with its increased mortality risk, is considered with a SOFA score ≥2. A quickSOFA can be performed bedside to immediately identify sepsis risk using the following criteria:

- Respiratory rate ≥22/min
- Altered mentation
- Systolic blood pressure ≤100 mm Hg

The Society of Critical Care Medicine (SCCM) task force 2016 recommended Sepsis SOFA score criteria as shown in the table below.

Sequential Organ Failure Assessment (SOFA) Score

SOFA score	0	1	2	3	4
Respiration PaO_2/FIO_2 (mm Hg) SaO_2/FIO_2	>400	<400 221–301	<300 142–220	<200 67–141	<100 <67
Coagulation Platelets $\times 10^3/mm^3$	>150	<150	<100	<50	<20
Liver Bilirubin (mg/dL)	<1.2	1.2–1.9	2.0–5.9	6.0–11.9	>12.0
Cardiovascular Hypotension	No hypotension	MAP <70	Dopamine </=5 or dobutamine (any)	Dopamine >5 or norepinephrine </=0.1	Dopamine >15 or norepinephrine >0.1
CNS Glasgow Coma Score	15	13–14	10–12	6–9	<6
Renal Creatinine (mg/dL) or urine output (mL/d)	<1.2	1.2–1.9	2.0-3.4	3.5-4.9 or <500	>5.0 or <200

Coding and Documentation Tip

Glasgow coma scale (GCS) score is one of the clinical criteria for organ dysfunction based on a sequential organ failure assessment (SOFA) score. However, the codes for GCS scores are not reported in sepsis cases. For fiscal 2021, the ICD-10-CM guidelines were revised to allow reporting of these codes only with trauma cases.

For fiscal 2021, guideline I.C.18.e was revised to read: "The coma scale codes (R40.2-) can be used in conjunction with traumatic brain injury codes. These codes are primarily for use by trauma registries, but they may be used in any setting where this information is collected."

This change in the guidelines is not intended to restrict use of the GCS in assessing patients. It is intended to limit the separate reporting of these symptom codes to the traumatic brain injuries and prevent their use in situations for which they were not intended.

Septic shock is considered a subset of sepsis with an increase in mortality to 40 percent due to profound circulatory, cellular, and metabolic abnormalities. A diagnosis of septic shock includes the clinical criteria of hypotension and hyperlactemia (when serum lactate information is available). ICD-10-CM currently recognizes sepsis as a systemic hematological infection due to either seeding from a localized infection or from direct introduction from an external or foreign body source. Severe sepsis is sepsis with acute organ dysfunction or SIRS due to an infectious process with acute organ dysfunction. When severe sepsis is present on admission and meets criteria as principal diagnosis, it is reported with the underlying infection or complication of care code sequenced first, then a code for any localized infection, followed by a code from subcategory R65.2 Severe sepsis, followed by codes for all documented acute organ dysfunction. Distributive septic shock is circulatory failure due to systemic infection, which releases histamine-causing vasodilation leading to hypotension despite adequate fluid resuscitation, in addition to other perfusion abnormalities (lactic acidosis, etc.). In ICD-10-CM, the presence of septic shock with severe sepsis in subcategory R65.2 is indicated by the fifth character 1 with shock, or with code T81.12X[A,D,S] Postprocedural septic shock, as a secondary code. A code for the precipitating postprocedural infection from the subcategory range T81.4Ø- to T81.43- (or O86.ØØ to O86.Ø3 if the infection is of an obstetric surgical wound) that identifies the site of the infection (unspecified site, superficial or deep incisional site, or organ and space surgical site) should be coded first, if known. An additional code is assigned from subcategory T81.44- for sepsis following a procedure or O86.Ø4 sepsis following an obstetrical procedure. Another additional code is assigned to identify the infectious agent. If the patient has severe sepsis, the appropriate code from subcategory R65.2 should also be assigned with the additional code(s) for any acute organ dysfunction.

Because of the mismatch of these new recommendations with the current ICD-10-CM codes, it is strongly advised that facilities have discussions with physician, CDI, and coding staff to educate decide how and when coding protocols will be handled to match these new definitions, understanding that there may also be denial impacts based on which sepsis criteria payers follow.

Excluded

- **Newborn sepsis, see category P36-.**
- **Obstetrical, see section OØØ–O9A.**

Physician documentation must validate the clinical scenario demonstrating the severity of illness through the history and physical, progress notes, review and comment on all consults, and review and comment on ancillary test results indicating improvement or worsening of patient status. Therapies should have a stated goal and the condition they target and measurement of their effectiveness to support clinical decision making should be documented. Development of a uniform tool that highlights key points of care may be an aid to documentation.

Long-term care hospital (LTCH): When transferred from an acute hospital for continued treatment of a condition that is resolving and no longer acute or now without clinical indicators, assign as a sequela with codes for both the resulting condition(s) and sequela. For example, continued antibiotic treatment for resolving severe sepsis and the patient is no longer septic, assign any documented consequential conditions (debility, etc.) and sequela of infectious disease (B94-) or sequela of complications of care with seventh character S.

Documentation Tip

Based on OCG 1.A.19, coders should never assign a code for sepsis based on clinical definition or criteria or clinical signs alone. Code assignment should be based strictly on physician documentation (regardless of the clinical criteria the physician used to arrive at that diagnosis).

Sepsis: *Suspected/presumptive/clinical/culture-negative:* Negative or inclusive blood cultures do not preclude a diagnosis of sepsis. The presence of one or more risk factors, the appropriate clinical presentation, and specific treatment in conjunction with physician confirmation validates the diagnosis.

Guideline I.C.1.d.1.i: "Negative or inconclusive blood cultures do not preclude a diagnosis of sepsis in patients with clinical evidence of the condition; however, the provider should be queried."

Some examples of underlying infections are:

- Systemic: sepsis (code to the identified organism):
  - bacterial: codes from category A41 Other sepsis
  - disseminated candida: B37.7 Candidal sepsis
  - herpesviral sepsis: BØØ.7 Disseminated herpesviral disease
- Due to/following a procedure code T81.4[Ø,1,2,3]X[A,D,S] followed by T81.44X[A,D,S] Sepsis following a procedure in addition to a code identifying the infectious agent
- Following infusion, transfusion, and therapeutic injection: a code from subcategory T8Ø.2 Infections following infusion, transfusion and therapeutic injection
- Due to prosthetic devices, implants, and grafts: codes from subcategories:

  T82.6 Infection and inflammatory reaction due to cardiac valve prosthesis

  T82.7 Infection and inflammatory reaction due to other cardiac and vascular devices, implants and grafts

T83.5	Infection and inflammatory reaction due to prosthetic device, implant and graft in urinary system
T83.6	Infection and inflammatory reaction due to prosthetic device, implant and graft in genital tract
T84.5	Infection and inflammatory reaction due to internal joint prosthesis
T84.6	Infection and inflammatory reaction due to internal fixation device
T84.7	Infection and inflammatory reaction due to other internal orthopedic prosthetic devices, implants and grafts
T85.7	Infection and inflammatory reaction due to other internal prosthetic devices, implants and grafts

Documentation Tip

Complications of care: The condition must be more than a routinely expected condition or event. The documentation must support that the condition is clinically significant with an indication that it is a complication, by demonstrating:

- **A cause-and-effect relationship between the care or procedure and the condition**
- **That the condition resulted in altering the course of a procedure or surgery**

The term "complication" does not have to be explicitly documented.

Coding Tip

For sepsis following a procedure, assign a code from subcategories T81.4Ø- to T81.43- Infection following a procedure, that identifies the surgical site of the infection first, if known. That code is followed by an additional code from subcategory T81.44- Sepsis following a procedure, with the appropriate seventh characters for the circumstances of the encounter. Use an additional code to identify the infectious agent.

For sepsis following an obstetric procedure, assign a code from O86.ØØ to O86.Ø3 Infection of obstetric surgical wound, that identifies the surgical site of the infection first, if known, followed by additional code O86.Ø4 Sepsis following an obstetrical procedure. Use an additional code to identify the infectious agent.

ICD-10-CM guideline I.C.1.d.1.a.iii states that a code is assigned for severe sepsis when the provider documents sepsis and an associated acute organ dysfunction or multiple organ dysfunction. Guideline I.C.1.d.1.a also states that a code from subcategory R65.2 Severe sepsis, is assigned when the provider documents "severe sepsis." A code for severe sepsis may also be assigned when the Alphabetic Index leads to a code for "severe sepsis." The conventions and instructions of the classification take precedence over guidelines. If acute organ dysfunction is present but not linked to severe sepsis or there are other conditions present, which may have caused the dysfunction, query the relationship.

Documentation Tip

Note that according to guideline I.C.1.d.2.a, septic shock generally refers to circulatory failure associated with severe sepsis, and, therefore, it represents a type of acute organ dysfunction. The acute organ dysfunction is inherent in this code. No other documentation of acute organ dysfunction is required if the physician documents septic shock. However, codes for any other additional acute organ dysfunction that is documented as associated should be assigned. In addition, the conditions listed in the tabular under subcategory R65.2-, Severe sepsis, are not a complete and comprehensive list. If there is any question or the documentation is unclear whether a specific condition is considered organ dysfunction/failure or is related to the sepsis, the physician should be queried for clarification.

Documentation Tip

When documentation and clinical indicators do not match, query the provider for clarification of the diagnosis.

Follow these coding guidelines for severe sepsis with a noninfectious condition that develops an infection:

- When a noninfectious condition leads to a subsequent infection, which then results in severe sepsis, assign a code from subcategory R65.2 without a code from subcategory R65.1.
- When the noninfectious condition develops a subsequent local infection that results in severe sepsis, sequence the noninfectious condition as principal diagnosis, followed by a code for sepsis, then the underlying local infection, followed by a code from subcategory R65.2.
- When the noninfectious condition and its associated local infection are both present on admission with the infection resulting in severe sepsis with POA=N and both meet the definition of principal diagnosis, sequence either the noninfectious condition or the associated local infection as principal, followed by a code for sepsis and a code from subcategory R65.2.

- When the noninfectious condition, with the associated local infection and severe sepsis are all present on admission, and all meet the definition of principal diagnosis, then any one can be sequenced as principal diagnosis, followed by a code from subcategory R65.2.
- With combined etiologies present (noninfectious and infectious), and it is not clear if SIRS is due to noninfectious condition or severe sepsis, query for clarification and if present on admission.

Coding and Documentation Tip

Since the principal diagnosis for COVID-19 with sepsis depends on the circumstances of admission, it is imperative to clarify whether the sepsis was present on admission (POA) and was chiefly responsible for the admission in order to use A41.89 Other specified sepsis as principal diagnosis. If sepsis clearly developed over the course of the admission and COVID-19 was POA, code first UØ7.1 COVID-19.

Documentation Tip

Code assignment cannot be based on ancillary test results, therapies, or clinical criteria alone. A diagnosis and its clinical significance must be supported by physician or other qualified healthcare professional documentation. When it is unclear or there is contradictory information, query the physician or other qualified healthcare professional for clarification.

Note: When documentation states SIRS and an infection is present, do not assume a link. Query the etiology of the SIRS; if no other information is available or forth coming, report a code from subcategory R65.1. In ICD-10-CM, SIRS does not equate to sepsis; documentation must state the etiology and only "severe sepsis due to infection" or "sepsis with acute organ dysfunction" is represented by codes for sepsis with the R65.2 subcategory.

When documentation states only SIRS (not sepsis) secondary to a localized infection such as pneumonia without organ dysfunction, code only the localized infection as there is no separate code or index entry for SIRS due to an infectious process in ICD-10-CM. If sepsis criteria appears to be met in the health record, query the provider for clarification (*AHA Coding Clinic*, Third Q, 2014, page 4).

Coding Tip

To preempt possible denial by external audit: diagnoses made within the record but not listed/included in the discharge summary, query the provider for concordance and inclusion into discharge summary. (Note: CMS reinforces that omission by provider of a consultant's diagnosis is not a conflict, but denials may be attempted.)

Coding/Reporting Criteria	Clinical Criteria	
1. Physical Evaluation *(routine/expected in italics)*	• Adult population current criteria: – must have a suspected infectious process – SIRS: Must have at least two of the four criteria indicated by an asterisk (*) - temperature: ≤ 36° C (100.4° F) or ≥ 38° C (96.8° F)* - tachycardia: heart rate: ≥ 90 bpm* - tachypnea/hyperventilation: Respiratory Rate: ≥ 20 breaths/min or $PaCO_2$ < 32 mmHg* - confusion/mental status changes - fever or hypothermia – sepsis-induced hypotension: (systolic bp < 90 mmHg or mean arterial pressure (MAP) < 70 mmHg or reduction in baseline bp by 40 mmHg) in the absence of other causes for hypotension - evidence of reduced organ perfusion w/o evidence of dehydration	- oliguria (with end-stage organ progression): urine output 0.5 mL for more than two hours despite adequate fluid resuscitation - hypoxemia (with end-stage organ progression) - acute lung injury with $PaO_2/FiO_2/250$ in the absence of pneumonia (PNA) as infection source - acute lung injury with $PaO_2/FiO_2/200$ in the presence of PNA as infection source - jaundice (with end-stage organ progression) - ileus - thrombocytopenia – disseminated intravascular coagulation (DIC)
2. Clinical Evaluation *(routine/expected in italics)*	• Leukocytosis: WBC: ≥ 12,000 cells/μL (12x109/L) or ≤ 4,000 cells/μL (4x109/L) or > 10% bands* • Creatinine: 2.0 mg/dL or 0.5 mg/dL rise for ARF • Acute kidney injury (AKI): 0.3 mg/dL rise • Bilirubin: 2 mg/dL • Platelet count: 100,000IL • Coagulopathy: international normalization ratio (INR) 1.5 • Sepsis: source of infection: suspected or confirmed source of infection • Arterial pH < 7.35/lactic metabolic acidosis • Positive blood culture (or culture negative with physician judgment) • CBC with differential • Cardiac enzymes • Blood/urine/wound cultures/analysis to evaluate for infection • Amylase • Interleukin-6 • Elevated plasma lactate level > 1.5 x normal • Plasma C-reactive protein more than two standard deviations (SD) above the normal value • Procalcitonin: able to differentiate between infectious and noninfectious SIRS: more than two SD above the normal value indicates sepsis/infection	• Plasma soluble triggering receptor expressed on myeloid cells 1 (sTREM-1) elevation • Elevated D Dimer • Hyperglycemia: plasma glucose 140 mg/dL or 7.7 μ/L in the absence of diabetes • Acute organ dysfunction/evidence: tests specific to organ system • Sepsis-induced hypotension (systolic bp < 90 mmHg or a reduction in baseline bp by 40 mmHg or < 70 mmHg) in the absence of other causes for hypotension – lactic acidosis – acute kidney injury – acute renal failure – acute lung injury – shock (NEC or specified) – acute liver/hepatic failure – acute respiratory failure – critical illness myopathy – critical illness polyneuropathy – disseminated intravascular coagulopathy – encephalopathy – multiple organ dysfunction (MOD) syndrome (evidence of ≥ organs failing)
3. Diagnostic Px *(routine/expected in italics)*	• Lumbar puncture	• Imaging will be directed towards causative condition or organ dysfunction
4. Therapeutic Tx *(routine/expected in italics)*	• Treatment is directed towards the cause, associated organ dysfunction and other conditions • Antibiotics or antifungals • IV fluids/electrolyte restoration: 30 mL/kg crystalloid • Vasopressor agents, inotropic agents and sympathomimetics for hypotension/central line	• Surgery as appropriate for the causative conditions • Low-dose steroids for refractory hypotension/anaphylaxis • Control of blood glucose levels (hyperglycemia) • Supplemental oxygen • Vent support • Plasma infusion for clotting abnormalities
5. Increased Nursing Care and/or Monitoring	• Continued treatment/monitoring of organ dysfunction	
6. Extends LOS	• Severe sepsis post-op as a complication of surgery	

Condition	Documentation Example	ICD-10-CM Corresponding Codes
Routine/Expected/ Integral/Inherent/ Incidental *(italics only)*	*NA*	*NA*
Principal Diagnosis	1. Patient admitted with COVID-19, treated for sepsis. **Query whether sepsis was present on admission (POA)**	1. If sepsis was POA, it can be reported as principal diagnosis, followed by UØ7.1 COVID-19. If it developed during the stay, UØ7.1 COVID-19, is coded first, followed by the appropriate sepsis code(s).
Comorbidity	1. Discharge Summary: Severe sepsis due to *Streptococcus pneumoniae* secondary to *Streptococcus pneumoniae* pneumonia, with acute respiratory failure, all present on admission; intubated and placed on vent in ED for respiratory failure; on mechanical vent for 80 hrs. **(Query response indicated acute respiratory failure due to severe sepsis.)**	1. Report A4Ø.3 Sepsis due to Streptococcus pneumonia, followed by J13 Pneumonia due to Streptococcus pneumonia; J96.ØØ Acute respiratory failure, unspecified whether with hypoxia or hypercapnia; R65.2Ø Severe sepsis without septic shock.
Complication of Care	1. IP Progress Note: Postprocedural infection with intraabdominal abscess causing severe sepsis with septic shock following partial pancreatectomy due to acute infectious gangrenous pancreatitis. Acute hepatic failure noted. **(Query whether the acute hepatic failure is due to the SIRS or the procedure.)**	1. Report T81.43XA Infection following a procedure, organ and space surgical site, followed by T81.44XA Sepsis following a procedure, initial encounter; A41.9 Sepsis, unspecified organism; T81.12XA Postprocedural septic shock, initial encounter; K65.1 Peritoneal abscess; and K85.92 Acute pancreatitis with infected necrosis, unspecified.
Poisoning or Adverse Effect of Medication/ Chemical	NA	NA

Additional References

AHA CC: 1Q, 2024, p. 19; 4Q, 2023, p. 88; 2Q, 2022, p. 5; 1Q, 2022, p. 35; 2Q, 2020, P. 17, 20; 3Q, 2019, p. 17; 2Q, 2019, p. 39; 1Q, 2019, p. 13-14; 4Q, 2018, p. 33, 89; 4Q, 2017, p. 98-99; 2Q, 2017, p. 8; 1Q, 2017, p. 51; 4Q, 2016, p. 147; 3Q, 2016, p. 8

CMS: Hospital Acquired Conditions (HAC) List https://www.cms.gov/medicare/medicare-fee-for-service-payment/hospitalacqcond/icd10_hacs

Sepsis Management: https://www.cdc.gov/sepsis/hcp/clinical-care/?

SOFA definition/criteria: https://www.sccm.org/Research/Quality/Sepsis-Definitions

Diagnoses

SIRS of Noninfectious Origin

R65.1Ø **Systemic inflammatory response syndrome [SIRS] of noninfectious origin without acute organ dysfunction** CC HCC

R65.11 **Systemic inflammatory response syndrome [SIRS] of noninfectious origin with acute organ dysfunction** MCC HCC

Associated terminology: SIRS due to noninfectious pancreatitis; SIRS due to burns; SIRS due to aspiration pneumonia without superimposed bacterial infection; SIRS due to medication; postoperative SIRS due to surgery

Discussion

Systemic inflammatory response syndrome (SIRS) is the body's inflammatory reaction in response to an assault by chemical, traumatic, or infectious stimuli. The first stage of the physiological response is directed at repair and protection; the second stage is homeostasis; if homeostasis is not achieved, during the third stage the system begins to self-destruct, which leads to end organ dysfunction. SIRS due to a noninfectious etiology is reported using subcategory R65.1 Systemic inflammatory response syndrome (SIRS) of noninfectious origin, when it meets clinical criteria and is supported by the clinical scenario. Documentation of "severe SIRS" implies acute end organ dysfunction; therefore, confirm any acute organ dysfunction and its etiology, whether the organ dysfunction is due to SIRS or due to another condition impacts reporting. Some populations with SIRS may not meet standard clinical criteria on admission: extremes of age, immunosuppressed patients, and diabetics may all present without routine signs and symptoms. Medications that a patient is on may also mask some of the symptoms.

Documentation Tip

When documentation and clinical criteria do not match, query the provider for clarification of the diagnosis.

When SIRS due to noninfectious condition is present with an associated infection which results in severe sepsis, only a code from subcategory R65.2 Severe sepsis, will be assigned and the sequencing will be determined by the circumstances of the admission and following official coding guidelines for chapters 1, 18, 19 and section II "Selection of Principal Diagnosis." See also the section for severe sepsis in this publication for further guidance regarding SIRS due to an infectious process.

For SIRS due to noninfectious condition (not all inclusive):

- Code first the underlying condition (without subsequent infection).
- Sequence R65.1Ø Systemic inflammatory response syndrome (SIRS) of noninfectious origin without acute organ dysfunction, or R65.11 Systemic inflammatory response syndrome (SIRS) of noninfectious origin with acute organ dysfunction, as additional code; these codes are never sequenced first.
- When R65.11 is assigned, report all codes for the documented associated acute organ dysfunctions; the link must be made between the SIRS and the acute organ dysfunction in order to assign R65.11; query when the etiology of the acute organ dysfunction is unclear.
- When a noninfectious condition leads to a subsequent infection, which then results in severe sepsis, assign a code from subcategory R65.2 Severe sepsis, without a code from subcategory R65.1 Systemic inflammatory response syndrome (SIRS) of noninfectious origin, as only one code from category R65 Symptoms and signs specifically associated with systemic inflammation and infection, should be assigned per encounter.
- When the noninfectious condition develops a subsequent local infection (present on admission=N), which results in severe sepsis, sequence the noninfectious condition as principal diagnosis, followed by a code for sepsis, then the underlying local infection, followed by a code from subcategory R65.2.
- When the noninfectious condition and its associated local infection are both present on admission with the infection resulting in severe sepsis, and both meet the definition of principal diagnosis, sequence either the noninfectious condition or the associated local infection as principal, followed by a code for sepsis and R65.2.
- When the noninfectious condition, the associated local infection, and severe sepsis are all present on admission, and all meet the definition of principal diagnosis, then any one can be sequenced as principal diagnosis, followed by R65.2.
- When combined etiologies are present (noninfectious and infectious), and it is not clear if SIRS is due to noninfectious condition or severe sepsis, query for clarification and if it was present on admission.

- When SIRS is due to an adverse reaction to medication, assign the presenting symptoms or nature of the adverse effect followed by the appropriate code from T36–T5Ø with fifth or sixth character 5 the drug causing the adverse effect.
- Common non-infectious causes of SIRS are:
  - adrenal insufficiency
  - cardiac tamponade
  - immunodeficiency
  - pulmonary embolism
  - dehydration
  - hemorrhage
  - trauma/serious injury
  - burn
  - pancreatitis, not due to infection
  - aspiration pneumonia
  - cholecystitis, not due to infection
  - cholelithiasis
  - diverticulitis, not due to infection
  - cholangitis, not due to infection
  - peritonitis, not due to infection
  - cirrhosis
  - ischemic bowel/mesentery
  - myocardial infarction
  - seizure
  - heatstroke
  - anaphylaxis
  - malignant neoplasm
  - complication of surgery
  - medication
  - drug abuse
  - transfusion reaction

Documentation Tip

Code assignment cannot be based on ancillary test results, therapies, or clinical criteria alone. A diagnosis and its clinical significance must be supported by physician or other qualified healthcare professional documentation. When it is unclear or there is contradictory information, query the physician or other qualified healthcare professional for clarification.

Note: When documentation states SIRS and an infection is present, do not assume a link. Query the etiology of the SIRS; if no other information is available or forth coming, report subcategory R65.1 Systemic inflammatory response syndrome (SIRS) of noninfectious origin. In ICD-10-CM, SIRS does not equate to sepsis; documentation must state the etiology and only "severe sepsis due to infection" or "sepsis with acute organ dysfunction" is represented by codes for sepsis and the R65.2 Severe sepsis, subcategory.

Coding Tip

To preempt possible denial by external audit: diagnoses made within the record but not listed/included in discharge summary, query the provider for concordance and inclusion into discharge summary. (Note: CMS reinforces that omission by provider of a consultants diagnosis is not a conflict, but denials may be attempted).

Coding/Reporting Criteria	Clinical Criteria	
1. Physical Evaluation *(routine/expected in italics)*	• Adult population criteria: – must have an inflammatory process • SIRS: Must have at least two of the four criteria indicated by an asterisk (*): – temperature: ≤ 36° C (100.4° F) or ≥ 38° C (96.8° F)* – tachycardia: heart rate: ≥ 90 bpm* – tachypnea/hyperventilation: respiratory rate: ≥ 20 breaths/min or $PaCO_2$ < 32 mmHg*	confusion/mental status changes – fever or hypothermia – evidence of reduced organ perfusion w/o evidence of dehydration – oliguria (with end-stage organ progression) – hypoxemia (with end-stage organ progression) – jaundice (with end-stage organ progression)
2. Clinical Evaluation *(routine/expected in italics)*	• Leukocytosis: WBC: ≥ 12,000 cells/μL (12x109/L) or ≤ 4,000 cells/μL (4x109/L) or > 10% bands* • Arterial pH < 7.35 (lactic metabolic acidosis) • CBC with differential • Cardiac enzymes • Blood/urinal cultures/analysis to evaluate for infection • Amylase • Interleukin-6 • Elevated plasma lactate level > 1.5 x normal • Procalcitonin: able to differentiate between infectious and noninfectious SIRS • Elevated D Dimer	• Acute organ dysfunction/evidence: tests specific to organ system: – hypotension – lactic acidosis – acute kidney injury – acute renal failure – acute lung injury – shock (NEC or specified) – acute liver/hepatic failure – acute respiratory failure – critical illness myopathy – critical illness polyneuropathy – disseminated intravascular coagulopathy (DIC) – encephalopathy – MOD syndrome (evidence of ≥ 2 organs failing)

Coding/Reporting Criteria	Clinical Criteria	
3. Diagnostic Px *(routine/expected in italics)*	• Lumbar puncture	• Imaging will be directed towards causative condition or organ dysfunction
4. Therapeutic Tx *(routine/expected in italics)*	• Treatment is directed towards the cause, associated organ dysfunction and other conditions • IV fluids/electrolyte restoration • Vasopressor agents, inotropic agents and sympathomimetics for hypotension/central line • Surgery as appropriate for causative conditions	• Low dose steroids for refractory hypotension/anaphylaxis • Control of blood glucose levels (hyperglycemia) • Supplemental oxygen • Vent support • Plasma infusion for clotting abnormalities
5. Increased Nursing Care and/or Monitoring	• Continued treatment/monitoring of organ dysfunction	
6. Extends LOS	• SIRS post-op as a complication of surgery	

Condition	Documentation Example	ICD-10-CM Corresponding Codes
Routine/Expected/ Integral/Inherent/ Incidental *(italics only)*	*NA*	*NA*
Principal Diagnosis	NA	NA
Comorbidity	1. Discharge Summary: An 80-year-old male with acute alcoholic intoxication with alcohol-induced acute pancreatitis; developed SIRS due to delayed presentation; pancreatitis treated with pain meds, IV fluids and npo with enteral feeding.	1. Report K85.20 Alcohol induced acute pancreatitis without necrosis or infection; F10.229 Alcohol dependence with intoxication, unspecified; R65.10 Systemic inflammatory response syndrome (SIRS) of noninfectious origin without acute organ dysfunction.
Complication of Care	1. IP Progress Note: Patient post-op day two from percutaneous transcatheter aortic valve implantation (TAVI), with leukocytosis, hyperventilation, tachycardia, fever; surgery-induced SIRS.	1. Report T81.89XA Other complications of procedures, not elsewhere classified, initial encounter, followed by R65.10 Systemic inflammatory response syndrome (SIRS) of noninfectious origin without acute organ dysfunction.
Poisoning or Adverse Effect of Medication/ Chemical	1. IP Admit Note: Admitted from OBS with tachycardia, fever, and leukocytosis; workup did not reveal any infectious process; patient had just started new med for COPD, Theophyl; final diagnosis SIRS as adverse effect of Theophyl, med held and symptoms resolved; new med prescribed.	1. Report codes for any one of the symptoms first, followed by T48.6X5A Adverse effect of antiasthmatics, initial encounter, and R65.10 Systemic inflammatory response syndrome (SIRS) of noninfectious origin without acute organ dysfunction, and J44.9 Chronic obstructive pulmonary disease, unspecified. • Adverse effect: nature of adverse drug effect: code for (adverse condition) followed by the code from T36–T50 with fifth or sixth character 5 to identify the drug. • Poisoning: Identify drug/chemical by the code from T36–T50 with fifth or sixth character of intent followed by a code for nature of adverse drug effect (manifestation).

Additional References

AHA CC: 2Q, 2019, p. 38; 3Q, 2014, p. 4

Syncope as Principal Diagnosis

R55 **Syncope and collapse; syncope (near) (pre) (cardiac) (heart) (vasoconstriction) (vasodepressor) (vasomotor) (vasovagal)**

Associated terminology: syncope of unknown cause; vasovagal attack; vasovagal response of unknown etiology; near syncope due to medication; presyncope possibly due to either stress or dehydration; drop attack

Diagnoses

Discussion

Syncope is a sudden, complete but brief loss of consciousness (LOC) due to insufficient cerebral blood flow or insufficient cerebral oxygen and/or glucose, with postural collapse followed by spontaneous, complete recovery. Near syncope is lightheadedness and a sense of an impending faint without LOC. Presyncope is lightheadedness with muscle weakness, dizziness, and blurred vision.

A detailed medical and medication history, account of the event, and physical exam should guide the workup to a suspected etiology or at least narrow the possibilities. Code R55 Syncope and collapse, is a sign or symptom code and is therefore not reported when workup demonstrates a definitive diagnosis or suspected etiology; in these instances the definitive diagnosis or suspected etiology is reported. Conditions that may cause syncope are cardiogenic, neurological, neurocardiogenic, metabolic derangement, orthostatic hypotension, hematological, or cerebrovascular.

Near or presyncope documented as vasovagal, etc., or of unknown etiology is reported as the principal diagnosis R55 Syncope and collapse, which in turn maps to MS-DRG 312 Syncope and Collapse.

MS-DRG 312 and acute inpatient "short-stays" (less than two days) are under scrutiny for medical necessity and proper patient status. It is suggested that facilities institute pre-billing internal reviews and case management protocols for patient status and medical necessity review. Facilities may write facility-specific admission status criteria and standards, which will be consistently followed throughout departments. When a patient presents to the ED with syncope, is determined to be noncritical, and requires a workup that will extend beyond the ED, then observation status may be considered as the next level. If after observation status limit is met, and either the decision is made for inpatient admission due to the need to treat the etiology or further workup is scheduled, or there is failure of observation, then physician orders and documentation of medical necessity is crucial. If in the physician's judgment inpatient treatment is required and not observation, then the reasons must be documented.

Coding Tip

For inpatient admissions, if the final diagnosis at the time of discharge is documented as syncope followed by two or more possible underlying causes, do not assign the symptom code R55 as principal diagnosis. Instead, follow guideline II.D, Two or more comparative or contrasting conditions, which states that in the rare instance that two or more contrasting or comparative diagnoses are documented as "either/or" they are coded as if they were confirmed. Either diagnosis may be sequenced first, if no further determination can be made as to which diagnosis should be the principal diagnosis, based on:

- **The circumstances of admission**
- **Diagnostic workup and/or therapy provided**
- **Alphabetic Index, tabular list, or another coding guideline**

For observation admissions, if the final diagnosis at the time of discharge is documented as syncope followed by two or more possible underlying causes, assign only R55 syncope as principal diagnosis, following guideline IV.H, which states: "Do not code diagnoses documented as "probable," "suspected,""questionable," "rule out," "compatible with," "consistent with," or "working diagnosis," or other similar terms indicating uncertainty. Rather, code the condition(s) to the highest degree of certainty for that encounter/visit, such as symptoms, signs, abnormal test results, or other reason for the visit."

The physician's order to admit and discharge as either observation or inpatient must contain the following three sets of information:

- Admitting physician order: must clearly state intent of status (OBS or IP), time, date, and signature
- Medical necessity criteria: must include each sign, symptom, condition, and diagnosis requiring the status type and relate them to the workup, history/comorbidities, risk of adverse event, impressions and medical decision making, and therapy

- Discharge order: must clearly state discharge from identified status (OBS or IP), time, date, and signature

Coding/Reporting Criteria	Clinical Criteria	
1. Physical Evaluation *(routine/expected in italics)*	• Syncope suspected if all are present: – complete loss of consciousness (LOC) – LOS rapid onset and short duration – recovery spontaneous, complete and w/o sequelae – postural tone lost (collapse)	• Motionless • Limp • Cool extremities • Weak pulse • Shallow breathing
2. Clinical Evaluation *(routine/expected in italics)*	• Evaluation will focus on w/u for underlying cause • Serum glucose • CBC • Serum electrolytes • Cardiac enzymes	• Total creatinine kinase • Urinalysis/dipstick • Stool guaiac test • Pregnancy test: females of child-bearing age
3. Diagnostic Px *(routine/expected in italics)*	• Vital signs • Neuro exam • Chest x-ray • CT head: neurological symptoms/head trauma with syncope event • CT chest/abdomen: suspected dissection, ruptured aneurysm, PE • MRI/MRA: vertebrobasilar vasculature • V/Q: suspected PE • Echocardiography: suspected heart structure abnormalities	• 12-lead ECG • Loop recorder • Head-up tilt table test: to confirm autonomic dysfunction • EEG: to rule in/out seizure • Stress test: suspect cardiac syncope or who have known or risk factors for coronary disease • Carotid sinus massage: to rule in/out carotid sinus syncope • Pulse oximetry
4. Therapeutic Tx *(routine/expected in italics)*	• Oxygen • Glucose administration • Pharmacological circulatory support • Defib or temporary pacing • TED stockings: orthostatic syncope • Mineralocorticoids	• Evaluate/adjust medications associated with hypotension • Increased fluid consumption • Cardiac arrhythmic syncope: antiarrhythmic drugs or pacer • Cardiac mechanical syncope: beta blocker, valve repair
5. Increased Nursing Care and/or Monitoring	• Education/reinforcement of steps to avoid syncope and cautions needed	
6. Extends LOS	• Continued workup	

Condition	Documentation Example	ICD-10-CM Corresponding Codes
Routine/Expected/ Integral/Inherent/ Incidental *(italics only)*	*NA*	*NA*
Principal Diagnosis	1. IP Discharge Summary Discharge Note: Final Dx: Syncope of unknown etiology in an 82-year-old male who lives alone; pacer check revealed functioning pacer; HF stable; history of CVA without sequela.	1. Report R55 Syncope and collapse; Z95.Ø Presence of cardiac pacemaker; I5Ø.9 HF, Z86.73 Personal history of transient ischemic attack (TIA), and cerebral infarction without residual deficits, h/o CVA w/o residual deficit; Z6Ø.2 Problems related to living alone.
Comorbidity	1. ED record: Dizziness and syncope with fall and left ankle fracture, syncope workup negative for cause and ankle strapped.	1. Report S82.892A Other fracture of left lower leg, initial encounter for closed fracture, followed by R55 Syncope and collapse; R42 Dizziness and giddiness; and W19.XXXA Unspecified fall, initial encounter.
Complication of Care	NA	NA
Poisoning or Adverse Effect of Medication/ Chemical	1. IP Discharge Summary Discharge Note: Patient presented after two days of experiencing syncopal episodes; began new antidepressant med prior to episodes, final dx: syncope due to hypersensitivity to antidepressant med, med discharged and new med/regimen began during stay.	1. Report R55 Syncope and collapse, followed by T43.2Ø5A Adverse effect of unspecified antidepressants, initial encounter adverse effect of antidepressant.

Transient Ischemic Attack

G45.Ø	**Vertebro-basilar artery syndrome**	CC
G45.1	**Carotid artery syndrome (hemispheric)**	CC
G45.2	**Multiple and bilateral precerebral artery syndromes**	CC
G45.3	**Amaurosis fugax**	CC
G45.4	**Transient global amnesia**	
G45.8	**Other transient cerebral ischemic attacks and related syndromes**	CC
G45.9	**Transient cerebral ischemic attack, unspecified**	CC
G97.8[1,2]	**Other [intraoperative, postprocedural] complications of nervous system**	CC

Associated terminology: transient ischemic attack (unspecified); TIA; cerebral artery spasm; transient cerebral ischemic syndrome (vertebra-basilar, carotid artery); multiple/bilateral precerebral artery syndrome; amaurosis fugax; transient global amnesia; intraoperative or postoperative TIA

Discussion

Transient ischemic attack (TIA) is a brief interruption of the blood flow of an intracerebral or precerebral artery that results in temporary neurological deficits that typically last less than one hour in duration (there are prolonged episodes but they will be without infarction). The interruption is due to a thrombus, embolism, occlusion, stricture, stenosis, or spasm that quickly resolves and causes no or minimal damage to the brain tissue. A diagnosis of TIA is made by history and clinical judgment when infarction, hemorrhage, seizure, or variant migraine is ruled out. There is a high probability of cerebral infarction/hemorrhage occurring after a TIA; therefore, the workup for the cause proceeds quickly and treatment begins promptly. Identified risk factors are also treated or management is prescribed.

Documentation Tip

When documentation and clinical criteria do not match, query the provider for clarification of the diagnosis.

The TIA syndromes represent arterial insufficiency or ischemia of the specified arteries. Insufficiency is caused by thrombus, embolism, occlusion, stricture, stenosis, or spasm. Mechanisms of the causes are atherosclerosis, sudden hypotension/orthostasis, or external or internal mechanical forces that exacerbate or occlude the arteries. Vertebrobasilar artery syndrome (VBS), also known as beauty parlor syndrome, affects the posterior circulation of the brain including the brainstem, cerebellum, and occipital cortex. Review of MRI results should distinguish between VBS/TIA or brainstem infarct. Carotid artery syndrome affects the anterior circulation of the brain, the anterior two-thirds of the cerebral hemisphere, including the deep white matter and the basal ganglia. Eagle syndrome or an elongated temporal bone styloid/calcified stylohyoid ligament can impinge on the carotid artery resulting in a TIA, known as eagle-elongated styloid-carotid syndrome.

Amaurosis fugax (AF) is a sudden, transient monocular total or partial vision loss caused by retinal artery ischemia. Vasospasm due to cocaine use can result in retinal artery ischemia. AF is also seen in carotid atherosclerosis when plaque dislodges and occludes the retinal artery. It also occurs in giant cell arteritis and sickle cell anemia. Evaluation should distinguish among the differential etiologies of circulatory, ocular, and neurologic in order to determine the best management plan.

Transient global amnesia is an episode of short term memory loss that does not involve a loss of personal or familial identities. It is usually accompanied by anxiety and there are a variety of precipitating causes and mechanisms and no consistent risk factors, with the exception of a history of migraines. The duration ranges from a few minutes to 24 hours and is not accompanied by any other neurological deficits. Seizure or postictal state or trauma must be ruled out as the cause. Perseveration is a common feature.

If the TIA or syndrome is stated as due to atherosclerosis, thrombosis, embolism, obstruction, stenosis, or occlusion of a precerebral artery, assign a code from category I65 Occlusion and stenosis of precerebral arteries, not resulting in cerebral infarction, only per the Excludes 1 (Not coded here) note. Assign the symptoms as additional codes to show that it was symptomatic.

Diagnoses

Documentation Tip

Code assignment cannot be based on ancillary test results, therapies, or clinical criteria alone. A diagnosis and its clinical significance must be supported by physician or other qualified healthcare professional documentation. When it is unclear or there is contradictory information, query the physician or other qualified healthcare professional for clarification.

A TIA or syndrome due to cerebral atherosclerosis, thrombosis, embolism, obstruction, stenosis, or occlusion, should be reported from category I66 Occlusion and stenosis of cerebral arteries, not resulting in cerebral infarction, and when appropriate with a code from category G45 Transient cerebral ischemic attacks and related syndromes, per the Excludes 2 (Not included here) note under the chapter.

When there is a final comparative or contrasting diagnosis of TIA versus CVA, either TIA or CVA, or other similar terminology, and the clinical evidence is suggestive of or consistent with one more than the other, query the physician if one or the other was suspected, possible, or probable.

Documentation Tip

Complications of care: The condition must be more than a routinely expected condition or event. The documentation must support that the condition is clinically significant with an indication that it is a complication, by demonstrating:

- **A cause-and-effect relationship between the care or procedure and the condition**
- **That the condition resulted in altering the course of a procedure or surgery**

The term "complication" does not have to be explicitly documented.

Coding/Reporting Criteria	Clinical Criteria	
1. Physical Evaluation *(routine/expected in italics)*	• Symptoms with abrupt onset vary and some reflect origin (cerebral/precerebral) and area of brain affected • Neurological deficits will affect contralateral side of ischemia at hemispheric site • Symptoms last less than one hour for infarct/hemorrhage and infarct/hemorrhage on imaging; if less than one hour/transient, suspect TIA w/o infarct/hemorrhage on imaging) • Syncope • Confusion, memory loss • Altered awareness • Weakness/paresis/numbness • Hemiplegia/quadriplegia • Hemisensory loss • Gaze preference • Neurological neglect • Facial droop	• Photophobia • Stiff neck/pain • Monocular/binocular blindness (amaurosis fugax) • Blurred vision or visual field defects: homonymous hemianopia • Eye movement abnormalities (diplopia or nystagmus) • Hyperglycemia • Dysphagia • Dysarthria or difficulty understanding speech • Vertigo • Ataxia • Aphasia • Headache (worst headache of my life, thunderclap) • Nausea/vomiting • New onset seizure • Acute neurological deficit
2. Clinical Evaluation *(routine/expected in italics)*	• CBC • Platelet count • Prothrombin time test (PT)/partial thromboplastin time test (PTT) • Fasting blood glucose	• Lipid profile • Homocysteine • Erythrocyte sedimentation rate (ESR) • Other tests as warranted for specific dx workup
3. Diagnostic Px *(routine/expected in italics)*	• Neurological exam/consult • CT: after 24 hours ischemic infarct visible; initial neuroimaging • Diffusion weighted MRI: follow-up to CT, esp. when initial CT is negative • Gradient echo MRI • Angiography	• Carotid duplex ultrasonography • ECG • Transesophageal echocardiography to evaluate cardiac etiology • Eye exam for amaurosis fugax • Toxicology screening

Coding/Reporting Criteria	Clinical Criteria
4. Therapeutic Tx *(routine/expected in italics)*	• Treatment depends on the cause • IV nicardipine; labetalol • Nimodipine to prevent vasospasm • Aspirin • Tissue plasminogen activator (tPA) administration (review ED record, transferring hospital records, ICU record, or radiology report): within three (or 4.5 hrs with certain criteria) of onset • Anticoagulation for thrombosis • Antiplatelet • Treat hypertension: – mean arterial pressure (MAP) > 130 mmHg – systolic BP > 185 mm Hg • Stents with or without percutaneous angioplasty/tPA: intracerebral or precerebral artery: atherosclerotic stenosis • Mechanical thrombectomy/embolectomy: Merci Retrieval System®, with or without tPA • Endarterectomy • Angioplasty • Arterial-vein bypass graft • Supportive measures • Treatment of complications: – physical therapy/occupational therapy – speech therapy – medications to control blood pressure, glucose, seizures
5. Increased Nursing Care and/or Monitoring	• TIA develops post admit
6. Extends LOS	• TIA due to complication of care

Condition	Documentation Example	ICD-10-CM Corresponding Codes
Routine/Expected/ Integral/Inherent/ Incidental *(italics only)*	*NA*	*NA*
Principal Diagnosis	1. IP Discharge Summary: A 70-year-old female woke up with left arm numbness and vertigo, which resolved by admit; in ED suspected left facial droop and patient complained of severe headache; workup for infarct/bleed negative; final diagnosis: TIA/CVA. **(Query if clinical indicators and results of workup are consistent with [suspected/probable] TIA or CVA.)** 2. IP Discharge Summary: patient admitted with TIA symptoms, infarct ruled out; TIA workup findings of cerebral atherosclerosis.	1. Code selection determined by the query response. 2. Report G45.9 Transient cerebral ischemic attack, unspecified; I67.2 Cerebral atherosclerosis.
Comorbidity	1. Discharge Note: Admitted due to syncope and transient right arm weakness; workup was negative for cerebral infarct; symptoms possibly due to either transient ischemic attack or basilar migraine.	1. Report both G45.9 Transient cerebral ischemic attack, unspecified and G43.1Ø9 Migraine with aura, not intractable, without status migrainosus. Either can be sequenced as principal diagnosis.
Complication of Care	1. IP Order for Admit: Postcardiac catheterization/PTCA TIA, PTCA performed for left coronary atherosclerosis with unstable angina.	1. Report G97.82 Other postprocedural complications and disorders of nervous system, followed by G45.9 Transient cerebral ischemic attack, unspecified; I25.11Ø Atherosclerotic heart disease of native coronary artery with unstable angina pectoris.
Poisoning or Adverse Effect of Medication/ Chemical	1. IP Discharge Summary: A 35-year-old female admitted due to TIA induced by crack cocaine use, accidental intent.	1. Report T4Ø.5X1A Poisoning by cocaine, accidental (unintentional), initial encounter, followed by G45.9 Transient cerebral ischemic attack, unspecified.

Additional References

AHA CC: 1Q, 2022, p. 34;1Q, 2023, p. 3; 2Q, 2018, p. 9

Urinary Tract Infection (Bacterial)

N39.Ø	**Urinary tract infection, site not specified**	CC HAC
N99.89	**Other postprocedural complications and disorders of genitourinary system**	
T83.51ØA	**Infection and inflammatory reaction due to cystostomy catheter, initial encounter**	CC
T83.511A	**Infection and inflammatory reaction due to indwelling urethral catheter, initial encounter**	CC HAC
T83.512A	**Infection and inflammatory reaction due to nephrostomy catheter, initial encounter**	CC
T83.518A	**Infection and inflammatory reaction due to other urinary catheter, initial encounter**	CC HAC
T83.59-	**Infection and inflammatory reaction due to prosthetic device, implant and graft in urinary system**	CC

Associated terminology: urinary tract infection, site not specified (bacterial); urinary tract infection due: to indwelling urinary catheter (bacterial), cystostomy, nephrostomy, or other urinary catheter (bacterial); urinary tract infection due to urinary system prosthetic device, implant, graft (bacterial)

Discussion

A bacterial urinary tract infection is evidenced by significant bacteriuria of colony-forming units (CFU) of greater than or equal to 105 per mL (100,000/mL) of a single organism with or without clinical signs or symptoms of an infection. The criteria can be modified depending on age or history of urinary instrumentation. Asymptomatic bacteriuria is significant bacteria, of one bacterial species, in urine (> 105 per mL) without symptoms or other abnormal findings.

The most common gram negative organism is *Escherichia coli*, which is the most common of all organisms. Other gram negative bacteria are *Klebsiella*, *Proteus mirabilis*, and *Pseudomonas aeruginosa*. The most common gram positive organisms are group D streptococci and *Staphylococcus saprophyticus*. In hospitalized patients, other organisms can be found: *Enterobacter*, *Serratia*, *Enterococcus faecalis*, and *Staphylococcus aureus*. The code that identifies the organism from categories B95–B97 Bacterial and viral infectious agents, will be reported as an additional diagnosis to identify the organism of an infection classified elsewhere. The descriptions stated as uncomplicated or complicated are characterized as:

- Uncomplicated UTI:
  - normal, unobstructed genitourinary tract
  - no history of recent instrumentation (catheterization, cystoscopy)
  - symptoms of lower urinary tract
  - young, sexually active female, male engaging in unprotected sex
  - uncircumcised male
- Complicated UTI:
  - the presence of anatomic, functional, metabolic abnormalities
  - causes of poor bladder emptying
  - obstruction
  - urinary instrumentation (catheterization, cystoscopy)
  - seeding of infection from another site
  - age
  - gender
  - associated infection
  - polymicrobial
  - multiresistant to drugs

- Indwelling urethral catheter (Foley) associated infection (intermittent or continuous irrigation):
  - CFU ≥ 102/mL of a single or two bacterial species is predominate
  - pyuria is expected with catheter presence
- Cystostomy-catheter-associated infection:
  - CFU ≥ 102/mL of a single or two bacterial species predominate
  - pyuria is expected with catheter presence

UTI due to poor self-catheterization technique or hygiene status post urostomy is reported using N99.89 Other postprocedural complications and disorders of genitourinary system, followed by N39.Ø Urinary tract infection, site not specified, and a code from B95–B97 Bacterial and viral infectious agents, to identify the organism, when known. Include a code from category Z93 Artificial opening status, to specify the type of urostomy.

When there is evidence that the site of the UTI can be further specified as pyelonephritis, cystitis, urethritis, etc., query the provider for specificity. When a specific site is confirmed, the code for the specific site is reported instead of N39.Ø. The term "urosepsis" must be queried as to the conditions it represents, either UTI or sepsis with UTI; there is no default code assignment in ICD-10-CM.

Colonization indicates a nonpathogenic state; assign carrier status code from subcategory Z22.3 Carrier of other specified bacterial diseases, for the identified organism(s). An abnormal (positive) urine culture without definitive diagnosis or further classification is reported using code R82.7 Abnormal findings on microbiological examination of urine. Contaminate, as indicated by mixed flora, each species at low levels or low CFU (usually < 103 CFU/mL), is not reported as a UTI. Normal flora is nonpathogenic species normally found at the site. Mixed flora at low pathogen count (102 to 104 mL) should be clinically evaluated if one or two species predominate, especially in the setting of certain patient characteristics (i.e., presence of [indwelling] catheter).

Fifty percent of those with a UTI recover within a few days or weeks without treatment. When treated, regimens range from a three-day course to five to 14 days, depending on the antibiotic prescribed.

Coding Tip

Hospital-acquired condition (HAC): CMS does not allow a code to increase MS-DRG reimbursement by acting as a CC or MCC with a present on admission (POA) value of N or U. The case will be paid as though these conditions were not reported.

A workup for a UTI is performed based on signs or symptoms and then antibiotics are started. If the results rule out a UTI, report the signs or symptoms that prompted the workup, not a code for the UTI. A condition that is ruled out, regardless of initiation of treatment, is reported with the signs or symptoms or condition that prompted the workup rather than the diagnosis.

Coding Tip

Pyuria is the presence of white blood cells or pus in the urine. It often occurs in urinary tract infections, though pyuria may also be present in autoimmune disease, inflammation, kidney stones, pneumonia, and tumors in the urinary tract. Pyuria is reported with code R82.81 and is excluded from code N39.Ø. Report code R82.81 when documentation indicates pyuria in the absence of infection in the urinary tract.

Documentation Tip

The term urosepsis is not identified by any code in ICD-10-CM. A query must be generated using appropriate clinical indicators to clarify if there is a diagnosis of urinary tract infection (UTI), sepsis, or another condition, which must be documented.

Coding/Reporting Criteria	Clinical Criteria	
1. Physical Evaluation *(routine/expected in italics)*	• *Asymptomatic (elderly)* • Symptoms vary depending on site of infection • Malaise • Low blood pressure • Anorexia • Tachypnea • Fever (> 38.0C or 100.3F, new or worsening) • Chills • Dysuria/burning on urination • Polyuria or passing frequent, small amounts of urine • Suprapubic/pelvic/abdominal pain: women • Costovertebral angle percussion tenderness on infected side • Rectal pain: men • Urethral discharge: men	• Nocturia • Pneumaturia • Nausea/vomiting • Flank pain • Foul-smelling, dark urine • Hematuria (microscopic) • Delirium/change in mental or functional status (elderly) • Presence of: – urinary catheter or recent instrumentation – cystostomy – pregnancy – diabetes mellitus – age – immunocompromised state – co-condition causing obstructive uropathy
2. Clinical Evaluation *(routine/expected in italics)*	• Urinalysis: clean-catch midstream-voided or via catheter for older women or women with vaginal bleeding/discharge or needle stick of catheter, or immediately after a catheter is removed – nitrates – WBC (leukocytes): > 10 WBCs/μL – leukocyte esterase	• Urine microscopy – RBC – WBC – bacteria • Urine culture • Antibiotic sensitivity/susceptibility test • Urethral swab if STD suspected; prior to voiding • Dipstick test
3. Diagnostic Px *(routine/expected in italics)*	• Cystourethrogram • Retrograde pyelogram • Renal scan	• Ultrasound of kidneys • Cystoscopy
4. Therapeutic Tx *(routine/expected in italics)*	• *Antibiotic prophylaxis* • Antibiotics • Analgesics • Antipyretics • Anticholinergics • Urinary catheterization for retention	• Surgery to address associated condition • Replace indwelling catheter or cystostomy tube • Cranberry juice: 50 mL of concentrate or 300mL juice/daily; not for all types of patients (avoid with anticoagulant use) • Increase total fluid intake
5. Increased Nursing Care and/or Monitoring	• Post admit develops hospital-acquired infection catheter-associated urinary tract infection (HAI CAUTI)	
6. Extends LOS	• Discharge delayed due to HAI CAUTI	

Condition	Documentation Example	ICD-10-CM Corresponding Codes
Routine/Expected/ Integral/Inherent/ Incidental *(italics only)*	1. *IP Progress Note: Administer prophylactic antibiotics prior to removal of urostomy catheter.* 2. *IP Discharge Summary: Foley replaced; previous catheter colonized with coagulase-negative staph, no antibiotic treatment necessary.* 3. *IP Progress Note: Patient is on antibiotic prophylaxis for chronic recurrent UTIs, continue during admission.*	1. *Long-term (current) prophylactic drug use, report a code from category Z79 Long term (current) drug therapy; report only when relevant to the encounter.* 2. *Colonization, without infection or bacteriuria/bacteremia, report a code from subcategory Z22.3 Carrier of other specified bacterial diseases, to identify organism; report only when relevant to the encounter.* 3. *Personal history codes report past conditions that no longer exist and are not receiving treatment, but have potential of recurrence and may require continued monitoring or alter the type of treatment currently ordered; report when relevant to the encounter.*

Condition	Documentation Example	ICD-10-CM Corresponding Codes
Principal Diagnosis	1. IP Discharge Summary: *E. coli* urinary tract infection with bacteremia in a 65-year-old female; co-infections treated with IV antibiotic regimen. 2. IP Discharge Summary: A 30-year-old female admitted with fever, chills, renal colic, hematuria, nausea and vomiting: workup reveals UTI with known right ureteral calculus with hydronephrosis, third encounter; treat with IV antibiotics; schedule outpatient removal of calculus.	1. Report N39.Ø Urinary tract infection, site not specified, followed by B96.2Ø Unspecified Escherichia coli [E. coli] as the cause of diseases classified elsewhere; and R78.81 Bacteremia. 2. Report N39.Ø Urinary tract infection, site not specified, followed by N13.2 Hydronephrosis with renal and ureteral calculus obstruction.
Comorbidity	1. IP Discharge Summary: A 70-year-old female admitted with nausea/vomiting and delirium; final diagnoses: Severe dehydration, *E. coli* UTI; IV hydration; po antibiotic; po antiemetic; monitor mental status with neuro checks. 2. IP Discharge Summary: 75-year old female with sepsis and UTI. **(Query if there is a causal link between sepsis and a localized infection if the documentation is unclear or missing.)**	1. Report E86.Ø followed by N39.Ø Urinary tract infection, site not specified; and B96.2Ø Unspecified Escherichia coli [E. coli] as the cause of diseases classified elsewhere. 2. Report A41.9 Sepsis, unspecified organism, followed by N39.Ø Urinary tract infection, site not specified.
Complication of Care	1. IP Discharge Summary: A debilitated 80-year-old male admitted from long-term care facility with methicillin-resistant *Staphylococcus aureus* (MRSA) UTI with indwelling Foley related to urinary incontinence; treated with IV antibiotics, catheter exchange. **(Query if there is a relationship between the UTI and the indwelling catheter and if so, can it be further specified.)**	1. If the physician query results in a link between the catheter and the UTI, report T83.511A Infection and inflammatory reaction due to indwelling urinary catheter, initial encounter, followed by N39.Ø Urinary tract infection, site not specified, in addition to the code B95.62 Methicillin resistant Staphylococcus aureus infection as the cause of diseases classified elsewhere. (If the organism code from category B95–B97 does not specify antibiotic resistance, include a code from category Z16.) • There must be a cause-and-effect relationship between the care provided and the condition and an indication in the documentation that it is a complication unless it is listed in the alphabetic index directly under the main term; the term "with" does not qualify as a link nor describe the nature of the relationship. • UTI/bacteriuria as a complication due to or resulting from device, implant, or graft, the complication code is sequenced first followed by a code for the specific complication and manifestation.
Poisoning or Adverse Effect of Medication/ Chemical	NA	NA

Additional References

AHA CC: 2Q, 2022, p. 7; 3Q, 2020, p. 25; 4Q, 2019, p. 16; 2Q, 2018, p. 21-22; 1Q, 2018, p. 1

American Society for Microbiology, *Journal of Clinical Microbiology*: http://JCM.asm.org

CDC: https://www.cdc.gov/uti/about/cauti-basics.html; https://www.cdc.gov/uti/about/

CMS: Hospital Acquired Conditions (HAC) List
https://www.cms.gov/medicare/medicare-fee-for-service-payment/hospitalacqcond/icd10_hacs

Infectious Disease Society of America: http://www.idsociety.org/

Diagnoses

Procedures

Bone Marrow/Stem Cell Transplant

Administration/New Technology—Transfusion. Putting in blood or blood products.

3Ø2* **Administration, Circulatory, Transfusion**

XW1* **New Technology, Anatomical Regions, Transfusion**

Procedure: bone marrow or stem cell transplant (infusion)

Discussion

Not all transplant procedures are defined the same way within the PCS classification. Some are reported using the root operation Transplantation while others, such as bone marrow and stem cells, are reported using the root operation Transfusion.

Coding Guideline B3.16: Transplantation vs. Administration

> Putting in a mature and functioning living body part taken from another individual or animal is coded to the root operation Transplantation. Putting in autologous or nonautologous cells is coded to the Administration section.

As described in the guideline above, most bone marrow and stem cell transplants will be captured in the Administration (3) section. But recently developed and/or emerging therapies will be captured in the New Technology (X) section. The blood and stem cell transplant-based products currently assigned in table XW1 include Betibeglogene autotemcel, Omidubicel, OTL-103, OTL-200, Lovotibeglogene autotemcel, and Exagamglogene autotemcel.

Bone marrow or peripheral blood stem cell transplantation is a process that includes mobilization, harvesting, and transplant of bone marrow or peripheral blood stem cells and the administration of high-dose chemotherapy or radiotherapy prior to the actual transplant. The bone marrow or peripheral stem cells are harvested from either a patient's (autologous) or donor's (allogeneic) bone marrow or peripheral blood for intravenous infusion.

Harvested bone marrow is usually obtained from a large bone of the donor. The donor is given general or regional anesthesia. A large-bore needle is inserted through the skin over the pelvic (hip) bone and into the bone marrow to draw the marrow out of the bone. The harvested bone marrow is then processed to remove blood and bone fragments. Harvested bone marrow may be cryopreserved. Purging is a process to remove certain types of cells, such as cancer cells and T-lymphocytes, from stem cells prior to infusion. After the bone marrow is processed, the processed marrow is infused into the bloodstream of the recipient through an intravenous catheter.

Hematopoietic stem cells are found in the bone marrow, in the bloodstream (peripheral blood stem cells) and in umbilical cord blood. Cells from each of these sources may be used in transplants.

An autologous transplant uses the patient's own bone marrow or stem cells for the transplant, while an allogeneic transplant uses a donor's bone marrow or stem cells. For stem cell harvesting from peripheral blood, the progenitor cells are collected by apheresis, often after the donor is given a hematopoietic growth factor to mobilize progenitor cells into the bloodstream. The patient is prepared in much the same way as when giving a regular blood donation. Whole blood is drawn out of one arm and put into an instrument called a cell separator. A special column in the separator sorts out the desired cells from the other cells, with the help of computerized calibration. The stem cells are collected while the remainder of the blood is returned to the donor through a tube and needle in the other arm. More than one collection session may be required to acquire the amount needed for transplantation. Blood-derived progenitor cells may also be harvested from placental and umbilical cord blood after delivery for transplantation to the neonate later in life or to others. Cord blood is also used to treat disease because it contains stem-progenitor cells. Harvesting is usually performed immediately after delivery of the baby. After the umbilical cord is clamped and separated from the baby, the physician inserts a syringe into the umbilical cord and blood is drawn. The recipient's immune system is first suppressed using radiation or chemotherapy. The harvested cord blood stem cells are injected into the recipient by intravenous drip therapy in a sterile environment.

---

* Indicates the ICD-10-PCS table where the remainder of the code is constructed.

Documentation must state:

In order to ensure accurate code assignment, review the documentation for specific information regarding the body part (peripheral vein, central vein), and the type of bone marrow/stem cell transplant used:

- Stem cells, cord blood
- Stem cells, hematopoietic
- Stem cells, embryonic
- Stem cells, T-cell depleted hematopoietic
- Hematopoietic stem/progenitor cells, genetically modified
- Nonautologous or allogeneic transplant uses bone marrow from a donor
- Autologous transplant uses the patient's own marrow that has been stored

Allogeneic and autologous stem cell transplants are covered under Medicare for specific diagnoses only, as outlined in the national coverage determination (NCD) for stem cell transplantation. For inpatient hospital claims, these cases are assigned to:

MS-DRG 014	Allogeneic Bone Marrow Transplant
MS-DRG 016 and 017	Autologous Bone Marrow Transplant

When bone marrow or peripheral blood stem cell transplantation is covered, all the necessary steps are included in coverage. When bone marrow or peripheral blood stem cell transplantation is not covered, none of the steps are covered.

Additional References

AHA CC: 1Q, 2023, p. 12; 4Q, 2022, p. 75-76; 4Q, 2019, p. 36; 4Q, 2016, p. 113

ICD-10-PCS Reference Manual, 2016 Edition, Centers for Medicare and Medicaid Services

Medicare Claims Processing Manual, Pub. 100-04, chap. 3, sec. 90.3

National Coverage Determination (NCD) for Stem Cell Transplantation (110.23): http://www.cms.gov/medicare-coverage-database/indexes/national-and-local-indexes.aspx

Bronchoalveolar Lavage (BAL)/Bronchial Washing

Drainage. Taking or letting out fluids and/or gases from a body part, the qualifier DIAGNOSTIC is used to identify drainage procedures that are biopsies

Approach (bronchoscopy). Via natural or artificial opening endoscopic

ØB9*	**Drainage/Respiratory System**
Procedure:	bronchoalveolar lavage (BAL) for biopsy of alveoli; biopsy of the bronchial tree, bronchial washing

Discussion

Bronchoscopy with alveolar lavage, or bronchoalveolar lavage, is a diagnostic procedure that uses repeated instillation and aspiration of lavage fluid to target specific smaller airways to obtain cells and noncellular components such as airway secretions from the epithelial surface of the lower respiratory tract for microbiological, cytological or immunological analysis.

In a bronchoalveolar lavage, the airway is anesthetized with a topical anesthetic and a flexible fiberoptic or rigid bronchoscope (a long, thin tube that has a close-focusing telescope on the end for viewing) is introduced Via Natural or Artificial Opening Endoscopic approach through the nasal or oral cavity, or a tracheostomy stoma. The bronchoscope is advanced through the nasal or oral cavity, or tracheostomy stoma past the larynx to inspect the bronchus. The procedure may employ fluoroscopic guidance.

After visualizing the bronchus, the practitioner samples alveolar lung tissue by irrigating with saline in small aliquots or subsets of the total fluid volume, followed by carefully suctioning the fluid. The suctioned fluid is sent for biopsy. The bronchoscope is removed. The root operation Drainage is used for this biopsy as the intent of the procedure is to withdraw fluid rather than tissue for diagnostic purposes.

As BAL involves washing out and sampling the alveoli of the lung, the lung body part values more appropriately capture the objective of the procedure.

Bronchial washing is a diagnostic procedure that uses repeated instillation and aspiration of lavage fluid to obtain cells and noncellular components such as airway secretions from the epithelial surface of the bronchial tree for microbiological, cytological, or immunological analysis.

Both bronchoalveolar lavage (BAL) and bronchial washing biopsies are performed with the same technique. The difference between them lies with the body part that is being biopsied. While the BAL removes fluid from the alveoli, which is considered part of the lung body part, the bronchial washing is performed only through the bronchus.

Coding Tip

Use the sixth character device value No Device (Z) since there is no drainage device left in after the procedure. Use the seventh character qualifier value Diagnostic (X) to identify the biopsy for BAL and bronchial washing.

Documentation Tip

When documentation does not state bronchoalveolar lavage or BAL, but does describe the use of a bronchoscope to instill saline and obtain a biopsy, ensure that the bronchial body parts involved are identified.

Additional References

AHA CC: 3Q, 2017, p. 15; 1Q, 2017, p. 51; 1Q, 2016, p. 26

* Indicates the ICD-10-PCS table where the remainder of the code is constructed.

Procedures

Control of Hemorrhage

Control. Stopping or attempting to stop, postprocedural or other acute bleeding.

Ø93*	**Control/Ear, Nose, Sinus**
ØW3*	**Control/Anatomical Regions, General**
ØX3*	**Control/Anatomical Regions, Upper Extremities**
ØY3*	**Control/Anatomical Regions, Lower Extremities**

Procedure: (initial) (successful) control of post-op or other acute bleed/hemorrhage (not requiring a more specific root operation procedure such as bypass, detachment, excision, extraction, reposition, replacement or resection), control of epistaxis

Discussion

ICD-10-PCS defines the root operation Control as, "stopping, or attempting to stop, postprocedural or other acute bleeding." Procedures that fall under root operation Control include:

- Ligation of arterial bleeders
- Cautery or fulguration of source of bleed
- Tamponade (i.e., balloon inflation)
- Vasopressin injection or infusion
- Silver nitrate instillation, irrigation, or chemical cautery with sticks
- Oversewing
- Absorbable Hemostats (i.e., SURGICEL®, Arista ™ AH)
- Bakri balloon

The site of the bleeding is most often coded as an anatomical region and not to a specific body part. For example, control of post-tonsillectomy hemorrhage is reported with ØW33XZZ Control bleeding in oral cavity and throat, external approach. The root operation Control is also included in one other body system outside of the Anatomical Regions; the Ear, Nose, Sinus (9) body system with only the body part of Nasal Mucosa and Soft Tissue as an option.

According to ICD-10-PCS guideline B3.7: "Control is the root operation coded when the procedure performed to achieve hemostasis, beyond what would be considered integral to the procedure, utilizes techniques (e.g., cautery, application of substances or pressure, suturing, or ligation or clipping of bleeding points at the site) that are not described by a more specific root operation definition, such as Bypass, Detachment, Excision, Extraction, Reposition, Replacement, or Resection. If a more specific root operation definition applies to the procedure performed, then the more specific root operation is coded instead of control."

Examples:

Silver nitrate cautery to treat acute nasal bleeding is coded to the root operation Control.

Liquid embolization of the right internal iliac artery to treat acute hematoma by stopping blood flow is coded to the root operation Occlusion.

Suctioning of residual blood to achieve hemostasis during a transbronchial cryobiopsy is considered integral to the cryobiopsy procedure and is not coded separately.

In most instances, Control is a root operation that will primarily be captured in the Anatomical Regions, General; Anatomical Regions, Upper Extremities; and Anatomical Regions, Lower Extremities body systems. This correlates with the explanation of Control because, in general, control of bleeding is performed on a broader body area than a more specific body site.

---

* Indicates the ICD-10-PCS table where the remainder of the code is constructed.

Example:
Successful control of a postoperative abdominal wall surgical hemorrhage is coded to Control of Abdominal Wall.

Only certain methods used to attain control of postoperative or acute bleeding can be captured with the root operation Control. These methods include but are not limited to packing, pressure balloon, cautery, suture, clipping, or drainage of the operative site. If Control of a general anatomical body part is unsuccessful and another root operation is performed on a more specific body part, then that root operation and body part are reported rather than Control.

Example:
After unsuccessful control of the postoperative hemorrhaging, the incision was reopened and a damaged portion of the inferior mesenteric vein was excised and reanastomosed. In this case the more definitive procedure of Excision, Inferior Mesenteric Vein is reported.

Unless it is specified as a complication of the procedure, control of intraoperative bleeding, rather than postoperative, is integral and inherent to the procedure and should not be coded separately.

Coding Tip

In the Medical and Surgical section, the root operation Control is included in one other body system outside of the Anatomical Regions; the Ear, Nose, Sinus (9) body system. This table is used to code control of bleeding from the nose (epistaxis) using body part value Nasal Mucosa and Soft Tissue (K) except when only packing is inserted to stop the bleeding. Packing is coded in the Placement (2) section with body part value Nasal (1).

Documentation Tip

Clarify the method used to Control bleeding or hemorrhage since certain methods are reported with the root operation Control while other more specific root operation may be employed if the initial control was unsuccessful. The more specific root operation may also change the body system and body part in addition to the root operation.

Additional References

AHA CC: 3Q, 2023, p. 5, 7; 2Q, 2023, p. 26; 4Q, 2021, p. 99; 3Q, 2019, p. 4; 4Q, 2018, p. 37, 38; 1Q, 2018, p. 19; 4Q, 2017, p. 105, 106; 4Q, 2016, p. 99-100; 1Q, 2015, p. 35; 3Q, 2013, p. 22; 2Q, 2013, p. 38

Debridement by Excision (Fascia, Muscle, Bone)

Excision. Cutting out or off, without replacement, a portion of a body part.

ØJB*	**Excision/Subcutaneous Tissue and Fascia**
ØKB*	**Excision/Muscles**
ØNB*	**Excision/Head and Facial Bones**
ØPB*	**Excision/Upper Bones**
ØQB*	**Excision/Lower Bones**

Procedure: debridement by excision of fascia or muscle or bone

Discussion

Procedures

In ICD-10-PCS, the root operation Excision describes a single, precise surgical objective, defined as "cutting out or off, without replacement, a portion of a body part."

Excision is coded when a portion of a body part is cut out or off using a sharp instrument. All root operations that employ cutting to accomplish the objective allow the use of any sharp instrument, including but not limited to: scalpel, wire, scissors (cutting), bone saw, laser scalpel, and electrocautery tip.

Debridement by excision of fascia/muscle/bone tissue is the definite cutting away and removal of tissue or excising tissue that is damaged, necrotic, devitalized, dead, infected, abscessed, ischemic, or has gross contamination, or with delayed healing or nonhealing or foreign material by a sharp instrument in order to promote healing of the tissue. Debridement is carried down to viable, bleeding tissue, when impaired vascularization is not present. It can be performed in the operating room, emergency department, or at bedside by physician, nurse, physical therapist, or physician assistant. The tissue does not require pathology exam.

The use of a sharp instrument does not ensure excision; the description of the procedure stating the definite cutting away of tissue or excising tissue and identification of the sharp instrument used is the only acceptable documentation that verifies the type of debridement.

Debridement is coded to the root operation that best describes the specific objective of the procedure performed and the deepest level of tissue removed. The body system for fascia is "subcutaneous tissue and fascia"; for muscle it is "muscles"; and for bone it is "head and facial bones" or "upper bones" or "lower bones." ICD-10-PCS coding guideline A10 states the word "and" when used in a code description, means "and/or." If tissue is excised for biopsy and then debridement is performed, code both procedures, even of the same tissue, following guidelines B3.2.c and B3.4. The biopsy will have the qualifier "diagnostic."

Fascia is connective tissue that is classified three ways:

- Superficial fascia is the deepest layer of subcutaneous tissue; the galea is the superficial fascia that attaches the scalp to the skull.
- Deep fascia is dense fibrous connective tissue also known as muscle fascia; this is the layer that covers, separates, and binds the muscles, bones, nerves, blood vessels, and internal organs.
- Visceral or parietal fascia is the connective tissue membrane that surrounds and suspends organs within their cavities.

Muscle is soft tissue and has three classifications:

- Skeletal muscle is "voluntary" meaning it is under conscious control and responsible for movement and maintaining posture.
- Cardiac muscle is "involuntary" meaning it is not under conscious control and found only in the heart and surrounding the pulmonary vein and superior vena cava.
- Smooth muscle is "involuntary" meaning it is not under conscious control and is within the walls of visceral organs (hollow tube organs), blood vessels, and some other structures.

* Indicates the ICD-10-PCS table where the remainder of the code is constructed.

Bone is dense connective tissue of several types: the two osseous tissues are: compact bone and trabecular bone.

- Compact bone is dense bone that comprises the hard, smooth outer layer.
- Trabecular bone is cancellous or spongy bone that constitutes the interior of the bone, making the bone lighter and allowing room for blood vessels and marrow.

The other tissues are: marrow, endosteum, periosteum, nerves, blood vessels, and cartilage.

Documentation must state:

- The diagnosis for which the procedure is being performed
- The term(s) that describe definite excision or cutting away are "excised" or "cut away"
- State if diagnostic or therapeutic
- Identify instrument and technique used
- Location of operative site
- Depth of tissue excised by identifying the tissue type excised (skin [epidermis or dermis], subcutaneous [adipose, fat, fascia], muscle, and/or bone)
- Description or nature of tissue pathology, characteristics of wound

Query

A query is indicated when only the term "sharp" is used to describe the type of debridement or when the term "excisional" is used without further description of definite excision or cutting away and of instrument or technique used. If the tissue type or tissue depth is not clear, a query is necessary in order to assign the procedure to the correct body system. The term "soft tissue" must be queried for specific tissue type when it cannot be further determined from the record.

Terms Denoting Excision	Excision Methods
Cut away	Scalpel
Excise	Scissors (not minor removal of loose fragments)
Trimming (not minor)	Blade
Escharectomy	Surgical knife

Coding Tip

***AHA Coding Clinic*, 2Q, 2023, page 30, provides guidance when both excisional and non-excisional debridement are performed at the same site. Report only the excisional debridement, as it is the more definitive procedure, even when the non-excisional debridement is performed at a deeper level.**

Documentation Tip

According to *AHA Coding Clinic*, 3Q, 2015, pages 3 to 5, physician documentation of "excisional debridement" alone is enough to code an excisional debridement. However, as part of a CDI review, the attainment of more specific documentation is desirable to alleviate potential denials and subsequent appeals.

Axial Skeleton	
Cranial-skull 0NB*	Base: temporal, occipital, ethmoid, sphenoid, nasal sinus, Vault: parietal, frontal, orbital roof
Cranial-facial 0NB*	Nose, zygomatic, maxilla, mandible, orbital floor, vomer, palatine, lacrimal, inferior nasal conchae
Cranial-auditory ossicles 09B*	Malleus, incus, stapes (skull base)
Hyoid 0NB*	Hyoid
Chest-thoracic cage 0PB*	Sternum (manubrium, body, xiphoid), ribs
Vertebral upper: 0PB* Lower: 0QB*	Upper: cervical, thoracic Lower: lumbar, sacrum, coccyx
Appendicular Skeleton	
Upper Bones, Excision Table 0PB* Clavicle Scapula-acromial process Humerus Ulna Radius Carpals Metacarpals Phalanges-fingers, thumb	Lower Bones, Excision Table 0QB* Pelvis-ilium, pubis, ischium Femur Patella Tibia-medial/posterior malleolus Fibula-lateral malleolus Tarsals Metatarsals Phalanges-toes

* Indicates the PCS table in which the code will be located.

Procedures

Additional References

AHA CC: 2Q, 2023, p. 30; 2Q, 2020, p. 26; 3Q, 2018, p. 17; 3Q, 2016, p. 20; 3Q, 2015, p. 3-8

Debridement by Excision (Skin, Subcutaneous Tissue, Nail)

Excision. Cutting out or off, without replacement, a portion of a body part.

ØHB* **Excision/Skin and Breast**

ØJB* **Excision/Subcutaneous Tissue and Fascia**

Procedure: debridement by excision of skin or subcutaneous tissue or nail

Discussion

In ICD-10-PCS, the root operation Excision describes a single, precise surgical objective, defined as "cutting out or off, without replacement, a portion of a body part."

Excision is coded when a portion of a body part is cut out or off using a sharp instrument. All root operations that employ cutting to accomplish the objective allow the use of any sharp instrument, including but not limited to: scalpel, scissors (cutting), bone saw, laser scalpel, electrocautery tip.

Debridement by excision of skin or subcutaneous or nail tissue is the definite cutting away and removal of tissue or excising tissue of a wound/ulcer that is damaged, necrotic, devitalized, dead, infected, abscessed, burned, ischemic, has gross contamination, slough, eschar, with delayed or nonhealing or foreign material by a sharp instrument in order to promote healing of the wound. Debridement is carried down to viable, bleeding tissue, when impaired vascularization is not present. It can be performed in the operating room, emergency department, or at bedside by physician, nurse, physical therapist, or physician assistant. The tissue does not require a pathology exam.

The use of a sharp instrument does not ensure excision; the description of the procedure stating the definite cutting away of tissue or excising tissue and identification of the sharp instrument used is the only acceptable documentation that verifies the type of debridement.

Debridement is coded to the root operation that best describes the specific objective of the procedure performed and the deepest level of tissue removed. The body system for skin is "skin and breast" and for subcutaneous tissue is "subcutaneous tissue and fascia." ICD-10-PCS coding guideline A10 states the word "and" when used in a code description, means "and/or." If tissue is excised for biopsy and then debridement is performed, code both procedures, even of the same tissue, following guidelines B3.2.c.and B3.4.

Skin (integument) is composed of two layers: the epidermis and dermis. The following describes the contents of skin:

- Epidermis: contains no blood vessels
- Dermis: connective tissue that has nerve endings, hair follicles, eccrine sweat glands, sebaceous glands, apocrine sweat glands, lymphatic vessels, nails and blood vessels

The subcutaneous tissue, also called the hypodermis or subcutis, contains the adipose (fat), connective tissue and fascia, which overlie the muscle. It contains superficial blood vessels and cutaneous nerves.

Documentation must state:

- The term that describes definite excision/cutting away: excised or cut away
- State if diagnostic (biopsy) or therapeutic
- Identify instrument and technique used
- Site of wound
- Depth of tissue excised by identifying the tissue type excised (skin [epidermis/dermis], subcutaneous [adipose, fat, fascia], muscle and/or bone)
- Description or nature of tissue pathology, characteristics of wound

* Indicates the ICD-10-PCS table where the remainder of the code is constructed.

Procedures

Query

A query is indicated when only the term "sharp" is used to describe the type of debridement or when the term "excisional" is used without further description of definite excision or cutting away, of instrument, or technique used. If the tissue type or tissue depth is not clear, a query is necessary in order to assign the procedure to the correct body system. The term "soft tissue" must be queried for specific tissue type when it cannot be further determined from the record.

Coding Tip

***AHA Coding Clinic*, 2Q, 2023, page 30, provides guidance when excisional and non-excisional debridement is performed at the same site. Report only the excisional debridement, as it is the more definitive procedure, even when the non-excisional debridement was performed at a deeper level.**

Documentation Tip

According to *AHA Coding Clinic*, 3Q, 2015, page 3 to 5, physician documentation of "excisional debridement" alone is enough to code an excisional debridement. However, as part of a CDI review, the attainment of more specific documentation is desirable to alleviate potential denials and subsequent appeals.

Terms Denoting Excision	Excision Methods
Cut away	Scalpel
Excise	Scissors (not minor removal of loose fragments)
Trimming (not minor)	Blade
Escharectomy	Surgical knife

Additional References

AHA CC: 2Q, 2023, p. 30; 1Q, 2018, p. 14; 3Q, 2015, p. 3-8

Debridement by Extraction (Muscle, Bone)

Extraction. Pulling or stripping out or off all or a portion of a body part by the use of force.

ØKD*	**Extraction/Muscle**
ØND*	**Extraction/Head and Facial Bones**
ØPD*	**Extraction/Upper Bones**
ØQD*	**Extraction/Lower Bones**

Procedure: debridement by extraction of muscle or bone

Discussion

Debridement by extraction is the pulling, stripping or scraping of tissue by force of a wound or tissue that is damaged, necrotic, devitalized, dead, infected, abscessed, burned, and ischemic, has gross contamination, or with delayed healing or nonhealing or foreign material by instrumentation in order to promote healing of the wound. Debridement is carried down to viable, bleeding tissue, when impaired vascularization is not present. It can be performed in the operating room, emergency department, or at bedside by physician, nurse, physical therapist, or physician assistant. The tissue does not require pathology exam.

The description of the procedure stating the technique or method used to remove tissue, identification of the instrument used, and depth of tissue involved are the only acceptable documentation that verify the type of debridement. The use of the terms "excisional" or "nonexcisional" alone are not adequate documentation.

Extraction is coded when the method employed to take out the body part is pulling, or stripping (scraping). Minor cutting, (such as trimming of loose fragments in non-excisional debridement) is included in Extraction if the objective of the procedure is met by pulling or stripping.

Non-excisional debridement is coded to Extraction. Examples of procedures coded as extraction include forceps removal of devitalized tissue, scraping with a scalpel or other sharp instrument, trimming of loose tissue fragments, and scrubbing.

Debridement is coded to the root operation that best describes the specific objective of the procedure performed and the deepest level of tissue removed. If tissue is excised for biopsy and then debridement is performed, code both procedures, even of the same tissue, following guidelines B3.2.c and B3.4. The biopsy will have the qualifier "diagnostic."

Muscle (deep fascia) is soft tissue and has three classifications:

- Skeletal muscle is "voluntary" meaning it is under conscious control and responsible for movement and maintaining posture.
- Cardiac muscle is "involuntary" meaning it is not under conscious control and found only in the heart and surrounding the pulmonary vein and superior vena cava.
- Smooth muscle is "involuntary" meaning it is not under conscious control and is within the walls of visceral organs (hollow tube organs), blood vessels, and some other structures.

Bone is dense connective tissue of several types. The two osseous tissues are compact bone and trabecular bone. Their features are as follows:

- Compact bone is dense bone that makes up the hard, smooth outer layer.
- Trabecular bone is cancellous or spongy bone that constitutes the interior of the bone, making the bone lighter and allowing room for blood vessels and marrow.

The other tissues are marrow, endosteum, periosteum, nerves, blood vessels, and cartilage.

* Indicates the ICD-10-PCS table where the remainder of the code is constructed.

Documentation must state:

- The diagnosis for which the procedure is being performed
- The term that describes the pulling, stripping, or scraping to remove tissue
- Approach
- Instrument and technique used
- Location of operative site
- Depth of tissue destroyed by identifying the tissue type treated (skin [epidermis/dermis], subcutaneous [adipose, fat, fascia], muscle and/or bone)
- Description or nature of tissue pathology, characteristics of wound

Query

A query is indicated when the description of the type of debridement is unclear or without further description of instrument or technique used. If the tissue type or tissue depth is not clear, a query is necessary in order to assign the procedure to the correct body system. The term "soft tissue" must be queried for specific tissue type when it cannot be further determined from the record.

Terms Denoting Extraction	Methods
abrasion, avulsion, brushing, curettage, decortication, dermabrasion, ligature, mechanical, neurexeresis, paring, phacoemulsification, phlebectomy, removal, scraping, shaving, snipping (minor), stripping, suction curettage	curette, forceps, suction device, Arobella Qoustic Wound Therapy System™, scissors (minor removal of loose fragments), rongeur, Versa Jet

Additional References

AHA CC: 4Q, 2017, pp. 41–42; 3Q, 2016, pp. 20–22; 3Q, 2015, pp. 3–8

Debridement by Extraction (Skin, Subcutaneous Tissue and Fascia, Nail)

Extraction. Pulling or stripping out or off all or a portion of a body part by the use of force.

ØHD*	**Extraction/Skin and Breast**
ØJD*	**Extraction/Subcutaneous Tissue and Fascia**

Procedure: debridement by extraction of skin or subcutaneous tissue or nail

Discussion

Debridement by extraction of skin or subcutaneous or nail tissue is the pulling, stripping, or scraping of tissue by force of a wound or ulcer that is damaged, necrotic, devitalized, dead, infected, abscessed, burned, ischemic, has gross contamination, slough, eschar, with delayed or nonhealing or foreign material by a instrumentation in order to promote healing of the wound. Debridement is carried down to viable, bleeding tissue, when impaired vascularization is not present. It can be performed in the operating room, emergency department, or at bedside by physician, nurse, physical therapist, or physician assistant. The tissue does not require pathology exam.

The description of the procedure stating the technique/method used to remove tissue, identification of the instrument used, and depth of the tissue involvement are the only acceptable documentation that verify the type of debridement. The terms "excisional" or "nonexcisional" alone are not adequate documentation.

Extraction is coded when the method employed to take out the body part is pulling, or stripping (scraping). Minor cutting, (such as trimming of loose fragments in non-excisional debridement) is included in Extraction if the objective of the procedure is met by pulling or stripping.

Non-excisional debridement is coded to Extraction. Examples of procedures coded as extraction include: forceps removal of devitalized tissue, scraping with a scalpel or other sharp instrument, trimming of loose tissue fragments, and scrubbing.

Debridement is coded to the root operation that best describes the specific objective of the procedure performed and the deepest level of tissue removed. The body system for skin is "skin and breast" and for subcutaneous tissue is "subcutaneous tissue and fascia." ICD-10-PCS coding guideline A10 states the word "and" when used in a code description, means "and/or." If tissue is excised for biopsy and then debridement is performed, code both procedures, even of the same tissue, following guidelines B3.2.c and B3.4.

Skin (integument) is composed of two layers: the epidermis and dermis. The following describes the contents of skin:

- Epidermis: contains no blood vessels
- Dermis: connective tissue that has nerve endings, hair follicles, eccrine sweat glands, sebaceous glands, apocrine sweat glands, lymphatic vessels, nails and blood vessels

The subcutaneous layer, also called the hypodermis or subcutis, contains adipose (fat), connective tissue and fascia, which overlie the muscle. It contains superficial blood vessels and cutaneous nerves.

Fascia is connective tissue that is classified three ways:

- Superficial fascia is the deepest layer of subcutaneous tissue; the galea is the superficial fascia that attaches the scalp to the skull.
- Deep fascia is dense fibrous connective tissue also known as muscle fascia; this is the layer that covers; separates; and binds the muscles, bones, nerves, blood vessels, and internal organs.
- Visceral or parietal fascia is the connective tissue membrane that surrounds and suspends organs within their cavities.

* Indicates the ICD-10-PCS table where the remainder of the code is constructed.

Documentation must state:

- The term that describes the pulling, stripping, or scraping to remove tissue
- Identify instrument and technique used
- Site of wound
- Depth of tissue removed by identifying the tissue type removed (skin [epidermis/dermis], subcutaneous [adipose, fat, fascia], muscle, and/or bone)
- Description or nature of tissue pathology, characteristics of wound

Query

A query is indicated when the description of the type of debridement is unclear or without further description of instrument or technique used. If the tissue type or tissue depth is not clear, a query is necessary in order to assign the procedure to the correct body system. The term "soft tissue" must be queried for specific tissue type when it cannot be further determined from the record.

Terms Denoting Extraction	Methods
abrasion, avulsion, brushing, curettage, decortication, dermabrasion, ligature, mechanical, neurexeresis, paring, phacoemulsification, phlebectomy, removal, scraping, shaving, snipping (minor), stripping, suction curettage	curette, forceps, suction device, Arobella Qoustic Wound Therapy System™, scissors (minor removal of loose fragments), rongeur, Versa Jet

Additional References

AHA CC: 1Q, 2023, p. 36; 4Q, 2019, p. 30; 3Q, 2016, p. 20-22; 1Q, 2016, p. 40; 3Q, 2015, p. 3-8; 1Q, 2015, p. 23

Fusion, Spinal

Fusion. Joining together portions of an articular body part rendering the articular body part immobile. The body part is joined together by fixation device, bone graft, or other means.

ØRG1*	**Fusion/Cervical Vertebral Joint**
ØRG2*	**Fusion/Cervical Vertebral Joints, 2 or more**
ØRG4*	**Fusion/Cervicothoracic Vertebral Joint**
ØRG6*	**Fusion/Thoracic Vertebral Joint**
ØRG7*	**Fusion/Thoracic Vertebral Joints, 2 to 7**
ØRG8*	**Fusion/Thoracic Vertebral Joints, 8 or more**
ØRGA*	**Fusion/Thoracolumbar Vertebral Joint**
ØSGØ*	**Fusion/Lumbar Vertebral Joint**
ØSG1*	**Fusion/Lumbar Vertebral Joints, 2 or more**
ØSG3*	**Fusion/Lumbosacral Joint**
ØSG5*	**Fusion/Sacrococcygeal Joint**
XRGA*	**Fusion/Thoracolumbar Vertebral Joint**
XRGB*	**Fusion/Lumbar Vertebral Joint**
XRGC*	**Fusion/Lumbar Vertebral Joints, 2 or more**
XRGD*	**Fusion/Lumbosacral Joint**

Procedure: occipital-cervical fusion, cervical fusion, cervicothoracic fusion, thoracic fusion, thoracolumbar fusion, lumbar fusion, lumbosacral fusion, anterior lumbar interbody fusion (ALIF), anteromedial (Smith-Robinson), extreme lateral interbody fusion (XLIF), direct lateral interbody fusion (DLIF), transpsoas interbody fusion, posterior or posterolateral fusion, posterior lumbar interbody fusion (PLIF), transforaminal lumbar interbody fusion (TLIF), axial lumbar interbody fusion (AxiaLIF), 360° fusion

Discussion

Spinal fusion, also known as spinal arthrodesis, fuses together one or more vertebral joints with bone graft, allograft implants or dowels, graft-filled titanium cages, or spacers, and in some cases is supplemented by screws, plates, and rods. Spinal arthrodesis may be performed to treat conditions such as herniated discs or degenerative, traumatic, or congenital lesions; or to stabilize fractures or dislocations of the spine. Codes identify the specific body parts for a single vertebral joint or multiple vertebral joints at each spine level where the procedure is performed (cervical, thoracic, or lumbar), the approach, and the spinal column fused (anterior, posterior) as well as devices.

* Indicates the ICD-10-PCS table where the remainder of the code is constructed.

Procedures

Coding Tip

Additional Procedures:

Plates, screws, and rods are often inserted to stabilize the fusion. These are considered inherent to the fusion procedure and are not reported separately.

Report separately any diskectomy performed—Excision for partial disc and Resection for total disc.

Laminectomy or Foraminotomy is only reported as an additional procedure if performed specifically for decompression of spinal nerve root or spinal cord (root operation Release). It is not reported if it is performed in order to access the site of the fusion.

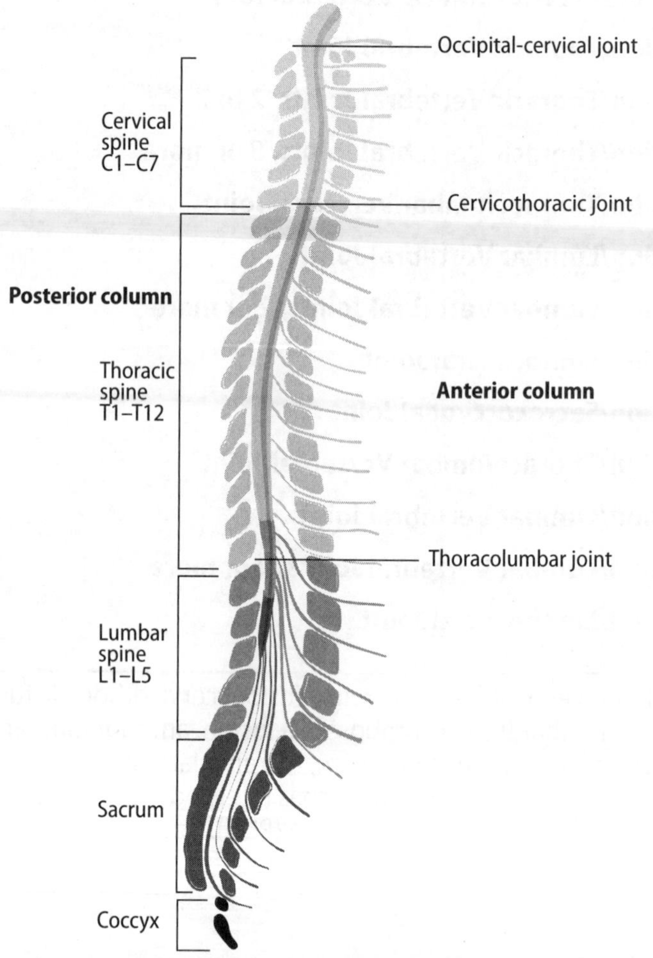

Body Part

The body part values identify the location and number of vertebral joints that are being fused. Several specific body part values (character 4) are provided in the fusion tables in order to identify whether a single joint, multiple joints, or a single joint that spans two anatomically different spinal levels are fused. Documentation must be specific to the precise vertebrae being fused.

Procedures

Approach

The approach value in the fifth-character position represents the method by which the vertebral joint was accessed and includes the choices of Open (Ø), Percutaneous (3), and Percutaneous Endoscopic (4).

Documentation Tip

Since the term "minimally invasive surgery" is not a specific PCS approach—it is vital that the description of the approach used is detailed and specific in order for the coder to discern the correct approach. For example, was it performed with tubular retractors and channels guided with the use of external fluoroscopy (Percutaneous) or were cameras/scopes inserted internally (Percutaneous endoscopic) to visualize the site? Was the site visualized and accessed using incisions that were smaller than traditional incisions (Open)?

Device

The device value supplies the type of device used to render the joint immobile. Because several different types of material can be used, alone or together, but only one device value per code can be assigned, guideline B3.10c provides a hierarchy of these materials to assist in proper code assignment. Interbody fusion devices are referred to as implants, cages or bone dowels and are only used to fuse the anterior column but can be placed via anterior, lateral, or posterior approach. Autologous tissue substitute also referred to as autograft is comprised from bone material taken from the patient's own body. Bone graft material may be bone chips obtained from the surrounding vertebra during the approach, also referred to as locally harvested bone graft. Alternatively, it may be harvested from a remote site, usually the iliac crest, through a separate incision. Nonautologous tissue substitute is often referred to as allograft which is cadaver bone obtained from a tissue bank. It is often mixed with demineralized bone substitute or bone morphogenetic proteins (BMP). Allograft is only coded if used without any autograft or interbody fusion device. There is no option for No Device for the spinal joint body parts in the Fusion tables as a spinal fusion requires graft material to be considered a fusion.

Coding Tip

Use the following hierarchy list when multiple devices are used. Devices are listed below from highest to lowest. Code to the highest value used.

- **Interbody Fusion Device (with bone graft or bone graft substitute)**
- **Autologous Tissue Substitute (alone or with nonautologous and/or with synthetic material)**
- **Nonautologous Tissue Substitute (alone or with synthetic)**
- **Synthetic Tissue Substitute**

When multiple vertebral joints are fused, each vertebral joint that uses a different device and/or a different qualifier is coded separately. (ICD-10-PCS Guidelines B3.10b and B3.10c.)

Coding and Documentation Tip

Two interbody fusion devices, nanotextured surface and radiolucent porous, have been removed from table XRG in the New Technology section. These devices should be coded in the Medical and Surgical section (Ø) using the device value Interbody Fusion Device (A) in the Fusion tables ØRG and ØSG.

Qualifier

For fusion codes created from the Medical and Surgical (Ø) section, the word "approach" is also used in the seventh-character qualifier value, referring to the anatomical access and fusion point. The qualifier values identify whether the anterior or posterior side of the spinal column was fused and whether the fusion was accomplished using an anterior or posterior approach. When the access is performed laterally (on the side), it is considered an anterior approach.

Documentation Tip

If both the anterior and posterior columns are fused in the same operative session, it is imperative that the documentation indicates if two separate incisions were made such as a posterior and anterior or posterior and lateral incision. This is often referred to as a 360° fusion. A fusion of both the anterior and posterior column performed using two separate incisions groups to a different DRG than one that is performed through a single incision.

Procedures

Coding Tip

In 360° fusion, both the anterior and posterior columns are fused. It is important to report with the appropriate qualifier (seventh character) whether these were performed using two separate incisions:

- **Anterior approach, anterior column (Ø), and**
- **Posterior approach, posterior column (1)**

Or through a single incision:

- **Posterior approach, anterior column (J), and**
- **Posterior approach, posterior column (1)**

Look for documentation noting that the patient was repositioned (e.g., from prone to supine). In some cases, a different surgeon may assist on one of the approaches (usually anterior).

The following table shows several common fusion techniques which are often referred to by their acronym. Note that all of these procedures use an interbody fusion device which can ONLY be used to fuse the anterior column of the spine.

Procedure	Approach	Device	Qualifier
ALIF—anterior lumbar interbody fusion	Supine, access front with open approach	Interbody fusion device	(0) Anterior approach Anterior column
AxiaLif—axial lumbar interbody fusion	On L5–S1—most often percutaneous with dilator tubes inserted in 1" incision by coccyx	Interbody fusion device	(J) Posterior approach Anterior column
DLIF—direct lateral interbody fusion	Lateral through side, more likely open approach although can be percutaneous or percutaneous endoscopic. Review carefully!	Interbody fusion device	(0) Anterior approach Anterior column
PLIF—posterior lumbar interbody fusion	Prone, access in back with open approach	Interbody fusion device	(J) Posterior approach Anterior column
TLIF—transforaminal lumbar interbody fusion	Prone position removal of facet joint to access through foramen—open approach	Interbody fusion device	(J) Posterior approach Anterior column
XLIF—Extreme lateral interbody fusion	Lateral through side, most likely to be percutaneous or percutaneous endoscopic. Review carefully!	Interbody fusion device	(0) Anterior approach Anterior column

Documentation must state:

- Patient positioning—where on the body the incision was made. Supine indicates anterior approach, prone indicates posterior approach, retroperitoneal or platysma muscle incision indicates lateral which is reported as anterior approach.
- Each level fused using the precise anatomical vertebrae involved
- Whether a device or graft material was used in EACH level. Root operation Fusion is reported only if an interbody fusion device/bone graft/allograft is used.
- The type of device or material used in each level of the fusion (e.g., interbody fusion device in L2–L3 but only autograft in L4–L5)
- For autograft used, it should state whether it is taken locally (from fusion site) or from a different operative site (e.g., iliac crest). Report an additional code for any autograft harvested from a different surgical location.
- Terms that describe the approach used—incision, channels, scopes
- Which column was fused—words such as vertebral body or disc space indicate anterior; terms such as vertebral foramen, spinal process, lamina, facets indicate posterior column.

Additional References

AHA CC: 2Q 2023, p. 25; 3Q, 2022, p. 21; 4Q, 2021, p. 68; 3Q, 2021, p. 25; 1Q, 2021, p. 53; 4Q, 2020, p. 93; 1Q, 2020, p. 33; 3Q, 2019, p. 35; 2Q, 2019, p. 19; 4Q, 2018, p. 43; 1Q, 2018, p. 22; 4Q, 2017, p. 76; 2Q, 2017, p. 23; 2Q, 2014, p. 7; 1Q, 2013, pp. 21–23, 29

Joint Replacement, Hip, Total, Partial, Revision and Spacers

Insertion. Putting in a nonbiological appliance that monitors, assists, performs, or prevents a physiological function but does not physically take the place of a body part.

Replacement. Putting in or on a biological or synthetic material that physically takes the place and/or function of all or a portion of a body part.

The body part may have been taken out or replaced, or may be taken out, physically eradicated, or rendered nonfunctional during the REPLACEMENT procedure. A REMOVAL procedure is coded for taking out the device used in a previous replacement procedure.

Removal. Taking out or off a device from a body part.

Revision. Correcting, to the extent possible, a portion of a malfunctioning device or the position of a displaced device.

ØSHB*	**Insertion/Hip Joint, Left**
ØSH9*	**Insertion/Hip Joint, Right**
ØSPE*	**Removal/Hip Joint, Acetabular Surface, Left**
ØSPA*	**Removal/Hip Joint, Acetabular Surface, Right**
ØSPS*	**Removal/Hip Joint, Femoral Surface, Left**
ØSPR*	**Removal/Hip Joint, Femoral Surface, Right**
ØSPB*	**Removal/Hip Joint, Left**
ØSP9*	**Removal/Hip Joint, Right**
ØSRE*	**Replacement/Hip Joint, Acetabular Surface, Left**
ØSRA*	**Replacement/Hip Joint, Acetabular Surface, Right**
ØSRS*	**Replacement/Hip Joint, Femoral Surface, Left**
ØSRR*	**Replacement/Hip Joint, Femoral Surface, Right**
ØSRB*	**Replacement/Hip Joint, Left**
ØSR9*	**Replacement/Hip Joint, Right**
ØSWE*	**Revision/Hip Joint, Acetabular Surface, Left**
ØSWA*	**Revision/Hip Joint, Acetabular Surface, Right**
ØSWS*	**Revision/Hip Joint, Femoral Surface, Left**
ØSWR*	**Revision/Hip Joint, Femoral Surface, Right**
ØSWB*	**Revision/Hip Joint, Left**
ØSW9*	**Revision/Hip Joint, Right**

Procedure:	total hip replacement, hip arthroplasty, partial hip replacement, hemiarthroplasty, replacement of acetabular surface, replacement of femoral surface, hip joint revision, insertion of articulating (antibiotic) or static (antibiotic) spacer, removal of articulating (antibiotic) or static (antibiotic) spacer

* Indicates the ICD-10-PCS table where the remainder of the code is constructed.

Procedures

Discussion

Hip replacement surgery is a reconstructive procedure performed on patients with painful hips due to osteoarthritis, rheumatoid arthritis, hip fracture, avascular necrosis/osteonecrosis, and bone tumors.

Surgeons often refer to a total hip replacement as a total arthroplasty and a partial hip replacement as a hemiarthroplasty. A total hip arthroplasty includes replacement of the femoral surface and the acetabulum, while a partial hip arthroplasty is the replacement of only the femoral or acetabular surface. The root operation Replacement is reported for a total or partial hip arthroplasty and includes any explantation or excision of the body part being replaced. Since the body parts in PCS are specific to right or left side, laterality is an important factor in the operative documentation.

The total or partial joint body parts are replaced with a prosthetic joint, which can be constructed from a variety of materials that make up the new bearing surface. The device, which is referred to as a synthetic substitute, is identified with the device value (character six) which specifies the type of material(s) used:

Total arthroplasty

- Synthetic Substitute, Metal
- Synthetic Substitute, Metal on Polyethylene
- Synthetic Substitute, Ceramic
- Synthetic Substitute, Ceramic on Polyethylene
- Synthetic Substitute, Oxidized Zirconium on Polyethylene
- Synthetic Substitute

Partial, Acetabular Surface

- Synthetic Substitute, Polyethylene
- Synthetic Substitute, Metal
- Synthetic Substitute, Ceramic
- Synthetic Substitute

Partial, Femoral Surface

- Synthetic Substitute, Metal
- Synthetic Substitute, Ceramic
- Synthetic Substitute

A cemented joint replacement uses epoxy cement to attach the joint to the bone. An uncemented joint prosthesis contains holes on its surface that allows the growth of the patient's natural bone to hold the device in place. The qualifier value (character seven) identifies whether the joint was cemented or uncemented with the value of No Qualifier (Z) is for use when documentation is insufficient to determine whether the synthetic joint prothesis is cemented or uncemented.

Documentation Tip

If the following information is not included in the operative report documentation, a query may be necessary to clarify:

- **Site and laterality of the joint replacement—total, acetabular or femoral surface only**
- **Type of material used in the bearing surface**
- **Cemented or uncemented**

Coding Tip

In cases of significant bone loss, additional support may be required to secure a hip replacement. In these cases, it is appropriate to report an additional code for any Supplement procedure performed, as well as any autograft harvest from a different surgical location. Autograft tissue harvested from the operative site, however, is not reported separately, according to ICD-10-PCS guideline B3.9.

Documentation Tip

The joint device may be removed and replaced with a new device, due to any number of reasons such as loosening, malfunction, wearing, fracture, error, pain. Although the operative report may refer to the procedure as a revision, the appropriate ICD-10-PCS root operations for reporting this procedure are Removal (of device) and Replacement. No query is necessary to clarify this language, as it is the coder's responsibility to determine what the documentation in the medical record equates to in the PCS definitions. (Official Coding Guideline A11)

Documentation Tip

Compared with traditional hip implants for hip replacement, a dual-mobility implant provides an additional bearing surface. A large polyethylene plastic femoral head fits inside a polished metal hip acetabular component, and an additional smaller metal or ceramic femoral head component is snap-fit within the polyethylene head. While there is no code to specifically capture dual-mobility hip replacements, in ICD-10-PCS coding the bearing surface reported is where the replacement femoral head meets the replacement acetabular socket. In the dual-mobility implant, the polyethylene femoral head bearing surface meets the metal acetabular socket, so the appropriate device value is 2 for metal on polyethylene. See *AHA Coding Clinic for ICD-10-CM*, third quarter 2020, page 33.

Coding Tip

The root operation Revision refers only to minor readjusting of a displaced device or correcting a malfunction by replacing a component such as a screw or pin, or recementing a loosened hip prosthesis without removing any of the components. It does not refer to the removal and replacement of the joint prosthesis or spacer.

Spacers

It is possible for the newly inserted prosthesis to develop infection. In this circumstance, it may be necessary to remove the total prosthesis and insert a temporary spacer filled with antibiotic which may need to be left in place for a period of months. There are two types of antibiotic spacers in the PCS classification:

- Spacer—this denotes a static spacer made from cement during the procedure that keeps the space open between the bones while treating the area with antibiotics but does not allow for joint movement. Available only in root operations Insertion and Removal table.
- Articulating spacer—These premade spacers which can be made of a variety of substances and include plastic or metal surfaces, allow for joint movement in addition to keeping the open space between bones and antibiotic treatment. Available only in root operations Replacement and Removal.

Since it is the device, not the body part that is now being replaced, two codes are needed. One code is reported for the removal of the prosthetic device, with the root operation Removal, the body part value of the original body part that the prosthesis replaced, and device value of synthetic substitute.

Another code is reported for the insertion of the static (antibiotic) spacer using root operation Insertion or in the case of an articulating (antibiotic) spacer, root operation Replacement. Replacement is used for the articulating spacer since it is more able to physically replace and perform the function of the joint.

After the infection is cleared, the spacer is removed and a new prosthesis is implanted. This is reported with two codes, one with the root operation of Removal and device value of Spacer or Articulating Spacer and the other with the root operation Replacement of the new prosthetic device with its appropriate device value. Although surgeons often refer to these staged procedures as an arthroplasty revision, the root operation Revision is not used.

Documentation Tip

It is important to clarify whether an articulating spacer or static spacer was used for the procedure as the function and cost of the articulating spacer is significantly different than a static spacer. An articulating spacer can often remain in place for years possibly saving the patient from further surgery. Different combinations of hip replacement and revision procedures, including those with articulating spacers and static spacers group to multiple different MS-DRGs with varying levels of reimbursement.

Additional References

AHA CC: 1Q, 2022, p. 39; 3Q, 2020, p. 33; 4Q, 2018, pp. 43–44; 4Q, 2017, pp. 38–39; 4Q, 2016, pp. 110–112; 3Q, 2016, p. 35; 3Q, 2015, p.18; 1Q, 2015, p. 30

Procedures

PICC/Central Venous Catheter/Vascular Access Device Insertion

Insertion. Putting in a nonbiological appliance that monitors, assists, performs or prevents a physiological function, but does not physically take the place of a body part.

Ø2HV*	**Insertion/Heart and Great Vessels/Superior Vena Cava**
Ø2H6*	**Insertion/Heart and Great Vessels/Right Atrium**
ØJH6ØWZ	**Insertion of Totally Implantable Vascular Access Device into Chest Subcutaneous Tissue and Fascia, Open Approach**
ØJH6[Ø,3]XZ	**Insertion of Tunneled Vascular Access Device into Chest Subcutaneous Tissue and Fascia, [Open, Percutaneous] Approach**

Procedure: peripherally-inserted central catheter (PICC), central venous catheter (CVC), vascular access device (VAD), nontunneled or tunneled, totally implantable vascular access device (TIVAD)

Discussion

Central venous catheter (CVC) lines or central venous access devices (CVAD) are for long-term use and may be inserted into the internal jugular vein of the neck, the subclavian vein in the upper chest under the clavicle, the femoral vein in the leg, groin, or the inferior vena cava. The CVC line terminates at or near to the heart in the superior vena cava, the right atrium or the cavoatrial junction that lies between them. The body part reported for the central (venous) catheter (CVC) insertion is the area where the tip resides—not the insertion site. CVC lines can have one, two, three, or more ports that can connect to IV tubing, medications, or monitors. Nontunneled catheters are inserted percutaneously, directly into a vein and are secured at the insertion site. Some are surgically tunneled under the skin, then into the vein to emerge at a distal exit site where they are secured. Procedures such as these are performed in the operating room or interventional radiology procedural suite.

A totally implanted venous access device (TIVAD) is a type of vascular access device (VAD) with a port that is implanted in a pocket created in the subcutaneous tissue. In a TIVAD, no part of the catheter system is brought out through the skin. Access to the vein is through skin puncture, via a special needle (Huber). VADs are used for blood sampling, medication administration, fluid administration, total parenteral nutrition (TPN), dialysis, transfusions, chemotherapy, cardiovascular, and fluid status monitoring.

Coding and Documentation Tip

Review the documentation for correct assignment of the ICD-10-PCS sixth character for device. Incorrect device reporting can lead to inappropriate reimbursement. Central venous and peripheral venous lines are generally not reported with sixth characters Ø Monitoring Device, Pressure Sensor, 2 Monitoring Device, D Intraluminal Device, or Y Other Device.

Common uses of central venous catheters or central lines are for medication and fluid administration. This is reported with device character 3 Infusion Device.

Common uses for PICC lines are chemotherapy, extended drug regimens such as antibiotics, and total parenteral nutrition (TPN). This is also reported with device character 3 Infusion Device.

* Indicates the ICD-10-PCS table where the remainder of the code is constructed.

Coding Tip

Vascular access device (VAD) is a broad category that includes both tunneled and nontunneled venous catheters and implantable ports. When coding a tunneled central venous catheter (CVAD) or totally implantable port (TIVAD) device, two codes are required, one code from table Ø2H Insertion Heart and Great Vessels, identifies the body part where the tip of the central line catheter resides (V Superior Vena Cava/6 Right Atrium) and the type of device (3 Infusion Device). The other code assigned, from table ØJH, identifies the Insertion of the access device into the Subcutaneous Tissue and Fascia, usually in the Chest, body part value 6. The device character from this table distinguishes between the tunneled and nontunneled device: The device value W Vascular Access Device, Totally Implantable, is reported for the TIVAD while the tunneled CVAD is represented by X Vascular Access Device, Tunneled.

A PICC is a CVC with entry sites usually in the superficial veins of the arms, legs, feet or hands or head, such as basilic or cephalic vein and terminates in the superior vena cava, the right atrium or the cavoatrial junction that lies between them. The body part reported for the peripherally inserted central (venous) catheter (PICC) insertion is the area where the tip resides—not the insertion site. Since these are often inserted by nurses, it is important to review nursing documentation for capture of this procedure in the documentation.

Peripherally inserted venous access device catheters (PVC) or midline catheters are inserted into peripheral veins of the hand or forearm and terminate before the level of the axillary line; therefore, they are considered short peripheral intravenous catheters, usually less than three inches for PVC and three to eight inches for midline. They perform the same functions as CVCs.

One way to distinguish a short PVC from a CVC is where the line terminates; the end placement of PVCs does not extend to the heart or enter the central veins. End placement of these types of catheters is reported with a code from table Ø5H Insertion, Upper Veins, with body part value corresponding to the body part with the end placement of the catheter.

Examples of CVCs/CVADs are:

- Cordis catheters
- Hickman® catheters
- BROVIAC® catheters
- GROSHONG® catheters
- Triple lumen catheters
- Double lumen catheters
- PICC
- Quinton™ catheter
- Umbilical venous catheter

Examples of TIVADs are:

- PORT-A-CATH®
- BardPort
- Infusaport
- Medi-port
- P.A.S. Port® peripheral vascular access system

Physicians must document, in the operative report, the intended use of the catheter and the anatomical site where the tip of the devices, such as peripherally inserted central catheter (PICC) lines and central venous catheters, end. This information is required to accurately select the body part character 4 and device character 6 in the ICD-10-PCS tables. Imaging reports can be used to identify end placement of the catheter for selecting the appropriate body part when the documentation by the provider does not specify. The initial insertion site (i.e., peripheral vein or central vein) is not reported. There is no character in the codes to distinguish between a central venous catheter insertion and a peripherally inserted central catheter.

Documentation Tip

According to *AHA Coding Clinic*, third quarter 2014, pages 5-6, when the provider's documentation does not specify the end placement of the catheter/infusion device, imaging reports may be used to identify the body part.

Coding Tip

According to *AHA Coding Clinic*, fourth quarter 2015, page 26, the cavoatrial junction is where the superior vena cava joins the wall of the right atrium. When the tip of the catheter is documented as ending in the cavoatrial junction, it is appropriate to assign body part character V Superior Vena Cava, instead of 6 Right Atrium.

A centrally inserted venous catheter inserted percutaneously into the right internal jugular vein and advanced to a final position in the superior vena cava is reported with ICD-10-PCS code Ø2HV33Z Insertion of infusion device into superior vena cava, percutaneous approach.

When coding a totally implantable vascular access device (Port-A-Cath) into the superior vena cava, code Ø2HV33Z for the percutaneous insertion of the CVC and code ØJH6ØWZ for the open insertion of the access port into the subcutaneous tissue of the chest.

Additional References

AHA CC: 4Q, 2017, pp. 63–64; 3Q, 2017, p. 11; 2Q, 2017, p. 24; 4Q, 2015, pp. 26–32; 2Q, 2015, p. 33; 3Q, 2014, p. 5; 4Q, 2013, p. 116; 3Q, 2013, p. 18

Release (Lysis) of Adhesions

Release. Freeing a body part from an abnormal physical constraint by cutting or by use of force.

Body part character. Assign the body part being freed and not the tissue being manipulated or cut to free the body part.

ØDN*	**Release/Gastrointestinal System**
ØFN*	**Release/Hepatobiliary System and Pancreas**
ØTN*	**Release/Urinary System**
ØUN*	**Release/Female Reproductive System**

Procedure: lysis of peritoneal adhesions; adhesiolysis; release of intestinal adhesions; lysis of pelvic adhesions; release of intestinal obstruction; enterolysis

Discussion

Adhesions are scar tissue that develops postsurgery as part of the healing process or after infection, injury, or other inflammatory process (i.e., appendicitis, peritonitis). When adhesions are symptomatic they cause pain, obstruction, and infertility. If present during surgery, adhesions can be an organized band that becomes an obstacle to and safe completion of that surgery. Lysis is the process of releasing these adhesions or scar tissue from the adjacent organs by cutting and freeing them.

It is common for minor adhesions to be present during many surgeries and their release is integral to the procedure. When adhesions and their lysis are documented as routine by terminology such as minor, easily or quickly lysed, integral, incidental, simple, several adhesions released or taken down, the diagnosis and procedure of lysis are not reported as they lack clinical significance.

Adhesions and lysis become clinically significant when they are documented as extensive, numerous, dense, obstructing, preventing access to organ removal, requiring lysis in order for the surgery to proceed or adding significant time and complexity to the main procedure.

Determination as to whether the adhesions and the lysis are significant enough to code and report must be made by the surgeon.

When intestinal bowel obstruction release is performed as a main procedure the associated treatment of "milking or running the bowel" (manual bowel decompression) is included in the procedure.

In ICD-10-PCS, the approach character for laparoscopic release is percutaneous endoscopic.

The objective of procedures represented in the root operation Release is to free a body part from abnormal constraint (i.e., adhesions). Release procedures are coded to the body part being freed, such as abdominal wall, peritoneum, colon, ureter, etc. The procedure can be performed on the area around a body part, on the attachments to a body part, or between subdivisions of a body part that are causing the abnormal constraint.

Documentation Tip

It is critical to clarify in the operative report the specific body part that is being freed, as the ICD-10-PCS root operation Release, which is used for lysis of adhesions, identifies the body part being released—NOT the body part that is incised or cut into in order to free another body part. A query must be generated if this information is not documented.

* Indicates the ICD-10-PCS table where the remainder of the code is constructed.

ICD-10-PCS guideline B3.2.a states: "During the same operative episode, multiple procedures are coded if: the same root operation is performed on different body parts as defined by distinct values of the body part character" and B3.2.b states "During the same operative episode, multiple procedures are coded if: The same root operation is repeated in multiple body parts, and those body parts are separate and distinct body parts classified to a single ICD-10-PCS body part value." Therefore, when release of adhesions of either the same body part that is represented by multiple characters or of a different body part is performed, each site is reported.

Additional References

AHA CC: 1Q, 2017, p. 35; 3Q, 2015, p.15; 1Q, 2014, p. 3

Right Heart Catheterization/Diagnostic with Right Heart Biopsy

Excision. Cutting out or off, without replacement, a portion of a body part. The qualifier Diagnostic is used to identify excision procedures that are biopsies.

Measurement. Determining the level of a physiological or physical function at a point in time.

Fluoroscopy. Single plane or bi-plane real time display of an image developed from the capture of external ionizing radiation on a fluorescent screen. The image may also be stored by either digital or analog means.

Ø2B*	**Excision/Heart and Great Vessels**
4AØ2*	**Measurement/Cardiac**
B21*	**Fluoroscopy/Heart**

Procedure: right heart catheterization with right heart biopsy

Discussion

Diagnostic right heart catheterization is performed via percutaneous insertion of a catheter into either the internal jugular, femoral vein, or radial artery. The catheter continues into one or more right cardiac chambers under fluoroscopic guidance for the purpose of obtaining blood samples for blood gas measurement and cardiac output (the amount of blood pumped by the heart per minute) measurement by Fick or other method. Right heart catheterization is most commonly used to assess right atrial (RA), right ventricular (RV), and pulmonary artery pressure and pulmonary artery occlusion pressure (PAOP). Indirect measurements of pressures in the left side of the heart can also be made by inflating a small balloon at the tip of the catheter. The pressure detected in front of the balloon is known as the pulmonary capillary "wedge" pressure (PCWP), or pulmonary artery occlusion pressure (PAOP). A right cardiac catheterization performed to measure the pressure or output in the heart is coded to Measurement, Cardiac 4AØ23N6.

The approach is percutaneous, as a procedure performed via a percutaneous approach (value 3) is one in which there is entry, by puncture or minor incision, of instrumentation through the skin or mucous membrane and any other body layers necessary to reach the site of the procedure. The access location for this approach is the skin or mucous membrane with nonvisualization instrumentation catheter used to reach the operative site. According to official guideline B5.4 Procedures performed percutaneously via a device placed for the procedure are coded to the approach Percutaneous.

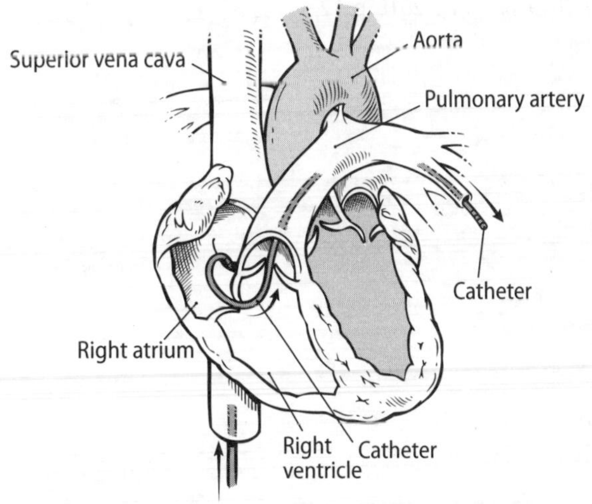

* Indicates the ICD-10-PCS table where the remainder of the code is constructed.

Procedures

A right heart (endomyocardial) biopsy requires intravascular placement of catheters into the right ventricle under fluoroscopic guidance and is performed either from the internal jugular, radial artery, or femoral vein. A sheath is first introduced in the vein and a pulmonary artery (PA) catheter is advanced into the right side of the heart and passed into the pulmonary artery. As the catheter is advanced into the pulmonary artery, the pressure measurements are done in the right atrium and right ventricle, to measure right heart pressures prior to obtaining biopsy specimens. After these pressure readings are obtained, a bioptome tissue biting forceps is advanced to the right ventricle and multiple specimens are obtained and sent to pathology.

This heart biopsy is reported with the root operation Excision and is used with a qualifier of diagnostic.

A right heart biopsy may be done to:

- Diagnose the cause of heart failure or heart disease, such as infectious dilated cardiomyopathy.
- Evaluate heart tissue after a heart transplant to assess for transplant rejection.
- Evaluate of heart and lung function prior to a heart transplant.

Right heart catheterization performed as the approach to the heart biopsy procedure, as well as any pressure measurements integral to the procedure, are not reported separately. However, if right heart catheterization is performed for diagnostic purposes or further evaluation, the cardiac catheterization may be coded and reported as measurement. Imaging guidance (fluoroscopy) done to assist in the performance of a procedure can be coded separately in the Imaging section.

A Swan-Ganz cardiac catheter is inserted into the right side of the heart to monitor pulmonary arterial pressures. This procedure is not considered a diagnostic cardiac catheterization.

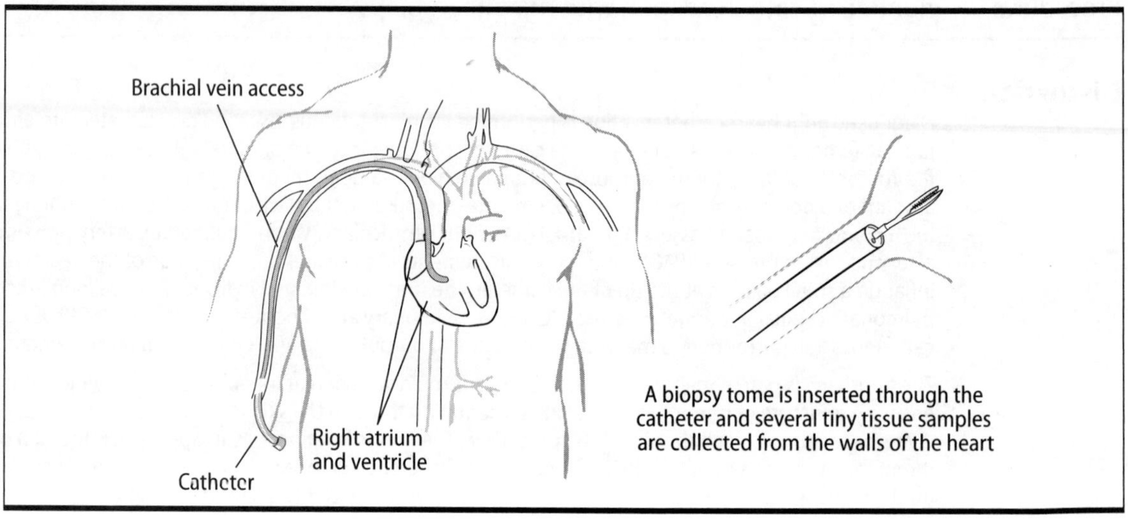

Additional References

AHA CC: 3Q, 2019, p. 32; 1Q, 2018, p. 12

Procedures

Tracheostomy and Ventilation

Tracheostomy. Bypass, respiratory system.

Tracheostomy tube. Bypass, tracheostomy device in respiratory system.

Ventilation, Mechanical. Extracorporeal or systemic assistance and performance (performance, respiratory) or (assistance, respiratory).

Endotracheal tube. Insertion, Trachea, Intraluminal Device, Endotracheal Airway.

Takedown of tracheostomy stoma. Repair (trachea) (skin).

Removal of tracheostomy tube or endotracheal tube. Removal, respiratory system, trachea, (tracheostomy device) (intraluminal device).

ØB1*	**Bypass/Respiratory System**
ØBH*	**Insertion/Respiratory System**
5A19*	**Performance/Respiratory**
5AØ9*	**Assistance/Respiratory**
ØBQ*	**Repair/Respiratory System**
ØBU*	**Supplement/Respiratory System**
ØWQ6*	**Repair/Anatomical Regions General/ Neck**
ØB21*	**Change/Trachea**

Procedure: tracheostomy; mechanical ventilation; endotracheal intubation; submental orotracheal intubation; continuous mandatory ventilation (CMV); continuous positive airway pressure (CPAP); intermittent positive pressure breathing (ventilation) (IPPB); positive end expiratory pressure (ventilation) (PEEP); synchronized intermittent mandatory ventilation (SIMV), noninvasive mechanical ventilation (NIMV); percutaneous transtracheal jet ventilation; minitracheostomy; percutaneous dilational tracheostomy (PDT); percutaneous tracheostomy; temporary tracheostomy; permanent tracheostomy; closure tracheostomy stoma; exchange tracheostomy tube

Discussion

Tracheostomy is made by vertical and/or horizontal incision of the anterior neck directly into the trachea at the cervical level to create a direct airway that bypasses the normal route of the nose and mouth. To maintain patency, the opening, stoma, or surgical fistula may be cannulated by inserting a tube and suturing it into position by securing with a tracheostomy tube tie. Tracheostomy can be temporary or permanent when the stoma requires development of skin flaps sutured to the edges of the tracheal opening and removal of small anterior portions of the tracheal rings. Tracheostomy can be performed open or percutaneous using a Seldinger technique modified with incorporation of progressive dilatation, as with the other newer techniques of Griggs and the Ciaglia Blue Rhino®. Percutaneous transtracheal jet ventilation (PTJV) employs a catheter that is placed percutaneously via a needle or surgical cricothyrotomy into the trachea and secured, then connected to an oxygen source through which the patient is oxygenated with jet ventilation maneuvers; it is used transiently or as an interim solution or during surgery. Decannulation is the removal of a tracheostomy tube to allow the stoma to close. When closure or takedown of the stoma is performed surgically, two codes will be reported, one each for the trachea and skin repair. Exchanging one tracheostomy tube for another is reported with the root operation Change, defined as taking out or off a device from a body part and replacing with an identical or similar device without cutting or puncturing the skin or mucus membrane.

* Indicates the ICD-10-PCS table where the remainder of the code is constructed.

Procedures

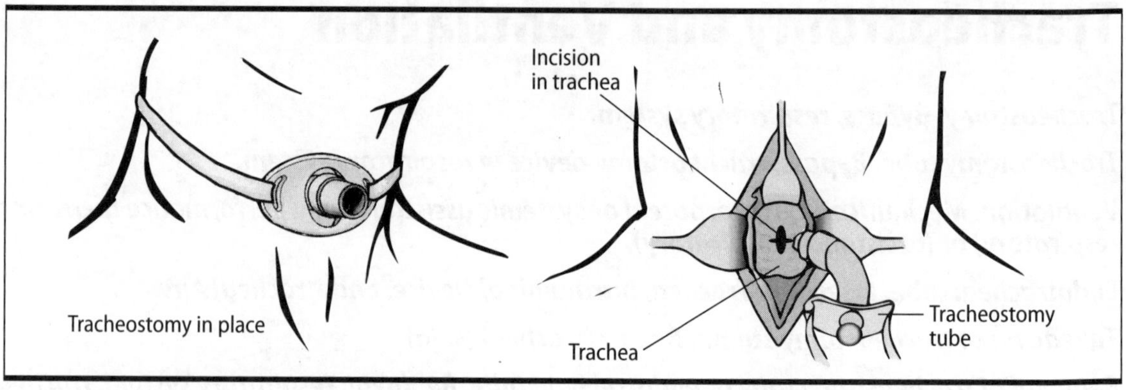

In ICD-10-PCS, the difference between modes of respiratory ventilation is the amount the mode takes over the physiological function by extracorporeal means. In other words, how much breathing is done by the patient versus how much is done by the machine. This is identified by the root operations:

- Performance: Completely taking over a physiological function by extracorporeal means. It replaces spontaneous breathing and the ventilatory effort is dependent on the machine.
- Assistance: Taking over a portion of a physiological function by extracorporeal means. The patient maintains spontaneous breathing and his or her own independent ventilator effort.

Both modes will identify the duration of the procedure in hours: < 24 consecutive hours, 24–96 consecutive hours, or > 96 consecutive hours. Calculation of duration guidelines:

- Count is done by hours, not number of days.
- Calculation should be based on multiple documents: physician orders must be verified with respiratory therapy notes and progress notes.
- Calculation begins at endotracheal intubation (ETT) or for tracheostomy (without preceding ETT) when ventilation is started.
- Stop time is at extubation for ETT or for tracheostomy when the ventilator is turned off or at discharge/transfer.
- The time of decannulation or ventilation stop or extubation must be documented, not just the order, as there may be hours delay between the two.
- Duration of consecutive hours means that if there is an interruption, for any reason, time must stop at the start of the interruption and then resume once ventilation begins again.
- Exception: When a patient self-extubates and is re-intubated and returned to ventilation, do not count as interruption: stop time is based on physician order and/or clinical indicators and actual discontinuation of ventilation, not interruptions of self-extubation.
- Ventilator weaning is counted in the duration hours. Weaning ends when the ventilator is turned off. A T-piece or trach-collar is used for a weaning trial to see if the patient can tolerate ventilator cessation and the time on it is also counted towards the duration.
- Postoperative extended period on ventilation for more than two days after surgery ends, report the code the ventilation and count the duration starting at 48 hours.
- Postoperative and continues on ventilation for less than two days for specified reason other than routine postsurgical maintenance, report the ventilation and the diagnosis that it is treating.
- Ventilation for airway protection is reported, even in the absence of a diagnosis of respiratory failure as certain conditions would necessitate ventilation due to the nature of the condition (i.e., neurological injury, etc.).

Ventilation may be delivered through:

- Invasive interface: Tracheostomy or endotracheal intubation
  - Tracheostomy is coded separately with the root operation Bypass and Tracheostomy Device.
  - Endotracheal intubation is coded separately with the root operation Insertion and Intraluminal Device, Endotracheal Airway EXCEPT when performed as an inherent part of the surgical procedure.
- Noninvasive interface: face mask, nasal mask, nasal pillow, oral mouthpiece, oronasal mask, without endotracheal tube or tracheostomy

Additional References

AHA CC: 4Q, 2023, 55; 3Q, 2023, 6; 4Q, 2020, p. 64; 1Q, 2020, p. 10; 1Q, 2018, p. 13; 4Q, 2014, p. 3-15

Transbronchial Biopsy of Lung, Lymph Node, Mediastinum via Bronchoscope (extraction) (suction catheter aspiration) (needle aspiration biopsy/Wang)

Biopsy. Extraction. Pulling or stripping out or off all or a portion of a body part by the use of force; with the qualifier diagnostic.

Approach (bronchoscopy). Via natural or artificial opening endoscopic.

ØBD*	**Extraction/Respiratory System**
Ø7D*	**Extraction/Lymphatic and Hemic Systems**

Procedure:	transbronchial lung biopsy (TBLBx); needle aspiration lung biopsy; Wang needle aspiration biopsy of thoracic lymph node; aspiration biopsy of mediastinum; TBLBx with transbronchial needle aspiration (TBNA) lymph node; TBLB with transbronchial catheter aspiration (TBCA); EUS-FNA lymph node; TBNA of lung; endobronchial needle biopsy of lung; transbronchial cryobiopsy

Discussion

Transbronchial lung biopsy (TBLBx) is performed via bronchoscopy, usually for a peripheral lung lesion or mass near the chest wall. Using forceps biopsy, four to 10 samples of alveolar tissue are obtained, with the desired specimen of at least one sample containing full thickness bronchial mucosa and some alveolar tissue. This is reported using the root operation Extraction. A forceps is a grasping tool used to pull, or exert traction, i.e., "extract." Similar to debridement procedures, a forceps is not an "excisional" tool.

Transbronchial biopsy using forceps punctured through the bronchus meets the definition of the root operation Extraction: Pulling or stripping out or off all or a portion of a body part by the use of force.

A higher diagnostic sampling of lung tissue is obtained when combined with suction catheter aspiration (TBCA) of lung tissue. A transbronchial needle/aspiration biopsy/Wang needle aspiration tissue biopsy, reported with root operation Extraction, may also be performed to sample lymph node, mediastinal tissue, paratracheal lesions, peribronchial lesions, or endobronchial submucosal tissue.

Often an endobronchial ultrasound (EBUS) will be performed to assist with a transbronchial needle aspiration (EBUS-TBNA). EBUS is less invasive than mediastinoscopy. Newer bronchoscopy techniques that are less invasive and allow access to more distant or smaller or earlier lung lesions include navigational electromagnetic bronchoscopy (ENB or EMN bronchoscopy) and autofluorescence bronchoscopy (Blue Light) or lung imaging fluorescence endoscopy (LIFE).

Endobronchial inspection during bronchoscopy is integral and precedes the biopsy forceps crossing through the segmental bronchus into the lung by puncturing the terminal bronchus. A transbronchial lung biopsy procedure is generally done with fluoroscopic guidance, as only the forceps puncture the bronchus and enter into the lung. There is no direct bronchoscopic visualization of the lung biopsy site, as the scope stays within the bronchus.

A newer technique used to obtain tissue samples is a transbronchial cryobiopsy. Transbronchial cryobiopsies use high-pressure gas cooling of a single use cryoprobe, which is inserted into the bronchoscope and punctured through the bronchus to the site of biopsy in the lung. The cryoprobe device freezes the targeted lung biopsy area, then pulls the specimen back through the scope to extract large frozen biopsy specimens. This allows extraction of larger samples of lung parenchyma without the crush artifact that can occur with forceps extraction. The cryoprobe and bronchoscope are removed in a pulling manner, meeting the definition for root operation Extraction—pulling or stripping out or off all or a portion of a body part by the use of force.

---

* Indicates the ICD-10-PCS table where the remainder of the code is constructed.

The intent of a lung biopsy is to obtain lung tissue; therefore, regardless of the tissue type or sample adequacy obtained, it is still reported as a lung biopsy. Inadvertent tissue is not reported as a biopsy of that tissue. Clinical correlation with pathology results should be made and discrepancies will require physician query to ensure the objective of the biopsy (i.e., lung or bronchus). In addition, when a needle biopsy is performed, close attention must be paid as to the structure being biopsied in order to report the appropriate body system and body part (e.g., lymph node, other extrinsic tissue, lung or bronchus). Thoracic lymph nodes are reported with a code using the appropriate body part value as noted in the ICD-10-PCS body part key. In the body part key, Lymphatic, Thorax includes the intercostal, mediastinal, parasternal, paratracheal, and tracheobronchial lymph nodes. The aortic lymph nodes include the para-aortic lymph nodes. These lymph nodes are indicated by the International Association for the Study of Lung Cancer (IASLC) mapping system:

- Supraclavicular zone nodes:
  - 1R/1L: right and left low cervical, supraclavicular, sternal notch (highest mediastinal nodes)
- Superior mediastinal nodes:
  - 2R/2L: right and left upper paratracheal
  - 3a: prevascular
  - 3p: retrotracheal
  - 4R/4L: right and left lower paratracheal (including azygos nodes)
- Aortic nodes:
  - 5: subaortic (A-P window)
  - 6: para-aortic (ascending aorta or phrenic)
- Inferior mediastinal nodes:
  - subcarinal zone: 7: subcarinal
  - lower zone: 8: paraesophageal (below carina); 9: pulmonary ligament
- N1 nodes:
  - hilar/interlobar zone: 10: (R/L) hilar (right and left tracheobronchial angle); 11: (R/L) interlobar
  - peripheral zone: 12: (R/L) lobar; 13: (R/L) segmental; 14: (R/L) subsegmental

There are two types of needle biopsies: fine needle biopsy, also called fine needle aspiration (FNA) and core needle biopsy. FNA uses a hollow, "fine" small-bore needle attached to a syringe to aspirate either fluid or tissue. A core biopsy uses a larger bore needle to remove a cylinder of tissue.

The root operation for transbronchial needle aspiration biopsy of lung tissue is Extraction. A needle aspiration biopsy involves placing a needle through tissue, applying suction and aspirating **tissue** for biopsy. Usually a needle used to biopsy tissue has a larger bore than a fine needle that obtains only fluid. The root operation Drainage is only used when **fluid or gas** is removed, for diagnostic or therapeutic purposes (i.e., collection of fluid or drainage of abscess). To determine the appropriate root operation, the full definition of the root operation as contained in the ICD-10-PCS Tables must be applied

Coding and Documentation Tip

ICD-10-PCS Guideline B3.4a:

"Biopsy procedures are coded using the root operations Excision, Extraction, or Drainage and the qualifier Diagnostic."

If there is insufficient documentation to determine the intent of the procedure or the type of tissue obtained in a biopsy, i.e., lymph fluid vs lymph tissue, query the surgeon.

The approach would be percutaneous endoscopic for an endobronchial ultrasound-guided transbronchial needle aspiration biopsy of a thoracic lymph node tissue via bronchoscopy.

In ICD-10-PCS, the percutaneous endoscopic approach is defined as entry, by puncture or minor incision, of instrumentation through the skin or mucous membrane and any other body layers necessary to reach and visualize the site of the procedure.

Assign the following ICD-10-PCS code for transbronchial endoscopic lymph node tissue needle biopsy: 07D74ZX Extraction of thorax lymphatic, percutaneous endoscopic approach, diagnostic.

It is expected that one or more biopsies will be obtained from an anatomical site, but code assignment is not based on the number of biopsies; therefore, report one biopsy code per anatomical site. When biopsies are taken from an additional anatomic site, then that additional site is also coded. For example, TBLB x2 from the right upper lung lobe is reported with one code (one unit with initial code: outpatient); if additional biopsies are taken from the right middle lobe, report one code for that site.

PCS coding guidelines B4.1a and B4.1b state that if a body part does not have its own designation, code the value of the whole body part. When terms with prefix "peri-" are combined with a whole body part to identify the site, and the site of the procedure is not further specified, code to the whole body part value. When a lesion or mass is stated as paratracheal, mediastinal, peribronchial, or extrinsic to respiratory system, further information is needed in order to report as accurately as possible. Waiting for pathology results is recommended in order to distinguish the tissue as lymph node or lymphocele, soft tissue, or other tissue type.

Additional References

AHA CC: 3Q, 2020, pp. 40-41; 4Q, 2018, p. 84; 4Q, 2017, p. 41; 1Q, 2014, p. 20, 26; 4Q, 2013, p. 111

MLN Matters

The IASLC Lymph Node Mapping: https://www.ncbi.nlm.nih.gov/pmc/articles/PMC4499584/

Procedures

Valve Replacement, Aortic

Replacement. Putting in or on a biological or synthetic material that physically takes the place and/or function of all or a portion of a body part.

The body part may have been taken out or replaced, or may be taken out, physically eradicated, or rendered nonfunctional during the Replacement procedure. A Removal procedure is coded for taking out the device used in a previous replacement procedure.

Ø2RF* **Replacement/Aortic Valve**

Optional:

5A1* **Extracorporeal or Systemic Assistance and Performance, Physiological Systems, Performance (cardiopulmonary bypass)**

8EØ2* **Other Procedures (robotic assisted procedure)**

X2A* **New Technology, Cardiovascular System, Assistance (cerebral embolic filtration)**

Procedure: open heart valve replacement, transcatheter aortic valve replacement (TAVR), transcatheter aortic valve implantation (TAVI), rapid deployment aortic valve replacement (RDAVR), cardiopulmonary bypass, cerebral embolic filtration

Discussion

The aortic valve regulates blood flow from the left ventricle to the aorta. The aortic valve has three leaflets (cusps): noncoronary (posterior semilunar), right coronary (semilunar), and left coronary (semilunar).

Insufficiency is a malfunction in the operation of the aortic valve leaflets, which results in failure of the valve to close properly, allowing regurgitation of blood from the aorta back into the left ventricle.

Stenosis is narrowing of the aortic valve, which may block blood flow into the aorta. These two conditions can occur alone or together. A common cause of aortic valve disorders in people older than age 65 is calcium deposits on the leaflets, causing stenosis and reducing the leaflet mobility. In severe cases of aortic stenosis and insufficiency, backflow of blood can accumulate in the lungs and prevent the necessary flow of blood to the brain or extremities.

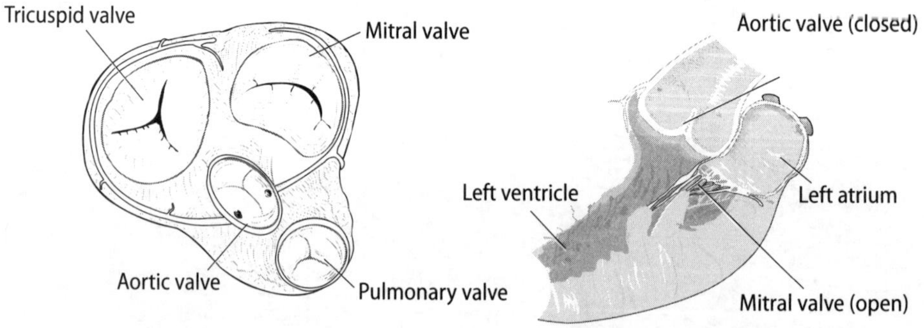

Overhead view of heart valves in closed position

Cutaway view of heart showing left-side valves

Aortic valve replacement may be performed through traditional open-heart surgery, which involves a sternotomy (incision) into the chest wall, or through minimally invasive methods that involve smaller incisions in the chest or a catheter inserted in the leg or chest (transcatheter aortic valve replacement, or TAVR). For proper coding,

* Indicates the ICD-10-PCS table where the remainder of the code is constructed.

documentation must distinctly indicate the technique or approach used to perform the procedure. The following descriptions help to discern between these techniques:

- Traditional Open approach: A large (6-8") incision is made, splitting the breastbone and removing the damaged valve and inserting the new valve through this incision. The PCS value of Open approach is reported.
- Minimally invasive approach: Smaller incision(s) are made in the chest avoiding splitting of the breastbone. Cameras and instrumentation are inserted to perform the procedure through these smaller incisions. Robotic assistance may be used. Because this procedure is still performed through the incision with endoscopic assistance, the PCS value of Open approach is reported, according to guideline B5.2 that states: "procedures performed using the open approach with percutaneous endoscopic assistance are coded to the approach Open."
- Transcatheter aortic valve replacement (TAVR/implantation [TAVI]): This technique uses a catheter instead of open surgery to replace a damaged aortic valve by inserting a fully collapsible valve replacement through a catheter. The new Zooplastic Tissue valve, which is made from cow or pig heart tissue (bovine or porcine), is wedged into the damaged valve and once it is expanded, takes over the function of the valve. The damaged valve is not typically removed. Access is usually achieved through the femoral artery; other access options include the subclavian artery, ascending aorta/transaortic (via small incision in the chest), and through the bottom of the heart (transapical).

Documentation Tip

In TAVR procedures performed via a small incision in the chest, the body part value of the code specifies the aortic valve, which is not visualized directly. The procedure is performed via a catheter inserted into the apex of the heart, so the appropriate approach value is Percutaneous. The qualifier Transapical is reported for this procedure vs a femoral artery access which is reported with No Qualifier. Documentation should denote the access location of the chest incision or via the femoral artery in the groin for appropriate qualifier selection.

- Rapid Deployment Aortic Valve Replacement (RDAVR): This type of valve replacement is performed either by standard open technique or minimally invasive open technique. Traditional aortic valve replacement involves excising the diseased aortic valve, and placing between 12 and 15 sutures through the aortic annulus and sewing the ring of the valve into place. Rapid deployment aortic valve replacement (RDAVR) uses a balloon expandable stent that allows precise positioning of the new valve with only three sutures, rather than the normal 12 to 15. The system uses a flexible deployment arm that allows optimal access to anatomy for valve deployment and suturing. This technique reduces the duration of cardiopulmonary bypass, and allows the use of smaller, less-invasive incisions.

Documentation Tip

A query to clarify type of valve device is unnecessary if the name brand is listed. The CDI or coder can match the name brand to the ICD-10-PCS value using the ICD-10-PCS Device Key or researching online if not listed in the Device Key. If a combination of synthetic (metal) and biologic (animal) tissue is used in the composition of the valve, report the biological (Zooplastic tissue).

Other procedures that may be performed during an aortic valve replacement and are coded separately include:

- Cardiopulmonary Bypass: Also known as artificial heart and lung or pump oxygenator, cardiopulmonary bypass is a form of extracorporeal (situated or occurring outside the body) circulation utilized to temporarily perform the complete functions of the heart and lungs during surgery and maintain the circulation of blood and the oxygen content of the body. This procedure is captured with 5A1221Z Performance of Cardiac Output, Continuous.
- Robotic Assisted: Robotic-assisted surgery expands the surgeon's abilities by augmenting them with miniaturized instruments combined with the use of robotic arms and high-definition 3D cameras that add precision at the surgical site. Common brands of robotic instrumentation are the DaVinci Surgical System® and Cyberknife®. The codes for Robotic Assisted Procedures are found in the Other Procedures Section (8EØ*).
- Cerebral Embolic Filtration: Embolic debris can be dislodged during transcatheter aortic valve replacements (TAVR), resulting in increased risk of stroke, dementia, and cognitive impairment. The Claret Medical Sentinel Cerebral Protection System protects the brain from this debris by inserting a dual filter in the innominate artery and left common carotid artery intraoperatively during the TAVR procedure. This percutaneous procedure is reported with code X2A5312 from the New Technology Section. Keystone Heart's TriGuard 3™ Cerebral Embolic Protection Device (CEPD) is a temporary, self-positioning polymeric mesh device that is positioned in the aortic arch intraoperatively during the TAVR procedure, using one of the two femoral artery access ports already established during the procedure. It uses a single filter that deploys rapidly and is intended to provide full coverage of all three major aortic vessels to decrease the risk of cerebral damage during TAVR by allowing maximal blood flow while diverting emboli toward the descending aorta. It is designed to accommodate variations in aortic arch anatomy and is removed upon completion of the procedure. This device is reported with code X2A6325, from the New Technology Section.

Documentation should state:

- Approach technique terminology—Sternotomy, large incision, cut breastbone (Open), Minimally invasive with small incisions into chest or mini thoracotomy with endoscopic assistance (Open), transcatheter (Percutaneous), TAVR/TAVI (Percutaneous)
- Device Type—mechanical (Synthetic Substitute) or biological tissue (Human = Autologous Tissue Substitute/Nonautologous Tissue Substitute) (Bovine/Porcine = Zooplastic Tissue). The ICD-10-PCS Device Key can be consulted for specific brand types.
- For TAVR/TAVI—access via femoral artery or transapical (chest incision, tip of heart)
- Use of cardiopulmonary bypass
- Use of cerebral embolic filtration, dual/single
- Review for any indications of Rapid Deployment device (see Documentation Tip)

Additional References

AHA CC: 2Q, 2024, p. 30; 4Q, 2022, p. 54; 1Q, 2021, p. 16; 4Q, 2019, p. 46; 1Q, 2019, p. 31; 3Q, 2018, p. 11; 1Q, 2017, p. 36; 4Q, 2016, p. 115–116; 3Q, 2013, p. 26

Whipple Procedure

Excision. Cutting out or off, without replacement, a portion of a body part.

Resection. Cutting out or off, without replacement, all of a body part.

ØDB*	**Gastrointestinal System, Excision**
ØDT*	**Gastrointestinal System, Resection**
ØFB*	**Hepatobiliary System and Pancreas, Excision**
ØFT*	**Hepatobiliary System and Pancreas, Resection**

Procedure: pancreaticoduodenectomy

Discussion

The Whipple procedure is an eponym for a pancreaticoduodenectomy named after an American surgeon, Allen Whipple, who first began performing these procedures in 1935. It is most often performed to treat pancreatic cancer in lieu of a total pancreatectomy. It can also be performed to treat other cancers, such as neuroendocrine tumors and ampullary or bile duct cancer. Other disorders of the pancreas, duodenum, or bile ducts such as pancreatitis, cysts, or trauma may be treated using the Whipple procedure.

The objective of the Whipple procedure is often the removal of the head of the pancreas; the procedure also involves excising multiple abdominal organs such as the tail of the pancreas, duodenum, stomach pylorus, common bile duct, and often the gallbladder and proximal jejunum. The reason for these multiple excisions is due to the pancreatic involvement with other digestive system organs. Anastomosis or reconnection after excision is necessary to restore normal digestive function and can include attaching the hepatic duct to the jejunum and the stomach to the jejunum. According to ICD-10-PCS official coding guideline B3.1b, the anastomosis of body parts that have been removed is inherent in closing the operative site and not reported separately.

There are multiple variations of the Whipple procedure that are dependent on the condition treated; two main techniques include conventional and pyloric sparing techniques. As the name indicates, in pyloric sparing technique no part of the stomach or stomach pylorus is removed, promoting better long-term nutritional status.

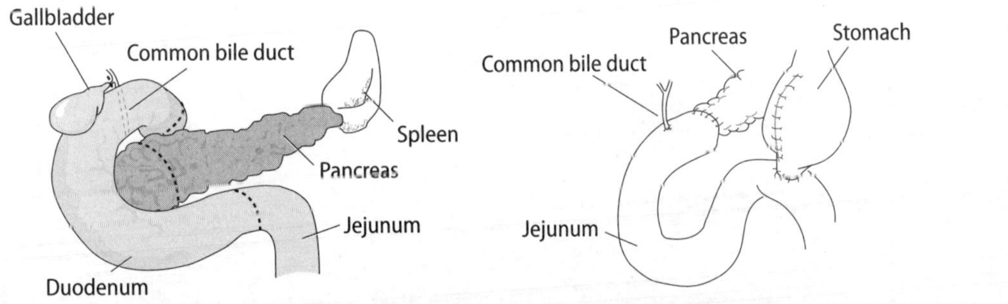

Coding Tip

Since the anastomosis of the organs is reconnecting rather than bypassing body parts, it is considered inherent to the Excision/Resection procedure and not coded separately. Guideline B3.1b.

Assign individual codes when the same procedure is performed on separate body parts. Guideline B3.2a.

* Indicates the ICD-10-PCS table where the remainder of the code is constructed.

Documentation must state:

- Because the root operation differs in the removal of these multiple body parts, it is critical that the documentation of the operative report clearly state whether each body part is partially (Excision) or totally (Resection) removed.
- With multiple body parts involved, specificity of each body part is necessary.
- The approach for the procedure may be open, percutaneous endoscopic, or a combination of both. Technique must be clearly described. Terminology such as "minimally invasive" is not enough. More appropriate terms include open, size of incision, clearly visualized, or laparoscopic, trocars, scopes, and insufflated. Often times a procedure will begin laparoscopically and convert to open. This should be clearly stated (e.g., inspection of the abdomen can be laparoscopic but the procedure done via Open approach).
- Robotic assisted surgery is reported with an additional code from table 8EØ and should be documented.

Additional References

AHA CC: 1Q, 2019, p. 3; 3Q, 2014, p. 32

Procedures

Appendix A. Query Guidelines, Examples, and Templates

According to the *ICD-10-CM Official Guidelines for Coding and Reporting*:

"A joint effort between the healthcare provider and the coder is essential to achieve complete and accurate documentation, code assignment, and reporting of diagnoses and procedures. These guidelines have been developed to assist both the healthcare provider and the coder in identifying those diagnoses that are to be reported. The importance of consistent, complete documentation in the medical record cannot be overemphasized. Without such documentation accurate coding cannot be achieved. The entire record should be reviewed to determine the specific reason for the encounter and the conditions treated."

The *ICD-10-PCS Official Guidelines for Coding and Reporting* contain similar language:

"A joint effort between the healthcare provider and the coder is essential to achieve complete and accurate documentation, code assignment, and reporting of diagnoses and procedures. These guidelines have been developed to assist both the healthcare provider and the coder in identifying those procedures that are to be reported. The importance of consistent, complete documentation in the medical record cannot be overemphasized. Without such documentation accurate coding cannot be achieved."

Centers for Medicare and Medicaid Services (CMS) Department of Health and Human Services, § 482.24 Conditions of participation: Medical record services, state:

"(c) Standard: Content of record. The medical record must contain information to justify admission and continued hospitalization, support the diagnosis, and describe the patient's progress and response to medications and services.

"(1) All patient medical record entries must be legible, complete, dated, timed, and authenticated in written or electronic form by the person responsible for providing or evaluating the service provided, consistent with hospital policies and procedures."

The need for a description of procedures is also required by the CMS Conditions of Participation for Hospitals Sec 482.51, which states: "An operative report describing techniques, findings, and tissues removed or altered must be written or dictated immediately following surgery and signed by the surgeon."

Medical record documentation entries must be consistent with all other parts of the record. When documentation entries conflict with other data within the record, clarification must be obtained when the information is used in the assignment of codes.

Queries should be used as a communication tool to clarify and improve the quality of health record documentation for all diseases, conditions or procedures, consistent for all payer types and not for revenue enhancement or optimization. Quality clinical documentation is necessary to meet regulatory agencies standards; ensure accurate and compliant diagnosis, procedure(s), MS-DRG, present on admission (POA), risk adjustment and other data assignments; provide accurate data to reporting agencies, research, and public health agencies; reduce risks of adverse events from incomplete or unclear documentation; ensure quality of patient care; and accurately reflect medical necessity and patient acuity levels.

The expansion of clinical documentation programs and new technologies such as electronic health record (EHR) "clinical alerts" and natural language understanding (NLU) or natural language processing (NLP) technologies have resulted in the need for prospective clinical documentation health record reviews.

Prospective reviews are performed before the provider sees the patient, with the goal of identifying chronic conditions using documentation from previous encounters, medication lists, abnormal laboratory values, etc. These new technologies can be used to prompt providers with "documentation alerts" to be more specific in their documentation, but these alerts still must be reviewed by a clinical documentation specialist and be compliant with best practices for clarifying documentation in the legal medical record.

Discussion of the challenges of avoiding leading queries and introducing new information when conducting prospective reviews, as well as examples, are included in the AHIMA Practice Brief "Prospective Clinical Documentation Integrity (CDI) Reviews and Query/Alert Practice Best Standards." This practice brief stresses the difference between documentation alerts designed to influence a provider's documentation versus a clinical alert for clinical decision-making at the time of entering the clinical information in the health record. It also stresses that the *ICD-10-CM Official Guidelines for Coding and Reporting*, Uniform Hospital Discharge Data Set (UHDDS) guidelines, and the practice brief "The Guidelines for Achieving a Compliant Query Practice Brief (2019 Update)" should still be followed.

Queries can be addressed to any licensed provider such as a physician, nurse practitioner, or physician assistant who is responsible for rendering direct patient care and diagnosis. It is appropriate to query nonphysician professionals (such as a wound nurse) only when that professional performs the service or procedure and official coding guidelines allow the use of this documentation for code assignment.

A query should properly identify the patient and the encounter and contain:

- Patient name
- Admission date (date of service)
- Medical record number
- Account number
- Date query initiated
- Name and contact information of the initiator of the query
- Date and signature of the responsible party making the entry (Note that every entry must have this information.)
- A statement of the issue. (List clinical indicators from the chart or ambiguous/unsubstantiated information.)

Queries for diagnoses and/or procedures are appropriate when record documentation:

- Is conflicting, imprecise, incomplete, illegible, unreliable, untimely, unclear, ambiguous, or inconsistent, including resolving conflicting documentation of diagnoses or procedures between the physician and other providers
- Describes or is associated with clinical indicators of a condition that meets Uniform Hospital Discharge Data Set (UHDDS) requirements but lacks a definitive statement of relationship to an underlying diagnosis or condition
- Describes a procedure that is inconsistent with the clinical test results from a procedure, including pathology and cytology reports
- Does not clearly document the reason for inpatient admission
- Does not clearly document the objective and extent of a procedure, including sufficient information to assign the appropriate root operation, body part, laterality, operative approach, devices, and other specific qualifier values
- Includes clinical indicators, diagnostic evaluation, and/or treatment not related to a specific condition or procedure
- Provides a documented diagnosis without underlying clinical validation/support
- Does not clearly establish a cause-and-effect relationship between medical conditions
- Documents signs, symptoms, or treatment without a related diagnosis
- Fails to document a diagnosis with the acuity or specificity required to assign other than a default or unspecified code
- Is unclear if a condition documented as "history of" is active or resolved and if it is relevant to the current encounter
- Is unclear for present on admission indicator assignment
- Fails to clarify if a diagnosis is ruled in or out at the time of discharge

Clinical coders and clinical documentation improvement (CDI) professionals should anticipate all of the clinically valid alternatives as possible answers and formulate the query question with those answers in mind.

Generally, there should be one question per query form. Coders should not ask multiple queries on the same form. Unrelated conditions should each have a separate query, but related conditions may be included in one query.

A question may be in two parts, or be worded to indicate "if A, then B, C, or other," or that a certain answer out of the possible answers may require a second follow-up question to clarify.

A clear concise query should be drafted that eliminates any need to re-query the physician for the same diagnosis or procedure clarification.

Query templates can be used to standardize information, but the clinical information in the query should be unique for each case. There are times when only a free-form query is appropriate. Free-form queries should be written in clear, concise, and precise language, and should not question a provider's clinical judgment.

Avoid the use of bold, highlighted, colored, or all capital letters in the body of the query. All typed content should be the same size, color, and style.

Avoid using a title in the header on query forms with the diagnosis anticipated in the physician response, such as:

- Acute blood loss anemia
- Acute respiratory failure
- Sepsis
- Aspiration pneumonia

Although open-ended queries are preferred, multiple choice and yes/no queries are acceptable in certain circumstances, especially with ICD-10-PCS procedure queries where the choices for code assignment are limited in the classification.

A multiple-choice format for diagnosis queries should include all clinically significant and reasonable choices as supported by the clinical indicators in the medical record, as well as "other,""unspecified" or "clinically undetermined," "not clinically significant," or "integral to" options, and include a blank line for the physician to add free text. It is recognized that occasionally there may be only one reasonable option.

Yes/no queries are permissible only when clarifying documentation that requires more specification, such as further validating a diagnosis already documented in the health record with interpretation by a provider, establishing or ruling-out a cause-and-effect relationship between documented conditions, or in determining POA status. If clinical indicators are present, but a diagnosis has not yet been documented, then a yes/no query would not be appropriate. As with any type of query, a yes/no query should present the documentation to be clarified with relevant clinical indicators, and in a format that is acceptable for a "yes" or "no" response from the provider. These types of queries should also include the option of "unable to determine."

Providing a new diagnosis is an option in a multiple-choice list, if it is supported and substantiated by the clinical indicators from the medical record documentation and is not introducing new information. New diagnoses cannot be derived from a yes/no query and should not be used in circumstances where clinical indicators of a condition are present but the condition/diagnosis has not yet been documented in the medical record.

Multiple-choice questions or questions requiring only a yes or no response are acceptable in the following circumstances:

- When confirming a diagnosis already present as an interpretation of a finding
- Establishing a cause and effect relationship between documented conditions such as manifestation/etiology, complications, and conditions/diagnostic findings
- Resolving conflicting practitioner documentation

A yes/no query for diagnoses should also include the additional options associated with multiple-choice queries (i.e., "other,""clinically undetermined,""not clinically significant," and "integral to").

A yes/no query for ICD-10-PCS procedures, on the other hand, does not need to include the additional options such as "other,""clinically undetermined,""not clinically significant," and "integral to," as the ICD-10-PCS classification does not provide options of unspecified, undetermined, or "other."

Note: ICD-10-PCS Convention A11 of the Official Coding and Reporting Guidelines states: "Many of the terms used to construct PCS codes are defined within the system. It is the coder's responsibility to determine what the documentation in the medical record equates to in the PCS definitions. The physician is not expected to use the terms used in PCS code descriptions, nor is the coder required to query the physician when the correlation between the documentation and the defined PCS terms is clear.

Example:

When the physician documents "partial resection" the coder can independently correlate "partial resection" to the root operation Excision without querying the physician for clarification."

This convention emphasizes the importance of coders and CDI staff proficiency in all PCS terms and definitions so that unnecessary queries are not requested.

The query should not lead or direct the provider to a specific response (i.e., sound presumptive, directive, prodding, or as if leading to an assumption) and should include a statement to the effect that the provider is requested to use his or her medical judgment without a specific answer in mind. The query should not be designed to require only a provider signature.

A query should not indicate a positive or negative effect on reimbursement such as complication/comorbidity (CC), major complication/comorbidity (MCC) designation, MS-DRG assignment or MS-DRG relative weights, or indicate any financial or quality reporting outcomes.

A query should not be performed for every discrepancy or unaddressed issue. Insignificant or irrelevant findings do not require a query regarding the assignment of an additional diagnosis code. The primary objective of the query process

Query Guidelines

should be improved clinical data. Documentation must meet the following additional diagnosis coding and reporting criteria:

- Clinical evaluation
- Therapeutic treatment
- Diagnostic procedure
- Increase length of stay
- Increase nursing care and/or monitoring

One additional reporting element is noted in the perinatal guidelines "has implications for future health care needs."

Although it is listed as a qualifier under the official coding guidelines for inpatient reporting of uncertain diagnoses, the term "possible" is vague and its use in a query is discouraged, unless the physician has documented it as such. A query may be used, however, to identify clinically relevant possible/probable diagnoses documented at the beginning or during the middle of hospitalization when not documented at the time of discharge.

Clinical information from a patient's past medical record may be referenced to support a query if it is pertinent to the current encounter; however, it is inappropriate to search documentation from previous records to query something that is not related to the present encounter.

There are two types of queries: retrospective and concurrent. A retrospective query is performed after discharge but prior to claim submission to review information that is lacking in the medical record. Concurrent queries are issued as an ongoing process of requesting clarification or additional information while the patient is still present.

Post-bill queries are initiated after the claim is submitted, usually a result of an audit or other internal quality monitoring. A post-bill query would be appropriate to correct an obvious error. Facilities should develop a policy regarding whether they will generate post-bill queries and the time frame for such queries, keeping in mind the following:

- Applying normal course of business guidelines
- Using payer-specific rules on rebilling time frames
- Requirements outlined in state law, regulation, or healthcare facility licensure standards as they relate to medical record completion guidelines
- Determining reliability of query response over time

For example, Centers for Medicare and Medicaid Services (CMS) CFR 482.24 Conditions of Participation: Medical record services, states that the medical record, including the discharge summary and the final diagnosis, must be complete within 30 days following discharge:

(vii) Discharge summary with outcome of hospitalization, disposition of case, and provisions for follow-up care.

(viii) Final diagnosis with completion of medical records within 30 days following discharge.

The Office of the Inspector General "Compliance Program Guidance for Hospitals" also indicates that all documentation should be done prior to billing and/or audit, and available for audit and review:

"With respect to reimbursement claims, a hospital's written policies and procedures should reflect and reinforce current Federal and State statutes and regulations regarding the submission of claims and Medicare cost reports. The policies must create a mechanism for the billing or reimbursement staff to communicate effectively and accurately with the clinical staff.

Policies and procedures should:

- Provide for proper and timely documentation of all physician and other professional services prior to billing to ensure that only accurate and properly documented services are billed
- Emphasize that claims should be submitted only when appropriate documentation supports the claims and only when such documentation is maintained and available for audit and review. The documentation, which may include patient records, should record the length of time spent in conducting the activity leading to the record entry, and the identity of the individual providing the service. The hospital should consult with its medical staff to establish other appropriate documentation guidelines
- State that, consistent with appropriate guidance from medical staff, physician and hospital records and medical notes used as a basis for a claim submission should be appropriately organized in a legible form so they can be audited and reviewed

- Indicate that the diagnosis and procedures reported on the reimbursement claim should be based on the medical record and other documentation, and that the documentation necessary for accurate code assignment should be available to coding staff…"

Organizational query retention policies should be developed consistent with statutory and/or regulatory guidelines. The policy and the query form should indicate if the query is part of the patient's permanent health record or stored as a separate business record. If the query form is not part of the health record, the policy should specify where it will be filed and the retention period. Also, if the form is not established as a permanent part of the medical record then the physician response to the query must be documented in the medical record, such as progress notes or discharge summary. If the record is complete, this should be appropriately documented, authenticated and signed as an addendum, with the current date, time, and reason for the additional information being added to the health record.

Queries that are stored as separate business records rather than as part of the permanent legal record are most likely subject to discovery as these documents are not considered privileged. Auditors may request copies of queries even if they are not considered part of the permanent legal record.

The Centers for Medicare and Medicaid Services (CMS) Recovery Audit Contractor (RAC) Scope of Work 2013 included this statement:

"Clinical validation is an additional process that may be performed along with DRG validation. Clinical validation involves a clinical review of the case to see whether or not the patient truly possesses the conditions that were documented in the medical record. Recovery Auditor clinicians shall review any information necessary to make a prepayment or post-payment claim determination. Clinical validation is performed by a clinician (RN, CMD or therapist). Clinical validation is beyond the scope of DRG (coding) validation, and the skills of a certified coder. This type of review can only be performed by a clinician or may be performed by a clinician with approved coding credentials."

Coding professionals should have at least enough basic clinical knowledge including medical terminology, anatomy of all body systems, pathophysiology, and pharmacology, and have the skill to communicate this information. It is crucial for coding professionals to develop their clinical knowledge by ongoing education so that they may learn what documentation to search for to refer questionable cases to clinical validators, consistent with ICD-10-CM Official Coding Guideline A.19., which indicates clinical validation is a separate function from the coding process and the codes assigned by the coding professional are based on the documentation by the physician, not on a particular clinical definition or specific criteria. This guideline underscores the need for a process of validating clinical conditions prior to completing the coding process. Each facility should establish specific criteria for the necessary credentials, education, and experience it will require of its clinical documentation improvement professionals and develop processes to ensure collaboration between clinical validators, coding professionals, and providers. Qualified clinical documentation specialists can include HIM professionals, physicians, nurses, and others with a clinical and/or coding background.

An effective query process will bridge the gap of communication between coders, clinical validators, and providers. This process is a best practice solution for physicians, coders, and healthcare organizations.

An effective query process positively impacts data integrity, reimbursement, and compliance by reducing inaccurate and incomplete documentation.

The following section includes examples of how physician queries may be completed for the diagnoses and procedures reviewed in this publication. A blank, generic query form is also included. As mentioned previously, the title of the query should not contain the anticipated diagnosis. The following example titles are only for the users' convenience for locating specific query examples in this chapter.

Additional References

AHIMA: "Clinical Documentation Improvement Toolkit (2016 version)" http://bok.ahima.org/Toolkit/CDI

AHIMA: "Clinical Validation: The Next Level of CDI (January 2019 Update)" http://bok.ahima.org/doc?oid=302679#.XV1tHuhKjcs

AHIMA Code of Ethics, Coding Standards, CDIP Standards: http://www.ahima.org/about/aboutahima?tabid=ethics

AHIMA e-HIM Work Group on Maintaining the Legal EHR,"Update: Maintaining a Legally Sound Health Record—Paper and Electronic." *Journal of AHIMA,* Vol. 76, no.10 November-December 2005, 64A-L

AHIMA Ethical Standards for Clinical Documentation Improvement (CDI) Professionals (2016): http://library.ahima.org/CDI_EthicalStandards#.WdKC1tLfPIV

AHIMA. "Guidance for Clinical Documentation Improvement Programs." *Journal of AHIMA* Vol. 81, no.5 (May 2010)

AHIMA "Guidelines for Achieving a Compliant ICD-10-PCS Query" (2019 Update) http://bok.ahima.org/doc?oid=302768#.XZzkWEZKjGh

American Health Information Management Association (AHIMA) and Association of Clinical Documentation Integrity Specialists (ACDIS) practice brief "Guidelines for Achieving a Compliant Query Practice (2022 Update)" December 2022
https://acdis.org/resources/guidelines-achieving-compliant-query-practice%E2%80%942022-update

AHIMA: "Prospective Clinical Documentation Integrity (CDI) Reviews and Query/Alert Practice Best Standards"
https://my.ahima.org/store/product?id=66670

AHIMA Standards of Ethical Coding

AHIMA: "Taking Coding to the Next Level through Clinical Validation"
http://bok.ahima.org/doc?oid=300246

American Academy of Professional Coders (AAPC) Medical Coding Code of Ethics:
https://www.aapc.com/AboutUs/code-of-ethics.aspx

Association of Clinical Documentation Improvement Specialists (ACDIS) Code of Ethics

Department of Health and Human Services, 42 CFR, Part 482, "Conditions of Participation for Hospitals"

Office of Inspector General (OIG). "Compliance Program Guidance for Hospitals and Office of Inspector General (OIG)," "Supplemental Compliance Program Guidance for Hospitals,"
https://oig.hhs.gov/compliance/compliance-guidance/index.asp

Acidosis Example

Request for Documentation Clarification

THIS FORM IS A PERMANENT PART OF THE MEDICAL RECORD

Dear Physician/PA/NP: ______________________________ or other responsible provider:

When responding to this query, please exercise your independent professional judgment. The fact that a question is asked does not imply that any particular answer is desired or expected. Please complete, sign, date, and time the query. Thank you for your assistance with clarification of this issue.

Please clarify the following documentation or clinical data noted in the medical record.

IP admit note states patient was admitted with nausea/vomiting and dehydration, altered level of consciousness, weak rapid pulse, with metabolic acidosis 7.1.

Urine dipstick highly positive for glucose, ketones.

Serum ketones present, anion gap >16.

Progress notes indicate patient is a known type 1 diabetic with serum glucose 400 mg/dl.

Patient was given rapid infusion of 1L of 0.9% NS over 30 min.

Insulin 10-20 unit bolus (0.15 u/kg), then 5-7 units/hr (0.1 unit/kg/hr).

CDI Analyst/Coder: ______________________________ Date: ____________ Time: ____________

MD/PA/NP Response (Check any that apply.)

Based on your medical judgment and review of the clinical indicators above, please clarify the diagnosis.

- ❑ Metabolic acidosis due to dehydration
- ❑ Metabolic acidosis due to diabetic ketoacidosis
- ❑ Metabolic acidosis due to other cause
- ❑ Metabolic acidosis due to unspecified cause
- ❑ Other ______________________________
- ❑ Unable to determine

Physician/PA/NP Printed Name: ____

Physician/PA/NP Signature: ______________________________ Date: ____________ Time: ____________

Acute Kidney Injury Example

Request for Documentation Clarification

THIS FORM IS A PERMANENT PART OF THE MEDICAL RECORD

Dear Physician/PA/NP: ______________________ or other responsible provider:

When responding to this query, please exercise your independent professional judgment. The fact that a question is asked does not imply that any particular answer is desired or expected. Please complete, sign, date, and time the query. Thank you for your assistance with clarification of this issue.

Please clarify the following documentation or clinical data noted in the medical record.

Pt admitted with severe volume depletion.

Renal insufficiency, renal failure, and AKI are documented interchangeably in the progress notes.

UO < 0.5 ml/kg/hr for > 12 hours.

Serum creatinine was 250 umol/L.

Hypovolemia was corrected with repeat boluses of 250–500 mL of 0.9% sodium chloride solution for a total of 2 liters over 2 hours.

Serum creatinine returned to within normal limits.

CDI Analyst/Coder: ______________________ Date: __________ Time: __________

MD/PA/NP Response (Check any that apply.)

Based on your medical judgment and review of the clinical indicators above, please clarify the diagnosis.

- ❑ Acute kidney injury (AKI)
- ❑ Acute kidney (renal) Insufficiency (AKI)
- ❑ Acute renal failure (ARF)
- ❑ Chronic renal Failure
- ❑ Acute kidney injury (AKI)/acute renal failure (ARF) on chronic kidney disease (CKD) (include CKD stage) ______________________
- ❑ Unspecified renal insufficiency
- ❑ Unspecified renal failure
- ❑ Dehydration
- ❑ Other ______________________
- ❑ Clinically unable to determine

Physician/PA/NP Printed Name: ______________________

Physician/PA/NP Signature: ______________________ Date: __________ Time: __________

Query Guidelines

Acute Myocardial Infarction Example

Request for Documentation Clarification

THIS FORM IS A PERMANENT PART OF THE MEDICAL RECORD

Dear Physician/PA/NP: ______________________ or other responsible provider:

When responding to this query, please exercise your independent professional judgment. The fact that a question is asked does not imply that any particular answer is desired or expected. Please complete, sign, date, and time the query. Thank you for your assistance with clarification of this issue.

Please clarify the following documentation or clinical data noted in the medical record.

Patient admitted for cardiac cath to evaluate CAD.

Procedure note and progress notes state acute MI during catheterization.

Troponins elevated.

ECG +

Aspirin, nitroglycerine (NTG), beta blocker, oxygen regimen started.

Discharge Summary: Cath performed, CAD, AMI

CDI Analyst/Coder: ______________________ Date: ____________ Time: ____________

MD/PA/NP Response (Check any that apply.)

Based on your medical judgment and review of the clinical indicators above, please clarify the diagnosis.

CHECK ALL THAT APPLY

- ☐ Non-ST elevation (NSTEMI) MI (Type 1) present prior to procedure
- ☐ ST elevation (STEMI) MI (Type 1) present prior to procedure
- ☐ Anterior wall, left main
- ☐ Anterior wall, LAD
- ☐ Anterior wall, other
- ☐ Inferior wall, RCA
- ☐ Inferior wall, other
- ☐ Left circumflex
- ☐ Other site
- ☐ Unspecified site
- ☐ Type 2 MI present prior to procedure (myocardial infarction due to demand ischemia or secondary to ischemic balance) with underlying cause (please specify underlying cause)______________________
- ☐ Any type of above MI (*check appropriate type/site above if known*) occurring during procedure due to disease process, not related to any current/past procedure.
- ☐ AMI (Type 4, 5) associated with/related to current or past procedure (CABG, stent restenosis, catheterization, stent thrombosis etc)
- ☐ Clinically undetermined—patient death before study (Type 3)
- ☐ Other (please specify)______________________

Physician/PA/NP Printed Name: ______________________

Physician/PA/NP Signature: ______________________ Date: ____________ Time: ____________

Acute Pulmonary Edema, Noncardiac Example

Request for Documentation Clarification

THIS FORM IS A PERMANENT PART OF THE MEDICAL RECORD

Dear Physician/PA/NP: ______________________________ or other responsible provider:

When responding to this query, please exercise your independent professional judgment. The fact that a question is asked does not imply that any particular answer is desired or expected. Please complete, sign, date, and time the query. Thank you for your assistance with clarification of this issue.

Please clarify the following documentation or clinical data noted in the medical record:

A chest radiograph taken immediately after PACU admission showed diffuse bilateral opacities.

Progress notes document postsurgical acute pulmonary edema; patient has no history of heart failure (HF).

Pt received supplemental 100% oxygen by non-rebreather mask (flow, 15 l/min), 10 mg furosemide intravenously, and bronchodilators.

Progress notes document rapid improvement of pulmonary edema with no need for pressure support ventilation.

CDI Analyst/Coder: ______________________________ Date: ____________ Time: ____________

MD/PA/NP Response (Check any that apply.)

Based on your medical judgment and review of the clinical indicators above, please clarify the diagnosis.

- ❑ Acute postoperative pulmonary edema due to the procedure—please specify cardiogenic or noncardiogenic and underlying cause ______________________________
- ❑ Acute postoperative pulmonary edema due to the anesthesia—please specify cardiogenic or noncardiogenic and underlying cause ______________________________
- ❑ Acute postoperative pulmonary edema unrelated to the procedure—please specify cardiogenic or noncardiogenic and underlying cause ______________________________
- ❑ Acute pulmonary edema due to unspecified cause
- ❑ Acute pulmonary edema of no clinical significance
- ❑ No acute pulmonary edema
- ❑ Clinically unable to determine
- ❑ Other ______________________________

Physician/PA/NP Printed Name: ______________________________

Physician/PA/NP Signature: ______________________________ Date: ____________ Time: ____________

Query Guidelines

AIDS Example

Request for Documentation Clarification

THIS FORM IS A PERMANENT PART OF THE MEDICAL RECORD

Dear Physician/PA/NP: ______________________________ or other responsible provider:

When responding to this query, please exercise your independent professional judgment. The fact that a question is asked does not imply that any particular answer is desired or expected. Please complete, sign, date, and time the query. Thank you for your assistance with clarification of this issue.

Please clarify the following documentation or clinical data noted in the medical record.

HIV history noted in History and Physical.

Admitted with recurrent *Candida* esophagitis with inability to swallow.

CDI Analyst/Coder: ______________________________ Date: ____________ Time: ____________

MD/PA/NP Response (Check any that apply.)

Based on your medical judgment and review of the clinical indicators above, please clarify the patient's HIV status.

- ❑ Asymptomatic HIV positive status without AIDS-Defining Illness or HIV-Related Illness
- ❑ HIV disease/AIDS: Meets the current CDC Definition of AIDS and/or History of or Current AIDS-Defining Illness or HIV-Related Disease
- ❑ Other (please specify)______________________________
- ❑ Unable to Determine

Physician/PA/NP Printed Name: ____

Physician/PA/NP Signature: ______________________________ Date: ____________ Time: ____________

Query Guidelines

Aspiration Pneumonia Example

Request for Documentation Clarification

THIS FORM IS A PERMANENT PART OF THE MEDICAL RECORD

Dear Physician/PA/NP: ______________________________ or other responsible provider:

When responding to this query, please exercise your independent professional judgment. The fact that a question is asked does not imply that any particular answer is desired or expected. Please complete, sign, date, and time the query. Thank you for your assistance with clarification of this issue.

Please clarify the following documentation or clinical data noted in the medical record:

Pt has history of CVA with dysphagia was admitted with diagnosis of pneumonia.

Chest radiology report revealed right upper lobe opacities consistent with aspiration pneumonia.

Patient was treated with IV Zosyn.

CDI Analyst/Coder: ______________________________ Date: ____________ Time: ____________

MD/PA/NP Response (Check any that apply.)

Based on your medical judgment and review of the clinical indicators above, please clarify the diagnosis to specify the type of pneumonia you are treating.

- ☐ Community-acquired pneumonia
- ☐ Aspiration pneumonia
- ☐ Gram negative pneumonia
- ☐ Health-care-acquired pneumonia, possible gram negative
- ☐ Pneumonia due to (specific organism) ____________________
- ☐ Pneumonia due to unknown organism
- ☐ Unable to determine
- ☐ Other ______________________________

Physician/PA/NP Printed Name: ______________________________

Physician/PA/NP Signature: ______________________________ Date: ____________ Time: ____________

Atelectasis Example

Request for Documentation Clarification

THIS FORM IS A PERMANENT PART OF THE MEDICAL RECORD

Dear Physician/PA/NP: ______________________________ or other responsible provider:

When responding to this query, please exercise your independent professional judgment. The fact that a question is asked does not imply that any particular answer is desired or expected. Please complete, sign, date and time the query. Thank you for your assistance with clarification of this issue.

Please clarify the following documentation or clinical data noted in the medical record:

Patient admitted with two rib fractures after falling from a horse.

Chest x-ray on admission showed two rib fractures and atelectasis.

Patient was treated with pain medication and started on incentive spirometry.

Follow-up chest x-ray showed stable rib fractures and resolved atelectasis.

CDI Analyst/Coder: ______________________________ Date: ______________ Time: ______________

MD/PA/NP Response (Check any that apply.)

Based on your medical judgment and review of the clinical indicators above, please clarify the clinical significance, if any, of the radiology findings of atelectasis.

- ❑ Chest x-ray finding of atelectasis is of clinical significance and required treatment in addition to that for the rib fractures
- ❑ Chest x-ray finding of atelectasis is of clinical significance but is integral to the rib fractures
- ❑ Chest x-ray finding of atelectasis is incidental/of no clinical significance
- ❑ Clinically unable to determine
- ❑ Other ______________________________

Physician/PA/NP Printed Name: ______________________________

Physician/PA/NP Signature: ______________________________ Date: ______________ Time: ______________

Bacteremia Example

Request for Documentation Clarification

THIS FORM IS A PERMANENT PART OF THE MEDICAL RECORD

Dear Physician/PA/NP: ______________________ or other responsible provider:

When responding to this query, please exercise your independent professional judgment. The fact that a question is asked does not imply that any particular answer is desired or expected. Please complete, sign, date, and time the query. Thank you for your assistance with clarification of this issue.

Please clarify the following documentation or clinical data noted in the medical record:

Pt with Port-A-Cath for chemotherapy admitted with fever and chills.

Blood cultures from the port were positive for coagulase negative *Staphylococcus.*

Blood cultures from the periphery were no growth.

Consult documents staph bacteremia.

The port was not removed.

Pt received IV Cipro 400mg q12h.

CDI Analyst/Coder: ______________________ Date: ____________ Time: ____________

MD/PA/NP Response (Check any that apply.)

Based on your medical judgment and review of the clinical indicators above, please clarify the clinical significance, if any, of the positive blood culture findings.

- ❑ Bacteremia due to infected Port-A-Cath
- ❑ Bacteremia due to other cause (please specify) ______________________
- ❑ Bacteremia is an insignificant laboratory finding
- ❑ Positive blood culture is contaminant
- ❑ Clinically unable to determine
- ❑ Other ______________________

Physician/PA/NP Printed Name: ______________________

Physician/PA/NP Signature: ______________________ Date: ____________ Time: ____________

Query Guidelines

Bone Marrow/Stem Cell Transplant Example

Request for Documentation Clarification

THIS FORM IS A PERMANENT PART OF THE MEDICAL RECORD

Dear Physician/PA/NP: ______________________________ or other responsible provider:

When responding to this query, please exercise your independent professional judgment. The fact that a question is asked does not imply that any particular answer is desired or expected. Please complete, sign, date and time the query. Thank you for your assistance with clarification of this issue.

Please clarify the following documentation or clinical data noted in the medical record:

Procedure report states bone marrow transplant was done without documentation of harvest or further information.

CDI Analyst/Coder: ______________________________ Date: ______________ Time: ______________

MD/PA/NP Response (Check any that apply.)

Based on your medical judgment and review of the clinical indicators above, please clarify the procedure performed.

TYPE

- ❑ Allogenic, Related
- ❑ Allogenic, Unrelated
- ❑ Allogenic, Unspecified
- ❑ Autologous transplant using the patient's own marrow that has been stored

ROUTE OF ADMINISTRATION

- ❑ Peripheral vein
- ❑ Central vein

APPROACH

- ❑ Open
- ❑ Percutaneous
- ❑ Other (please specify) ______________________________

Physician/PA/NP Printed Name: ____

Physician/PA/NP Signature: ______________________________ Date: ______________ Time: ______________

Bronchoalveolar Lavage (BAL)/Bronchial Washing Example

Request for Documentation Clarification

THIS FORM IS A PERMANENT PART OF THE MEDICAL RECORD

Dear Physician/PA/NP: ______________________________ or other responsible provider:

When responding to this query, please exercise your independent professional judgment. The fact that a question is asked does not imply that any particular answer is desired or expected. Please complete, sign, date and time the query. Thank you for your assistance with clarification of this issue.

Please clarify the following documentation or clinical data noted in the medical record:

Procedure report states bronchoscope was used to instill saline to obtain a biopsy, but does not identify the specific body parts involved/sampled.

CDI Analyst/Coder: ______________________________ Date: ____________ Time: ____________

MD/PA/NP Response (Check any that apply.)

Based on your medical judgment and review of the clinical indicators above, could you please clarify the procedure performed?

- ❑ Bronchoalveolar lavage of alveolar lung tissue
- ❑ Bronchial washing within the bronchial tree
- ❑ Other (please describe in detail instruments used, tissue removed and intent of procedure)
  ____
  ____
  ____

Physician/PA/NP Printed Name: ____

Physician/PA/NP Signature: ______________________________ Date: ____________ Time: ____________

Query Guidelines

Cerebral Edema Example

Request for Documentation Clarification

THIS FORM IS A PERMANENT PART OF THE MEDICAL RECORD

Dear Physician/PA/NP: ______________________ or other responsible provider:

When responding to this query, please exercise your independent professional judgment. The fact that a question is asked does not imply that any particular answer is desired or expected. Please complete, sign, date, and time the query. Thank you for your assistance with clarification of this issue.

Please clarify the following documentation or clinical data noted in the medical record.

Pt admitted with ischemic cerebral infarction.

CT scan in follow up on day 2 shows increasing vasogenic cerebral edema causing mass effect.

Patient treated with thrombolytics and IV mannitol and high dose steroids.

CDI Analyst/Coder: ______________________ Date: __________ Time: __________

MD/PA/NP Response (Check any that apply.)

Based on your medical judgment and review of the clinical indicators above, please clarify the clinical significance of the abnormal CT findings of vasogenic cerebral edema causing mass effect.

- ☐ Finding of vasogenic cerebral edema is clinically significant
- ☐ Finding of vasogenic cerebral edema is clinically insignificant/incidental finding
- ☐ Clinically unable to determine
- ☐ Other ______________________

Physician/PA/NP Printed Name: ______________________

Physician/PA/NP Signature: ______________________ Date: __________ Time: __________

Query Guidelines

Cerebrovascular Accident Example

Request for Documentation Clarification

THIS FORM IS A PERMANENT PART OF THE MEDICAL RECORD

Dear Physician/PA/NP: ______________________ or other responsible provider:

When responding to this query, please exercise your independent professional judgment. The fact that a question is asked does not imply that any particular answer is desired or expected. Please complete, sign, date, and time the query. Thank you for your assistance with clarification of this issue.

Please clarify the following documentation or clinical data noted in the medical record.

Patient with thrombotic cerebral infarction, treated with Merci® Retrieval System thrombectomy and tPA.

Postprocedure imaging demonstrated hemorrhage at the infarction site.

Progress notes indicate follow-up imaging was ordered to follow the size of the hemorrhage.

CDI Analyst/Coder: ______________________ Date: ____________ Time: ____________

MD/PA/NP Response (Check any that apply.)

Based on your medical judgment and review of the clinical indicators above, please clarify the diagnostic findings.

- ❑ Cerebral hemorrhage due to spontaneous conversion of the thrombotic infarct
- ❑ Cerebral hemorrhage due to tPA administration
- ❑ Cerebral hemorrhage as a complication of the thrombectomy procedure
- ❑ Cerebral hemorrhage of other etiology ____________________
- ❑ Imaging findings of cerebral hemorrhage are clinically insignificant
- ❑ Other ______________________________
- ❑ Unable to determine

Physician/PA/NP Printed Name: ______________________________________

Physician/PA/NP Signature: ______________________ Date: ____________ Time: ____________

Chest Pain Example

Request for Documentation Clarification

THIS FORM IS A PERMANENT PART OF THE MEDICAL RECORD

Dear Physician/PA/NP: ______________________________ or other responsible provider:

When responding to this query, please exercise your independent professional judgment. The fact that a question is asked does not imply that any particular answer is desired or expected. Please complete, sign, date, and time the query. Thank you for your assistance with clarification of this issue.

Please clarify the following documentation or clinical data noted in the medical record.

Physician documentation in the progress notes indicates chest pain without further description or documentation of etiology.

CDI Analyst/Coder: ______________________________ Date: ______________ Time: ______________

MD/PA/NP Response (Check any that apply.)

Based on your medical judgment and review of the clinical indicators above, please clarify the possible underlying cause of the chest pain, if known.

- ❑ Coronary artery disease
- ❑ Unstable angina
- ❑ Angina
- ❑ Cardiac arrhythmia (specify type if known) ______________________________
- ❑ Gastroesophageal reflux disease
- ❑ Gastritis
- ❑ Esophagitis
- ❑ Pleuritic
- ❑ Musculoskeletal
- ❑ Costochondritis
- ❑ Stress/anxiety
- ❑ Psychogenic chest pain
- ❑ Chest pain—etiology undetermined
- ❑ Patient does not have chest pain
- ❑ Other ______________________________
- ❑ Clinically unable to determine

Physician/PA/NP Printed Name: ______________________________

Physician/PA/NP Signature: ______________________________ Date: ______________ Time: ______________

Query Guidelines

Chronic Obstructive Pulmonary Disease (COPD)—Exacerbation with Asthma/Bronchitis Example

Request for Documentation Clarification

THIS FORM IS A PERMANENT PART OF THE MEDICAL RECORD

Dear Physician/PA/NP: ______________________________ or other responsible provider:

When responding to this query, please exercise your independent professional judgment. The fact that a question is asked does not imply that any particular answer is desired or expected. Please complete, sign, date, and time the query. Thank you for your assistance with clarification of this issue.

Please clarify the following documentation or clinical data noted in the medical record:

Patient admitted with COPD exacerbation with exacerbation of asthma.

Patient was treated with IV corticosteroids, nebulizers with Bi-PAP and oxygen ordered.

CDI Analyst/Coder: ______________________________ Date: ____________ Time: ____________

MD/PA/NP Response (Check any that apply.)

Based on your medical judgment and review of the clinical indicators above, please clarify the diagnosis.

- ❑ Mild intermittent asthma with acute exacerbation with COPD exacerbation
- ❑ Mild persistent asthma with acute exacerbation with COPD exacerbation
- ❑ Moderate persistent asthma with acute exacerbation with COPD exacerbation
- ❑ Severe persistent asthma with acute exacerbation with COPD exacerbation
- ❑ Unspecified asthma with acute exacerbation with COPD exacerbation
- ❑ Other asthma with COPD exacerbation ______________________________
- ❑ Other ______________________________
- ❑ Unable to determine

Physician/PA/NP Printed Name: ______________________________

Physician/PA/NP Signature: ______________________________ Date: ____________ Time: ____________

Coagulopathy Example

Request for Documentation Clarification

THIS FORM IS A PERMANENT PART OF THE MEDICAL RECORD

Dear Physician/PA/NP: ______________________________ or other responsible provider:

When responding to this query, please exercise your independent professional judgment. The fact that a question is asked does not imply that any particular answer is desired or expected. Please complete, sign, date, and time the query. Thank you for your assistance with clarification of this issue.

Please clarify the following documentation or clinical data noted in the medical record.

Patient admitted with epistaxis documented by the ED physician as coagulopathy due to Coumadin toxicity.

Patient is on Coumadin prophylaxis for atrial fibrillation.

Progress notes document Coumadin was taken as prescribed and prothrombin times were within normal limits.

CDI Analyst/Coder: ______________________________ Date: ______________ Time: ______________

MD/PA/NP Response (Check any that apply.)

Based on your medical judgment and review of the clinical indicators above, please clarify the diagnosis.

- ❑ Epistaxis as an adverse effect of Coumadin taken as prescribed
- ❑ Epistaxis as a toxic effect of Coumadin taken incorrectly (overdose)
- ❑ Epistaxis due to other cause (specify cause) ______________________
- ❑ Other ____
- ❑ Unable to determine

Physician/PA/NP Printed Name: ____

Physician/PA/NP Signature: ______________________________ Date: ______________ Time: ______________

Query Guidelines

Control of Hemorrhage Example

Request for Documentation Clarification

THIS FORM IS A PERMANENT PART OF THE MEDICAL RECORD

Dear Physician/PA/NP: ______________________ or other responsible provider:

When responding to this query, please exercise your independent professional judgment. The fact that a question is asked does not imply that any particular answer is desired or expected. Please complete, sign, date, and time the query. Thank you for your assistance with clarification of this issue.

Please clarify the following documentation or clinical data noted in the medical record.

According to the operative report, the patient underwent laparoscopic appendectomy. After the appendix was removed, bleeding was noted from the site of the laparoscopic port. The surgery was converted to an open approach and the bleeding was controlled. The operative report, however, does not describe the site of the hemorrhage and the surgical technique used.

CDI Analyst/Coder: ______________________ Date: __________ Time: __________

MD/PA/NP Response (Check any that apply.)

Based on your medical judgment and review of the clinical indicators above, could you please clarify the procedure performed?

Site of hemorrhage:

- ❑ Abdominal wall
- ❑ Abdominal/peritoneal cavity
- ❑ Abdominal/pelvic cavity
- ❑ Retroperitoneum
- ❑ Other (please specify) ______________________

Method of control:

- ❑ Packing
- ❑ Pressure
- ❑ Fibrin glue/Gelfoam/Surgicel
- ❑ Vessel ligation using sutures/clamps/clips (specify site)______________________
- ❑ Coagulation/cautery
- ❑ Excision (specify site)
- ❑ Other (please specify) ______________________

Physician/PA/NP Printed Name: ______________________

Physician/PA/NP Signature: ______________________ Date: __________ Time: __________

COVID-19 Example

Request for Documentation Clarification

THIS FORM IS A PERMANENT PART OF THE MEDICAL RECORD

Dear Physician/PA/NP: ______________________ or other responsible provider:

When responding to this query, please exercise your independent professional judgment. The fact that a question is asked does not imply that any particular answer is desired or expected. Please complete, sign, date, and time the query. Thank you for your assistance with clarifying this issue.

Please clarify the following documentation or clinical data noted in the medical record.

Patient with possible recent exposure to COVID-19 presented from nursing home with fever of 102.1, cough, shortness of breath, tachycardia and rising WBC. Chest x-ray with bilateral opacities. Was admitted for pneumonia with suspected COVID-19 infection. Chest CT revealed rounded ground-glass opacities in both lower lungs. Treatments included supplemental oxygen, remdesivir, fluids, and antibiotics. COVID-19 test results not available at discharge.

CDI Analyst/Coder: ______________________ Date: ____________ Time: ____________

MD/PA/NP Response (Check any that apply.)

Based on your medical judgment and review of the clinical indicators above, please clarify the diagnosis.

- ❑ Viral pneumonia due to COVID-19
- ❑ Viral pneumonia without COVID-19 (please specify virus if known)______________________
- ❑ Viral pneumonia due to COVID-19 with superimposed bacterial pneumonia (please specify bacterial organism if known) ______________________
- ❑ Viral and bacterial pneumonia without COVID-19 (please specify virus and bacterial organism if known) ______________________
- ❑ Bacterial pneumonia and COVID-19 (please specify bacterial organism if known) ______________________
- ❑ Bacterial pneumonia without COVID-19 (please specify bacterial organism if known) ______________________
- ❑ Community-acquired pneumonia
- ❑ Aspiration pneumonia
- ❑ Other pneumonia (specify) ______________________
- ❑ Pneumonia, unspecified
- ❑ COVID-19 only
- ❑ Unable to determine
- ❑ Other condition (please specify) ______________________

Physician/PA/NP Printed Name: ______________________

Physician/PA/NP Signature: ______________________ Date: ____________ Time: ____________

Debridement by Excision (Subcutaneous Tissue, and Fascia or Muscle) Example

Request for Documentation Clarification

THIS FORM IS A PERMANENT PART OF THE MEDICAL RECORD

Dear Physician/PA/NP: ______________________ or other responsible provider:

When responding to this query, please exercise your independent professional judgment. The fact that a question is asked does not imply that any particular answer is desired or expected. Please complete, sign, date, and time the query. Thank you for your assistance with clarification of this issue.

Please clarify the following documentation or clinical data noted in the medical record:

Operative report states excisional debridement down to muscle

CDI Analyst/Coder: ______________________ Date: ____________ Time: ____________

Excisional debridement is coded to the root operation Excision. Definition: Cutting out or off, without replacement, a portion of a body part. Example: Cutting or excising tissue using a scalpel or laser

Nonexcisional debridement is coded to the root operation Extraction. Definition: Pulling or stripping out or off all or a portion of a body part by the use of force. Example: Scraping with a knife, scalpel or rongeur; forceps, tongs, pick-ups, and other grasping or scraping devices, stripping, scrubbing, brushing, pulsed lavage, mechanical lavage, mechanical irrigation, high-pressure irrigation, Versajet™ debridement.

MD/PA/NP Response (Check any that apply.)

Based on your medical judgment and review of the clinical indicators above, please clarify the debridement procedure performed.

- ❑ Debridement by excision (excisional: cutting out or off) was performed using ______________________ instrumentation, involving the following tissue depth:
  - ❑ skin
  - ❑ subcutaneous tissue
  - ❑ fascia
  - ❑ tendon
  - ❑ muscle
  - ❑ bone
- ❑ Debridement by extraction (nonexcisional: pulling or stripping out by the use of force) was performed using ______________________ instrumentation, involving the following tissue depth:
  - ❑ skin
  - ❑ subcutaneous tissue
  - ❑ fascia
  - ❑ tendon
  - ❑ muscle
  - ❑ bone

Physician/PA/NP Printed Name: ______________________

Physician/PA/NP Signature: ______________________ Date: ____________ Time: ____________

Query Guidelines

Debridement by Extraction (Fascia) Example

Request for Documentation Clarification

THIS FORM IS A PERMANENT PART OF THE MEDICAL RECORD

Dear Physician/PA/NP: ______________________ or other responsible provider:

When responding to this query, please exercise your independent professional judgment. The fact that a question is asked does not imply that any particular answer is desired or expected. Please complete, sign, date, and time the query. Thank you for your assistance with clarification of this issue.

Please clarify the following documentation or clinical data noted in the medical record:

Operative report states debridement of fascia of right leg to remove debris and nonviable tissue of a highly contaminated deep wound.

CDI Analyst/Coder: ______________________ Date: __________ Time: __________

Excisional debridement is coded to the root operation Excision. Definition: Cutting out or off, without replacement, a portion of a body part. Example: Cutting or excising tissue using a scalpel or laser.

Nonexcisional debridement is coded to the root operation Extraction—Definition: Pulling or stripping out or off all or a portion of a body part by the use of force. Example: Scraping with a knife, scalpel or rongeur; forceps, tongs, pick-ups, and other grasping or scraping devices, stripping, scrubbing, brushing, pulsed lavage, mechanical lavage, mechanical irrigation, high-pressure irrigation, Versajet™ debridement.

MD/PA/NP Response (Check any that apply.)

Based on your medical judgment and review of the clinical indicators above, please clarify the debridement procedure performed.

- ❑ Debridement by excision (excisional: Cutting out or off) was performed using ______________ instrumentation, involving the following tissue depth:
  - ❑ Skin
  - ❑ Subcutaneous tissue
  - ❑ Fascia
  - ❑ Tendon
  - ❑ Muscle
  - ❑ Bone
- ❑ Debridement by extraction (nonexcisional: Pulling or stripping out by the use of force) was performed using ______________ instrumentation, involving the following tissue depth:
  - ❑ Skin
  - ❑ Subcutaneous tissue
  - ❑ Fascia
  - ❑ Tendon
  - ❑ Muscle
  - ❑ Bone

Physician/PA/NP Printed Name: ______________________________

Physician/PA/NP Signature: ______________________ Date: __________ Time: __________

Query Guidelines

Deep Vein Thrombosis of Upper and Lower Extremities Example

Request for Documentation Clarification

THIS FORM IS A PERMANENT PART OF THE MEDICAL RECORD

Dear Physician/PA/NP: ______________________ or other responsible provider:

When responding to this query, please exercise your independent professional judgment. The fact that a question is asked does not imply that any particular answer is desired or expected. Please complete, sign, date, and time the query. Thank you for your assistance with clarification of this issue.

Please clarify the following documentation or clinical data noted in the medical record:

History and physical states left femoral acute peripheral vascular disease.

Imaging noted thrombus in the left femoral vein treated with tPA on the first day of admission followed by AngioJet thrombectomy on day 2.

Interventional radiology report documents thrombus.

CDI Analyst/Coder: ______________________ Date: __________ Time: __________

MD/PA/NP Response (Check any that apply.)

Based on your medical judgment and review of the clinical indicators above, please clarify the diagnosis.

- ☐ Acute deep left femoral vein thrombosis
- ☐ Chronic deep left femoral vein thrombosis
- ☐ Left femoral acute peripheral vascular disease
- ☐ Unspecified left femoral peripheral vascular disease
- ☐ Other left femoral peripheral vascular disease ______________________
- ☐ Other ______________________
- ☐ Unable to determine

Physician/PA/NP Printed Name: ______________________________________

Physician/PA/NP Signature: ______________________ Date: __________ Time: __________

Query Guidelines

Dehydration as Principal Diagnosis Example

Request for Documentation Clarification

THIS FORM IS A PERMANENT PART OF THE MEDICAL RECORD

Dear Physician/PA/NP: ______________________ or other responsible provider:

When responding to this query, please exercise your independent professional judgment. The fact that a question is asked does not imply that any particular answer is desired or expected. Please complete, sign, date, and time the query. Thank you for your assistance with clarification of this issue.

Please clarify the following documentation or clinical data noted in the medical record:

Patient was admitted with dehydration and orthostatic hypotension.

ED physician documents dehydration with hypotension.

Cardiology consult documents iatrogenic hypotension due to adverse effect of medication Catapres.

Patient was treated with IV hydration and medication was adjusted.

CDI Analyst/Coder: ______________________ Date: __________ Time: __________

MD/PA/NP Response (Check any that apply.)

Based on your medical judgment and review of the clinical indicators above, please clarify the diagnosis.

- ❑ Orthostatic hypotension due to dehydration
- ❑ Orthostatic hypotension due to adverse effect of Catapres
- ❑ Orthostatic hypotension due to incorrect dosage of Catapres
- ❑ Orthostatic hypotension due to both dehydration and adverse effect of Catapres
- ❑ Orthostatic hypotension due to both dehydration and incorrect dosage of Catapres
- ❑ Orthostatic hypotension due to other cause (specify)__________
- ❑ Orthostatic hypotension due to unknown cause
- ❑ Other ______________________
- ❑ Clinically unable to determine

Physician/PA/NP Printed Name: ______________________________

Physician/PA/NP Signature: ______________________ Date: __________ Time: __________

Diabetic Ketoacidosis Example

Request for Documentation Clarification

THIS FORM IS A PERMANENT PART OF THE MEDICAL RECORD

Dear Physician/PA/NP: ______________________________ or other responsible provider:

When responding to this query, please exercise your independent professional judgment. The fact that a question is asked does not imply that any particular answer is desired or expected. Please complete, sign, date, and time the query. Thank you for your assistance with clarification of this issue.

Please clarify the following documentation or clinical data noted in the medical record:

Progress note indicates newly diagnosed diabetic with ketoacidosis and stupor.

Initial laboratory findings blood glucose 500 mg/dL, pH 6.9, bicarbonate 9mEq/L, anion gap 13

Glasgow coma scale total score 8 on arrival in ED

CDI Analyst/Coder: ______________________________ Date: ____________ Time: ____________

MD/PA/NP Response (Check any that apply.)

Based on your medical judgment and review of the clinical indicators above, could you please clarify the clinical significance of the laboratory findings and/or diagnosis?

- ❑ Diabetes mellitus due to underlying condition with ketoacidosis without coma (specify underlying condition) ______________________________
- ❑ Diabetes mellitus due to underlying condition with ketoacidosis with coma (specify underlying condition) ______________________________
- ❑ Drug or chemical induced diabetes mellitus with ketoacidosis without coma (specify drug or chemical) ______________________________
- ❑ Drug or chemical induced diabetes mellitus with ketoacidosis with coma (specify drug or chemical) ______________________________
- ❑ Type 1 diabetes mellitus with ketoacidosis without coma
- ❑ Type 1 diabetes mellitus with ketoacidosis with coma
- ❑ Type 2 diabetes mellitus with ketoacidosis without coma
- ❑ Type 2 diabetes mellitus with ketoacidosis with coma
- ❑ Other specified diabetes mellitus with ketoacidosis without coma (specify other type) ____________________
- ❑ Other specified diabetes mellitus with ketoacidosis with coma (specify other type) ____________________
- ❑ Unable to determine
- ❑ Other ______________________________

Physician/PA/NP Printed Name: ______________________________

Physician/PA/NP Signature: ______________________________ Date: ____________ Time: ____________

Query Guidelines

Empyema, Pleural or Pyothorax Example

Request for Documentation Clarification

THIS FORM IS A PERMANENT PART OF THE MEDICAL RECORD

Dear Physician/PA/NP: ______________________ or other responsible provider:

When responding to this query, please exercise your independent professional judgment. The fact that a question is asked does not imply that any particular answer is desired or expected. Please complete, sign, date, and time the query. Thank you for your assistance with clarification of this issue.

Please clarify the following documentation or clinical data noted in the medical record:

Patient was admitted with pneumonia.

Radiology report on admission shows either an empyema or pulmonary abscess.

IV piperacillin and tazobactam administered.

CDI Analyst/Coder: ______________________ Date: __________ Time: __________

MD/PA/NP Response (Check any that apply.)

Based on your medical judgment and review of the clinical indicators above, please clarify the clinical significance of the radiology findings and/or diagnosis, if any.

- ☐ Empyema______________________
- ☐ Pulmonary (lung abscess)
- ☐ Pleural abscess
- ☐ Other ______________________
- ☐ Clinically unable to determine

Physician/PA/NP Printed Name: ______________________

Physician/PA/NP Signature: ______________________ Date: __________ Time: __________

Query Guidelines

Encephalopathy Example

Request for Documentation Clarification

THIS FORM IS A PERMANENT PART OF THE MEDICAL RECORD

Dear Physician/PA/NP: ______________________ or other responsible provider:

When responding to this query, please exercise your independent professional judgment. The fact that a question is asked does not imply that any particular answer is desired or expected. Please complete, sign, date, and time the query. Thank you for your assistance with clarification of this issue.

Please clarify the following documentation or clinical data noted in the medical record.

Progress notes document altered mental status due to dehydration, encephalopathy, and alteration in consciousness.

Patient was noted to return quickly back to baseline after rehydration.

CDI Analyst/Coder: ______________________ Date: __________ Time: __________

MD/PA/NP Response (Check any that apply.)

Based on your medical judgment and review of the clinical indicators above, please clarify the nature, chronicity, and underlying cause of the altered mental status.

Nature (check all that apply):

- ❑ Dementia
- ❑ Delirium
- ❑ Psychosis
- ❑ Obtundation
- ❑ Stupor
- ❑ Coma
- ❑ Vegetative state
- ❑ Other: ______________________
- ❑ Unable to determine

Chronicity (check all that apply):

- ❑ Acute
- ❑ Chronic
- ❑ Acute on chronic
- ❑ Other: ______________________
- ❑ Unable to determine

Underlying cause (check all that apply):

- ❑ Alzheimer's disease
- ❑ Encephalopathy (indicate type and underlying medical illness) ______________________ ______________________
- ❑ Lewy body dementia
- ❑ Acute stroke
- ❑ Late effect of stroke
- ❑ Transient ischemic attack
- ❑ Generalized cerebral ischemia
- ❑ Seizure disorder (state its nature and whether status epilepticus is present or symptoms are intractable) ______________________
- ❑ Normal pressure hydrocephalus
- ❑ Psychiatric illness (indicate type)______________________
- ❑ Other: ______________________
- ❑ Unable to determine

Physician/PA/NP Printed Name: ______________________

Physician/PA/NP Signature: ______________________ Date: __________ Time: __________

Fusion, Spinal Example

Request for Documentation Clarification

THIS FORM IS A PERMANENT PART OF THE MEDICAL RECORD

Dear Physician/PA/NP: ______________________________ or other responsible provider:

When responding to this query, please exercise your independent professional judgment. The fact that a question is asked does not imply that any particular answer is desired or expected. Please complete, sign, date, and time the query. Thank you for your assistance with clarification of this issue.

Please clarify the following documentation or clinical data noted in the medical record:

Lumbar spinal fusion was performed.

CDI Analyst/Coder: ______________________________ Date: ____________ Time: ____________

MD/PA/NP Response (Check any that apply.)

Based on your medical judgment and review of the clinical indicators above, please clarify the procedure performed. Please use a separate column for each level performed using different device, approach location, and/or column. Check all that apply.

LEVEL OF FUSION ❑ Thoracolumbar ❑ Lumbar ❑ 1-2 ❑ 2-3 ❑ 3-4 ❑ 4-5 ❑ Lumbosacral	LEVEL OF FUSION ❑ Thoracolumbar ❑ Lumbar ❑ 1-2 ❑ 2-3 ❑ 3-4 ❑ 4-5 ❑ Lumbosacral	LEVEL OF FUSION ❑ Thoracolumbar ❑ Lumbar ❑ 1-2 ❑ 2-3 ❑ 3-4 ❑ 4-5 ❑ Lumbosacral
DEVICE check each that apply ❑ Interbody Fusion Device ❑ Autologous (autograft) bone graft—If not locally obtained state harvest site: ____________ ❑ Nonautologous (Allogenic) bone graft ❑ Synthetic	DEVICE check each that apply ❑ Interbody Fusion Device ❑ Autologous (autograft) bone graft—if not locally obtained state harvest site: ____________ ❑ Nonautologous (Allogenic) bone graft ❑ Synthetic	DEVICE check each that apply ❑ Interbody Fusion Device ❑ Autologous (autograft) bone graft—if not locally obtained state harvest site: ____________ ❑ Nonautologous (Allogenic) bone graft ❑ Synthetic
APPROACH ACCESS ❑ Anterior ❑ Lateral ❑ Posterior	APPROACH ACCESS ❑ Anterior ❑ Lateral ❑ Posterior	APPROACH ACCESS ❑ Anterior ❑ Lateral ❑ Posterior
COLUMN FUSED ❑ Anterior ❑ Posterior ❑ Both Anterior and Posterior	COLUMN FUSED ❑ Anterior ❑ Posterior ❑ Both Anterior and Posterior	COLUMN FUSED ❑ Anterior ❑ Posterior ❑ Both Anterior and Posterior

Physician/PA/NP Printed Name: ____

Physician/PA/NP Signature: ______________________________ Date: ____________ Time: ____________

Gastrointestinal Hemorrhage Example

Request for Documentation Clarification

THIS FORM IS A PERMANENT PART OF THE MEDICAL RECORD

Dear Physician/PA/NP: ______________________________ or other responsible provider:

When responding to this query, please exercise your independent professional judgment. The fact that a question is asked does not imply that any particular answer is desired or expected. Please complete, sign, date, and time the query. Thank you for your assistance with clarification of this issue.

Please clarify the following documentation or clinical data noted in the medical record.

Patient admitted from ED with diagnosis of GI bleed.

EGD was performed which identified gastric erosions and healed duodenal ulcer without stigmata of bleeding.

Biopsy was positive for Helicobacter pylori.

CDI Analyst/Coder: ______________________________ Date: ____________ Time: ____________

MD/PA/NP Response (Check Any that Apply)

Based on your medical judgment and review of the clinical indicators above, please clarify the diagnosis.

- ❑ Gastrointestinal bleed from gastric erosions
- ❑ Gastrointestinal bleed from healed duodenal ulcer
- ❑ Gastrointestinal bleed due to other etiology ______________________________
- ❑ Gastrointestinal bleed due to unknown etiology
- ❑ Other
- ❑ Unable to determine

Physician/PA/NP Printed Name: ______________________________

Physician/PA/NP Signature: ______________________________ Date: ____________ Time: ____________

Heart Failure (Nonrheumatic) Example

Request for Documentation Clarification

THIS FORM IS A PERMANENT PART OF THE MEDICAL RECORD

Dear Physician/PA/NP: ______________________ or other responsible provider:

When responding to this query, please exercise your independent professional judgment. The fact that a question is asked does not imply that any particular answer is desired or expected. Please complete, sign, date, and time the query. Thank you for your assistance with clarification of this issue.

Please clarify the following documentation or clinical data noted in the medical record:

Per history and physical and progress notes, patient has chronic decompensated congestive heart failure, treated with IV Lasix.

Echocardiogram report documents interpretation of systolic dysfunction and is maintained.

CDI Analyst/Coder: ______________________ Date: __________ Time: __________

MD/PA/NP Response (Check any that apply.)

Based on your medical judgment and review of the clinical indicators above, please clarify the diagnosis.

- ❑ Acute systolic heart failure
- ❑ Chronic systolic heart failure
- ❑ Acute on chronic systolic heart failure
- ❑ Acute diastolic heart failure
- ❑ Chronic diastolic heart failure
- ❑ Acute on chronic diastolic heart failure
- ❑ Acute combined systolic and diastolic heart failure
- ❑ Chronic combined systolic and diastolic heart failure
- ❑ Acute on chronic combined systolic and diastolic heart failure
- ❑ Left heart failure (ventricular)
- ❑ Right heart failure ❑ Acute ❑ Chronic ❑ Acute on chronic
- ❑ Right heart failure due to left heart failure
- ❑ Biventricular heart failure
- ❑ High output heart failure
- ❑ End stage heart failure (stage D)
- ❑ Unspecified congestive heart failure
- ❑ Patient does NOT have acute or chronic congestive heart failure
- ❑ Other ______________________
- ❑ Unable to determine

Physician/PA/NP Printed Name: ______________________________________

Physician/PA/NP Signature: ______________________ Date: __________ Time: __________

Query Guidelines

Hepatic Encephalopathy Example

Request for Documentation Clarification

THIS FORM IS A PERMANENT PART OF THE MEDICAL RECORD

Dear Physician/PA/NP: ______________________ or other responsible provider:

When responding to this query, please exercise your independent professional judgment. The fact that a question is asked does not imply that any particular answer is desired or expected. Please complete, sign, date, and time the query. Thank you for your assistance with clarification of this issue.

Please clarify the following documentation or clinical data noted in the medical record.

Pt admitted with hepatic coma due to liver failure per ED physician.

Progress notes document hepatic failure.

Discharge summary documents hepatitis with hepatic failure and hepatic encephalopathy.

CDI Analyst/Coder: ______________________ Date: __________ Time: __________

MD/PA/NP Response (Check any that apply.)

Based on your medical judgment and review of the clinical indicators above, please clarify the underlying cause of the hepatitis with hepatic failure, hepatic encephalopathy with coma diagnosis.

- ❑ Alcoholic hepatic failure
- ❑ Alcoholic hepatitis
- ❑ Toxic liver disease with hepatic necrosis
- ❑ Acute or subacute hepatic failure
- ❑ Chronic hepatic failure
- ❑ Hepatic failure, unspecified
- ❑ Hepatic failure due to drugs
- ❑ Hepatorenal failure
- ❑ Infectious hepatitis
- ❑ Acute viral hepatitis A
- ❑ Acute viral hepatitis B with delta-agent
- ❑ Acute viral hepatitis B without delta-agent
- ❑ Unspecified viral hepatitis B
- ❑ Acute viral hepatitis C
- ❑ Unspecified viral hepatitis C
- ❑ Unspecified viral hepatitis
- ❑ Other ______________________
- ❑ Clinically unable to determine

Physician/PA/NP Printed Name: ______________________________________

Physician/PA/NP Signature: ______________________ Date: __________ Time: __________

Hypernatremia Example

Request for Documentation Clarification

THIS FORM IS A PERMANENT PART OF THE MEDICAL RECORD

Dear Physician/PA/NP: ______________________ or other responsible provider:

When responding to this query, please exercise your independent professional judgment. The fact that a question is asked does not imply that any particular answer is desired or expected. Please complete, sign, date, and time the query. Thank you for your assistance with clarification of this issue.

Please clarify the following documentation or clinical data noted in the medical record:

Progress note indicates "↑" NA, oral fluid replacement and monitor.

Initial laboratory finding of serum sodium of 147; repeat value down to 140.

CDI Analyst/Coder: ______________________ Date: __________ Time: __________

MD/PA/NP Response (Check any that apply.)

Based on your medical judgment and review of the clinical indicators above, please clarify the clinical significance of the laboratory finding and/or diagnosis.

- ❑ Hypernatremia
- ❑ Dehydration
- ❑ Clinically insignificant laboratory finding
- ❑ Unable to determine
- ❑ Other ______________________

Physician/PA/NP Printed Name: ______________________

Physician/PA/NP Signature: ______________________ Date: __________ Time: __________

Hyponatremia Example

Request for Documentation Clarification

THIS FORM IS A PERMANENT PART OF THE MEDICAL RECORD

Dear Physician/PA/NP: ______________________ or other responsible provider:

When responding to this query, please exercise your independent professional judgment. The fact that a question is asked does not imply that any particular answer is desired or expected. Please complete, sign, date, and time the query. Thank you for your assistance with clarification of this issue.

Please clarify the following documentation or clinical data noted in the medical record:

Progress note indicates sodium decreased at 129, decrease fluid intake and change IV fluids to normal saline and monitor.

Initial laboratory finding of serum sodium of 147; repeat value down to 140.

CDI Analyst/Coder: ______________________ Date: __________ Time: __________

MD/PA/NP Response (Check any that apply.)

Based on your medical judgment and review of the clinical indicators above, please clarify the clinical significance of the laboratory finding and/or diagnosis.

- ☐ Hyponatremia
- ☐ Clinically insignificant laboratory finding
- ☐ Unable to determine
- ☐ Other ______________________

Physician/PA/NP Printed Name: ______________________

Physician/PA/NP Signature: ______________________ Date: __________ Time: __________

Iatrogenic (Intraoperative) Puncture or Laceration (Tear) (Rent) Example

Request for Documentation Clarification

THIS FORM IS A PERMANENT PART OF THE MEDICAL RECORD

Dear Physician/PA/NP: ______________________ or other responsible provider:

When responding to this query, please exercise your independent professional judgment. The fact that a question is asked does not imply that any particular answer is desired or expected. Please complete, sign, date, and time the query. Thank you for your assistance with clarification of this issue.

Please clarify the following documentation or clinical data noted in the medical record:

During the cholecystectomy, the operative report states a 3 cm liver laceration occurred during the procedure, which was repaired along with hemostasis by electrocautery.

> 250 cc EBL

CDI Analyst/Coder: ______________________________ Date: ____________ Time: ____________

MD/PA/NP Response (Check any that apply.)

Based on your medical judgment and review of the clinical indicators above, please clarify if this laceration and repair were:

- ❑ Unexpected and complicated the procedure performed
- ❑ Not routinely expected but integral/inherent to the procedure performed
- ❑ Routinely expected and integral/inherent to the procedure performed
- ❑ Incidental and without clinical significance
- ❑ Unable to determine
- ❑ Other ______________________________

Physician/PA/NP Printed Name: ____

Physician/PA/NP Signature: ______________________________ Date: ____________ Time: ____________

Query Guidelines

Ileus Example

Request for Documentation Clarification

THIS FORM IS A PERMANENT PART OF THE MEDICAL RECORD

Dear Physician/PA/NP: ______________________ or other responsible provider:

When responding to this query, please exercise your independent professional judgment. The fact that a question is asked does not imply that any particular answer is desired or expected. Please complete, sign, date, and time the query. Thank you for your assistance with clarification of this issue.

Please clarify the following documentation or clinical data noted in the medical record:

On post-op day 4 after adhesiolysis for SBO due to adhesions, patient had follow up abdominal x-ray that was positive for ileus.

Patient had absent bowel sounds, was made NPO and NG tube inserted.

Progress notes document ileus resolved.

CDI Analyst/Coder: ______________________ Date: __________ Time: __________

A diminished return of bowel function is expected in the postoperative period for some patients, and an ileus can have different relationships to the procedure and may not be related to any procedure whatsoever. Please complete this form indicating if any ileus exists and if so, how it should be classified.

MD/PA/NP (Check any that apply.)

Based on your medical judgment and review of the clinical indicators above, please clarify the diagnosis.

- ☐ There is no Ileus
- ☐ Ileus is present but is clinically insignificant
- ☐ Ileus is present but is an expected outcome of the surgical procedure
- ☐ Ileus is present but is unrelated to the procedure
- ☐ Ileus is present and is not an expected outcome of the surgical procedure
- ☐ Ileus due to a complication that occurred during the surgical procedure
- ☐ Ileus was present prior to procedure and unrelated
- ☐ Ileus present prior to procedure and due to disease
- ☐ Ileus occurred after the procedure due to preexisting disease
- ☐ Ileus due to adhesions
- ☐ Ileus due to anesthesia
- ☐ Ileus due to immobility
- ☐ Ileus due to medications
- ☐ Ileus due to other etiology ______________________
- ☐ Ileus due to unknown etiology
- ☐ Clinically unable to determine
- ☐ Other ______________________

Physician/PA/NP Printed Name: ______________________

Physician/PA/NP Signature: ______________________ Date: __________ Time: __________

Intra-op or Post-op Hematoma/Hemorrhage/ Seroma (Not Due to Device, Implant, or Graft) Example

Request for Documentation Clarification

THIS FORM IS A PERMANENT PART OF THE MEDICAL RECORD

Dear Physician/PA/NP: ______________________________ or other responsible provider:

When responding to this query, please exercise your independent professional judgment. The fact that a question is asked does not imply that any particular answer is desired or expected. Please complete, sign, date, and time the query. Thank you for your assistance with clarification of this issue.

Please clarify the following documentation or clinical data noted in the medical record:

Post-op day one progress note states slight oozing at suture line, controlled with two suture tacks.

CDI Analyst/Coder: ________________________________ Date: ______________ Time: ______________

MD/PA/NP Response (Check any that apply.)

Based on your medical judgment and review of the clinical indicators above, please clarify the clinical significance.

- ❑ Unexpected and complicated the procedure performed
- ❑ Not routinely expected but integral/inherent to the procedure performed
- ❑ Routinely expected and integral/inherent to the procedure performed
- ❑ Incidental and without clinical significance
- ❑ Unable to determine
- ❑ Other ______________________________

Physician/PA/NP Printed Name: ____

Physician/PA/NP Signature: ______________________________ Date: ______________ Time: ______________

Intravenous/Dialysis Line/Catheter Infections Example

Request for Documentation Clarification

THIS FORM IS A PERMANENT PART OF THE MEDICAL RECORD

Dear Physician/PA/NP: ______________________ or other responsible provider:

When responding to this query, please exercise your independent professional judgment. The fact that a question is asked does not imply that any particular answer is desired or expected. Please complete, sign, date, and time the query. Thank you for your assistance with clarification of this issue.

Please clarify the following documentation or clinical data noted in the medical record:

Patient has documented cellulitis at his CVC catheter site.

Progress notes also state fever and chills.

CDI Analyst/Coder: ______________________ Date: ____________ Time: ____________

MD/PA/NP Response (Check any that apply.)

Based on your medical judgment and review of the clinical indicators above, please clarify the diagnosis.

- ❑ Localized central line site infection
- ❑ Infected central line
- ❑ Central line associated blood stream infection
- ❑ Unknown
- ❑ Unable to determine
- ❑ Other ______________________

Physician/PA/NP Printed Name: ______________________

Physician/PA/NP Signature: ______________________ Date: ____________ Time: ____________

Joint Replacement, Hip, Total Example

Request for Documentation Clarification

THIS FORM IS A PERMANENT PART OF THE MEDICAL RECORD

Dear Physician/PA/NP: ______________________ or other responsible provider:

When responding to this query, please exercise your independent professional judgment. The fact that a question is asked does not imply that any particular answer is desired or expected. Please complete, sign, date, and time the query. Thank you for your assistance with clarification of this issue.

Please clarify the following documentation or clinical data noted in the medical record:

According to the operative report, patient had a right total hip arthroplasty, but the procedure report fails to document the type of material used in the bearing surface, and whether the prosthesis was cemented or uncemented.

CDI Analyst/Coder: ______________________ Date: __________ Time: __________

MD/PA/NP Response (Check any that apply.)

Based on your medical judgment and review of the clinical indicators above, could you please clarify the procedure performed?

- ❑ Metal
- ❑ Metal on Polyethylene
- ❑ Ceramic
- ❑ Ceramic on Polyethylene
- ❑ Oxidized Zirconium on Polyethylene
- ❑ Cemented
- ❑ Uncemented
- ❑ Unable to determine
- ❑ Other______________________

Physician/PA/NP Printed Name: ______________________

Physician/PA/NP Signature: ______________________ Date: __________ Time: __________

Malnutrition Example

Request for Documentation Clarification

THIS FORM IS A PERMANENT PART OF THE MEDICAL RECORD

Dear Physician/PA/NP: ______________________ or other responsible provider:

When responding to this query, please exercise your independent professional judgment. The fact that a question is asked does not imply that any particular answer is desired or expected. Please complete, sign, date, and time the query. Thank you for your assistance with clarification of this issue.

Please clarify the following documentation or clinical data noted in the medical record:

Protein-calorie malnutrition is documented in the progress notes.

Nutrition consultation was ordered and nutritional supplements (Ensure) were given.

CDI Analyst/Coder: ______________________ Date: __________ Time: __________

MD/PA/NP Response (Check any that apply.)

Based on your medical judgment and review of the clinical indicators above, please clarify the diagnosis.

- ❑ Severe malnutrition not otherwise specified
- ❑ Severe protein-calorie malnutrition
- ❑ Malnutrition of moderate degree
- ❑ Malnutrition of mild degree
- ❑ Other protein-calorie malnutrition ______________
- ❑ Unspecified protein-calorie malnutrition
- ❑ Malnutrition, not otherwise specified
- ❑ Unable to determine
- ❑ Other ______________________

Physician/PA/NP Printed Name: ______________________________

Physician/PA/NP Signature: ______________________ Date: __________ Time: __________

Mechanical Ventilation Example

Request for Documentation Clarification

THIS FORM IS A PERMANENT PART OF THE MEDICAL RECORD

Dear Physician/PA/NP: ______________________________ or other responsible provider:

When responding to this query, please exercise your independent professional judgment. The fact that a question is asked does not imply that any particular answer is desired or expected. Please complete, sign, date, and time the query. Thank you for your assistance with clarification of this issue.

Please clarify the following documentation or clinical data noted in the medical record:

Patient with history of COPD under treatment underwent CABG for symptomatic CAD.

Patient was maintained on mechanical ventilation for 46 hours post-op.

CDI Analyst/Coder: ______________________________ Date: ____________ Time: ____________

MD/PA/NP Response (Check any that apply.)

Based on your medical judgment and review of the clinical indicators above, please clarify the reason for the continued mechanical ventilation.

- ❑ Mechanical ventilation was done for routine maintenance after surgery
- ❑ Mechanical ventilation was continued after routine surgical maintenance for COPD
- ❑ Mechanical ventilation due to continued sedation from anesthesia
- ❑ Mechanical ventilation due to slow wean from anesthesia
- ❑ Mechanical ventilation due to acute respiratory failure due to the surgery (i.e., complication)
- ❑ Unable to determine
- ❑ Other ______________________________

Physician/PA/NP Printed Name: ______________________________

Physician/PA/NP Signature: ______________________________ Date: ____________ Time: ____________

Poisoning and Toxic Effects of Illicit Drugs, Prescribed Drugs, Nonprescribed Drugs, Alcohol, Chemicals, and Other Substances Example

Request for Documentation Clarification

THIS FORM IS A PERMANENT PART OF THE MEDICAL RECORD

Dear Physician/PA/NP: ______________________________ or other responsible provider:

When responding to this query, please exercise your independent professional judgment. The fact that a question is asked does not imply that any particular answer is desired or expected. Please complete, sign, date, and time the query. Thank you for your assistance with clarification of this issue.

Please clarify the following documentation or clinical data noted in the medical record:

ED record states the patient experienced severe chest pain within 30 min after snorting cocaine.

Acute transmural inferior myocardial infarction documented on ECG and noted in progress notes.

ED final diagnosis is "cocaine-induced acute coronary syndrome."

Toxicology screen was positive for cocaine.

CDI Analyst/Coder: ______________________________ Date: ____________ Time: ____________

MD/PA/NP Response (Check any that apply.)

Based on your medical judgment and review of the clinical indicators above, please clarify cause and effect relationship, if any, and the diagnosis.

- ❑ Cocaine-induced acute coronary syndrome
- ❑ Cocaine-induced acute transmural inferior myocardial infarction
- ❑ Other acute transmural inferior myocardial infarction
- ❑ Other acute coronary syndrome ____________________
- ❑ Unspecified acute transmural inferior myocardial infarction
- ❑ Unable to determine
- ❑ Other ______________________________

Physician/PA/NP Printed Name: ____

Physician/PA/NP Signature: ______________________________ Date: ____________ Time: ____________

Pleural Effusion Example

Request for Documentation Clarification

THIS FORM IS A PERMANENT PART OF THE MEDICAL RECORD

Dear Physician/PA/NP: ______________________ or other responsible provider:

When responding to this query, please exercise your independent professional judgment. The fact that a question is asked does not imply that any particular answer is desired or expected. Please complete, sign, date, and time the query. Thank you for your assistance with clarification of this issue.

Please clarify the following documentation or clinical data noted in the medical record:

Patient with lung cancer, history of heart failure and pneumonia had thoracentesis for analysis of pleural effusion.

CDI Analyst/Coder: ______________________ Date: __________ Time: __________

MD/PA/NP Response (Check any that apply.)

Based on your medical judgment and review of the clinical indicators above, please clarify the etiology/underlying cause of the pleural effusion.

- ❑ Chylous pleural effusion
- ❑ Encysted pleurisy
- ❑ Malignant pleural effusion
- ❑ Pleural effusion due to heart failure
- ❑ Parapneumonic pleural effusion
- ❑ Pleural effusion due to nephrotic syndrome
- ❑ Pleurisy with effusion
- ❑ Tuberculous pleural effusion
- ❑ Other pleural effusion (specify)______________________
- ❑ Clinically unable to determine
- ❑ Other ______________________

Physician/PA/NP Printed Name: ______________________

Physician/PA/NP Signature: ______________________ Date: __________ Time: __________

Postoperative Anemia Example

Request for Documentation Clarification

THIS FORM IS A PERMANENT PART OF THE MEDICAL RECORD

Dear Physician/PA/NP: ______________________________ or other responsible provider:

When responding to this query, please exercise your independent professional judgment. The fact that a question is asked does not imply that any particular answer is desired or expected. Please complete, sign, date, and time the query. Thank you for your assistance with clarification of this issue.

Please clarify the following documentation or clinical data noted in the medical record:

Patient underwent a laparoscopic-assisted transvaginal hysterectomy for severe menometrorrhagia with EBL 1000 ml.

Hemoglobin was 11.5 g/dL before surgery and 9.0 g/dL after surgery.

Patient received 2 units PRBC postoperatively.

Progress notes document anemia.

CDI Analyst/Coder: ______________________________ Date: ______________ Time: ______________

MD/PA/NP Response (Check any that apply.)

Based on your medical judgment and review of the clinical indicators above, please clarify the diagnosis.

- ❑ Acute blood loss anemia in the postoperative period, not due to surgery
- ❑ Acute on chronic blood loss anemia
- ❑ Agranulocytic anemia
- ❑ Anemia of chronic disease
- ❑ Aplastic anemia
- ❑ Chronic blood loss anemia
- ❑ Dilutional anemia
- ❑ Hemolytic anemia
- ❑ Iron deficiency anemia
- ❑ Nutritional/pernicious anemia
- ❑ Postoperative (due to surgery) blood loss anemia (expected)
- ❑ Postoperative (due to surgery) blood loss anemia (unexpected)
- ❑ Refractory anemia
- ❑ Unspecified anemia
- ❑ Other (please specify)______________________________
- ❑ Clinically unable to determine

Physician/PA/NP Printed Name: ____

Physician/PA/NP Signature: ______________________________ Date: ______________ Time: ______________

Postoperative (Postprocedural) (Wound) Infection Example

Request for Documentation Clarification

THIS FORM IS A PERMANENT PART OF THE MEDICAL RECORD

Dear Physician/PA/NP: ______________________ or other responsible provider:

When responding to this query, please exercise your independent professional judgment. The fact that a question is asked does not imply that any particular answer is desired or expected. Please complete, sign, date, and time the query. Thank you for your assistance with clarification of this issue.

Please clarify the following documentation or clinical data noted in the medical record:

S/P right total knee replacement admitted due to cellulitis at the surgical site.

CT scan indicates the abscess is in the superficial tissues only and does not track to the prosthesis.

Prosthesis is not being removed at this time.

CDI Analyst/Coder: ______________________ Date: __________ Time: __________

MD/PA/NP Response (Check any that apply.)

Based on your medical judgment and review of the clinical indicators above, please clarify the diagnosis.

- ❑ Cellulitis related to the knee replacement procedure—surgical wound infection
  - ❑ Superficial, skin and/or subcutaneous tissue, stitch abscess
  - ❑ Deep incisional (intra-muscular abscess)
  - ❑ Other surgical site
- ❑ Cellulitis related to the knee replacement procedure—infected knee prosthesis
- ❑ Cellulitis was unrelated to the surgical procedure
- ❑ Other (please specify) ______________________
- ❑ Clinically unable to determine

Physician/PA/NP Printed Name: ______________________

Physician/PA/NP Signature: ______________________ Date: __________ Time: __________

Query Guidelines

Pressure (Decubitus) Ulcer Example

Request for Documentation Clarification

THIS FORM IS A PERMANENT PART OF THE MEDICAL RECORD

Dear Physician/PA/NP: ______________________ or other responsible provider:

When responding to this query, please exercise your independent professional judgment. The fact that a question is asked does not imply that any particular answer is desired or expected. Please complete, sign, date, and time the query. Thank you for your assistance with clarification of this issue.

Please clarify the following documentation or clinical data noted in the medical record:

Discharge summary and History & Physical identify left ischial pressure ulcer.

Wound care notes state left ischial pressure ulcer routine dressing changes and Silvadene ordered.

Progress note documents full-thickness skin loss, involving damage to subcutaneous tissue.

CDI Analyst/Coder: ______________________ Date: ____________ Time: ____________

MD/PA/NP Response (Check any that apply.)

Based on your medical judgment and review of the clinical indicators above, please clarify the pressure ulcer stage.

- ❑ Stage 1—Pre-ulcer skin changes limited to persistent focal edema
- ❑ Stage 2—Abrasion, blister, partial thickness skin loss involving epidermis and/or dermis
- ❑ Stage 3—Full thickness skin loss involving damage or necrosis of subcutaneous tissue
- ❑ Stage 4—Necrosis of soft tissues through to underlying muscle, tendon, or bone
- ❑ Pressure ulcer—unspecified stage
- ❑ Pressure ulcer—unstageable
- ❑ Pressure-induced deep tissue injury/damage
- ❑ Other ______________________
- ❑ Clinically unable to determine

Physician/PA/NP Printed Name: ______________________________________

Physician/PA/NP Signature: ______________________ Date: ____________ Time: ____________

Pulmonary and Respiratory Insufficiency or Distress Example

Request for Documentation Clarification

THIS FORM IS A PERMANENT PART OF THE MEDICAL RECORD

Dear Physician/PA/NP: ______________________ or other responsible provider:

When responding to this query, please exercise your independent professional judgment. The fact that a question is asked does not imply that any particular answer is desired or expected. Please complete, sign, date, and time the query. Thank you for your assistance with clarification of this issue.

Please clarify the following documentation or clinical data noted in the medical record:

Patient with hx of COPD and tobacco abuse underwent CABG x3 for CAD.

Pulmonary consult was ordered for ventilation management.

Ventilator weaning and extubation were within 48 hours of surgery.

Progress note by pulmonary consult states "postoperative respiratory insufficiency, ready for extubation" without symptoms or etiology documented.

CDI Analyst/Coder: ______________________ Date: __________ Time: __________

MD/PA/NP Response (Check any that apply.)

Based on your medical judgment and review of the clinical indicators above, please clarify the diagnosis of postoperative respiratory insufficiency.

- ❑ Acute postoperative pulmonary/respiratory insufficiency integral to reversal from anesthesia
- ❑ Acute postoperative pulmonary/respiratory insufficiency integral to the surgical procedure
- ❑ Acute postoperative pulmonary/respiratory insufficiency integral to patient's chronic condition(s)
- ❑ Chronic postoperative pulmonary/respiratory insufficiency integral to reversal from anesthesia
- ❑ Chronic postoperative pulmonary/respiratory insufficiency integral to the surgical procedure
- ❑ Chronic postoperative pulmonary/respiratory insufficiency integral to patient's chronic condition(s)
- ❑ Other respiratory insufficiency ______________________
- ❑ Postoperative respiratory insufficiency of no clinical significance
- ❑ Unexpected postoperative respiratory insufficiency of clinical significance not integral to the procedure
- ❑ No postoperative respiratory insufficiency
- ❑ Clinically unable to determine
- ❑ Other ______________________

Physician/PA/NP Printed Name: ______________________

Physician/PA/NP Signature: ______________________ Date: __________ Time: __________

Release (Lysis) of Adhesions Example

Request for Documentation Clarification

THIS FORM IS A PERMANENT PART OF THE MEDICAL RECORD

Dear Physician/PA/NP: ______________________ or other responsible provider:

When responding to this query, please exercise your independent professional judgment. The fact that a question is asked does not imply that any particular answer is desired or expected. Please complete, sign, date, and time the query. Thank you for your assistance with clarification of this issue.

Please clarify the following documentation or clinical data noted in the medical record.

Operative report indicates that during surgery for obstructed ventral hernia intestinal adhesions were noted and released in addition to the hernia repair.

CDI Analyst/Coder: ______________________ Date: __________ Time: __________

MD/PA/NP Response (Check any that apply.)

Based on your medical judgment and review of the clinical indicators above, please clarify the clinical significance of the lysis of adhesions.

- ❑ Lysis of adhesions not clinically significant—incidental/integral to the procedure
- ❑ Lysis of adhesions clinically significant—added to the complexity/difficulty of the procedure
- ❑ Other ______________________
- ❑ Clinically unable to determine

Physician/PA/NP Printed Name: ______________________

Physician/PA/NP Signature: ______________________ Date: __________ Time: __________

Query Guidelines

Respiratory Failure Example

Request for Documentation Clarification

THIS FORM IS A PERMANENT PART OF THE MEDICAL RECORD

Dear Physician/PA/NP: ______________________________ or other responsible provider:

When responding to this query, please exercise your independent professional judgment. The fact that a question is asked does not imply that any particular answer is desired or expected. Please complete, sign, date, and time the query. Thank you for your assistance with clarification of this issue.

Please clarify the following documentation or clinical data noted in the medical record:

Patient admitted with COPD exacerbation.

Patient was on supplemental oxygen at home prn.

Progress notes document both "severe respiratory distress" and "respiratory failure."

Oxygen saturation on admission was 88 percent on room air, respiratory rate of 30, and arterial blood gas (ABG) results of pO^2 45, pCO^2 50, pH 7.32, with Bi-PAP and oxygen ordered.

CDI Analyst/Coder: ______________________________ Date: ______________ Time: ______________

MD/PA/NP Response (Check any that apply.)

Based on your medical judgment and review of the clinical indicators above, please clarify the diagnosis.

- ❑ Acute respiratory distress integral to COPD exacerbation
- ❑ Acute respiratory insufficiency
- ❑ Chronic respiratory insufficiency
- ❑ Acute hypoxic respiratory failure
- ❑ Acute hypercapnic respiratory failure
- ❑ Chronic hypoxic respiratory failure
- ❑ Chronic hypercapnic respiratory failure
- ❑ Acute on chronic hypoxic respiratory failure
- ❑ Acute on chronic hypercapnic respiratory failure
- ❑ Other ______________________________
- ❑ Clinically unable to determine

Physician/PA/NP Printed Name: ____

Physician/PA/NP Signature: ______________________________ Date: ______________ Time: ______________

Query Guidelines

Sepsis Example

Request for Documentation Clarification

THIS FORM IS A PERMANENT PART OF THE MEDICAL RECORD

Dear Physician/PA/NP: ______________________________ or other responsible provider:

When responding to this query, please exercise your independent professional judgment. The fact that a question is asked does not imply that any particular answer is desired or expected. Please complete, sign, date, and time the query. Thank you for your assistance with clarification of this issue.

Please clarify the following documentation or clinical data noted in the medical record:

Pt admitted with diagnosis of sepsis with HR of 120, BP of 80/40, T 37.5, on Levophed IV, with acute kidney injury (AKI) and encephalopathy" documented on admission.
Progress notes document "sepsis with all cultures negative at 72 hours."

CDI Analyst/Coder: ______________________________ Date: ______________ Time: ______________

MD/PA/NP Response (Check any that apply.)

Based on your medical judgment and review of the clinical indicators above, please clarify the diagnosis of sepsis.

- ❑ Sepsis
  - ❑ Specify organism(s)_______________
  - ❑ Unspecified
  - ❑ Unable to determine
  - ❑ Other (Please specify) ______________________
- ❑ Systemic Inflammatory Response Syndrome (SIRS)
  - ❑ Due to infectious process (please specify infectious origin) ______________________
  - ❑ Noninfectious origin (please specify noninfectious origin) ______________________
  - ❑ Unspecified
  - ❑ Unable to determine
  - ❑ Other (please specify) ______________________
- ❑ Severe sepsis
  - ❑ Acute organ failure
    - ❑ Acute renal failure
    - ❑ Acute respiratory failure
    - ❑ Acute hepatic failure
    - ❑ Other organ failure (please specify organ/system)_______________
    - ❑ Unable to determine
    - ❑ Other (please specify)____________________
- ❑ Sepsis ruled out

Infectious/noninfectious process

- ❑ Present on admission
- ❑ Not present on admission

Sepsis

- ❑ Present on admission
- ❑ Not present on admission

Physician/PA/NP Printed Name: ____

Physician/PA/NP Signature: ______________________________ Date: ______________ Time: ______________

SIRS of Noninfectious Origin Example

Request for Documentation Clarification

THIS FORM IS A PERMANENT PART OF THE MEDICAL RECORD

Dear Physician/PA/NP: ______________________________ or other responsible provider:

When responding to this query, please exercise your independent professional judgment. The fact that a question is asked does not imply that any particular answer is desired or expected. Please complete, sign, date, and time the query. Thank you for your assistance with clarification of this issue.

Please clarify the following documentation or clinical data noted in the medical record:

Pt admitted with SIRS due to gallstone pancreatitis.

Patient did receive pre-op IV antibiotics prior to cholecystectomy.

CDI Analyst/Coder: ______________________________ Date: ____________ Time: ____________

MD/PA/NP Response (Check any that apply.)

Based on your medical judgment and review of the clinical indicators above, please clarify the term "SIRS" and if it is of infectious or noninfectious origin.

- ❑ Severe sepsis with associated acute organ dysfunction
- ❑ Sepsis with acute organ dysfunction
- ❑ Sepsis with multiple organ dysfunctions
- ❑ Systemic inflammatory response syndrome (SIRS) due to infectious process with acute organ dysfunction (specify infectious process) ______________________________
- ❑ Systemic inflammatory response syndrome (SIRS) due to infectious process without acute organ dysfunction (specify infectious process) ______________________________
- ❑ Severe sepsis without septic shock
- ❑ Severe sepsis with septic shock
- ❑ Severe sepsis unspecified
- ❑ Systemic inflammatory response syndrome (SIRS) of noninfectious origin with acute organ dysfunction (specify noninfectious origin) ______________________________
- ❑ Systemic inflammatory response syndrome (SIRS) of noninfectious origin without acute organ dysfunction (specify noninfectious origin) ______________________________
- ❑ Systemic inflammatory response syndrome (SIRS) not otherwise specified
- ❑ Other specified sepsis ______________________________
- ❑ Clinically unable to determine
- ❑ Other ______________________________

Physician/PA/NP Printed Name: ______________________________

Physician/PA/NP Signature: ______________________________ Date: ____________ Time: ____________

Query Guidelines

Syncope as Principal Diagnosis Example

Request for Documentation Clarification

THIS FORM IS A PERMANENT PART OF THE MEDICAL RECORD

Dear Physician/PA/NP: ______________________ or other responsible provider:

When responding to this query, please exercise your independent professional judgment. The fact that a question is asked does not imply that any particular answer is desired or expected. Please complete, sign, date and time the query. Thank you for your assistance with clarification of this issue.

Please clarify the following documentation or clinical data noted in the medical record:

ER physician documents on admit order "syncopal episode complicated by anemia."

History and physical states patient was admitted for syncope.

The history and physical also states patient has breast cancer and is receiving weekly chemotherapy treatments.

Discharge summary states anemia due to chemotherapy, and hypotension.

Progress notes indicate patient is treated with three units PRBCs.

CDI Analyst/Coder: ______________________ Date: __________ Time: __________

MD/PA/NP Response (Check any that apply.)

Based on your medical judgment and review of the clinical indicators above, please clarify the diagnosis.

- ❑ Syncope due to anemia due to chemotherapy
- ❑ Syncope due to hypotension (specify type/cause) ______________
- ❑ Syncope due to other cause (specify) ______________
- ❑ Syncope due to unknown cause
- ❑ Clinically unable to determine
- ❑ Other ______________________

Physician/PA/NP Printed Name: ______________________

Physician/PA/NP Signature: ______________________ Date: __________ Time: __________

Query Guidelines

Transbronchial Biopsy of Lung, via Bronchoscope Example

Request for Documentation Clarification

THIS FORM IS A PERMANENT PART OF THE MEDICAL RECORD

Dear Physician/PA/NP: ______________________________ or other responsible provider:

When responding to this query, please exercise your independent professional judgment. The fact that a question is asked does not imply that any particular answer is desired or expected. Please complete, sign, date, and time the query. Thank you for your assistance with clarification of this issue.

Please clarify the following documentation or clinical data noted in the medical record:

Procedure report states transbronchial lung biopsy to rule out lung cancer, but pathology report does not identify lung or alveolar tissue.

CDI Analyst/Coder: ______________________________ Date: ____________ Time: ____________

MD/PA/NP Response (Check any that apply.)

Based on your medical judgment and review of the clinical indicators above, please clarify the procedure performed.

Transbronchial biopsy of:

- ❑ Main bronchus, right
- ❑ Upper lobe bronchus, right
- ❑ Middle lobe bronchus, right
- ❑ Lower lobe bronchus, right
- ❑ Main bronchus, left
- ❑ Upper lobe bronchus, left
- ❑ Lingula bronchus
- ❑ Lower lobe bronchus, left

Transbronchial lung biopsy, performed via puncture through the bronchus, of:

- ❑ Upper lung lobe, right
- ❑ Middle lung lobe, right
- ❑ Lower lung lobe, right
- ❑ Lung, right
- ❑ Upper lung lobe, left
- ❑ Lung lingula
- ❑ Lower lung lobe, left
- ❑ Lung, left
- ❑ Lungs, bilateral

❑ Other (please describe in detail instruments used, tissue removed, and intent of procedure)

____

____

Physician/PA/NP Printed Name: ______________________________

Physician/PA/NP Signature: ______________________________ Date: ____________ Time: ____________

Query Guidelines

Transient Ischemic Attack Example

Request for Documentation Clarification

THIS FORM IS A PERMANENT PART OF THE MEDICAL RECORD

Dear Physician/PA/NP: ________________ or other responsible provider:

When responding to this query, please exercise your independent professional judgment. The fact that a question is asked does not imply that any particular answer is desired or expected. Please complete, sign, date, and time the query. Thank you for your assistance with clarification of this issue.

Please clarify the following documentation or clinical data noted in the medical record:

Patient admitted with slurred speech and confusion; workup revealed critical stenosis of the left carotid artery and endarterectomy is scheduled for next week.

Discharge summary states final diagnosis is TIA.

CDI Analyst/Coder: ________________ Date: __________ Time: __________

MD/PA/NP Response (Check any that apply)

Based on your medical judgment and review of the clinical indicators above, please clarify the etiology of the TIA:

- ❑ Transient ischemic attack due to left critical stenosis of the left carotid artery
- ❑ Transient ischemic attack due to other cause (please specify) ________________
- ❑ Transient ischemic attack due to unknown cause
- ❑ Clinically unable to determine
- ❑ Other ________________

Physician/PA/NP Printed Name: ________________

Physician/PA/NP Signature: ________________ Date: __________ Time: __________

Urinary Tract Infection (Bacterial) Example

Request for Documentation Clarification

THIS FORM IS A PERMANENT PART OF THE MEDICAL RECORD

Dear Physician/PA/NP: ______________________________ or other responsible provider:

When responding to this query, please exercise your independent professional judgment. The fact that a question is asked does not imply that any particular answer is desired or expected. Please complete, sign, date, and time the query. Thank you for your assistance with clarification of this issue.

Please clarify the following documentation or clinical data noted in the medical record:

Pt presented with hematuria and groin pain.

History and physical notes pt had Foley catheter inserted five days ago for BPH/urinary retention.

Temp 102, HR 95, RR 22 and BP 120/70.

Urine culture was positive for *E. coli*.

Treated with IV Cipro.

History and physical documents UTI.

Discharge summary *E. coli*, UTI.

Patient's Foley catheter was changed and emphasis placed on catheter care at discharge.

CDI Analyst/Coder: ______________________________ Date: ____________ Time: ____________

MD/PA/NP Response (Check any that apply.)

Based on your medical judgment and review of the clinical indicators above, please clarify the diagnosis.

- ❑ *E. coli* UTI related to/due to/caused by the Foley catheter
- ❑ *E. coli* UTI unrelated to Foley catheter—due to other etiology (please specify) ______________________
- ❑ *E. coli* UTI of unknown etiology
- ❑ Clinically unable to determine
- ❑ Other ______________________________

Physician/PA/NP Printed Name: ____

Physician/PA/NP Signature: ______________________________ Date: ____________ Time: ____________

Query Guidelines

Valve Replacement, Aortic Example

Request for Documentation Clarification

THIS FORM IS A PERMANENT PART OF THE MEDICAL RECORD

Dear Physician/PA/NP: ______________________________ or other responsible provider:

When responding to this query, please exercise your independent professional judgment. The fact that a question is asked does not imply that any particular answer is desired or expected. Please complete, sign, date, and time the query. Thank you for your assistance with clarification of this issue.

Please clarify the following documentation or clinical data noted in the medical record:

Patient is here for aortic valve replacement. SAPIAN valve deployed and properly seated, procedure was concluded.

CDI Analyst/Coder: ______________________________ Date: ________ Time: __________

MD/PA/NP Response (Check any that apply.)

Based on your medical judgment and review of the clinical indicators above, please clarify the procedure performed.

APPROACH

- ❑ Open sternotomy with breastbone cracked
- ❑ Mini thoracotomy with endoscopic assistance
- ❑ Small chest incisions with endoscopic assistance
- ❑ Transcatheter with access through femoral artery
- ❑ Transcatheter through chest and apex of heart (transapical)
- ❑ Other ______________________________

Check any additional procedures performed

- ❑ Cardiopulmonary bypass
- ❑ Cerebral embolic filtration dual (innominate artery and left common carotid artery)
- ❑ Cerebral embolic filtration single (aortic arch)
- ❑ Rapid deployment device
- ❑ Other ______________________________

Physician/PA/NP Printed Name: ______________________________

Physician/PA/NP Signature: ______________________________ Date: __________ Time: __________

Query Guidelines

Whipple Procedure Example

Request for Documentation Clarification

THIS FORM IS A PERMANENT PART OF THE MEDICAL RECORD

Dear Physician/PA/NP: ______________________ or other responsible provider:

When responding to this query, please exercise your independent professional judgment. The fact that a question is asked does not imply that any particular answer is desired or expected. Please complete, sign, date, and time the query. Thank you for your assistance with clarification of this issue.

Please clarify the following documentation or clinical data noted in the medical record:

Patient with pancreatic cancer here for Whipple procedure. We removed a portion of the pancreas and small bowel with clean margins. Performed biopsies to ensure cancer had not spread to other body parts.

CDI Analyst/Coder: ______________________ Date: __________ Time: __________

MD/PA/NP Response (Check any that apply.)

Based on your medical judgment and review of the clinical indicators above, please clarify the procedure performed.

BODY PART REMOVED (Check all that apply)

- ❑ Pancreas, partial (e.g. head of pancreas)
- ❑ Pancreas, total
- ❑ Stomach pylorus, partial
- ❑ Stomach pylorus, total
- ❑ Other portion of stomach
- ❑ Duodenum, partial
- ❑ Duodenum, total (with anastomosis to jejunum)
- ❑ Jejunum, partial
- ❑ Gallbladder, if partial—was it for biopsy? ❑ Yes ❑ No
- ❑ Gallbladder, total
- ❑ Common bile duct, if partial—was it for biopsy? ❑ Yes ❑ No
- ❑ Common bile duct, total
- ❑ Other (including biopsies) ______________________

APPROACH

- ❑ Open laparotomy
- ❑ Open laparotomy with laparoscopic (endoscopic) assistance
- ❑ Entirely laparoscopic
- ❑ Laparoscopic converted to Open

Was robotic assistance used: ❑ Yes ❑ No

Physician/PA/NP Printed Name: ______________________

Physician/PA/NP Signature: ______________________ Date: __________ Time: __________

Query Guidelines

Blank Template

Request for Documentation Clarification

THIS FORM IS A PERMANENT PART OF THE MEDICAL RECORD

Dear Physician/PA/NP: ______________________________ or other responsible provider:

When responding to this query, please exercise your independent professional judgment. The fact that a question is asked does not imply that any particular answer is desired or expected. Please complete, sign, date, and time the query. Thank you for your assistance with clarification of this issue.

Please clarify the following documentation or clinical data noted in the medical record:

CDI Analyst/Coder: ______________________________ Date: ______________ Time: ______________

MD/PA/NP Response (Check any that apply.)

Based on your medical judgment and review of the clinical indicators above, please clarify the diagnosis.

❑ [Place multiple choice options here.]

Physician/PA/NP Printed Name: ______________________________

Physician/PA/NP Signature: ______________________________ Date: ______________ Time: ______________

Query Guidelines

Yes/No Query Template

Request for Documentation Clarification

THIS FORM IS A PERMANENT PART OF THE MEDICAL RECORD

Dear Physician/PA/NP: ______________________________ or other responsible provider:

When responding to this query, please exercise your independent professional judgment. The fact that a question is asked does not imply that any particular answer is desired or expected. Please complete, sign, date, and time the query. Thank you for your assistance with clarification of this issue.

Please clarify the following documentation or clinical data noted in the medical record:

The patient was admitted to inpatient status on February 10th. On February 13th, provider notes indicated that the patient has a Stage 3 pressure ulcer to the right heel.

CDI Analyst/Coder: ______________________________ Date: ______________ Time: ______________

MD/PA/NP Response (Check any that apply.)

Based on your medical judgment and review of the clinical indicators above, please clarify present on admission (POA) status of the Stage 3 right heel pressure ulcer.

- ❑ Yes, the Stage 3 right heel pressure ulcer was POA
- ❑ No, the Stage 3 right heel pressure ulcer was not POA
- ❑ Clinically unable to determine POA status of Stage 3 right heel pressure ulcer
- ❑ Other (please specify)______________________________

Physician/PA/NP Printed Name: ______________________________

Physician/PA/NP Signature: ______________________________ Date: ______________ Time: ______________

Query Guidelines

Appendix B. 2025 ICD-10-CM Official Guidelines for Coding and Reporting

Narrative changes effective October 1, 2024 appear in **bold** text

Narrative changes effective April 1, 2024 appear in shaded text

Items underlined have been moved within the guidelines since the April 2024, FY 2024 version

Italics are used to indicate revisions to heading changes

The Centers for Medicare and Medicaid Services (CMS) and the National Center for Health Statistics (NCHS), two departments within the U.S. Federal Government's Department of Health and Human Services (DHHS) provide the following guidelines for coding and reporting using the International Classification of Diseases, 10th Revision, Clinical Modification (ICD-10-CM). These guidelines should be used as a companion document to the official version of the ICD-10-CM as published on the NCHS website. The ICD-10-CM is a morbidity classification published by the United States for classifying diagnoses and reason for visits in all health care settings. The ICD-10-CM is based on the ICD-10, the statistical classification of disease published by the World Health Organization (WHO).

These guidelines have been approved by the four organizations that make up the Cooperating Parties for the ICD-10-CM: the American Hospital Association (AHA), the American Health Information Management Association (AHIMA), CMS, and NCHS.

These guidelines are a set of rules that have been developed to accompany and complement the official conventions and instructions provided within the ICD-10-CM itself. The instructions and conventions of the classification take precedence over guidelines. These guidelines are based on the coding and sequencing instructions in the Tabular List and Alphabetic Index of ICD-10-CM, but provide additional instruction. Adherence to these guidelines when assigning ICD-10-CM diagnosis codes is required under the Health Insurance Portability and Accountability Act (HIPAA). The diagnosis codes (Tabular List and Alphabetic Index) have been adopted under HIPAA for all healthcare settings. A joint effort between the healthcare provider and the coder is essential to achieve complete and accurate documentation, code assignment, and reporting of diagnoses and procedures. These guidelines have been developed to assist both the healthcare provider and the coder in identifying those diagnoses that are to be reported. The importance of consistent, complete documentation in the medical record cannot be overemphasized. Without such documentation accurate coding cannot be achieved. The entire record should be reviewed to determine the specific reason for the encounter and the conditions treated.

The term encounter is used for all settings, including hospital admissions. In the context of these guidelines, the term provider is used throughout the guidelines to mean physician or any qualified health care practitioner who is legally accountable for establishing the patient's diagnosis. Only this set of guidelines, approved by the Cooperating Parties, is official.

The guidelines are organized into sections. Section I includes the structure and conventions of the classification and general guidelines that apply to the entire classification, and chapter-specific guidelines that correspond to the chapters as they are arranged in the classification. Section II includes guidelines for selection of principal diagnosis for non-outpatient settings. Section III includes guidelines for reporting additional diagnoses in non-outpatient settings. Section IV is for outpatient coding and reporting. It is necessary to review all sections of the guidelines to fully understand all of the rules and instructions needed to code properly.

ICD-10-CM Official Guidelines

Section I. Conventions, general coding guidelines and chapter specific guidelines

The conventions, general guidelines and chapter-specific guidelines are applicable to all health care settings unless otherwise indicated. The conventions and instructions of the classification take precedence over guidelines.

A. Conventions for the ICD-10-CM

The conventions for the ICD-10-CM are the general rules for use of the classification independent of the guidelines. These conventions are incorporated within the Alphabetic Index and Tabular List of the ICD-10-CM as instructional notes.

1. **The Alphabetic Index and Tabular List**
   The ICD-10-CM is divided into the Alphabetic Index, an alphabetical list of terms and their corresponding code, and the Tabular List, a structured list of codes divided into chapters based on body system or condition. The Alphabetic Index consists of the following parts: the Index of Diseases and Injury, the Index of External Causes of Injury, the Table of Neoplasms and the Table of Drugs and Chemicals.

   See Section I.C.2. Neoplasms

   See Section I.C.19. Adverse effects, poisoning, underdosing and toxic effects

2. **Format and Structure:**
   The ICD-10-CM Tabular List contains categories, subcategories and codes. Characters for categories, subcategories and codes may be either a letter or a number. All categories are 3 characters. A three-character category that has no further subdivision is equivalent to a code. Subcategories are either 4 or 5 characters. Codes may be 3, 4, 5, 6 or 7 characters. That is, each level of subdivision after a category is a subcategory. The final level of subdivision is a code. Codes that have applicable 7th characters are still referred to as codes, not subcategories. A code that has an applicable 7th character is considered invalid without the 7th character.

   The ICD-10-CM uses an indented format for ease in reference.

3. **Use of codes for reporting purposes**
   For reporting purposes only codes are permissible, not categories or subcategories, and any applicable 7th character is required.

4. **Placeholder character**
   The ICD-10-CM utilizes a placeholder character "X". The "X" is used as a placeholder at certain codes to allow for future expansion. An example of this is at the poisoning, adverse effect and underdosing codes, categories T36-T50. Where a placeholder exists, the X must be used in order for the code to be considered a valid code.

5. **7th Characters**
   Certain ICD-10-CM categories have applicable 7th characters. The applicable 7th character is required for all codes within the category, or as the notes in the Tabular List instruct. The 7th character must always be the 7th character in the data field. If a code that requires a 7th character is not 6 characters, a placeholder X must be used to fill in the empty characters.

6. **Abbreviations**
   a. **Alphabetic Index abbreviations**
      NEC "Not elsewhere classifiable"

      This abbreviation in the Alphabetic Index represents "other specified." When a specific code is not available for a condition, the Alphabetic Index directs the coder to the "other specified" code in the Tabular List.

      NOS "Not otherwise specified"

      This abbreviation is the equivalent of unspecified.

   b. **Tabular List abbreviations**
      NEC "Not elsewhere classifiable"

      This abbreviation in the Tabular List represents "other specified". When a specific code is not available for a condition, the Tabular List includes an NEC entry under a code to identify the code as the "other specified" code.

      NOS "Not otherwise specified"

      This abbreviation is the equivalent of unspecified.

7. **Punctuation**
   [ ] Brackets are used in the Tabular List to enclose synonyms, alternative wording or explanatory phrases. Brackets are used in the Alphabetic Index to identify manifestation codes.

( ) Parentheses are used in both the Alphabetic Index and Tabular List to enclose supplementary words that may be present or absent in the statement of a disease or procedure without affecting the code number to which it is assigned. The terms within the parentheses are referred to as nonessential modifiers. The nonessential modifiers in the Alphabetic Index to Diseases apply to subterms following a main term except when a nonessential modifier and a subentry are mutually exclusive, the subentry takes precedence. For example, in the **ICD-10-CM** Alphabetic Index under the main term Enteritis, "acute" is a nonessential modifier and "chronic" is a subentry. In this case, the nonessential modifier "acute" does not apply to the subentry "chronic".

: Colons are used in the Tabular List after an incomplete term which needs one or more of the modifiers following the colon to make it assignable to a given category.

8. Use of "and".
See Section I.A.14. Use of the term "And"

9. Other and Unspecified codes

a. "Other" codes
Codes titled "other" or "other specified" are for use when the information in the medical record provides detail for which a specific code does not exist. Alphabetic Index entries with NEC in the line designate "other" codes in the Tabular List. These Alphabetic Index entries represent specific disease entities for which no specific code exists, so the term is included within an "other" code.

b. "Unspecified" codes
Codes titled "unspecified" are for use when the information in the medical record is insufficient to assign a more specific code. For those categories for which an unspecified code is not provided, the "other specified" code may represent both other and unspecified.

See Section I.B.18. Use of Signs/Symptom/Unspecified Codes

10. Includes Notes
This note appears immediately under a three-character code title to further define, or give examples of, the content of the category.

11. Inclusion terms
List of terms is included under some codes. These terms are the conditions for which that code is to be used. The terms may be synonyms of the code title, or, in the case of "other specified" codes, the terms are a list of the various conditions assigned to that code. The inclusion terms are not necessarily exhaustive. Additional terms found only in the Alphabetic Index may also be assigned to a code.

12. Excludes Notes
The ICD-10-CM has two types of excludes notes. Each type of note has a different definition for use, but they are all similar in that they indicate that codes excluded from each other are independent of each other.

a. Excludes1
A type 1 Excludes note is a pure excludes note. It means "NOT CODED HERE!" An Excludes1 note indicates that the code excluded should never be used at the same time as the code above the Excludes1 note. An Excludes1 is used when two conditions cannot occur together, such as a congenital form versus an acquired form of the same condition.

An exception to the Excludes1 definition is the circumstance when the two conditions are unrelated to each other. If it is not clear whether the two conditions involving an Excludes1 note are related or not, query the provider. For example, code F45.8, Other somatoform disorders, has an Excludes1 note for "sleep related teeth grinding (G47.63)," because "teeth grinding" is an inclusion term under F45.8. Only one of these two codes should be assigned for teeth grinding. However psychogenic dysmenorrhea is also an inclusion term under F45.8, and a patient could have both this condition and sleep related teeth grinding. In this case, the two conditions are clearly unrelated to each other, and so it would be appropriate to report F45.8 and G47.63 together.

b. Excludes2
A type 2 Excludes note represents "Not included here." An excludes2 note indicates that the condition excluded is not part of the condition represented by the code, but a patient may have both conditions at the same time. When an Excludes2 note appears under a code, it is acceptable to use both the code and the excluded code together, when appropriate.

13. Etiology/manifestation convention ("code first", "use additional code" and "in diseases classified elsewhere" notes)
Certain conditions have both an underlying etiology and multiple body system manifestations due to the underlying etiology. For such conditions, the ICD-10-CM has a coding convention that requires the underlying condition be sequenced first, if applicable, followed by the manifestation. Wherever such a combination exists, there is a "use additional code" note at the etiology code, and a "code first" note at the

ICD-10-CM Official Guidelines

manifestation code. These instructional notes indicate the proper sequencing order of the codes, etiology followed by manifestation.

In most cases the manifestation codes will have in the code title, "in diseases classified elsewhere." Codes with this title are a component of the etiology/ manifestation convention. The code title indicates that it is a manifestation code. "In diseases classified elsewhere" codes are never permitted to be used as first listed or principal diagnosis codes. They must be used in conjunction with an underlying condition code and they must be listed following the underlying condition. See category FØ2, Dementia in other diseases classified elsewhere, for an example of this convention.

There are manifestation codes that do not have "in diseases classified elsewhere" in the title. For such codes, there is a "use additional code" note at the etiology code and a "code first" note at the manifestation code, and the rules for sequencing apply.

In addition to the notes in the Tabular List, these conditions also have a specific Alphabetic Index entry structure. In the Alphabetic Index both conditions are listed together with the etiology code first followed by the manifestation codes in brackets. The code in brackets is always to be sequenced second.

An example of the etiology/manifestation convention is dementia with Parkinson's disease. In the Alphabetic Index, a code from category G2Ø is listed first, followed by code FØ2.8Ø or FØ2.81- in brackets. A code from category G2Ø- represents the underlying etiology, Parkinson's disease, and must be sequenced first, whereas codes FØ2.8Ø and FØ2.81- represent the manifestation of dementia in diseases classified elsewhere, with or without behavioral disturbance.

"Code first" and "Use additional code" notes are also used as sequencing rules in the classification for certain codes that are not part of an etiology/ manifestation combination.

See Section I.B.7. Multiple coding for a single condition.

14. "And"

The word "and" should be interpreted to mean either "and" or "or" when it appears in a title.

For example, cases of "tuberculosis of bones", "tuberculosis of joints" and "tuberculosis of bones and joints" are classified to subcategory A18.Ø, Tuberculosis of bones and joints.

15. "With"

The word "with" or "in" should be interpreted to mean "associated with" or "due to" when it appears in a code title, the Alphabetic Index (either under a main term or subterm), or an instructional note in the Tabular List. The classification presumes a causal relationship between the two conditions linked by these terms in the Alphabetic Index or Tabular List. These conditions should be coded as related even in the absence of provider documentation explicitly linking them, unless the documentation clearly states the conditions are unrelated or when another guideline exists that specifically requires a documented linkage between two conditions (e.g., sepsis guideline for "acute organ dysfunction that is not clearly associated with the sepsis").

For conditions not specifically linked by these relational terms in the classification or when a guideline requires that a linkage between two conditions be explicitly documented, provider documentation must link the conditions in order to code them as related.

The word "with" in the Alphabetic Index is sequenced immediately following the main term or subterm, not in alphabetical order.

16. "See" and "See Also"

The "see" instruction following a main term in the Alphabetic Index indicates that another term should be referenced. It is necessary to go to the main term referenced with the "see" note to locate the correct code.

A "see also" instruction following a main term in the Alphabetic Index instructs that there is another main term that may also be referenced that may provide additional Alphabetic Index entries that may be useful. It is not necessary to follow the "see also" note when the original main term provides the necessary code.

17. "Code also" note

A "code also" note instructs that two codes may be required to fully describe a condition, but this note does not provide sequencing direction. The sequencing depends on the circumstances of the encounter.

18. Default codes

A code listed next to a main term in the ICD-10-CM Alphabetic Index is referred to as a default code. The default code represents that condition that is most commonly associated with the main term or is the unspecified code for the condition. If a condition is documented in a medical record (for example, appendicitis) without any additional information, such as acute or chronic, the default code should be assigned.

19. **Code assignment and Clinical Criteria**
The assignment of a diagnosis code is based on the provider's diagnostic statement that the condition exists. The provider's statement that the patient has a particular condition is sufficient. Code assignment is not based on clinical criteria used by the provider to establish the diagnosis. If there is conflicting medical record documentation, query the provider.

B. General Coding Guidelines

1. **Locating a code in the ICD-10-CM**
To select a code in the classification that corresponds to a diagnosis or reason for visit documented in a medical record, first locate the term in the Alphabetic Index, and then verify the code in the Tabular List. Read and be guided by instructional notations that appear in both the Alphabetic Index and the Tabular List.

It is essential to use both the Alphabetic Index and Tabular List when locating and assigning a code. The Alphabetic Index does not always provide the full code. Selection of the full code, including laterality and any applicable 7th character can only be done in the Tabular List. A dash (-) at the end of an Alphabetic Index entry indicates that additional characters are required. Even if a dash is not included at the Alphabetic Index entry, it is necessary to refer to the Tabular List to verify that no 7th character is required.

2. **Level of Detail in Coding**
Diagnosis codes are to be used and reported at their highest number of characters available and to the highest level of specificity documented in the medical record.

ICD-10-CM diagnosis codes are composed of codes with 3, 4, 5, 6 or 7 characters. Codes with three characters are included in ICD-10-CM as the heading of a category of codes that may be further subdivided by the use of fourth and/or fifth characters and/or sixth characters, which provide greater detail.

A three-character code is to be used only if it is not further subdivided. A code is invalid if it has not been coded to the full number of characters required for that code, including the 7th character, if applicable.

3. **Code or codes from AØØ.Ø through T88.9, ZØØ-Z99.8, UØØ-U85**
The appropriate code or codes from A00.0 through T88.9, Z00-Z99.8, and U00-U85 must be used to identify diagnoses, symptoms, conditions, problems, complaints or other reason(s) for the encounter/visit.

4. **Signs and symptoms**
Codes that describe symptoms and signs, as opposed to diagnoses, are acceptable for reporting purposes when a related definitive diagnosis has not been established (confirmed) by the provider. Chapter 18 of ICD-10-CM, Symptoms, Signs, and Abnormal Clinical and Laboratory Findings, Not Elsewhere Classified (codes R00.0-R99) contains many, but not all, codes for symptoms.

See Section I.B.18. Use of Signs/Symptom/Unspecified Codes

5. **Conditions that are an integral part of a disease process**
Signs and symptoms that are associated routinely with a disease process should not be assigned as additional codes, unless otherwise instructed by the classification.

6. **Conditions that are not an integral part of a disease process**
Additional signs and symptoms that may not be associated routinely with a disease process should be coded when present.

7. **Multiple coding for a single condition**
In addition to the etiology/manifestation convention that requires two codes to fully describe a single condition that affects multiple body systems, there are other single conditions that also require more than one code. "Use additional code" notes are found in the Tabular List at codes that are not part of an etiology/manifestation pair where a secondary code is useful to fully describe a condition. The sequencing rule is the same as the etiology/manifestation pair, "use additional code" indicates that a secondary code should be added, if known.

For example, for bacterial infections that are not included in chapter 1, a secondary code from category B95, Streptococcus, Staphylococcus, and Enterococcus, as the cause of diseases classified elsewhere, or B96, Other bacterial agents as the cause of diseases classified elsewhere, may be required to identify the bacterial organism causing the infection. A "use additional code" note will normally be found at the infectious disease code, indicating a need for the organism code to be added as a secondary code.

"Code first" notes are also under certain codes that are not specifically manifestation codes but may be due to an underlying cause. When there is a "code first" note and an underlying condition is present, the underlying condition should be sequenced first, if known.

"Code, if applicable, any causal condition first" notes indicate that this code may be assigned as a principal diagnosis when the causal condition is unknown or not applicable. If a causal condition is known, then the code for that condition should be sequenced as the principal or first-listed diagnosis.

Multiple codes may be needed for sequela, complication codes and obstetric codes to more fully describe a condition. See the specific guidelines for these conditions for further instruction.

8. Acute and Chronic Conditions

If the same condition is described as both acute (subacute) and chronic, and separate subentries exist in the Alphabetic Index at the same indentation level, code both and sequence the acute (subacute) code first.

9. Combination Code

A combination code is a single code used to classify:

Two diagnoses, or

A diagnosis with an associated secondary process (manifestation)

A diagnosis with an associated complication

Combination codes are identified by referring to subterm entries in the Alphabetic Index and by reading the inclusion and exclusion notes in the Tabular List.

Assign only the combination code when that code fully identifies the diagnostic conditions involved or when the Alphabetic Index so directs. Multiple coding should not be used when the classification provides a combination code that clearly identifies all of the elements documented in the diagnosis. When the combination code lacks necessary specificity in describing the manifestation or complication, an additional code should be used as a secondary code.

10. Sequela (Late Effects)

A sequela is the residual effect (condition produced) after the acute phase of an illness or injury has terminated. There is no time limit on when a sequela code can be used. The residual may be apparent early, such as in cerebral infarction, or it may occur months or years later, such as that due to a previous injury. Examples of sequela include: scar formation resulting from a burn, deviated septum due to a nasal fracture, and infertility due to tubal occlusion from old tuberculosis. Coding of sequela generally requires two codes sequenced in the following order: the condition or nature of the sequela is sequenced first. The sequela code is sequenced second.

An exception to the above guidelines are those instances where the code for the sequela is followed by a manifestation code identified in the Tabular List and title, or the sequela code has been expanded (at the fourth, fifth or sixth character levels) to include the manifestation(s). The code for the acute phase of an illness or injury that led to the sequela is never used with a code for the late effect.

See Section I.C.9. Sequelae of cerebrovascular disease

See Section I.C.15. Sequelae of complication of pregnancy, childbirth and the puerperium

See Section I.C.19. Application of 7th characters for Chapter 19

11. Impending or Threatened Condition

Code any condition described at the time of discharge as "impending" or "threatened" as follows:

If it did occur, code as confirmed diagnosis.

If it did not occur, reference the Alphabetic Index to determine if the condition has a subentry term for "impending" or "threatened" and also reference main term entries for "Impending" and for "Threatened."

If the subterms are listed, assign the given code.

If the subterms are not listed, code the existing underlying condition(s) and not the condition described as impending or threatened.

12. Reporting Same Diagnosis Code More than Once

Each unique ICD-10-CM diagnosis code may be reported only once for an encounter. This applies to bilateral conditions when there are no distinct codes identifying laterality or two different conditions classified to the same ICD-10-CM diagnosis code.

13. Laterality

Some ICD-10-CM codes indicate laterality, specifying whether the condition occurs on the left, right or is bilateral. If no bilateral code is provided and the condition is bilateral, assign separate codes for both the left and right side. If the side is not identified in the medical record, assign the code for the unspecified side.

When a patient has a bilateral condition and each side is treated during separate encounters, assign the "bilateral" code (as the condition still exists on both sides), including for the encounter to treat the first side.

For the second encounter for treatment after one side has previously been treated and the condition no longer exists on that side, assign the appropriate unilateral code for the side where the condition still exists (e.g., cataract surgery performed on each eye in separate encounters). The bilateral code would not be assigned for the subsequent encounter, as the patient no longer has the condition in the previously-treated site. If the treatment on the first side did not completely resolve the condition, then the bilateral code would still be appropriate.

When laterality is not documented by the patient's provider, code assignment for the affected side may be based on medical record documentation from other clinicians. If there is conflicting medical record documentation regarding the affected side, the patient's provider should be queried for clarification. Codes for "unspecified" side should rarely be used, such as when the documentation in the record is insufficient to determine the affected side and it is not possible to obtain clarification.

14. **Documentation by Clinicians Other than the Patient's Provider**
Code assignment is based on the documentation by the patient's provider (i.e., physician or other qualified healthcare practitioner legally accountable for establishing the patient's diagnosis). There are a few exceptions when code assignment may be based on medical record documentation from clinicians who are not the patient's provider (i.e., physician or other qualified healthcare practitioner legally accountable for establishing the patient's diagnosis). In this context, "clinicians" other than the patient's provider refer to healthcare professionals permitted, based on regulatory or accreditation requirements or internal hospital policies, to document in a patient's official medical record.

These exceptions include codes for:

- Body Mass Index (BMI)
- Depth of non-pressure chronic ulcers
- Pressure ulcer stage
- Coma scale
- NIH stroke scale (NIHSS)
- Social determinants of health (SDOH) classified to Chapter 21
- Laterality
- Blood alcohol level
- Underimmunization status

This information is typically, or may be, documented by other clinicians involved in the care of the patient (e.g., a dietitian often documents the BMI, a nurse often documents the pressure ulcer stages, and an emergency medical technician often documents the coma scale). However, the associated diagnosis (such as overweight, obesity, acute stroke, pressure ulcer, or a condition classifiable to category F1Ø, Alcohol related disorders) must be documented by the patient's provider. If there is conflicting medical record documentation, either from the same clinician or different clinicians, the patient's provider should be queried for clarification.

The BMI, coma scale, NIHSS, blood alcohol level codes, codes for social determinants of health and underimmunization status should only be reported as secondary diagnoses.

See Section I.C.21.c.17. for additional information regarding coding social determinants of health.

15. **Syndromes**
Follow the Alphabetic Index guidance when coding syndromes. In the absence of Alphabetic Index guidance, assign codes for the documented manifestations of the syndrome. Additional codes for manifestations that are not an integral part of the disease process may also be assigned when the condition does not have a unique code.

16. **Documentation of Complications of Care**
Code assignment is based on the provider's documentation of the relationship between the condition and the care or procedure, unless otherwise instructed by the classification. The guideline extends to any complications of care, regardless of the chapter the code is located in. It is important to note that not all conditions that occur during or following medical care or surgery are classified as complications. There must be a cause-and-effect relationship between the care provided and the condition, and the documentation must support that the condition is clinically significant. It is not necessary for the provider to explicitly document the term "complication." For example, if the condition alters the course of the surgery as documented in the operative report, then it would be appropriate to report a complication code. Query the provider for clarification if the documentation is not clear as to the relationship between the condition and the care or procedure.

17. Borderline Diagnosis

If the provider documents a "borderline" diagnosis at the time of discharge, the diagnosis is coded as confirmed, unless the classification provides a specific entry (e.g., borderline diabetes). If a borderline condition has a specific index entry in ICD-10-CM, it should be coded as such. Since borderline conditions are not uncertain diagnoses, no distinction is made between the care setting (inpatient versus outpatient). Whenever the documentation is unclear regarding a borderline condition, coders are encouraged to query for clarification.

18. Use of Sign/Symptom/Unspecified Codes

Sign/symptom and "unspecified" codes have acceptable, even necessary, uses. While specific diagnosis codes should be reported when they are supported by the available medical record documentation and clinical knowledge of the patient's health condition, there are instances when signs/symptoms or unspecified codes are the best choices for accurately reflecting the healthcare encounter. Each healthcare encounter should be coded to the level of certainty known for that encounter.

As stated in the introductory section of these official coding guidelines, a joint effort between the healthcare provider and the coder is essential to achieve complete and accurate documentation, code assignment, and reporting of diagnoses and procedures. The importance of consistent, complete documentation in the medical record cannot be overemphasized. Without such documentation accurate coding cannot be achieved. The entire record should be reviewed to determine the specific reason for the encounter and the conditions treated.

If a definitive diagnosis has not been established by the end of the encounter, it is appropriate to report codes for sign(s) and/or symptom(s) in lieu of a definitive diagnosis. When sufficient clinical information isn't known or available about a particular health condition to assign a more specific code, it is acceptable to report the appropriate "unspecified" code (e.g., a diagnosis of pneumonia has been determined, but not the specific type). Unspecified codes should be reported when they are the codes that most accurately reflect what is known about the patient's condition at the time of that particular encounter. It would be inappropriate to select a specific code that is not supported by the medical record documentation or conduct medically unnecessary diagnostic testing in order to determine a more specific code.

19. Coding for Healthcare Encounters in Hurricane Aftermath

a. Use of External Cause of Morbidity Codes

An external cause of morbidity code should be assigned to identify the cause of the injury(ies) incurred as a result of the hurricane. The use of external cause of morbidity codes is supplemental to the application of ICD-10-CM codes. External cause of morbidity codes are never to be recorded as a principal diagnosis (first-listed in non-inpatient settings). The appropriate injury code should be sequenced before any external cause codes. The external cause of morbidity codes capture how the injury or health condition happened (cause), the intent (unintentional or accidental; or intentional, such as suicide or assault), the place where the event occurred, the activity of the patient at the time of the event, and the person's status (e.g., civilian, military). They should not be assigned for encounters to treat hurricane victims' medical conditions when no injury, adverse effect or poisoning is involved. External cause of morbidity codes should be assigned for each encounter for care and treatment of the injury. External cause of morbidity codes may be assigned in all health care settings. For the purpose of capturing complete and accurate ICD-10-CM data in the aftermath of the hurricane, a healthcare setting should be considered as any location where medical care is provided by licensed healthcare professionals.

b. Sequencing of External Causes of Morbidity Codes

Codes for cataclysmic events, such as a hurricane, take priority over all other external cause codes except child and adult abuse and terrorism and should be sequenced before other external cause of injury codes. Assign as many external cause of morbidity codes as necessary to fully explain each cause. For example, if an injury occurs as a result of a building collapse during the hurricane, external cause codes for both the hurricane and the building collapse should be assigned, with the external causes code for hurricane being sequenced as the first external cause code. For injuries incurred as a direct result of the hurricane, assign the appropriate code(s) for the injuries, followed by the code X37.0-, Hurricane (with the appropriate 7th character), and any other applicable external cause of injury codes. Code X37.0- also should be assigned when an injury is incurred as a result of flooding caused by a levee breaking related to the hurricane. Code X38.-, Flood (with the appropriate 7th character), should be assigned when an injury is from flooding resulting directly from the storm. Code X36.0.-, Collapse of dam or man-made structure, should not be assigned when the cause of the collapse is due to the hurricane. Use of code X36.0- is limited to collapses of man-made structures due to earth surface movements, not due to storm surges directly from a hurricane.

c. Other External Causes of Morbidity Code Issues

For injuries that are not a direct result of the hurricane, such as an evacuee that has incurred an injury as a result of a motor vehicle accident, assign the appropriate external cause of morbidity code(s) to describe the cause of the injury, but do not assign code X37.0-, Hurricane. If it is not clear whether the injury was a direct result of the hurricane, assume the injury is due to the hurricane and assign code X37.0-, Hurricane, as well as any other applicable external cause of morbidity codes. In addition to code X37.0-, Hurricane, other possible applicable external cause of morbidity codes include:

X3Ø-, Exposure to excessive natural heat

X31-, Exposure to excessive natural cold

X38-, Flood

d. Use of Z codes

Z codes (other reasons for healthcare encounters) may be assigned as appropriate to further explain the reasons for presenting for healthcare services, including transfers between healthcare facilities, or provide additional information relevant to a patient encounter. The ICD-10-CM Official Guidelines for Coding and Reporting identify which codes maybe assigned as principal or first-listed diagnosis only, secondary diagnosis only, or principal/first-listed or secondary (depending on the circumstances). Possible applicable Z codes include:

Z59.Ø-, Homelessness

Z59.1, Inadequate housing

Z59.5, Extreme poverty

Z75.1, Person awaiting admission to adequate facility elsewhere

Z75.3, Unavailability and inaccessibility of health-care facilities

Z75.4, Unavailability and inaccessibility of other helping agencies

Z76.2, Encounter for health supervision and care of other healthy infant and child

Z99.12, Encounter for respirator [ventilator] dependence during power failure

The external cause of morbidity codes and the Z codes listed above are not an all-inclusive list. Other codes may be applicable to the encounter based upon the documentation. Assign as many codes as necessary to fully explain each healthcare encounter. Since patient history information may be very limited, use any available documentation to assign the appropriate external cause of morbidity and Z codes.

C. Chapter-Specific Coding Guidelines

In addition to general coding guidelines, there are guidelines for specific diagnoses and/or conditions in the classification. Unless otherwise indicated, these guidelines apply to all health care settings. Please refer to Section II for guidelines on the selection of principal diagnosis.

1. Chapter 1: Certain Infectious and Parasitic Diseases (AØØ-B99), UØ7.1, UØ9.9

a. Human Immunodeficiency Virus (HIV) Infections

1) Code only confirmed cases

Code only confirmed cases of HIV infection/illness. This is an exception to the hospital inpatient guideline Section II, H.

In this context, "confirmation" does not require documentation of positive serology or culture for HIV; the provider's diagnostic statement that the patient is HIV positive or has an HIV-related illness is sufficient.

2) Selection and sequencing of HIV codes

(a) Patient admitted for HIV-related condition

If a patient is admitted for an HIV-related condition, the principal diagnosis should be B2Ø, Human immunodeficiency virus [HIV] disease followed by additional diagnosis codes for all reported HIV-related conditions.

An exception to this guideline is if the reason for admission is hemolytic-uremic syndrome associated with HIV disease. Assign code D59.31, Infection- associated hemolytic-uremic syndrome, followed by code B2Ø, Human immunodeficiency virus [HIV] disease.

(b) Patient with HIV disease admitted for unrelated condition

If a patient with HIV disease is admitted for an unrelated condition (such as a traumatic injury), the code for the unrelated condition (e.g., the nature of injury code) should be the principal diagnosis. Other diagnoses would be B2Ø followed by additional diagnosis codes for all reported HIV-related conditions.

(c) Whether the patient is newly diagnosed
Whether the patient is newly diagnosed or has had previous admissions/encounters for HIV conditions is irrelevant to the sequencing decision.

(d) Asymptomatic human immunodeficiency virus
Z21, Asymptomatic human immunodeficiency virus [HIV] infection status, is to be applied when the patient without any documentation of symptoms is listed as being "HIV positive," "known HIV," "HIV test positive," or similar terminology. Do not use this code if the term "AIDS" or "HIV disease" is used or if the patient is treated for any HIV-related illness or is described as having any condition(s) resulting from his/her HIV positive status; use B2Ø in these cases.

(e) Patients with inconclusive HIV serology
Patients with inconclusive HIV serology, but no definitive diagnosis or manifestations of the illness, may be assigned code R75, Inconclusive laboratory evidence of human immunodeficiency virus [HIV].

(f) Previously diagnosed HIV-related illness
Patients with any known prior diagnosis of an HIV-related illness should be coded to B2Ø. Once a patient has developed an HIV-related illness, the patient should always be assigned code B2Ø on every subsequent admission/encounter. Patients previously diagnosed with any HIV illness (B2Ø) should never be assigned to R75 or Z21, Asymptomatic human immunodeficiency virus [HIV] infection status.

(g) HIV Infection in Pregnancy, Childbirth and the Puerperium
During pregnancy, childbirth or the puerperium, a patient admitted (or presenting for a health care encounter) because of an HIV-related illness should receive a principal diagnosis code of O98.7-, Human immunodeficiency [HIV] disease complicating pregnancy, childbirth and the puerperium, followed by B2Ø and the code(s) for the HIV-related illness(es). Codes from Chapter 15 always take sequencing priority.

Patients with asymptomatic HIV infection status admitted (or presenting for a health care encounter) during pregnancy, childbirth, or the puerperium should receive codes of O98.7- and Z21.

(h) Encounters for testing for HIV
If a patient is being seen to determine his/her HIV status, use code Z11.4, Encounter for screening for human immunodeficiency virus [HIV]. Use additional codes for any associated high-risk behavior, if applicable.

If a patient with signs or symptoms is being seen for HIV testing, code the signs and symptoms. An additional counseling code Z71.7, Human immunodeficiency virus [HIV] counseling, may be used if counseling is provided during the encounter for the test.

When a patient returns to be informed of his/her HIV test results and the test result is negative, use code Z71.7, Human immunodeficiency virus [HIV] counseling.

If the results are positive, see previous guidelines and assign codes as appropriate.

(i) HIV managed by antiretroviral medication
If a patient with documented HIV disease, HIV-related illness or AIDS is currently managed on antiretroviral medications, assign code B2Ø, Human immunodeficiency virus [HIV] disease. Code Z79.899, Other long term (current) drug therapy, may be assigned as an additional code to identify the long-term (current) use of antiretroviral medications.

(j) Encounter for HIV Prophylaxis Measures
When a patient is seen for administration of pre-exposure prophylaxis medication for HIV, assign code Z29.81, Encounter for HIV pre-exposure prophylaxis. Pre-exposure prophylaxis (PrEP) is intended to prevent infection in people who are at risk for getting HIV through sex or injection drug use. Any risk factors for HIV should also be coded.

b. Infectious agents as the cause of diseases classified to other chapters
Certain infections are classified in chapters other than Chapter 1 and no organism is identified as part of the infection code. In these instances, it is necessary to use an additional code from Chapter 1 to identify the organism. A code from category B95, Streptococcus, Staphylococcus, and Enterococcus as the cause of diseases classified to other chapters, B96, Other bacterial agents as the cause of diseases classified to other chapters, or B97, Viral agents as the cause of diseases classified to other chapters, is to be used as an additional code to identify the organism. An instructional note will be found at the infection code advising that an additional organism code is required.

c. Infections resistant to antibiotics

Many bacterial infections are resistant to current antibiotics. It is necessary to identify all infections documented as antibiotic resistant. Assign a code from category Z16, Resistance to antimicrobial drugs, following the infection code only if the infection code does not identify drug resistance.

d. Sepsis, Severe Sepsis, and Septic Shock Infections resistant to antibiotics

1) Coding of Sepsis and Severe Sepsis

(a) Sepsis

For a diagnosis of sepsis, assign the appropriate code for the underlying systemic infection. If the type of infection or causal organism is not further specified, assign code A41.9, Sepsis, unspecified organism.

A code from subcategory R65.2, Severe sepsis, should not be assigned unless severe sepsis or an associated acute organ dysfunction is documented.

(i) Negative or inconclusive blood cultures and sepsis

Negative or inconclusive blood cultures do not preclude a diagnosis of sepsis in patients with clinical evidence of the condition; however, the provider should be queried.

(ii) Urosepsis

The term urosepsis is a nonspecific term. It is not to be considered synonymous with sepsis. It has no default code in the Alphabetic Index. Should a provider use this term, he/she must be queried for clarification.

(iii) Sepsis with organ dysfunction

If a patient has sepsis and associated acute organ dysfunction or multiple organ dysfunction (MOD), follow the instructions for coding severe sepsis.

(iv) Acute organ dysfunction that is not clearly associated with the sepsis

If a patient has sepsis and an acute organ dysfunction, but the medical record documentation indicates that the acute organ dysfunction is related to a medical condition other than the sepsis, do not assign a code from subcategory R65.2, Severe sepsis. An acute organ dysfunction must be associated with the sepsis in order to assign the severe sepsis code. If the documentation is not clear as to whether an acute organ dysfunction is related to the sepsis or another medical condition, query the provider.

(b) Severe sepsis

The coding of severe sepsis requires a minimum of 2 codes: first a code for the underlying systemic infection, followed by a code from subcategory R65.2, Severe sepsis. If the causal organism is not documented, assign code A41.9, Sepsis, unspecified organism, for the infection. Additional code(s) for the associated acute organ dysfunction are also required.

Due to the complex nature of severe sepsis, some cases may require querying the provider prior to assignment of the codes.

2) Septic shock

Septic shock generally refers to circulatory failure associated with severe sepsis, and therefore, it represents a type of acute organ dysfunction.

For cases of septic shock, the code for the systemic infection should be sequenced first, followed by code R65.21, Severe sepsis with septic shock or code T81.12, Postprocedural septic shock.

Any additional codes for the other acute organ dysfunctions should also be assigned. As noted in the sequencing instructions in the Tabular List, the code for septic shock cannot be assigned as a principal diagnosis.

3) Sequencing of severe sepsis

If severe sepsis is present on admission, and meets the definition of principal diagnosis, the underlying systemic infection should be assigned as principal diagnosis followed by the appropriate code from subcategory R65.2 as required by the sequencing rules in the Tabular List. A code from subcategory R65.2 can never be assigned as a principal diagnosis.

When severe sepsis develops during an encounter (it was not present on admission), the underlying systemic infection and the appropriate code from subcategory R65.2 should be assigned as secondary diagnoses.

Severe sepsis may be present on admission, but the diagnosis may not be confirmed until sometime after admission. If the documentation is not clear whether severe sepsis was present on admission, the provider should be queried.

For infection-associated hemolytic-uremic syndrome with severe sepsis, see guideline I.C.1.d.9.

4) Sepsis or severe sepsis with a localized infection

If the reason for admission is sepsis or severe sepsis and a localized infection, such as pneumonia or cellulitis, a code(s) for the underlying systemic infection should be assigned first and the code for the localized infection should be assigned as a secondary diagnosis. If the patient has severe sepsis, a code from subcategory R65.2 should also be assigned as a secondary diagnosis. If the patient is admitted with a localized infection, such as pneumonia, and sepsis/severe sepsis doesn't develop until after admission, the localized infection should be assigned first, followed by the appropriate sepsis/severe sepsis codes.

For hemolytic-uremic syndrome associated with sepsis, see guideline I.C.1.d.9.

5) Sepsis due to a postprocedural infection

(a) Documentation of causal relationship

As with all postprocedural complications, code assignment is based on the provider's documentation of the relationship between the infection and the procedure.

(b) Sepsis due to a postprocedural infection

For sepsis following a postprocedural wound (surgical site) infection, a code from T81.41 to T81.43, Infection following a procedure, T81.49, Infection following a procedure, other surgical site, or a code from O86.ØØ to O86.Ø3, Infection of obstetric surgical wound, or code O86.Ø9, Infection of obstetric surgical wound, other surgical site, that identifies the site of the infection should be sequenced first, if known. Assign an additional code for sepsis following a procedure (T81.44) or sepsis following an obstetrical procedure (O86.Ø4). Use an additional code to identify the infectious agent. If the patient has severe sepsis, the appropriate code from subcategory R65.2 should also be assigned with the additional code(s) for any acute organ dysfunction.

For infections following infusion, transfusion, therapeutic injection, or immunization, a code from subcategory T8Ø.2, Infections following infusion, transfusion, and therapeutic injection, or code T88.Ø-, Infection following immunization, should be coded first, followed by the code for the specific infection. If the patient has severe sepsis, the appropriate code from subcategory R65.2 should also be assigned, with the additional codes(s) for any acute organ dysfunction.

(c) Postprocedural infection and postprocedural septic shock

If a postprocedural infection has resulted in postprocedural septic shock, assign the codes indicated above for sepsis due to a postprocedural infection, followed by code T81.12-, Postprocedural septic shock. Do not assign code R65.21, Severe sepsis with septic shock. Additional code(s) should be assigned for any acute organ dysfunction.

6) Sepsis and severe sepsis associated with a noninfectious process (condition)

In some cases, a noninfectious process (condition) such as trauma, may lead to an infection which can result in sepsis or severe sepsis. If sepsis or severe sepsis is documented as associated with a noninfectious condition, such as a burn or serious injury, and this condition meets the definition for principal diagnosis, the code for the noninfectious condition should be sequenced first, followed by the code for the resulting infection. If severe sepsis is present, a code from subcategory R65.2 should also be assigned with any associated organ dysfunction(s) codes. It is not necessary to assign a code from subcategory R65.1, Systemic inflammatory response syndrome (SIRS) of non-infectious origin, for these cases.

If the infection meets the definition of principal diagnosis, it should be sequenced before the non-infectious condition. When both the associated non-infectious condition and the infection meet the definition of principal diagnosis, either may be assigned as principal diagnosis.

Only one code from category R65, Symptoms and signs specifically associated with systemic inflammation and infection, should be assigned. Therefore, when a non-infectious condition leads to an infection resulting in severe sepsis, assign the appropriate code from subcategory R65.2, Severe sepsis. Do not additionally assign a code from subcategory R65.1, Systemic inflammatory response syndrome (SIRS) of non-infectious origin.

See Section I.C.18. SIRS due to non-infectious process

7) Sepsis and septic shock complicating abortion, pregnancy, childbirth, and the puerperium

See Section I.C.15. Sepsis and septic shock complicating abortion, pregnancy, childbirth and the puerperium

8) Newborn sepsis

See Section I.C.16. f. Bacterial sepsis of Newborn

9) Hemolytic-uremic syndrome associated with sepsis

If the reason for admission is hemolytic-uremic syndrome that is associated with sepsis, assign code D59.31, Infection-associated hemolytic-uremic syndrome, as the principal diagnosis. Codes for the underlying systemic infection and any other conditions (such as severe sepsis) should be assigned as secondary diagnoses.

e. Methicillin Resistant Staphylococcus aureus (MRSA) Conditions

1) Selection and sequencing of MRSA codes

(a) Combination codes for MRSA infection

When a patient is diagnosed with an infection that is due to methicillin resistant *Staphylococcus aureus* (MRSA), and that infection has a combination code that includes the causal organism (e.g., sepsis, pneumonia) assign the appropriate combination code for the condition (e.g., code A41.Ø2, Sepsis due to Methicillin resistant Staphylococcus aureus or code J15.212, Pneumonia due to Methicillin resistant Staphylococcus aureus). Do not assign code B95.62, Methicillin resistant Staphylococcus aureus infection as the cause of diseases classified elsewhere, as an additional code, because the combination code includes the type of infection and the MRSA organism. Do not assign a code from subcategory Z16.11, Resistance to penicillins, as an additional diagnosis.

See Section C.1. for instructions on coding and sequencing of sepsis and severe sepsis.

(b) Other codes for MRSA infection

When there is documentation of a current infection (e.g., wound infection, stitch abscess, urinary tract infection) due to MRSA, and that infection does not have a combination code that includes the causal organism, assign the appropriate code to identify the condition along with code B95.62, Methicillin resistant Staphylococcus aureus infection as the cause of diseases classified elsewhere for the MRSA infection. Do not assign a code from subcategory Z16.11, Resistance to penicillins.

(c) Methicillin susceptible Staphylococcus aureus (MSSA) and MRSA colonization

The condition or state of being colonized or carrying MSSA or MRSA is called colonization or carriage, while an individual person is described as being colonized or being a carrier.

Colonization means that MSSA or MSRA is present on or in the body without necessarily causing illness. A positive MRSA colonization test might be documented by the provider as "MRSA screen positive" or "MRSA nasal swab positive".

Assign code Z22.322, Carrier or suspected carrier of Methicillin resistant Staphylococcus aureus, for patients documented as having MRSA colonization. Assign code Z22.321, Carrier or suspected carrier of Methicillin susceptible Staphylococcus aureus, for patients documented as having MSSA colonization. Colonization is not necessarily indicative of a disease process or as the cause of a specific condition the patient may have unless documented as such by the provider.

(d) MRSA colonization and infection

If a patient is documented as having both MRSA colonization and infection during a hospital admission, code Z22.322, Carrier or suspected carrier of Methicillin resistant Staphylococcus aureus, and a code for the MRSA infection may both be assigned.

f. Zika virus infections

1) Code only confirmed cases

Code only a confirmed diagnosis of Zika virus (A92.5, Zika virus disease) as documented by the provider. This is an exception to the hospital inpatient guideline Section II, H. In this context, "confirmation" does not require documentation of the type of test performed; the provider's diagnostic statement that the condition is confirmed is sufficient. This code should be assigned regardless of the stated mode of transmission.

If the provider documents "suspected", "possible" or "probable" Zika, do not assign code A92.5. Assign a code(s) explaining the reason for encounter (such as fever, rash, or joint pain) or Z2Ø.821, Contact with and (suspected) exposure to Zika virus.

g. Coronavirus infections

1) COVID-19 infection (infection due to SARS-CoV-2)

(a) Code only confirmed cases

Code only a confirmed diagnosis of the 2019 novel coronavirus disease (COVID-19) as documented by the provider, or documentation of a positive COVID-19 test result. For a confirmed diagnosis, assign code UØ7.1, COVID-19. This is an exception to the hospital inpatient guideline Section II, H. In this context, "confirmation" does not require documentation of a positive test result for COVID-19; the provider's documentation that the individual has COVID-19 is sufficient.

If the provider documents "suspected," "possible," "probable," or "inconclusive" COVID-19, do not assign code UØ7.1. Instead, code the signs and symptoms reported. See guideline I.C.1.g.1.g.

(b) Sequencing of codes

When COVID-19 meets the definition of principal diagnosis, code UØ7.1, COVID-19, should be sequenced first, followed by the appropriate codes for associated manifestations, except when another guideline requires that certain codes be sequenced first, such as obstetrics, sepsis, or transplant complications.

For a COVID-19 infection that progresses to sepsis, see Section I.C.1.d. Sepsis, Severe Sepsis, and Septic Shock

See Section I.C.15.s. for COVID-19 infection in pregnancy, childbirth, and the puerperium

See Section I.C.16.h. for COVID-19 infection in newborn

For a COVID-19 infection in a lung transplant patient, see Section I.C.19.g.3.a. Transplant complications other than kidney.

(c) Acute respiratory manifestations of COVID-19

When the reason for the encounter/admission is a respiratory manifestation of COVID-19, assign code UØ7.1, COVID-19, as the principal/first-listed diagnosis and assign code(s) for the respiratory manifestation(s) as additional diagnoses.

The following conditions are examples of common respiratory manifestations of COVID-19.

(i) Pneumonia

For a patient with pneumonia confirmed as due to COVID-19, assign codes UØ7.1, COVID-19, and J12.82, Pneumonia due to coronavirus disease 2019.

(ii) Acute bronchitis

For a patient with acute bronchitis confirmed as due to COVID-19, assign codes UØ7.1, and J2Ø.8, Acute bronchitis due to other specified organisms.

Bronchitis not otherwise specified (NOS) due to COVID-19 should be coded using code UØ7.1 and J4Ø, Bronchitis, not specified as acute or chronic.

(iii) Lower respiratory infection

If the COVID-19 is documented as being associated with a lower respiratory infection, not otherwise specified (NOS), or an acute respiratory infection, NOS, codes UØ7.1 and J22, Unspecified acute lower respiratory infection, should be assigned.

If the COVID-19 is documented as being associated with a respiratory infection, NOS, codes UØ7.1 and J98.8, Other specified respiratory disorders, should be assigned.

(iv) Acute respiratory distress syndrome

For acute respiratory distress syndrome (ARDS) due to COVID-19, assign codes UØ7.1, and J8Ø, Acute respiratory distress syndrome.

(v) Acute respiratory failure

For acute respiratory failure due to COVID-19, assign code UØ7.1, and code J96.Ø-, Acute respiratory failure.

(d) Non-respiratory manifestations of COVID-19

When the reason for the encounter/admission is a non-respiratory manifestation (e.g., viral enteritis) of COVID-19, assign code UØ7.1, COVID-19, as the principal/first-listed diagnosis and assign code(s) for the manifestation(s) as additional diagnoses.

(e) Exposure to COVID-19

For asymptomatic individuals with actual or suspected exposure to COVID-19, assign code Z20.822, Contact with and (suspected) exposure to COVID-19.

For symptomatic individuals with actual or suspected exposure to COVID-19 and the infection has been ruled out, or test results are inconclusive or unknown, assign code Z20.822, Contact with and (suspected) exposure to COVID-19. See guideline I.C.21.c.1, Contact/Exposure, for additional guidance regarding the use of category Z20 codes.

If COVID-19 is confirmed, see guideline I.C.1.g.1.a.

(f) Screening for COVID-19

For screening for COVID-19, including preoperative testing, assign code Z11.52, Encounter for screening for COVID-19.

(g) Signs and symptoms without definitive diagnosis of COVID-19

For patients presenting with any signs/symptoms associated with COVID-19 (such as fever, etc.) but a definitive diagnosis has not been established, assign the appropriate code(s) for each of the presenting signs and symptoms such as:

- R05.1, Acute cough, or R05.9, Cough, unspecified
- R06.02 Shortness of breath
- R50.9 Fever, unspecified

If a patient with signs/symptoms associated with COVID-19 also has an actual or suspected contact with or exposure to COVID-19, assign Z20.822, Contact with and (suspected) exposure to COVID-19, as an additional code.

(h) Asymptomatic individuals who test positive for COVID-19

For asymptomatic individuals who test positive for COVID-19, see guideline I.C.1.g.1.a. Although the individual is asymptomatic, the individual has tested positive and is considered to have the COVID-19 infection.

(i) Personal history of COVID-19

For patients with a history of COVID-19, assign code Z86.16, Personal history of COVID-19.

(j) Follow-up visits after COVID-19 infection has resolved

For individuals who previously had COVID-19, without residual symptom(s) or condition(s), and are being seen for follow-up evaluation, and COVID-19 test results are negative, assign codes Z09, Encounter for follow-up examination after completed treatment for conditions other than malignant neoplasm, and Z86.16, Personal history of COVID-19.

For follow-up visits for individuals with symptom(s) or condition(s) related to a previous COVID-19 infection, see guideline I.C.1.g.1.m.

See Section I.C.21.c.8, Factors influencing health states and contact with health services, Follow-up

(k) Encounter for antibody testing

For an encounter for antibody testing that is not being performed to confirm a current COVID-19 infection, nor is a follow-up test after resolution of COVID-19, assign Z01.84, Encounter for antibody response examination.

Follow the applicable guidelines above if the individual is being tested to confirm a current COVID-19 infection.

For follow-up testing after a COVID-19 infection, see guideline I.C.1.g.1.j.

(l) Multisystem Inflammatory Syndrome

For individuals with multisystem inflammatory syndrome (MIS) and COVID-19, assign code U07.1, COVID-19, as the principal/first-listed diagnosis and assign code M35.81, Multisystem inflammatory syndrome, as an additional diagnosis.

If an individual with a history of COVID-19 develops MIS, assign codes M35.81, Multisystem inflammatory syndrome, and U09.9, Post COVID-19 condition, unspecified.

If an individual with a known or suspected exposure to COVID-19, and no current COVID-19 infection or history of COVID-19, develops MIS, assign codes M35.81, Multisystem inflammatory syndrome, and Z20.822, Contact with and (suspected) exposure to COVID-19.

Additional codes should be assigned for any associated complications of MIS.

(m) Post COVID-19 Condition

For sequela of COVID-19, or associated symptoms or conditions that develop following a previous COVID-19 infection, assign a code(s) for the specific symptom(s) or condition(s) related to the previous COVID-19 infection, if known, and code UØ9.9, Post COVID-19 condition, unspecified.

Code UØ9.9 should not be assigned for manifestations of an active (current) COVID-19 infection.

If a patient has a condition(s) associated with a previous COVID-19 infection and develops a new active (current) COVID-19 infection, code UØ9.9 may be assigned in conjunction with code UØ7.1, COVID-19, to identify that the patient also has a condition(s) associated with a previous COVID-19 infection. Code(s) for the specific condition(s) associated with the previous COVID-19 infection and code(s) for manifestation(s) of the new active (current) COVID-19 infection should also be assigned.

(n) Underimmunization for COVID-19 Status

Code Z28.31Ø, Unvaccinated for COVID-19, may be assigned when the patient has not received a COVID-19 vaccine of any type. Code Z28.311, Partially vaccinated for COVID-19, may be assigned when the patient has been partially vaccinated for COVID-19 as per the recommendations of the Centers for Disease Control and Prevention (CDC) in place at the time of the encounter. For information, visit the CDC's website https://www.cdc.gov/coronavirus/2Ø19-ncov/vaccines/.

See Section I.B.14. for underimmunization documentation by clinicians other than patient's provider.

2. Chapter 2: Neoplasms (CØØ-D49)
General Guidelines

Chapter 2 of the ICD-10-CM contains the codes for most benign and all malignant neoplasms. Certain benign neoplasms, such as prostatic adenomas, may be found in the specific body system chapters. To properly code a neoplasm, it is necessary to determine from the record if the neoplasm is benign, in-situ, malignant, or of uncertain histologic behavior. If malignant, any secondary (metastatic) sites should also be determined.

Primary malignant neoplasms overlapping site boundaries

A primary malignant neoplasm that overlaps two or more contiguous (next to each other) sites should be classified to the subcategory/code .8 ('overlapping lesion'), unless the combination is specifically indexed elsewhere. For multiple neoplasms of the same site that are not contiguous such as tumors in different quadrants of the same breast, codes for each site should be assigned.

Malignant neoplasm of ectopic tissue

Malignant neoplasms of ectopic tissue are to be coded to the site of origin mentioned, e.g., ectopic pancreatic malignant neoplasms involving the stomach are coded to malignant neoplasm of pancreas, unspecified (C25.9).

The neoplasm table in the Alphabetic Index should be referenced first. However, if the histological term is documented, that term should be referenced first, rather than going immediately to the Neoplasm Table, in order to determine which column in the Neoplasm Table is appropriate. For example, if the documentation indicates "adenoma," refer to the term in the Alphabetic Index to review the entries under this term and the instructional note to "see also neoplasm, by site, benign." The table provides the proper code based on the type of neoplasm and the site. It is important to select the proper column in the table that corresponds to the type of neoplasm. The Tabular List should then be referenced to verify that the correct code has been selected from the table and that a more specific site code does not exist.

See Section I.C.21. Factors influencing health status and contact with health services, Status, for information regarding Z15.0, codes for genetic susceptibility to cancer.

a. Admission/Encounter for treatment of primary site

If the malignancy is chiefly responsible for occasioning the patient admission/encounter and treatment is directed at the primary site, designate the primary malignancy as the principal/first-listed diagnosis.

The only exception to this guideline is if the administration of chemotherapy, immunotherapy or external beam radiation therapy is chiefly responsible for occasioning the admission/encounter. In that case, assign the appropriate Z51.-- code as the first-listed or principal diagnosis, and the underlying diagnosis or problem for which the service is being performed as a secondary diagnosis.

ICD-10-CM Official Guidelines

for the malignancy is sequenced as the principal or first-listed diagnosis followed by code D63.Ø, Anemia in neoplastic disease.

5) **Complication from surgical procedure for treatment of a neoplasm**
When an encounter is for treatment of a complication resulting from a surgical procedure performed for the treatment of the neoplasm, designate the complication as the principal/first-listed diagnosis. See the guideline regarding the coding of a current malignancy versus personal history to determine if the code for the neoplasm should also be assigned.

6) **Pathologic fracture due to a neoplasm**
When an encounter is for a pathological fracture due to a neoplasm, and the focus of treatment is the fracture, a code from subcategory M84.5, Pathological fracture in neoplastic disease, should be sequenced first, followed by the code for the neoplasm.

If the focus of treatment is the neoplasm with an associated pathological fracture, the neoplasm code should be sequenced first, followed by a code from M84.5 for the pathological fracture.

m. **Current malignancy versus personal history of malignancy**
When a primary malignancy has been excised but further treatment, such as an additional surgery for the malignancy, radiation therapy or chemotherapy is directed to that site, the primary malignancy code should be used until treatment is completed.

When a primary malignancy has been previously excised or eradicated from its site, there is no further treatment (of the malignancy) directed to that site, and there is no evidence of any existing primary malignancy at that site, a code from category Z85, Personal history of malignant neoplasm, should be used to indicate the former site of the malignancy.

Codes from subcategories Z85.Ø – Z85.85 should only be assigned for the former site of a primary malignancy, not the site of a secondary malignancy. Code Z85.89 may be assigned for the former site(s) of either a primary or secondary malignancy.
See Section I.C.21. Factors influencing health status and contact with health services, History (of)

n. **Leukemia, Multiple Myeloma, and Malignant Plasma Cell Neoplasms in remission versus personal history**
The categories for leukemia, and category C9Ø, Multiple myeloma and malignant plasma cell neoplasms, have codes indicating whether or not the leukemia has achieved remission. There are also codes Z85.6, Personal history of leukemia, and Z85.79, Personal history of other malignant neoplasms of lymphoid, hematopoietic and related tissues. If the documentation is unclear as to whether the leukemia has achieved remission, the provider should be queried.

See Section I.C.21. Factors influencing health status and contact with health services, History (of)

o. **Aftercare following surgery for neoplasm**
See Section I.C.21. Factors influencing health status and contact with health services, Aftercare

p. **Follow-up care for completed treatment of a malignancy**
See Section I.C.21. Factors influencing health status and contact with health services, Follow-up

q. **Prophylactic organ removal for prevention of malignancy**
See Section I.C. 21, Factors influencing health status and contact with health services, Prophylactic organ removal

r. **Malignant neoplasm associated with transplanted organ**
A malignant neoplasm of a transplanted organ should be coded as a transplant complication. Assign first the appropriate code from category T86.-, Complications of transplanted organs and tissue, followed by code C8Ø.2, Malignant neoplasm associated with transplanted organ. Use an additional code for the specific malignancy.

s. **Breast Implant Associated Anaplastic Large Cell Lymphoma**
Breast implant associated anaplastic large cell lymphoma (BIA-ALCL) is a type of lymphoma that can develop around breast implants. Assign code C84.7A, Anaplastic large cell lymphoma, ALK-negative, breast, for BIA-ALCL **or C84.7B, Anaplastic large cell lymphoma, ALK-negative, in remission, for BIA-ALCL in remission**. Do not assign a complication code from chapter 19.

t. **Secondary malignant neoplasm of lymphoid tissue**
When a malignant neoplasm of lymphoid tissue metastasizes beyond the lymph nodes, a code from categories C81-C85 with a final character identifying "extranodal and solid organ sites" **should be assigned** rather than a code for the secondary neoplasm of the affected solid organ. For example, for metastasis of diffuse large B-cell lymphoma to the lung, brain and left adrenal gland, assign code C83.39**8**, Diffuse large B-cell lymphoma **of other** extranodal and solid organ sites.

3. Chapter 3: Disease of the blood and blood-forming organs and certain disorders involving the immune mechanism (D5Ø-D89)

Reserved for future guideline expansion

4. Chapter 4: Endocrine, Nutritional, and Metabolic Diseases (EØØ-E89)

a. Diabetes mellitus

The diabetes mellitus codes are combination codes that include the type of diabetes mellitus, the body system affected, and the complications affecting that body system. As many codes within a particular category as are necessary to describe all of the complications of the disease may be used. They should be sequenced based on the reason for a particular encounter. Assign as many codes from categories E08 – E13 as needed to identify all of the associated conditions that the patient has.

1) Type of diabetes

The age of a patient is not the sole determining factor, though most type 1 diabetics develop the condition before reaching puberty. For this reason, type 1 diabetes mellitus is also referred to as juvenile diabetes.

(a) Presymptomatic Type 1 Diabetes Mellitus

Codes E1Ø.A-, Type 1 diabetes mellitus, presymptomatic, are assigned for early-stage type 1 diabetes that predates the onset of symptoms.

2) Type of diabetes mellitus not documented

If the type of diabetes mellitus is not documented in the medical record the default is E11.-, Type 2 diabetes mellitus.

3) Diabetes mellitus and the use of insulin, oral hypoglycemics, and injectable non-insulin drugs

If the documentation in a medical record does not indicate the type of diabetes but does indicate that the patient uses insulin, code E11-, Type 2 diabetes mellitus, should be assigned. Additional code(s) should be assigned from category Z79 to identify the long-term (current) use of insulin, oral hypoglycemic drugs, or injectable non-insulin antidiabetic, as follows:

If the patient is treated with both oral hypoglycemic drugs and insulin, both code Z79.4, Long term (current) use of insulin, and code Z79.84, Long term (current) use of oral hypoglycemic drugs, should be assigned.

If the patient is treated with both insulin and an injectable non-insulin antidiabetic drug, assign codes Z79.4, Long term (current) use of insulin, and Z79.85, Long-term (current) use of injectable non-insulin antidiabetic drugs.

If the patient is treated with both oral hypoglycemic drugs and an injectable non-insulin antidiabetic drug, assign codes Z79.84, Long term (current) use of oral hypoglycemic drugs, and Z79.85, Long-term (current) use of injectable non-insulin antidiabetic drugs.

Code Z79.4 should not be assigned if insulin is given temporarily to bring a type 2 patient's blood sugar under control during an encounter.

4) Diabetes mellitus in pregnancy and gestational diabetes

See Section I.C.15. Diabetes mellitus in pregnancy.

See Section I.C.15. Gestational (pregnancy induced) diabetes

5) Complications due to insulin pump malfunction

(a) Underdose of insulin due to insulin pump failure

An underdose of insulin due to an insulin pump failure should be assigned to a code from subcategory T85.6, Mechanical complication of other specified internal and external prosthetic devices, implants and grafts, that specifies the type of pump malfunction, as the principal or first-listed code, followed by code T38.3X6-, Underdosing of insulin and oral hypoglycemic [antidiabetic] drugs. Additional codes for the type of diabetes mellitus and any associated complications due to the underdosing should also be assigned.

(b) Overdose of insulin due to insulin pump failure

The principal or first-listed code for an encounter due to an insulin pump malfunction resulting in an overdose of insulin, should also be T85.6-, Mechanical complication of other specified internal and external prosthetic devices, implants and grafts, followed by code T38.3X1-, Poisoning by insulin and oral hypoglycemic [antidiabetic] drugs, accidental (unintentional).

6) Secondary diabetes mellitus

Codes under categories EØ8, Diabetes mellitus due to underlying condition, EØ9, Drug or chemical induced diabetes mellitus, and E13, Other specified diabetes mellitus, identify complications/manifestations associated with secondary diabetes mellitus. Secondary diabetes is always caused by another condition or event (e.g., cystic fibrosis, malignant neoplasm of pancreas, pancreatectomy, adverse effect of drug, or poisoning).

(a) Secondary diabetes mellitus and the use of insulin, oral hypoglycemic drugs, or injectable non-insulin drugs

For patients with secondary diabetes mellitus who routinely use insulin, oral hypoglycemic drugs, or injectable non-insulin drugs, additional code(s) from category Z79 should be assigned to identify the long-term (current) use of insulin, oral hypoglycemic drugs, or non-injectable non-insulin drugs as follows:

If the patient is treated with both oral hypoglycemic drugs and insulin, both code Z79.4, Long term (current) use of insulin, and code Z79.84, Long term (current) use of oral hypoglycemic drugs, should be assigned.

If the patient is treated with both insulin and an injectable non-insulin antidiabetic drug, assign codes Z79.4, Long-term (current) use of insulin, and Z79.85, Long-term (current) use of injectable non-insulin antidiabetic drugs.

If the patient is treated with both oral hypoglycemic drugs and an injectable non-insulin antidiabetic drug, assign codes Z79.84, Long-term (current) use of oral hypoglycemic drugs, and Z79.85, Long-term (current) use of injectable non-insulin antidiabetic drugs.

Code Z79.4 should not be assigned if insulin is given temporarily to bring a secondary diabetic patient's blood sugar under control during an encounter.

(b) Assigning and sequencing secondary diabetes codes and its causes

The sequencing of the secondary diabetes codes in relationship to codes for the cause of the diabetes is based on the Tabular List instructions for categories EØ8, EØ9 and E13.

(i) Secondary diabetes mellitus due to pancreatectomy

For postpancreatectomy diabetes mellitus (lack of insulin due to the surgical removal of all or part of the pancreas), assign code E89.1, Postprocedural hypoinsulinemia.

Assign a code from category E13 as the principal or first-listed diagnosis and a code from subcategory Z9Ø.41, Acquired absence of pancreas, as an additional code.

(ii) Secondary diabetes due to drugs

Secondary diabetes may be caused by an adverse effect of correctly administered medications, poisoning or sequela of poisoning.

See section I.C.19.e. for coding of adverse effects and poisoning, and section I.C.20 for external cause code reporting.

5. Chapter 5: Mental, Behavioral and Neurodevelopmental disorders (FØ1-F99)

a. Pain disorders related to psychological factors

Assign code F45.41, for pain that is exclusively related to psychological disorders. As indicated by the Excludes 1 note under category G89, a code from category G89 should not be assigned with code F45.41.

Code F45.42, Pain disorders with related psychological factors, should be used with a code from category G89, Pain, not elsewhere classified, if there is documentation of a psychological component for a patient with acute or chronic pain.

See Section I.C.6. Pain

b. Mental and behavioral disorders due to psychoactive substance use

1) In Remission

Selection of codes describing "in remission" for categories F1Ø-F19, Mental and behavioral disorders due to psychoactive substance use (categories F1Ø-F19 with -.11, -.21, -.91) requires the provider's clinical judgment and are assigned only on the basis of provider documentation (as defined in the Official Guidelines for Coding and Reporting), unless otherwise instructed by the classification.

Mild substance use disorders in early or sustained remission are classified to the appropriate codes for substance abuse in remission, and moderate or severe substance use disorders in early or sustained remission are classified to the appropriate codes for substance dependence in remission.

2) Psychoactive Substance Use, Abuse and Dependence
When the provider documentation refers to use, abuse and dependence of the same substance (e.g. alcohol, opioid, cannabis, etc.), only one code should be assigned to identify the pattern of use based on the following hierarchy:

- If both use and abuse are documented, assign only the code for abuse
- If both abuse and dependence are documented, assign only the code for dependence
- If use, abuse and dependence are all documented, assign only the code for dependence
- If both use and dependence are documented, assign only the code for dependence.

3) Psychoactive Substance Use, Unspecified
As with all other unspecified diagnoses, the codes for unspecified psychoactive substance use (F1Ø.9-, F11.9-, F12.9-, F13.9-, F14.9-, F15.9-, F16.9-, F18.9-, F19.9-) should only be assigned based on provider documentation and when they meet the definition of a reportable diagnosis (see Section III, Reporting Additional Diagnoses). These codes are to be used only when the psychoactive substance use is associated with a substance related disorder (chapter 5 disorders such as sexual dysfunction, sleep disorder, or a mental or behavioral disorder) or medical condition, and such a relationship is documented by the provider.

4) Medical Conditions Due to Psychoactive Substance Use, Abuse and Dependence
Medical conditions due to substance use, abuse, and dependence are not classified as substance-induced disorders. Assign the diagnosis code for the medical condition as directed by the Alphabetical Index along with the appropriate psychoactive substance use, abuse or dependence code. For example, for alcoholic pancreatitis due to alcohol dependence, assign the appropriate code from subcategory K85.2, Alcohol induced acute pancreatitis, and the appropriate code from subcategory F1Ø.2, such as code F1Ø.2Ø, Alcohol dependence, uncomplicated. It would not be appropriate to assign code F1Ø.288, Alcohol dependence with other alcohol-induced disorder.

5) Blood Alcohol Level
A code from category Y9Ø, Evidence of alcohol involvement determined by blood alcohol level, may be assigned when this information is documented and the patient's provider has documented a condition classifiable to category F1Ø, Alcohol related disorders. The blood alcohol level does not need to be documented by the patient's provider in order for it to be coded.

See Section I.B.14. for blood alcohol level documentation by clinicians other than patient's provider.

c. Factitious Disorder
Factitious disorder imposed on self or Munchausen's syndrome is a disorder in which a person falsely reports or causes his or her own physical or psychological signs or symptoms. For patients with documented factitious disorder on self or Munchausen's syndrome, assign the appropriate code from subcategory F68.1-, Factitious disorder imposed on self.

Munchausen's syndrome by proxy (MSBP) is a disorder in which a caregiver (perpetrator) falsely reports or causes an illness or injury in another person (victim) under his or her care, such as a child, an elderly adult, or a person who has a disability. The condition is also referred to as "factitious disorder imposed on another" or "factitious disorder by proxy." The perpetrator, not the victim, receives this diagnosis. Assign code F68.A, Factitious disorder imposed on another, to the perpetrator's record. For the victim of a patient suffering from MSBP, assign the appropriate code from categories T74, Adult and child abuse, neglect and other maltreatment, confirmed, or T76, Adult and child abuse, neglect and other maltreatment, suspected.

See Section I.C.19.f. Adult and child abuse, neglect and other maltreatment

d. Dementia
The ICD-10-CM classifies dementia (categories F01, F02, and F03) on the basis of the etiology and severity (unspecified, mild, moderate or severe). Selection of the appropriate severity level requires the provider's clinical judgment and codes should be assigned only on the basis of provider documentation (as defined in the *Official Guidelines for Coding and Reporting*), unless otherwise instructed by the classification. If the documentation does not provide information about the severity of the dementia, assign the appropriate code for unspecified severity.

If a patient is admitted to an inpatient acute care hospital or other inpatient facility setting with dementia at one severity level and it progresses to a higher severity level, assign one code for the highest severity level reported during the stay.

6. Chapter 6: Diseases of the Nervous System (GØØ-G99)

a. Dominant/nondominant side

Codes from category G81, Hemiplegia and hemiparesis, and subcategories G83.1, Monoplegia of lower limb, G83.2, Monoplegia of upper limb, and G83.3, Monoplegia, unspecified, identify whether the dominant or nondominant side is affected. Should the affected side be documented, but not specified as dominant or nondominant, and the classification system does not indicate a default, code selection is as follows:

- For ambidextrous patients, the default should be dominant.
- If the left side is affected, the default is non-dominant.
- If the right side is affected, the default is dominant.

b. Pain - Category G89

1) General coding information

Codes in category G89, Pain, not elsewhere classified, may be used in conjunction with codes from other categories and chapters to provide more detail about acute or chronic pain and neoplasm-related pain, unless otherwise indicated below.

If the pain is not specified as acute or chronic, post-thoracotomy, postprocedural, or neoplasm-related, do not assign codes from category G89.

A code from category G89 should not be assigned if the underlying (definitive) diagnosis is known, unless the reason for the encounter is pain control/ management and not management of the underlying condition.

When an admission or encounter is for a procedure aimed at treating the underlying condition (e.g., spinal fusion, kyphoplasty), a code for the underlying condition (e.g., vertebral fracture, spinal stenosis) should be assigned as the principal diagnosis. No code from category G89 should be assigned.

(a) Category G89 Codes as Principal or First-Listed Diagnosis

Category G89 codes are acceptable as principal diagnosis or the first-listed code:

- When pain control or pain management is the reason for the admission/encounter (e.g., a patient with displaced intervertebral disc, nerve impingement and severe back pain presents for injection of steroid into the spinal canal). The underlying cause of the pain should be reported as an additional diagnosis, if known.
- When a patient is admitted for the insertion of a neurostimulator for pain control, assign the appropriate pain code as the principal or first-listed diagnosis. When an admission or encounter is for a procedure aimed at treating the underlying condition and a neurostimulator is inserted for pain control during the same admission/encounter, a code for the underlying condition should be assigned as the principal diagnosis and the appropriate pain code should be assigned as a secondary diagnosis.

(b) Use of Category G89 Codes in Conjunction with Site Specific Pain Codes

(i) Assigning Category G89 and Site-Specific Pain Codes

Codes from category G89 may be used in conjunction with codes that identify the site of pain (including codes from chapter 18) if the category G89 code provides additional information. For example, if the code describes the site of the pain, but does not fully describe whether the pain is acute or chronic, then both codes should be assigned.

(ii) Sequencing of Category G89 Codes with Site-Specific Pain Codes

The sequencing of category G89 codes with site-specific pain codes (including chapter 18 codes), is dependent on the circumstances of the encounter/admission as follows:

- If the encounter is for pain control or pain management, assign the code from category G89 followed by the code identifying the specific site of pain (e.g., encounter for pain management for acute neck pain from trauma is assigned code G89.11, Acute pain due to trauma, followed by code M54.2, Cervicalgia, to identify the site of pain).
- If the encounter is for any other reason except pain control or pain management, and a related definitive diagnosis has not been established (confirmed) by the provider,

ICD-10-CM Official Guidelines

assign the code for the specific site of pain first, followed by the appropriate code from category G89.

2) Pain due to devices, implants and grafts
See Section I.C.19. Pain due to medical devices

3) Postoperative Pain
The provider's documentation should be used to guide the coding of postoperative pain, as well as *Section III. Reporting Additional Diagnoses* and *Section IV. Diagnostic Coding and Reporting in the Outpatient Setting.*

The default for post-thoracotomy and other postoperative pain not specified as acute or chronic is the code for the acute form.

Routine or expected postoperative pain immediately after surgery should not be coded.

(a) Postoperative pain not associated with specific postoperative complication
Postoperative pain not associated with a specific postoperative complication is assigned to the appropriate postoperative pain code in category G89.

(b) Postoperative pain associated with specific postoperative complication
Postoperative pain associated with a specific postoperative complication (such as painful wire sutures) is assigned to the appropriate code(s) found in Chapter 19, Injury, poisoning, and certain other consequences of external causes. If appropriate, use additional code(s) from category G89 to identify acute or chronic pain (G89.18 or G89.28).

4) Chronic pain
Chronic pain is classified to subcategory G89.2. There is no time frame defining when pain becomes chronic pain. The provider's documentation should be used to guide use of these codes.

5) Neoplasm Related Pain
Code G89.3 is assigned to pain documented as being related, associated or due to cancer, primary or secondary malignancy, or tumor. This code is assigned regardless of whether the pain is acute or chronic.

This code may be assigned as the principal or first-listed code when the stated reason for the admission/encounter is documented as pain control/pain management. The underlying neoplasm should be reported as an additional diagnosis.

When the reason for the admission/encounter is management of the neoplasm and the pain associated with the neoplasm is also documented, code G89.3 may be assigned as an additional diagnosis. It is not necessary to assign an additional code for the site of the pain.

See Section I.C.2. for instructions on the sequencing of neoplasms for all other stated reasons for the admission/encounter (except for pain control/pain management).

6) Chronic pain syndrome
Central pain syndrome (G89.Ø) and chronic pain syndrome (G89.4) are different than the term "chronic pain," and therefore codes should only be used when the provider has specifically documented this condition.

See Section I.C.5. Pain disorders related to psychological factors

7. Chapter 7: Diseases of the Eye and Adnexa (HØØ-H59)

a. Glaucoma

1) Assigning Glaucoma Codes
Assign as many codes from category H4Ø, Glaucoma, as needed to identify the type of glaucoma, the affected eye, and the glaucoma stage.

2) Bilateral glaucoma with same type and stage
When a patient has bilateral glaucoma and both eyes are documented as being the same type and stage, and there is a code for bilateral glaucoma, report only the code for the type of glaucoma, bilateral, with the seventh character for the stage.

When a patient has bilateral glaucoma and both eyes are documented as being the same type and stage, and the classification does not provide a code for bilateral glaucoma (i.e. subcategories H4Ø.1Ø, and H4Ø.2Ø) report only one code for the type of glaucoma with the appropriate seventh character for the stage.

3) **Bilateral glaucoma stage with different types or stages**
When a patient has bilateral glaucoma and each eye is documented as having a different type or stage, and the classification distinguishes laterality, assign the appropriate code for each eye rather than the code for bilateral glaucoma.

When a patient has bilateral glaucoma and each eye is documented as having a different type, and the classification does not distinguish laterality (i.e., subcategories H4Ø.1Ø, and H4Ø.2Ø), assign one code for each type of glaucoma with the appropriate seventh character for the stage.

When a patient has bilateral glaucoma and each eye is documented as having the same type, but different stage, and the classification does not distinguish laterality (i.e., subcategories H4Ø.1Ø and H4Ø.2Ø), assign a code for the type of glaucoma for each eye with the seventh character for the specific glaucoma stage documented for each eye.

4) **Patient admitted with glaucoma and stage evolves during the admission**
If a patient is admitted with glaucoma and the stage progresses during the admission, assign the code for highest stage documented.

5) **Indeterminate stage glaucoma**
Assignment of the seventh character "4" for "indeterminate stage" should be based on the clinical documentation. The seventh character "4" is used for glaucomas whose stage cannot be clinically determined. This seventh character should not be confused with the seventh character "Ø", unspecified, which should be assigned when there is no documentation regarding the stage of the glaucoma.

b. **Blindness**
If "blindness" or "low vision" of both eyes is documented but the visual impairment category is not documented, assign code H54.3, Unqualified visual loss, both eyes. If "blindness" or "low vision" in one eye is documented but the visual impairment category is not documented, assign a code from H54.6-, Unqualified visual loss, one eye. If "blindness" or "visual loss" is documented without any information about whether one or both eyes are affected, assign code H54.7, Unspecified visual loss.

8. **Chapter 8: Diseases of the Ear and Mastoid Process (H6Ø-H95)**
Reserved for future guideline expansion

9. **Chapter 9: Diseases of the Circulatory System (IØØ-I99)**

a. **Hypertension**
The classification presumes a causal relationship between hypertension and heart involvement and between hypertension and kidney involvement, as the two conditions are linked by the term "with" in the Alphabetic Index. These conditions should be coded as related even in the absence of provider documentation explicitly linking them, unless the documentation clearly states the conditions are unrelated.

For hypertension and conditions not specifically linked by relational terms such as "with," "associated with" or "due to" in the classification, provider documentation must link the conditions in order to code them as related.

1) **Hypertension with Heart Disease**
Hypertension with heart conditions classified to I5Ø.- or I51.4- I51.7, I51.89, I51.9, are assigned to a code from category I11, Hypertensive heart disease. Use additional code(s) from category I5Ø, Heart failure, to identify the type(s) of heart failure in those patients with heart failure.

The same heart conditions (I5Ø.-, I51.4-I51.7, I51.89, I51.9) with hypertension are coded separately if the provider has documented they are unrelated to the hypertension. Sequence according to the circumstances of the admission/encounter.

2) **Hypertensive Chronic Kidney Disease**
Assign codes from category I12, Hypertensive chronic kidney disease, when both hypertension and a condition classifiable to category N18, Chronic kidney disease (CKD), are present. CKD should not be coded as hypertensive if the provider indicates the CKD is not related to the hypertension.

The appropriate code from category N18 should be used as a secondary code with a code from category I12 to identify the stage of chronic kidney disease.

See Section I.C.14. Chronic kidney disease.

If a patient has hypertensive chronic kidney disease and acute renal failure, the acute renal failure should also be coded. Sequence according to the circumstances of the admission/encounter.

3) Hypertensive Heart and Chronic Kidney Disease
Assign codes from combination category I13, Hypertensive heart and chronic kidney disease, when there is hypertension with both heart and kidney involvement. If heart failure is present, assign an additional code from category I50 to identify the type of heart failure.

The appropriate code from category N18, Chronic kidney disease, should be used as a secondary code with a code from category I13 to identify the stage of chronic kidney disease.

See Section I.C.14. Chronic kidney disease.

The codes in category I13, Hypertensive heart and chronic kidney disease, are combination codes that include hypertension, heart disease and chronic kidney disease. The Includes note at I13 specifies that the conditions included at I11 and I12 are included together in I13. If a patient has hypertension, heart disease and chronic kidney disease, then a code from I13 should be used, not individual codes for hypertension, heart disease and chronic kidney disease, or codes from I11 or I12.

For patients with both acute renal failure and chronic kidney disease, the acute renal failure should also be coded. Sequence according to the circumstances of the admission/encounter.

4) Hypertensive Cerebrovascular Disease
For hypertensive cerebrovascular disease, first assign the appropriate code from categories I60-I69, followed by the appropriate hypertension code.

5) Hypertensive Retinopathy
Subcategory H35.0, Background retinopathy and retinal vascular changes, should be used along with a code from categories I10-I15, in the Hypertensive diseases section, to include the systemic hypertension. The sequencing is based on the reason for the encounter.

6) Hypertension, Secondary
Secondary hypertension is due to an underlying condition. Two codes are required: one to identify the underlying etiology and one from category I15 to identify the hypertension. Sequencing of codes is determined by the reason for admission/encounter.

7) Hypertension, Transient
Assign code R03.0, Elevated blood pressure reading without diagnosis of hypertension, unless patient has an established diagnosis of hypertension. Assign code O13.-, Gestational [pregnancy-induced] hypertension without significant proteinuria, or O14.-, Pre-eclampsia, for transient hypertension of pregnancy.

8) Hypertension, Controlled
This diagnostic statement usually refers to an existing state of hypertension under control by therapy. Assign the appropriate code from categories I10-I15, Hypertensive diseases.

9) Hypertension, Uncontrolled
Uncontrolled hypertension may refer to untreated hypertension or hypertension not responding to current therapeutic regimen. In either case, assign the appropriate code from categories I10-I15, Hypertensive diseases.

10) Hypertensive Crisis
Assign a code from category I16, Hypertensive crisis, for documented hypertensive urgency, hypertensive emergency or unspecified hypertensive crisis. Code also any identified hypertensive disease (I10-I15). The sequencing is based on the reason for the encounter.

11) Pulmonary Hypertension
Pulmonary hypertension is classified to category I27, Other pulmonary heart diseases. For secondary pulmonary hypertension (I27.1, I27.2-), code also any associated conditions or adverse effects of drugs or toxins. The sequencing is based on the reason for the encounter, except for adverse effects of drugs (See Section I.C.19.e.).

12) Hypertension, Resistant
Resistant hypertension refers to blood pressure of a patient with hypertension that remains above goal in spite of the use of antihypertensive medications. Assign code I1A.0, Resistant hypertension, as an additional code when apparent treatment resistant hypertension, treatment resistant hypertension, or true resistant hypertension is documented by the provider. A code for the specific type of existing hypertension is sequenced first, if known.

b. Atherosclerotic Coronary Artery Disease and Angina
ICD-10-CM has combination codes for atherosclerotic heart disease with angina pectoris. The subcategories for these codes are I25.11, Atherosclerotic heart disease of native coronary artery with

angina pectoris and I25.7, Atherosclerosis of coronary artery bypass graft(s) and coronary artery of transplanted heart with angina pectoris.

When using one of these combination codes it is not necessary to use an additional code for angina pectoris. A causal relationship can be assumed in a patient with both atherosclerosis and angina pectoris, unless the documentation indicates the angina is due to something other than the atherosclerosis.

If a patient with coronary artery disease is admitted due to an acute myocardial infarction (AMI), the AMI should be sequenced before the coronary artery disease.

See Section I.C.9. Acute myocardial infarction (AMI)

c. Intraoperative and Postprocedural Cerebrovascular Accident

Medical record documentation should clearly specify the cause- and-effect relationship between the medical intervention and the cerebrovascular accident in order to assign a code for intraoperative or postprocedural cerebrovascular accident.

Proper code assignment depends on whether it was an infarction or hemorrhage and whether it occurred intraoperatively or postoperatively. If it was a cerebral hemorrhage, code assignment depends on the type of procedure performed.

d. Sequelae of Cerebrovascular Disease

1) Category I69, Sequelae of Cerebrovascular disease

Category I69 is used to indicate conditions classifiable to categories I6Ø-I67 as the causes of sequela (neurologic deficits), themselves classified elsewhere. These "late effects" include neurologic deficits that persist after initial onset of conditions classifiable to categories I6Ø-I67. The neurologic deficits caused by cerebrovascular disease may be present from the onset or may arise at any time after the onset of the condition classifiable to categories I6Ø-I67.

Codes from category I69, Sequelae of cerebrovascular disease, that specify hemiplegia, hemiparesis and monoplegia identify whether the dominant or nondominant side is affected. Should the affected side be documented, but not specified as dominant or nondominant, and the classification system does not indicate a default, code selection is as follows:

- For ambidextrous patients, the default should be dominant.
- If the left side is affected, the default is non-dominant.
- If the right side is affected, the default is dominant.

2) Codes from category I69 with codes from I6Ø-I67

Codes from category I69 may be assigned on a health care record with codes from I6Ø-I67, if the patient has a current cerebrovascular disease and deficits from an old cerebrovascular disease.

3) Codes from category I69 and Personal history of transient ischemic attack (TIA) and cerebral infarction (Z86.73)

Codes from category I69 should not be assigned if the patient does not have neurologic deficits.

See Section I.C.21.4. History (of) for use of personal history codes

e. Acute myocardial infarction (AMI)

1) Type 1 ST elevation myocardial infarction (STEMI) and non-ST elevation myocardial infarction (NSTEMI)

The ICD-10-CM codes for type 1 acute myocardial infarction (AMI) identify the site, such as anterolateral wall or true posterior wall. Subcategories I21.Ø-I21.2 and code I21.3 are used for type 1 ST elevation myocardial infarction (STEMI). Code I21.4, Non-ST elevation (NSTEMI) myocardial infarction, is used for type 1 non-ST elevation myocardial infarction (NSTEMI) and nontransmural MIs.

If a type 1 NSTEMI evolves to STEMI, assign the STEMI code. If a type 1 STEMI converts to NSTEMI due to thrombolytic therapy, it is still coded as STEMI.

For encounters occurring while the myocardial infarction is equal to, or less than, four weeks old, including transfers to another acute setting or a postacute setting, and the myocardial infarction meets the definition for "other diagnoses" (see Section III, Reporting Additional Diagnoses), codes from category I21 may continue to be reported. For encounters after the 4-week time frame and the patient is still receiving care related to the myocardial infarction, the appropriate aftercare code should be assigned, rather than a code from category I21. For old or healed myocardial infarctions not requiring further care, code I25.2, Old myocardial infarction, may be assigned.

2) **Acute myocardial infarction, unspecified**
Code I21.9, Acute myocardial infarction, unspecified, is the default for unspecified acute myocardial infarction or unspecified type. If only type 1 STEMI or transmural MI without the site is documented, assign code I21.3, ST elevation (STEMI) myocardial infarction of unspecified site.

3) **AMI documented as nontransmural or subendocardial but site provided**
If an AMI is documented as nontransmural or subendocardial, but the site is provided, it is still coded as a subendocardial AMI.

See Section I.C.21.3. for information on coding status post administration of tPA in a different facility within the last 24 hours.

4) **Subsequent acute myocardial infarction**
A code from category I22, Subsequent ST elevation (STEMI) and non-ST elevation (NSTEMI) myocardial infarction, is to be used when a patient who has suffered a type 1 or unspecified AMI has a new AMI within the 4 week time frame of the initial AMI. A code from category I22 must be used in conjunction with a code from category I21. The sequencing of the I22 and I21 codes depends on the circumstances of the encounter.

Do not assign code I22 for subsequent myocardial infarctions other than type 1 or unspecified. For subsequent type 2 AMI assign only code I21.A1. For subsequent type 4 or type 5 AMI, assign only code I21.A9.

If a subsequent myocardial infarction of one type occurs within 4 weeks of a myocardial infarction of a different type, assign the appropriate codes from category I21 to identify each type. Do not assign a code from I22. Codes from category I22 should only be assigned if both the initial and subsequent myocardial infarctions are type 1 or unspecified.

5) **Other Types of Myocardial Infarction**
The ICD-10-CM provides codes for different types of myocardial infarction. Type 1 myocardial infarctions are assigned to codes I21.Ø-I21.4.

Type 2 myocardial infarction (myocardial infarction due to demand ischemia or secondary to ischemic imbalance) is assigned to code I21.A1, Myocardial infarction type 2 with the underlying cause coded first**, if applicable**. Do not assign code I24.89, Other forms of acute ischemic heart disease, for the demand ischemia. If a type 2 AMI is described as NSTEMI or STEMI, only assign code I21.A1. Codes I21.Ø1-I21.4 should only be assigned for type 1 AMIs.

Acute myocardial infarctions type 3, 4a, 4b, 4c and 5 are assigned to code I21.A9, Other myocardial infarction type.

The "Code also" and "Code first" notes should be followed related to complications, and for coding of postprocedural myocardial infarctions during or following cardiac surgery.

6) **Myocardial Infarction with Coronary Microvascular Dysfunction**
Coronary microvascular dysfunction (CMD) is a condition that impacts the microvasculature by restricting microvascular flow and increasing microvascular resistance. Code I21.B, Myocardial infarction with coronary microvascular dysfunction, is assigned for myocardial infarction with coronary microvascular disease, myocardial infarction with coronary microvascular dysfunction, and myocardial infarction with non-obstructive coronary arteries (MINOCA) with microvascular disease.

10. Chapter 10: Diseases of the Respiratory System (JØØ-J99), UØ7.Ø

a. Chronic Obstructive Pulmonary Disease [COPD] and Asthma

1) **Acute exacerbation of chronic obstructive bronchitis and asthma**
The codes in categories J44 and J45 distinguish between uncomplicated cases and those in acute exacerbation. An acute exacerbation is a worsening or a decompensation of a chronic condition. An acute exacerbation is not equivalent to an infection superimposed on a chronic condition, though an exacerbation may be triggered by an infection.

b. Acute Respiratory Failure

1) **Acute respiratory failure as principal diagnosis**
A code from subcategory J96.Ø, Acute respiratory failure, or subcategory J96.2, Acute and chronic respiratory failure, may be assigned as a principal diagnosis when it is the condition established after study to be chiefly responsible for occasioning the admission to the hospital, and the selection is supported by the Alphabetic Index and Tabular List. However, chapter-specific coding guidelines (such as obstetrics, poisoning, HIV, newborn) that provide sequencing direction take precedence.

2) **Acute respiratory failure as secondary diagnosis**
Respiratory failure may be listed as a secondary diagnosis if it occurs after admission, or if it is present on admission, but does not meet the definition of principal diagnosis.

3) **Sequencing of acute respiratory failure and another acute condition**
When a patient is admitted with respiratory failure and another acute condition, (e.g., myocardial infarction, cerebrovascular accident, aspiration pneumonia), the principal diagnosis will not be the same in every situation. This applies whether the other acute condition is a respiratory or nonrespiratory condition. Selection of the principal diagnosis will be dependent on the circumstances of admission. If both the respiratory failure and the other acute condition are equally responsible for occasioning the admission to the hospital, and there are no chapter-specific sequencing rules, the guideline regarding two or more diagnoses that equally meet the definition for principal diagnosis (Section II, C.) may be applied in these situations.

If the documentation is not clear as to whether acute respiratory failure and another condition are equally responsible for occasioning the admission, query the provider for clarification.

c. **Influenza due to certain identified influenza viruses**
Code only confirmed cases of influenza due to certain identified influenza viruses (category JØ9), and due to other identified influenza virus (category J1Ø). This is an exception to the hospital inpatient guideline Section II, H. (Uncertain Diagnosis).

In this context, "confirmation" does not require documentation of positive laboratory testing specific for avian or other novel influenza A or other identified influenza virus. However, coding should be based on the provider's diagnostic statement that the patient has avian influenza, or other novel influenza A, for category JØ9, or has another particular identified strain of influenza, such as H1N1 or H3N2, but not identified as novel or variant, for category J1Ø.

If the provider records "suspected" or "possible" or "probable" avian influenza, or novel influenza, or other identified influenza, then the appropriate influenza code from category J11, Influenza due to unidentified influenza virus, should be assigned. A code from category JØ9, Influenza due to certain identified influenza viruses, should not be assigned nor should a code from category J1Ø, Influenza due to other identified influenza virus.

d. **Ventilator associated Pneumonia**

1) **Documentation of Ventilator associated Pneumonia**
As with all procedural or postprocedural complications, code assignment is based on the provider's documentation of the relationship between the condition and the procedure.

Code J95.851, Ventilator associated pneumonia, should be assigned only when the provider has documented ventilator associated pneumonia (VAP). An additional code to identify the organism (e.g., Pseudomonas aeruginosa, code B96.5) should also be assigned. Do not assign an additional code from categories J12-J18 to identify the type of pneumonia.

Code J95.851 should not be assigned for cases where the patient has pneumonia and is on a mechanical ventilator and the provider has not specifically stated that the pneumonia is ventilator-associated pneumonia. If the documentation is unclear as to whether the patient has a pneumonia that is a complication attributable to the mechanical ventilator, query the provider.

2) **Ventilator associated Pneumonia Develops after Admission**
A patient may be admitted with one type of pneumonia (e.g., code J13, Pneumonia due to Streptococcus pneumonia) and subsequently develop VAP. In this instance, the principal diagnosis would be the appropriate code from categories J12-J18 for the pneumonia diagnosed at the time of admission. Code J95.851, Ventilator associated pneumonia, would be assigned as an additional diagnosis when the provider has also documented the presence of ventilator associated pneumonia.

e. **Vaping-related disorders**
For patients presenting with condition(s) related to vaping, assign code UØ7.Ø, Vaping-related disorder, as the principal diagnosis. For lung injury due to vaping, assign only code UØ7.Ø. Assign additional codes for other manifestations, such as acute respiratory failure (subcategory J96.Ø-) or pneumonitis (code J68.Ø).

Associated respiratory signs and symptoms due to vaping, such as cough, shortness of breath, etc., are not coded separately, when a definitive diagnosis has been established. However, it would be appropriate to code separately any gastrointestinal symptoms, such as diarrhea and abdominal pain.

See Section I.C.1.g.1.c.i. for Pneumonia confirmed as due to COVID-19

ICD-10-CM Official Guidelines

11. Chapter 11: Diseases of the Digestive System (KØØ-K95)

Reserved for future guideline expansion

12. Chapter 12: Diseases of the Skin and Subcutaneous Tissue (LØØ-L99)

a. Pressure ulcer stage codes

1) Pressure ulcer stages

Codes in category L89, Pressure ulcer, identify the site and stage of the pressure ulcer.

The ICD-10-CM classifies pressure ulcer stages based on severity, which is designated by stages 1-4, deep tissue pressure injury, unspecified stage, and unstageable.

Assign as many codes from category L89 as needed to identify all the pressure ulcers the patient has, if applicable.

See Section I.B.14. for pressure ulcer stage documentation by clinicians other than patient's provider.

2) Unstageable pressure ulcers

Assignment of the code for unstageable pressure ulcer (L89.--Ø) should be based on the clinical documentation. These codes are used for pressure ulcers whose stage cannot be clinically determined (e.g., the ulcer is covered by eschar or has been treated with a skin or muscle graft). This code should not be confused with the codes for unspecified stage (L89.--9). When there is no documentation regarding the stage of the pressure ulcer, assign the appropriate code for unspecified stage (L89.-- 9).

If during an encounter, the stage of an unstageable pressure ulcer is revealed after debridement, assign only the code for the stage revealed following debridement.

3) Documented pressure ulcer stage

Assignment of the pressure ulcer stage code should be guided by clinical documentation of the stage or documentation of the terms found in the Alphabetic Index. For clinical terms describing the stage that are not found in the Alphabetic Index, and there is no documentation of the stage, the provider should be queried.

4) Patients admitted with pressure ulcers documented as healed

No code is assigned if the documentation states that the pressure ulcer is completely healed at the time of admission.

5) Pressure ulcers documented as healing

Pressure ulcers described as healing should be assigned the appropriate pressure ulcer stage code based on the documentation in the medical record. If the documentation does not provide information about the stage of the healing pressure ulcer, assign the appropriate code for unspecified stage.

If the documentation is unclear as to whether the patient has a current (new) pressure ulcer or if the patient is being treated for a healing pressure ulcer, query the provider.

For ulcers that were present on admission but healed at the time of discharge, assign the code for the site and stage of the pressure ulcer at the time of admission.

6) Patient admitted with pressure ulcer evolving into another stage during the admission

If a patient is admitted to an inpatient hospital with a pressure ulcer at one stage and it progresses to a higher stage, two separate codes should be assigned: one code for the site and stage of the ulcer on admission and a second code for the same ulcer site and the highest stage reported during the stay.

7) Pressure-induced deep tissue damage

For pressure-induced deep tissue damage or deep tissue pressure injury, assign only the appropriate code for pressure-induced deep tissue damage (L89.--6).

b. Non-Pressure Chronic Ulcers

1) Patients admitted with non-pressure ulcers documented as healed

No code is assigned if the documentation states that the non-pressure ulcer is completely healed at the time of admission.

2) Non-pressure ulcers documented as healing

Non-pressure ulcers described as healing should be assigned the appropriate non-pressure ulcer code based on the documentation in the medical record. If the documentation does not provide information about the severity of the healing non-pressure ulcer, assign the appropriate code for unspecified severity.

If the documentation is unclear as to whether the patient has a current (new) non-pressure ulcer or if the patient is being treated for a healing non-pressure ulcer, query the provider.

For ulcers that were present on admission but healed at the time of discharge, assign the code for the site and severity of the non-pressure ulcer at the time of admission.

3) **Patient admitted with non-pressure ulcer that progresses to another severity level during the admission**
If a patient is admitted to an inpatient hospital with a non-pressure ulcer at one severity level and it progresses to a higher severity level, two separate codes should be assigned: one code for the site and severity level of the ulcer on admission and a second code for the same ulcer site and the highest severity level reported during the stay.

See Section I.B.14. for pressure ulcer stage documentation by clinicians other than patient's provider

13. Chapter 13: Diseases of the Musculoskeletal System and Connective Tissue (MØØ-M99)

a. Site and laterality
Most of the codes within Chapter 13 have site and laterality designations. The site represents the bone, joint or the muscle involved. For some conditions where more than one bone, joint or muscle is usually involved, such as osteoarthritis, there is a "multiple sites" code available. For categories where no multiple site code is provided and more than one bone, joint or muscle is involved, multiple codes should be used to indicate the different sites involved.

1) **Bone versus joint**
For certain conditions, the bone may be affected at the upper or lower end, (e.g., avascular necrosis of bone, M87, Osteoporosis, M8Ø, M81). Though the portion of the bone affected may be at the joint, the site designation will be the bone, not the joint.

b. Acute traumatic versus chronic or recurrent musculoskeletal conditions
Many musculoskeletal conditions are a result of previous injury or trauma to a site, or are recurrent conditions. Bone, joint or muscle conditions that are the result of a healed injury are usually found in chapter 13. Recurrent bone, joint or muscle conditions are also usually found in chapter 13. Any current, acute injury should be coded to the appropriate injury code from chapter 19. Chronic or recurrent conditions should generally be coded with a code from chapter 13. If it is difficult to determine from the documentation in the record which code is best to describe a condition, query the provider.

c. Coding of Pathologic Fractures
7th character A is for use as long as the patient is receiving active treatment for the fracture. While the patient may be seen by a new or different provider over the course of treatment for a pathological fracture, assignment of the 7th character is based on whether the patient is undergoing active treatment and not whether the provider is seeing the patient for the first time.

7th character D is to be used for encounters after the patient has completed active treatment for the fracture and is receiving routine care for the fracture during the healing or recovery phase. The other 7th characters, listed under each subcategory in the Tabular List, are to be used for subsequent encounters for treatment of problems associated with the healing, such as malunions, nonunions, and sequelae.

Care for complications of surgical treatment for fracture repairs during the healing or recovery phase should be coded with the appropriate complication codes.

See Section I.C.19. Coding of traumatic fractures.

d. Osteoporosis
Osteoporosis is a systemic condition, meaning that all bones of the musculoskeletal system are affected. Therefore, site is not a component of the codes under category M81, Osteoporosis without current pathological fracture. The site codes under category M8Ø, Osteoporosis with current pathological fracture, identify the site of the fracture, not the osteoporosis.

1) **Osteoporosis without pathological fracture**
Category M81, Osteoporosis without current pathological fracture, is for use for patients with osteoporosis who do not currently have a pathologic fracture due to the osteoporosis, even if they have had a fracture in the past. For patients with a history of osteoporosis fractures, status code Z87.31Ø, Personal history of (healed) osteoporosis fracture, should follow the code from M81.

2) **Osteoporosis with current pathological fracture**
Category M8Ø, Osteoporosis with current pathological fracture, is for patients who have a current pathologic fracture at the time of an encounter. The codes under M8Ø identify the site of the fracture. A code from category M8Ø, not a traumatic fracture code, should be used for any patient

with known osteoporosis who suffers a fracture, even if the patient had a minor fall or trauma, if that fall or trauma would not usually break a normal, healthy bone.

e. Multisystem Inflammatory Syndrome

See Section I.C.1.g.1.l. for Multisystem Inflammatory Syndrome

14. Chapter 14: Diseases of Genitourinary System (NØØ-N99)

a. Chronic kidney disease

1) Stages of chronic kidney disease (CKD)

The ICD-10-CM classifies CKD based on severity. The severity of CKD is designated by stages 1-5. Stage 2, code N18.2, equates to mild CKD; stage 3, codes N18.3Ø-N18.32, equate to moderate CKD; and stage 4, code N18.4, equates to severe CKD. Code N18.6, End stage renal disease (ESRD), is assigned when the provider has documented end-stage renal disease (ESRD).

If both a stage of CKD and ESRD are documented, assign code N18.6 only.

2) Chronic kidney disease and kidney transplant status

Patients who have undergone kidney transplant may still have some form of chronic kidney disease (CKD) because the kidney transplant may not fully restore kidney function. Therefore, the presence of CKD alone does not constitute a transplant complication. Assign the appropriate N18 code for the patient's stage of CKD and code Z94.Ø, Kidney transplant status. If a transplant complication such as failure or rejection or other transplant complication is documented, see section I.C.19.g for information on coding complications of a kidney transplant. If the documentation is unclear as to whether the patient has a complication of the transplant, query the provider.

3) Chronic kidney disease with other conditions

Patients with CKD may also suffer from other serious conditions, most commonly diabetes mellitus and hypertension. The sequencing of the CKD code in relationship to codes for other contributing conditions is based on the conventions in the Tabular List.

See I.C.9. Hypertensive chronic kidney disease.

See I.C.19. Chronic kidney disease and kidney transplant complications.

15. Chapter 15: Pregnancy, Childbirth, and the Puerperium (OØØ-O9A)

a. General Rules for Obstetric Cases

1) Codes from chapter 15 and sequencing priority

Obstetric cases require codes from chapter 15, codes in the range OØØ-O9A, Pregnancy, Childbirth, and the Puerperium. Chapter 15 codes have sequencing priority over codes from other chapters. Additional codes from other chapters may be used in conjunction with chapter 15 codes to further specify conditions. Should the provider document that the pregnancy is incidental to the encounter, then code Z33.1, Pregnant state, incidental, should be used in place of any chapter 15 codes. It is the provider's responsibility to state that the condition being treated is not affecting the pregnancy.

2) Chapter 15 codes used only on the maternal record

Chapter 15 codes are to be used only on the maternal record, never on the record of the newborn.

3) Final character for trimester

The majority of codes in Chapter 15 have a final character indicating the trimester of pregnancy. The timeframes for the trimesters are indicated at the beginning of the chapter. If trimester is not a component of a code, it is because the condition always occurs in a specific trimester, or the concept of trimester of pregnancy is not applicable. Certain codes have characters for only certain trimesters because the condition does not occur in all trimesters, but it may occur in more than just one.

Assignment of the final character for trimester should be based on the provider's documentation of the trimester (or number of weeks) for the current admission/encounter. This applies to the assignment of trimester for pre-existing conditions as well as those that develop during or are due to the pregnancy. The provider's documentation of the number of weeks may be used to assign the appropriate code identifying the trimester.

Whenever delivery occurs during the current admission, and there is an "in childbirth" option for the obstetric complication being coded, the "in childbirth" code should be assigned. When the classification does not provide an obstetric code with an "in childbirth" option, it is appropriate to assign a code describing the current trimester.

4) Selection of trimester for inpatient admissions that encompass more than one trimester
In instances when a patient is admitted to a hospital for complications of pregnancy during one trimester and remains in the hospital into a subsequent trimester, the trimester character for the antepartum complication code should be assigned on the basis of the trimester when the complication developed, not the trimester of the discharge. If the condition developed prior to the current admission/encounter or represents a pre-existing condition, the trimester character for the trimester at the time of the admission/encounter should be assigned.

5) Unspecified trimester
Each category that includes codes for trimester has a code for "unspecified trimester." The "unspecified trimester" code should rarely be used, such as when the documentation in the record is insufficient to determine the trimester and it is not possible to obtain clarification.

6) 7th character for fetus identification
Where applicable, a 7th character is to be assigned for certain categories (O31, O32, O33.3-O33.6, O35, O36, O4Ø, O41, O6Ø.1, O6Ø.2, O64, and O69) to identify the fetus for which the complication code applies.

Assign 7th character "Ø":

- For single gestations
- When the documentation in the record is insufficient to determine the fetus affected and it is not possible to obtain clarification.
- When it is not possible to clinically determine which fetus is affected.

7) Completed weeks of gestation
In ICD-10-CM, "completed" weeks of gestation refers to full weeks. For example, if the provider documents gestation at 39 weeks and 6 days, the code for 39 weeks of gestation should be assigned, as the patient has not yet reached 40 completed weeks.

b. Selection of OB Principal or First-listed Diagnosis

1) Routine outpatient prenatal visits
For routine outpatient prenatal visits when no complications are present, a code from category Z34, Encounter for supervision of normal pregnancy, should be used as the first-listed diagnosis. These codes should not be used in conjunction with chapter 15 codes.

2) Supervision of High-Risk Pregnancy
Codes from category OØ9, Supervision of high-risk pregnancy, are intended for use only during the prenatal period. For complications during the labor or delivery episode as a result of a high-risk pregnancy, assign the applicable complication codes from Chapter 15. If there are no complications during the labor or delivery episode, assign code O8Ø, Encounter for full-term uncomplicated delivery.

For routine prenatal outpatient visits for patients with high-risk pregnancies, a code from category OØ9, Supervision of high-risk pregnancy, should be used as the first-listed diagnosis. Secondary chapter 15 codes may be used in conjunction with these codes if appropriate.

3) Episodes when no delivery occurs
In episodes when no delivery occurs, the principal diagnosis should correspond to the principal complication of the pregnancy which necessitated the encounter. Should more than one complication exist, all of which are treated or monitored, any of the complication codes may be sequenced first.

4) When a delivery occurs
When an obstetric patient is admitted and delivers during that admission, the condition that prompted the admission should be sequenced as the principal diagnosis. If multiple conditions prompted the admission, sequence the one most related to the delivery as the principal diagnosis. A code for any complication of the delivery should be assigned as an additional diagnosis. In cases of cesarean delivery, if the patient was admitted with a condition that resulted in the performance of a cesarean procedure, that condition should be selected as the principal diagnosis. If the reason for the admission was unrelated to the condition resulting in the cesarean delivery, the condition related to the reason for the admission should be selected as the principal diagnosis.

5) Outcome of delivery
A code from category Z37, Outcome of delivery, should be included on every maternal record when a delivery has occurred. These codes are not to be used on subsequent records or on the newborn record.

c. Pre-existing conditions versus conditions due to the pregnancy

Certain categories in Chapter 15 distinguish between conditions of the mother that existed prior to pregnancy (pre-existing) and those that are a direct result of pregnancy. When assigning codes from Chapter 15, it is important to assess if a condition was pre-existing prior to pregnancy or developed during or due to the pregnancy in order to assign the correct code.

Categories that do not distinguish between pre-existing and pregnancy-related conditions may be used for either. It is acceptable to use codes specifically for the puerperium with codes complicating pregnancy and childbirth if a condition arises postpartum during the delivery encounter.

d. Pre-existing hypertension in pregnancy

Category O1Ø, Pre-existing hypertension complicating pregnancy, childbirth and the puerperium, includes codes for hypertensive heart and hypertensive chronic kidney disease. When assigning one of the O10 codes that includes hypertensive heart disease or hypertensive chronic kidney disease, it is necessary to add a secondary code from the appropriate hypertension category to specify the type of heart failure or chronic kidney disease.

See Section I.C.9. Hypertension.

e. Fetal Conditions Affecting the Management of the Mother

1) Codes from categories O35 and O36

Codes from categories O35, Maternal care for known or suspected fetal abnormality and damage, and O36, Maternal care for other fetal problems, are assigned only when the fetal condition is actually responsible for modifying the management of the mother, i.e., by requiring diagnostic studies, additional observation, special care, or termination of pregnancy. The fact that the fetal condition exists does not justify assigning a code from this series to the mother's record.

2) In utero surgery

In cases when surgery is performed on the fetus, a diagnosis code from category O35, Maternal care for known or suspected fetal abnormality and damage, should be assigned identifying the fetal condition. Assign the appropriate procedure code for the procedure performed.

No code from Chapter 16, the perinatal codes, should be used on the mother's record to identify fetal conditions. Surgery performed in utero on a fetus is still to be coded as an obstetric encounter.

f. HIV Infection in Pregnancy, Childbirth and the Puerperium

During pregnancy, childbirth or the puerperium, a patient admitted because of an HIV-related illness should receive a principal diagnosis from subcategory O98.7-, Human immunodeficiency [HIV] disease complicating pregnancy, childbirth and the puerperium, followed by the code(s) for the HIV-related illness(es).

Patients with asymptomatic HIV infection status admitted during pregnancy, childbirth, or the puerperium should receive codes of O98.7- and Z21, Asymptomatic human immunodeficiency virus [HIV] infection status.

g. Diabetes mellitus in pregnancy

Diabetes mellitus is a significant complicating factor in pregnancy. Pregnant patients who are diabetic should be assigned a code from category O24, Diabetes mellitus in pregnancy, childbirth, and the puerperium, first, followed by the appropriate diabetes code(s) (E08-E13) from Chapter 4.

h. Long term use of insulin and oral hypoglycemics

See section I.C.4.a.3 for information on the long-term use of insulin and oral hypoglycemics.

i. Gestational (pregnancy induced) diabetes

Gestational (pregnancy induced) diabetes can occur during the second and third trimester of pregnancy in patients who were not diabetic prior to pregnancy. Gestational diabetes can cause complications in the pregnancy similar to those of pre-existing diabetes mellitus. It also puts the patient at greater risk of developing diabetes after the pregnancy.

Codes for gestational diabetes are in subcategory O24.4, Gestational diabetes mellitus. No other code from category O24, Diabetes mellitus in pregnancy, childbirth, and the puerperium, should be used with a code from O24.4.

The codes under subcategory O24.4 include diet controlled, insulin controlled, and controlled by oral hypoglycemic drugs. If a patient with gestational diabetes is treated with both diet and insulin, only the code for insulin-controlled is required. If a patient with gestational diabetes is treated with both diet and oral hypoglycemic medications, only the code for "controlled by oral hypoglycemic drugs" is required. Codes Z79.4, Long-term (current) use of insulin, Z79.84, Long-term (current) use of oral hypoglycemic drugs, and Z79.85, Long-term (current) use of injectable non-insulin antidiabetic drugs, should not be assigned with codes from subcategory O24.4.

An abnormal glucose tolerance in pregnancy is assigned a code from subcategory O99.81, Abnormal glucose complicating pregnancy, childbirth, and the puerperium.

j. Sepsis and septic shock complicating abortion, pregnancy, childbirth and the puerperium

When assigning a chapter 15 code for sepsis complicating abortion, pregnancy, childbirth, and the puerperium, a code for the specific type of infection should be assigned as an additional diagnosis. If severe sepsis is present, a code from subcategory R65.2, Severe sepsis, and code(s) for associated organ dysfunction(s) should also be assigned as additional diagnoses.

k. Puerperal sepsis

Code O85, Puerperal sepsis, should be assigned with a secondary code to identify the causal organism (e.g., for a bacterial infection, assign a code from category B95-B96, Bacterial infections in conditions classified elsewhere). A code from category A4Ø, Streptococcal sepsis, or A41, Other sepsis, should not be used for puerperal sepsis. If applicable, use additional codes to identify severe sepsis (R65.2-) and any associated acute organ dysfunction.

Code O85 should not be assigned for sepsis following an obstetrical procedure (See Section I.C.1.d.5.b., Sepsis due to a postprocedural infection).

l. Alcohol, tobacco and drug use during pregnancy, childbirth and the puerperium

1) Alcohol use during pregnancy, childbirth and the puerperium

Codes under subcategory O99.31, Alcohol use complicating pregnancy, childbirth, and the puerperium, should be assigned for any pregnancy case when a patient uses alcohol during the pregnancy or postpartum. A secondary code from category F1Ø, Alcohol related disorders, should also be assigned to identify manifestations of the alcohol use.

2) Tobacco use during pregnancy, childbirth and the puerperium

Codes under subcategory O99.33, Smoking (tobacco) complicating pregnancy, childbirth, and the puerperium, should be assigned for any pregnancy case when a patient uses any type of tobacco product during the pregnancy or postpartum.

A secondary code from category F17, Nicotine dependence, should also be assigned to identify the type of nicotine dependence.

3) Drug use during pregnancy, childbirth and the puerperium

Codes under subcategory O99.32, Drug use complicating pregnancy, childbirth, and the puerperium, should be assigned for any pregnancy case when a patient uses drugs during the pregnancy or postpartum. This can involve illegal drugs, or inappropriate use or abuse of prescription drugs. Secondary code(s) from categories F11-F16 and F18-F19 should also be assigned to identify manifestations of the drug use.

m. Poisoning, toxic effects, adverse effects and underdosing in a pregnant patient

A code from subcategory O9A.2, Injury, poisoning and certain other consequences of external causes complicating pregnancy, childbirth, and the puerperium, should be sequenced first, followed by the appropriate injury, poisoning, toxic effect, adverse effect or underdosing code, and then the additional code(s) that specifies the condition caused by the poisoning, toxic effect, adverse effect or underdosing.

See Section I.C.19. Adverse effects, poisoning, underdosing and toxic effects.

n. Normal Delivery, Code O8ø

1) Encounter for full term uncomplicated delivery

Code O8Ø should be assigned when a patient is admitted for a full-term normal delivery and delivers a single, healthy infant without any complications antepartum, during the delivery, or postpartum during the delivery episode. Code O8Ø is always a principal diagnosis. It is not to be used if any other code from chapter 15 is needed to describe a current complication of the antenatal, delivery, or postnatal period. Additional codes from other chapters may be used with code O8Ø if they are not related to or are in any way complicating the pregnancy.

2) Uncomplicated delivery with resolved antepartum complication

Code O8Ø may be used if the patient had a complication at some point during the pregnancy, but the complication is not present at the time of the admission for delivery.

3) Outcome of delivery for O8Ø

Z37.Ø, Single live birth, is the only outcome of delivery code appropriate for use with O8Ø.

ICD-10-CM Official Guidelines

o. The Peripartum and Postpartum Periods

1) Peripartum and Postpartum periods

The postpartum period begins immediately after delivery and continues for six weeks following delivery. The peripartum period is defined as the last month of pregnancy to five months postpartum.

2) Peripartum and postpartum complication

A postpartum complication is any complication occurring within the six-week period.

3) Pregnancy-related complications after 6-week period

Chapter 15 codes may also be used to describe pregnancy-related complications after the peripartum or postpartum period if the provider documents that a condition is pregnancy related.

4) Admission for routine postpartum care following delivery outside hospital

When the mother delivers outside the hospital prior to admission and is admitted for routine postpartum care and no complications are noted, code Z39.Ø, Encounter for care and examination of mother immediately after delivery, should be assigned as the principal diagnosis.

5) Pregnancy associated cardiomyopathy

Pregnancy associated cardiomyopathy, code O9Ø.3, is unique in that it may be diagnosed in the third trimester of pregnancy but may continue to progress months after delivery. For this reason, it is referred to as peripartum cardiomyopathy. Code O9Ø.3 is only for use when the cardiomyopathy develops as a result of pregnancy in a patient who did not have pre-existing heart disease.

p. Code O94, Sequelae of complication of pregnancy, childbirth, and the puerperium

1) Code O94

Code O94, Sequelae of complication of pregnancy, childbirth, and the puerperium, is for use in those cases when an initial complication of a pregnancy develops a sequela or sequelae requiring care or treatment at a future date.

2) After the initial postpartum period

This code may be used at any time after the initial postpartum period.

3) Sequencing of Code O94

This code, like all sequela codes, is to be sequenced following the code describing the sequelae of the complication.

q. Termination of Pregnancy and Spontaneous abortions

1) Abortion with Liveborn Fetus

When an attempted termination of pregnancy results in a liveborn fetus, assign code Z33.2, Encounter for elective termination of pregnancy and a code from category Z37, Outcome of Delivery.

2) Retained Products of Conception following an abortion

Subsequent encounters for retained products of conception following a spontaneous abortion or elective termination of pregnancy, without complications are assigned OØ3.4, Incomplete spontaneous abortion without complication, or code OØ7.4, Failed attempted termination of pregnancy without complication. This advice is appropriate even when the patient was discharged previously with a discharge diagnosis of complete abortion. If the patient has a specific complication associated with the spontaneous abortion or elective termination of pregnancy in addition to retained products of conception, assign the appropriate complication code (e.g., OØ3.-, OØ4.-, OØ7.-) instead of code OØ3.4 or OØ7.4.

3) Complications leading to abortion

Codes from Chapter 15 may be used as additional codes to identify any documented complications of the pregnancy in conjunction with codes in categories in OØ4, OØ7 and OØ8.

4) Hemorrhage following elective abortion

For hemorrhage post elective abortion, assign code OØ4.6, Delayed or excessive hemorrhage following (induced) termination of pregnancy. Do not assign code O72.1, Other immediate postpartum hemorrhage, as this code should not be assigned for post abortion conditions.

r. Abuse in a pregnant patient

For suspected or confirmed cases of abuse of a pregnant patient, a code(s) from subcategories O9A.3, Physical abuse complicating pregnancy, childbirth, and the puerperium, O9A.4, Sexual abuse complicating pregnancy, childbirth, and the puerperium, and O9A.5, Psychological abuse complicating pregnancy, childbirth, and the puerperium, should be sequenced first, followed by the appropriate codes (if applicable) to identify any associated current injury due to physical abuse, sexual abuse, and the perpetrator of abuse.

See Section I.C.19. Adult and child abuse, neglect and other maltreatment.

s. COVID-19 infection in pregnancy, childbirth, and the puerperium

During pregnancy, childbirth or the puerperium, when COVID-19 is the reason for admission/encounter, code O98.5-, Other viral diseases complicating pregnancy, childbirth and the puerperium, should be sequenced as the principal/first-listed diagnosis, and code U07.1, COVID-19, and the appropriate codes for associated manifestation(s) should be assigned as additional diagnoses. Codes from Chapter 15 always take sequencing priority.

If the reason for admission/encounter is unrelated to COVID-19 but the patient tests positive for COVID-19 during the admission/encounter, the appropriate code for the reason for admission/encounter should be sequenced as the principal/first-listed diagnosis, and codes O98.5- and U07.1, as well as the appropriate codes for associated COVID-19 manifestations, should be assigned as additional diagnoses.

16. Chapter 16: Certain Conditions Originating in the Perinatal Period (PØØ-P96)

For coding and reporting purposes the perinatal period is defined as before birth through the 28th day following birth. The following guidelines are provided for reporting purposes.

a. General Perinatal Rules

1) Use of Chapter 16 Codes

Codes in this chapter are never for use on the maternal record. Codes from Chapter 15, the obstetric chapter, are never permitted on the newborn record. Chapter 16 codes may be used throughout the life of the patient if the condition is still present.

2) Principal Diagnosis for Birth Record

When coding the birth episode in a newborn record, assign a code from category Z38, Liveborn infants according to place of birth and type of delivery, as the principal diagnosis. A code from category Z38 is assigned only once, to a newborn at the time of birth. If a newborn is transferred to another institution, a code from category Z38 should not be used at the receiving hospital.

A code from category Z38 is used only on the newborn record, not on the mother's record.

3) Use of Codes from other Chapters with Codes from Chapter 16

Codes from other chapters may be used with codes from chapter 16 if the codes from the other chapters provide more specific detail. Codes for signs and symptoms may be assigned when a definitive diagnosis has not been established. If the reason for the encounter is a perinatal condition, the code from chapter 16 should be sequenced first.

4) Use of Chapter 16 Codes after the Perinatal Period

Should a condition originate in the perinatal period, and continue throughout the life of the patient, the perinatal code should continue to be used regardless of the patient's age.

5) Birth process or community acquired conditions

If a newborn has a condition that may be either due to the birth process or community acquired and the documentation does not indicate which it is, the default is due to the birth process and the code from Chapter 16 should be used. If the condition is community-acquired, a code from Chapter 16 should not be assigned.

For COVID-19 infection in a newborn, see guideline I.C.16.h.

6) Code all clinically significant conditions

All clinically significant conditions noted on routine newborn examination should be coded. A condition is clinically significant if it requires:

- clinical evaluation; or
- therapeutic treatment; or
- diagnostic procedures; or
- extended length of hospital stay; or
- increased nursing care and/or monitoring; or
- has implications for future health care needs

Note: The perinatal guidelines listed above are the same as the general coding guidelines for "additional diagnoses," except for the final point regarding implications for future health care needs. Codes should be assigned for conditions that have been specified by the provider as having implications for future health care needs.

b. Observation and Evaluation of Newborns for Suspected Conditions not Found

1) Use of ZØ5 codes

Assign a code from category ZØ5, Observation and evaluation of newborn for suspected diseases and conditions ruled out, to identify those instances when a healthy newborn is evaluated for a suspected condition/disease that is determined after study not to be present. Do not use a code from category ZØ5 when the patient is documented to have signs or symptoms of a suspected problem; in such cases code the sign or symptom.

2) ZØ5 on other than the birth record

A code from category ZØ5 may also be assigned as a principal or first-listed code for readmissions or encounters when the code from category Z38 code no longer applies. Codes from category ZØ5 are for use only for healthy newborns and infants for which no condition after study is found to be present.

3) ZØ5 on a birth record

A code from category ZØ5 is to be used as a secondary code after the code from category Z38, Liveborn infants according to place of birth and type of delivery.

c. Coding Additional Perinatal Diagnoses

1) Assigning codes for conditions that require treatment

Assign codes for conditions that require treatment or further investigation, prolong the length of stay, or require resource utilization.

2) Codes for conditions specified as having implications for future health care needs

Assign codes for conditions that have been specified by the provider as having implications for future health care needs.

Note: This guideline should not be used for adult patients.

d. Prematurity and Fetal Growth Retardation

Providers utilize different criteria in determining prematurity. A code for prematurity should not be assigned unless it is documented. Assignment of codes in categories P05, Disorders of newborn related to slow fetal growth and fetal malnutrition, and P07, Disorders of newborn related to short gestation and low birth weight, not elsewhere classified, should be based on the recorded birth weight and estimated gestational age.

When both birth weight and gestational age are available, two codes from category PØ7 should be assigned, with the code for birth weight sequenced before the code for gestational age.

e. Low birth weight and immaturity status

Codes from category PØ7, Disorders of newborn related to short gestation and low birth weight, not elsewhere classified, are for use for a child or adult who was premature or had a low birth weight as a newborn and this is affecting the patient's current health status.

See Section I.C.21. Factors influencing health status and contact with health services, Status.

f. Bacterial Sepsis of Newborn

Category P36, Bacterial sepsis of newborn, includes congenital sepsis. If a perinate is documented as having sepsis without documentation of congenital or community acquired, the default is congenital and a code from category P36 should be assigned. If the P36 code includes the causal organism, an additional code from category B95, Streptococcus, Staphylococcus, and Enterococcus as the cause of diseases classified elsewhere, or B96, Other bacterial agents as the cause of diseases classified elsewhere, should not be assigned. If the P36 code does not include the causal organism, assign an additional code from category B96. If applicable, use additional codes to identify severe sepsis (R65.2-) and any associated acute organ dysfunction.

g. Stillbirth

Code P95, Stillbirth, is only for use in institutions that maintain separate records for stillbirths. No other code should be used with P95. Code P95 should not be used on the mother's record.

h. COVID-19 Infection in Newborn

For a newborn that tests positive for COVID-19, assign code U07.1, COVID-19, and the appropriate codes for associated manifestation(s) in neonates/newborns in the absence of documentation indicating a specific type of transmission. For a newborn that tests positive for COVID-19 and the provider documents the condition was contracted in utero or during the birth process, assign codes P35.8, Other congenital viral diseases, and U07.1, COVID-19. When coding the birth episode in a newborn record, the appropriate code from category Z38, Liveborn infants according to place of birth and type of delivery, should be assigned as the principal diagnosis.

17. Chapter 17: Congenital malformations, deformations, and chromosomal abnormalities (QØØ-Q99)

Assign an appropriate code(s) from categories Q00-Q99, Congenital malformations, deformations, and chromosomal abnormalities when a malformation/deformation or chromosomal abnormality is documented. A malformation/deformation/or chromosomal abnormality may be the principal/first-listed diagnosis on a record or a secondary diagnosis.

When a malformation/deformation or chromosomal abnormality does not have a unique code assignment, assign additional code(s) for any manifestations that may be present.

When the code assignment specifically identifies the malformation/deformation or chromosomal abnormality, manifestations that are an inherent component of the anomaly should not be coded separately. Additional codes should be assigned for manifestations that are not an inherent component.

Codes from Chapter 17 may be used throughout the life of the patient. If a congenital malformation or deformity has been corrected, a personal history code should be used to identify the history of the malformation or deformity. Although present at birth, a malformation/deformation/or chromosomal abnormality may not be identified until later in life. Whenever the condition is diagnosed by the provider, it is appropriate to assign a code from codes Q00-Q99. For the birth admission, the appropriate code from category Z38, Liveborn infants, according to place of birth and type of delivery, should be sequenced as the principal diagnosis, followed by any congenital anomaly codes, Q00-Q99.

18. Chapter 18: Symptoms, signs, and abnormal clinical and laboratory findings, not elsewhere classified (RØØ-R99)

Chapter 18 includes symptoms, signs, abnormal results of clinical or other investigative procedures, and ill-defined conditions regarding which no diagnosis classifiable elsewhere is recorded. Signs and symptoms that point to a specific diagnosis have been assigned to a category in other chapters of the classification.

a. Use of symptom codes

Codes that describe symptoms and signs are acceptable for reporting purposes when a related definitive diagnosis has not been established (confirmed) by the provider.

b. Use of a symptom code with a definitive diagnosis code

Codes for signs and symptoms may be reported in addition to a related definitive diagnosis when the sign or symptom is not routinely associated with that diagnosis, such as the various signs and symptoms associated with complex syndromes. The definitive diagnosis code should be sequenced before the symptom code.

Signs or symptoms that are associated routinely with a disease process should not be assigned as additional codes, unless otherwise instructed by the classification.

c. Combination codes that include symptoms

ICD-10-CM contains a number of combination codes that identify both the definitive diagnosis and common symptoms of that diagnosis. When using one of these combination codes, an additional code should not be assigned for the symptom.

d. Repeated falls

Code R29.6, Repeated falls, is for use for encounters when a patient has recently fallen and the reason for the fall is being investigated.

Code Z91.81, History of falling, is for use when a patient has fallen in the past and is at risk for future falls. When appropriate, both codes R29.6 and Z91.81 may be assigned together.

e. Coma

Code R40.20, Unspecified coma, should be assigned when the underlying cause of the coma is not known, or the cause is a traumatic brain injury and the coma scale is not documented in the medical record.

Do not report codes for unspecified coma, individual or total Glasgow coma scale scores for a patient with a medically induced coma or a sedated patient.

1) Coma Scale

The coma scale codes (R4Ø.21- to R4Ø.24-) can be used in conjunction with traumatic brain injury codes. These codes cannot be used with code R4Ø.2A, Nontraumatic coma due to underlying condition. They are primarily for use by trauma registries, but they may be used in any setting where this information is collected. The coma scale codes should be sequenced after the diagnosis code(s).

These codes, one from each subcategory, are needed to complete the scale. The 7th character indicates when the scale was recorded. The 7th character should match for all three codes.

At a minimum, report the initial score documented on presentation at your facility. This may be a score from the emergency medicine technician (EMT) or in the emergency department. If desired, a facility may choose to capture multiple coma scale scores.

Assign code R40.24-, Glasgow coma scale, total score, when only the total score is documented in the medical record and not the individual score(s).

If multiple coma scores are captured within the first 24 hours after hospital admission, assign only the code for the score at the time of admission. ICD-10-CM does not classify coma scores that are reported after admission but less than 24 hours later.

See Section I.B.14. for coma scale documentation by clinicians other than patient's provider

f. **Functional quadriplegia**
GUIDELINE HAS BEEN DELETED EFFECTIVE OCTOBER 1, 2017

g. **SIRS due to Non-Infectious Process**
The systemic inflammatory response syndrome (SIRS) can develop as a result of certain non-infectious disease processes, such as trauma, malignant neoplasm, or pancreatitis. When SIRS is documented with a noninfectious condition, and no subsequent infection is documented, the code for the underlying condition, such as an injury, should be assigned, followed by code R65.10, Systemic inflammatory response syndrome (SIRS) of non-infectious origin without acute organ dysfunction, or code R65.11, Systemic inflammatory response syndrome (SIRS) of non-infectious origin with acute organ dysfunction. If an associated acute organ dysfunction is documented, the appropriate code(s) for the specific type of organ dysfunction(s) should be assigned in addition to code R65.11. If acute organ dysfunction is documented, but it cannot be determined if the acute organ dysfunction is associated with SIRS or due to another condition (e.g., directly due to the trauma), the provider should be queried.

h. **Death NOS**
Code R99, Ill-defined and unknown cause of mortality, is only for use in the very limited circumstance when a patient who has already died is brought into an emergency department or other healthcare facility and is pronounced dead upon arrival. It does not represent the discharge disposition of death.

i. **NIHSS Stroke Scale**
The NIH stroke scale (NIHSS) codes (R29.7- -) can be used in conjunction with acute stroke codes (I60–I63) to identify the patient's neurological status and the severity of the stroke. The stroke scale codes should be sequenced after the acute stroke diagnosis code(s).

At a minimum, report the initial score documented. If desired, a facility may choose to capture multiple stroke scale scores.

See Section I.B.14. for NIHSS stroke scale documentation by clinicians other than patient's provider

19. **Chapter 19: Injury, poisoning, and certain other consequences of external causes (S00-T88)**

a. **Application of 7th Characters in Chapter 19**
Most categories in chapter 19 have a 7th character requirement for each applicable code. Most categories in this chapter have three 7th character values (with the exception of fractures): A, initial encounter, D, subsequent encounter and S, sequela. Categories for traumatic fractures have additional 7th character values. While the patient may be seen by a new or different provider over the course of treatment for an injury, assignment of the 7th character is based on whether the patient is undergoing active treatment and not whether the provider is seeing the patient for the first time.

For complication codes, active treatment refers to treatment for the condition described by the code, even though it may be related to an earlier precipitating problem. For example, code T84.50XA, Infection and inflammatory reaction due to unspecified internal joint prosthesis, initial encounter, is used when active treatment is provided for the infection, even though the condition relates to the prosthetic device, implant or graft that was placed at a previous encounter.

7th character "A", initial encounter is used for each encounter where the patient is receiving active treatment for the condition.

7th character "D" subsequent encounter is used for encounters after the patient has completed active treatment of the condition and is receiving routine care for the condition during the healing or recovery phase.

The aftercare Z codes should not be used for aftercare for conditions such as injuries or poisonings, where 7th characters are provided to identify subsequent care. For example, for aftercare of an injury, assign the acute injury code with the 7th character "D" (subsequent encounter).

7th character "S", sequela, is for use for complications or conditions that arise as a direct result of a condition, such as scar formation after a burn. The scars are sequelae of the burn. When using 7th character "S", it is necessary to use both the injury code that precipitated the sequela and the code for the sequela itself. The "S" is added only to the injury code, not the sequela code. The 7th character "S" identifies the injury responsible for the sequela. The specific type of sequela (e.g. scar) is sequenced first, followed by the injury code.

See Section I.B.10. Sequelae, (Late Effects)

b. Coding of Injuries

When coding injuries, assign separate codes for each injury unless a combination code is provided, in which case the combination code is assigned. Codes from category TØ7, Unspecified multiple injuries should not be assigned in the inpatient setting unless information for a more specific code is not available. Traumatic injury codes (SØØ-T14.9) are not to be used for normal, healing surgical wounds or to identify complications of surgical wounds.

The code for the most serious injury, as determined by the provider and the focus of treatment, is sequenced first.

1) Superficial injuries

Superficial injuries such as abrasions or contusions are not coded when associated with more severe injuries of the same site.

2) Primary injury with damage to nerves/blood vessels

When a primary injury results in minor damage to peripheral nerves or blood vessels, the primary injury is sequenced first with additional code(s) for injuries to nerves and spinal cord (such as category SØ4), and/or injury to blood vessels (such as category S15). When the primary injury is to the blood vessels or nerves, that injury should be sequenced first.

3) Iatrogenic injuries

Injury codes from Chapter 19 should not be assigned for injuries that occur during, or as a result of, a medical intervention. Assign the appropriate complication code(s).

c. Coding of Traumatic Fractures

The principles of multiple coding of injuries should be followed in coding fractures. Fractures of specified sites are coded individually by site in accordance with both the provisions within categories S02, S12, S22, S32, S42, S49, S52, S59, S62, S72, S79, S82, S89, S92 and the level of detail furnished by medical record content.

A fracture not indicated as open or closed should be coded to closed. A fracture not indicated whether displaced or not displaced should be coded to displaced.

More specific guidelines are as follows:

1) Initial vs. subsequent encounter for fractures

Traumatic fractures are coded using the appropriate 7th character for initial encounter (A, B, C) for each encounter where the patient is receiving active treatment for the fracture. The appropriate 7th character for initial encounter should also be assigned for a patient who delayed seeking treatment for the fracture or nonunion.

Fractures are coded using the appropriate 7th character for subsequent care for encounters after the patient has completed active treatment of the fracture and is receiving routine care for the fracture during the healing or recovery phase.

Care for complications of surgical treatment for fracture repairs during the healing or recovery phase should be coded with the appropriate complication codes.

Care of complications of fractures, such as malunion and nonunion, should be reported with the appropriate 7th character for subsequent care with nonunion (K, M, N,) or subsequent care with malunion (P, Q, R).

Malunion/nonunion: The appropriate 7th character for initial encounter should also be assigned for a patient who delayed seeking treatment for the fracture or nonunion.

The open fracture designations in the assignment of the 7th character for fractures of the forearm, femur and lower leg, including ankle are based on the Gustilo open fracture classification. When the Gustilo classification type is not specified for an open fracture, the 7th character for open fracture type I or II should be assigned (B, E, H, M, Q).

A code from category M8Ø, not a traumatic fracture code, should be used for any patient with known osteoporosis who suffers a fracture, even if the patient had a minor fall or trauma, if that fall or trauma would not usually break a normal, healthy bone.

See Section I.C.13. Osteoporosis.

The aftercare Z codes should not be used for aftercare for traumatic fractures. For aftercare of a traumatic fracture, assign the acute fracture code with the appropriate 7th character.

2) Multiple fractures sequencing
Multiple fractures are sequenced in accordance with the severity of the fracture.

3) Physeal fractures
For physeal fractures, assign only the code identifying the type of physeal fracture. Do not assign a separate code to identify the specific bone that is fractured.

d. Coding of Burns and Corrosions
The ICD-10-CM makes a distinction between burns and corrosions. The burn codes are for thermal burns, except sunburns, that come from a heat source, such as a fire or hot appliance. The burn codes are also for burns resulting from electricity and radiation. Corrosions are burns due to chemicals. The guidelines are the same for burns and corrosions.

Current burns (T20-T25) are classified by depth, extent and by agent (X code). Burns are classified by depth as first degree (erythema), second degree (blistering), and third degree (full-thickness involvement). Burns of the eye and internal organs (T26-T28) are classified by site, but not by degree.

1) Sequencing of burn and related condition codes
Sequence first the code that reflects the highest degree of burn when more than one burn is present.

a.When the reason for the admission or encounter is for treatment of external multiple burns, sequence first the code that reflects the burn of the highest degree.

b.When a patient has both internal and external burns, the circumstances of admission govern the selection of the principal diagnosis or first-listed diagnosis.

c.When a patient is admitted for burn injuries and other related conditions such as smoke inhalation and/or respiratory failure, the circumstances of admission govern the selection of the principal or first-listed diagnosis.

2) Burns of the same anatomic site
Classify burns of the same anatomic site and on the same side but of different degrees to the subcategory identifying the highest degree recorded in the diagnosis (e.g., for second and third degree burns of right thigh, assign only code T24.311-).

3) Non-healing burns
Non-healing burns are coded as acute burns.

Necrosis of burned skin should be coded as a non-healed burn.

4) Infected burn
For any documented infected burn site, use an additional code for the infection.

5) Assign separate codes for each burn site
When coding burns, assign separate codes for each burn site. Category T3Ø, Burn and corrosion, body region unspecified is extremely vague and should rarely be used.

Codes for burns of "multiple sites" should only be assigned when the medical record documentation does not specify the individual sites.

6) Burns and corrosions classified according to extent of body surface involved
Assign codes from category T31, Burns classified according to extent of body surface involved, or T32, Corrosions classified according to extent of body surface involved, for acute burns or corrosions when the site of the burn or corrosion is not specified or when there is a need for additional data. It is advisable to use category T31 as additional coding when needed to provide data for evaluating burn mortality, such as that needed by burn units. It is also advisable to use category T31 as an additional code for reporting purposes when there is mention of a third-degree burn involving 20 percent or more of the body surface. Codes from categories T31 and T32 should not be used for sequelae of burns or corrosions.

Categories T31 and T32 are based on the classic "rule of nines" in estimating body surface involved: head and neck are assigned nine percent, each arm nine percent, each leg 18 percent, the anterior trunk 18 percent, posterior trunk 18 percent, and genitalia one percent. Providers may change these percentage assignments where necessary to accommodate infants and children who have proportionately larger heads than adults, and patients who have large buttocks, thighs, or abdomen that involve burns.

7) **Encounters for treatment of sequela of burns**
Encounters for the treatment of the late effects of burns or corrosions (i.e., scars or joint contractures) should be coded with a burn or corrosion code with the 7th character "S" for sequela.

8) **Sequelae with a late effect code and current burn**
When appropriate, both a code for a current burn or corrosion with 7th character "A" or "D" and a burn or corrosion code with 7th character "S" may be assigned on the same record (when both a current burn and sequelae of an old burn exist). Burns and corrosions do not heal at the same rate and a current healing wound may still exist with sequela of a healed burn or corrosion.

See Section I.B.10. Sequela (Late Effects)

9) **Use of an external cause code with burns and corrosions**
An external cause code should be used with burns and corrosions to identify the source and intent of the burn, as well as the place where it occurred.

e. **Adverse Effects, Poisoning, Underdosing and Toxic Effects**
Codes in categories T36-T65 are combination codes that include the substance that was taken as well as the intent. No additional external cause code is required for poisonings, toxic effects, adverse effects and underdosing codes.

1) **Do not code directly from the Table of Drugs**
Do not code directly from the Table of Drugs and Chemicals. Always refer back to the Tabular List.

2) **Use as many codes as necessary to describe**
Use as many codes as necessary to describe completely all drugs, medicinal or biological substances.

3) **If the same code would describe the causative agent**
If the same code would describe the causative agent for more than one adverse reaction, poisoning, toxic effect or underdosing, assign the code only once.

4) **If two or more drugs, medicinal or biological substances**
If two or more drugs, medicinal or biological substances are taken, code each individually unless a combination code is listed in the Table of Drugs and Chemicals.

If multiple unspecified drugs, medicinal or biological substances were taken, assign the appropriate code from subcategory T5Ø.91, Poisoning by, adverse effect of and underdosing of multiple unspecified drugs, medicaments and biological substances.

5) **The occurrence of drug toxicity is classified in ICD-10-CM as follows:**

(a) **Adverse Effect**
When coding an adverse effect of a drug that has been correctly prescribed and properly administered, assign the appropriate code for the nature of the adverse effect followed by the appropriate code for the adverse effect of the drug (T36-T5Ø). The code for the drug should have a 5th or 6th character "5" (for example T36.ØX5-) Examples of the nature of an adverse effect are tachycardia, delirium, gastrointestinal hemorrhaging, vomiting, hypokalemia, hepatitis, renal failure, or respiratory failure.

(b) **Poisoning**
When coding a poisoning or reaction to the improper use of a medication (e.g., overdose, wrong substance given or taken in error, wrong route of administration), first assign the appropriate code from categories T36-T5Ø. The poisoning codes have an associated intent as their 5th or 6th character (accidental, intentional self-harm, assault and undetermined). If the intent of the poisoning is unknown or unspecified, code the intent as accidental intent. The undetermined intent is only for use if the documentation in the record specifies that the intent cannot be determined. Use additional code(s) for all manifestations of poisonings.

If there is also a diagnosis of abuse or dependence of the substance, the abuse or dependence is assigned as an additional code.

Examples of poisoning include:

(i) Error was made in drug prescription
Errors made in drug prescription or in the administration of the drug by provider, nurse, patient, or other person.

(ii) Overdose of a drug intentionally taken
If an overdose of a drug was intentionally taken or administered and resulted in drug toxicity, it would be coded as a poisoning.

(iii) Nonprescribed drug taken with correctly prescribed and properly administered drug
If a nonprescribed drug or medicinal agent was taken in combination with a correctly prescribed and properly administered drug, any drug toxicity or other reaction resulting from the interaction of the two drugs would be classified as a poisoning.

(iv) Interaction of drug(s) and alcohol
When a reaction results from the interaction of a drug(s) and alcohol, this would be classified as poisoning.

See Section I.C.4. if poisoning is the result of insulin pump malfunctions.

For Sequela (Late Effects) see Section I.B.10.

(c) Underdosing

Underdosing refers to taking less of a medication than is prescribed by a provider or a manufacturer's instruction. Discontinuing the use of a prescribed medication on the patient's own initiative (not directed by the patient's provider) is also classified as an underdosing. For underdosing, assign the code from categories T36-T5Ø (fifth or sixth character "6").

Documentation of a change in the patient's condition is not required in order to assign an underdosing code. Documentation that the patient is taking less of a medication than is prescribed or discontinued the prescribed medication is sufficient for code assignment.

Codes for underdosing should never be assigned as principal or first-listed codes. If a patient has a relapse or exacerbation of the medical condition for which the drug is prescribed because of the reduction in dose, then the medical condition itself should be coded.

Noncompliance (Z91.12-, Z91.13-, Z91.14- and Z91.A4-) or complication of care (Y63.6-Y63.9) codes are to be used with an underdosing code to indicate intent, if known.

(d) Toxic Effects

When a harmful substance is ingested or comes in contact with a person, this is classified as a toxic effect. The toxic effect codes are in categories T51-T65. When coding a toxic effect, assign the toxic effect code first, followed by codes for all associated manifestations of the toxic effect.

Toxic effect codes have an associated intent: accidental, intentional self-harm, assault and undetermined.

For Sequela (Late Effects) see Section I.B.10. Sequela

f. Adult and child abuse, neglect and other maltreatment

Sequence first the appropriate code from categories T74, Adult and child abuse, neglect and other maltreatment, confirmed, or T76, Adult and child abuse, neglect and other maltreatment, suspected, for abuse, neglect and other maltreatment, followed by any accompanying mental health or injury code(s).

If the documentation in the medical record states abuse or neglect, it is coded as confirmed (T74.-). It is coded as suspected if it is documented as suspected (T76.-).

For cases of confirmed abuse or neglect an external cause code from the assault section (X92-Y09) should be added to identify the cause of any physical injuries. A perpetrator code (Y07) should be added when the perpetrator of the abuse is known. For suspected cases of abuse or neglect, do not report external cause or perpetrator code.

If a suspected case of abuse, neglect or mistreatment is ruled out during an encounter code Z04.71, Encounter for examination and observation following alleged physical adult abuse, ruled out, or code Z04.72, Encounter for examination and observation following alleged child physical abuse, ruled out, should be used, not a code from T76.

If a suspected case of alleged rape or sexual abuse is ruled out during an encounter code Z04.41, Encounter for examination and observation following alleged adult rape or code Z04.42, Encounter for examination and observation following alleged child rape, should be used, not a code from T76.

If a suspected case of forced sexual exploitation or forced labor exploitation is ruled out during an encounter, code Z04.81, Encounter for examination and observation of victim following forced sexual exploitation, or code Z04.82, Encounter for examination and observation of victim following forced labor exploitation, should be used, not a code from T76.

See Section I.C.15. Abuse in a pregnant patient.

g. Complications of care

1) General guidelines for complications of care

(a) Documentation of complications of care

See Section I.B.16. for information on documentation of complications of care.

2) Pain due to medical devices

Pain associated with devices, implants or grafts left in a surgical site (for example painful hip prosthesis) is assigned to the appropriate code(s) found in Chapter 19, Injury, poisoning, and certain other consequences of external causes. Specific codes for pain due to medical devices are found in the T code section of the ICD-10-CM. Use additional code(s) from category G89 to identify acute or chronic pain due to presence of the device, implant or graft (G89.18 or G89.28).

3) Transplant complications

(a) Transplant complications other than kidney

Codes under category T86, Complications of transplanted organs and tissues, are for use for both complications and rejection of transplanted organs. A transplant complication code is only assigned if the complication affects the function of the transplanted organ. Two codes are required to fully describe a transplant complication: the appropriate code from category T86 and a secondary code that identifies the complication.

Pre-existing conditions or conditions that develop after the transplant are not coded as complications unless they affect the function of the transplanted organs.

See I.C.21. for transplant organ removal status

See I.C.2. for malignant neoplasm associated with transplanted organ.

See I.C.1.d.4. for sequencing of sepsis due to infection in transplanted organ

(b) Kidney transplant complications

Patients who have undergone kidney transplant may still have some form of chronic kidney disease (CKD) because the kidney transplant may not fully restore kidney function. Code T86.1- should be assigned for documented complications of a kidney transplant, such as transplant failure or rejection or other transplant complication. Code T86.1- should not be assigned for post kidney transplant patients who have chronic kidney (CKD) unless a transplant complication such as transplant failure or rejection is documented. If the documentation is unclear as to whether the patient has a complication of the transplant, query the provider.

Conditions that affect the function of the transplanted kidney, other than CKD, should be assigned a code from subcategory T86.1, Complications of transplanted organ, Kidney, and a secondary code that identifies the complication.

For patients with CKD following a kidney transplant, but who do not have a complication such as failure or rejection, *see section I.C.14. Chronic kidney disease and kidney transplant status.*

See I.C.1.d.4. for sequencing of sepsis due to infection in transplanted organ

4) Complication codes that include the external cause

As with certain other T codes, some of the complications of care codes have the external cause included in the code. The code includes the nature of the complication as well as the type of procedure that caused the complication. No external cause code indicating the type of procedure is necessary for these codes.

5) Complications of care codes within the body system chapters

Intraoperative and postprocedural complication codes are found within the body system chapters with codes specific to the organs and structures of that body system. These codes should be sequenced first, followed by a code(s) for the specific complication, if applicable.

Complication codes from the body system chapters should be assigned for intraoperative and postprocedural complications (e.g., the appropriate complication code from chapter 9 would be assigned for a vascular intraoperative or postprocedural complication) unless the complication is specifically indexed to a T code in chapter 19.

20. Chapter 20: External Causes of Morbidity (VØØ-Y99)
The external causes of morbidity codes should never be sequenced as the first-listed or principal diagnosis.

External cause codes are intended to provide data for injury research and evaluation of injury prevention strategies. These codes capture how the injury or health condition happened (cause), the intent (unintentional or accidental; or intentional, such as suicide or assault), the place where the event occurred the activity of the patient at the time of the event, and the person's status (e.g., civilian, military).

There is no national requirement for mandatory ICD-10-CM external cause code reporting. Unless a provider is subject to a state-based external cause code reporting mandate or these codes are required by a particular payer, reporting of ICD-10-CM codes in Chapter 20, External Causes of Morbidity, is not required. In the absence of a mandatory reporting requirement, providers are encouraged to voluntarily report external cause codes, as they provide valuable data for injury research and evaluation of injury prevention strategies.

a. General External Cause Coding Guidelines

1) Used with any code in the range of AØØ.Ø-T88.9, ZØØ-Z99
An external cause code may be used with any code in the range of AØØ.Ø-T88.9, ZØØ-Z99, classification that represents a health condition due to an external cause. Though they are most applicable to injuries, they are also valid for use with such things as infections or diseases due to an external source, and other health conditions, such as a heart attack that occurs during strenuous physical activity.

2) External cause code used for length of treatment
Assign the external cause code, with the appropriate 7th character (initial encounter, subsequent encounter or sequela) for each encounter for which the injury or condition is being treated.

Most categories in chapter 20 have a 7th character requirement for each applicable code. Most categories in this chapter have three 7th character values: A, initial encounter, D, subsequent encounter and S, sequela. While the patient may be seen by a new or different provider over the course of treatment for an injury or condition, assignment of the 7th character for external cause should match the 7th character of the code assigned for the associated injury or condition for the encounter.

3) Use the full range of external cause codes
Use the full range of external cause codes to completely describe the cause, the intent, the place of occurrence, and if applicable, the activity of the patient at the time of the event, and the patient's status, for all injuries, and other health conditions due to an external cause.

4) Assign as many external cause codes as necessary
Assign as many external cause codes as necessary to fully explain each cause. If only one external code can be recorded, assign the code most related to the principal diagnosis.

5) The selection of the appropriate external cause code
The selection of the appropriate external cause code is guided by the Alphabetic Index of External Causes and by Inclusion and Exclusion notes in the Tabular List.

6) External cause code can never be a principal diagnosis
An external cause code can never be a principal (first-listed) diagnosis.

7) Combination external cause codes
Certain of the external cause codes are combination codes that identify sequential events that result in an injury, such as a fall which results in striking against an object. The injury may be due to either event or both. The combination external cause code used should correspond to the sequence of events regardless of which caused the most serious injury.

8) No external cause code needed in certain circumstances
No external cause code from Chapter 20 is needed if the external cause and intent are included in a code from another chapter (e.g., T36.ØX1-, Poisoning by penicillins, accidental (unintentional)).

b. Place of Occurrence Guideline
Codes from category Y92, Place of occurrence of the external cause, are secondary codes for use after other external cause codes to identify the location of the patient at the time of injury or other condition.

Generally, a place of occurrence code is assigned only once, at the initial encounter for treatment. However, in the rare instance that a new injury occurs during hospitalization, an additional place of occurrence code may be assigned. No 7th characters are used for Y92.

Do not use place of occurrence code Y92.9 if the place is not stated or is not applicable.

c. Activity Code

Assign a code from category Y93, Activity code, to describe the activity of the patient at the time the injury or other health condition occurred.

An activity code is used only once, at the initial encounter for treatment. Only one code from Y93 should be recorded on a medical record.

The activity codes are not applicable to poisonings, adverse effects, misadventures or sequela.

Do not assign Y93.9, Unspecified activity, if the activity is not stated.

A code from category Y93 is appropriate for use with external cause and intent codes if identifying the activity provides additional information about the event.

d. Place of Occurrence, Activity, and Status Codes Used with other External Cause Code

When applicable, place of occurrence, activity, and external cause status codes are sequenced after the main external cause code(s). Regardless of the number of external cause codes assigned, generally there should be only one place of occurrence code, one activity code, and one external cause status code assigned to an encounter. However, in the rare instance that a new injury occurs during hospitalization, an additional place of occurrence code may be assigned.

e. If the Reporting Format Limits the Number of External Cause Codes

If the reporting format limits the number of external cause codes that can be used in reporting clinical data, report the code for the cause/intent most related to the principal diagnosis. If the format permits capture of additional external cause codes, the cause/intent, including medical misadventures, of the additional events should be reported rather than the codes for place, activity, or external status.

f. Multiple External Cause Coding Guidelines

More than one external cause code is required to fully describe the external cause of an illness or injury. The assignment of external cause codes should be sequenced in the following priority:

If two or more events cause separate injuries, an external cause code should be assigned for each cause. The first-listed external cause code will be selected in the following order:

External codes for child and adult abuse take priority over all other external cause codes.

See Section I.C.19., Child and Adult abuse guidelines.

External cause codes for terrorism events take priority over all other external cause codes except child and adult abuse.

External cause codes for cataclysmic events take priority over all other external cause codes except child and adult abuse and terrorism.

External cause codes for transport accidents take priority over all other external cause codes except cataclysmic events, child and adult abuse and terrorism.

Activity and external cause status codes are assigned following all causal (intent) external cause codes.

The first-listed external cause code should correspond to the cause of the most serious diagnosis due to an assault, accident, or self-harm, following the order of hierarchy listed above.

g. Child and Adult Abuse Guideline

Adult and child abuse, neglect and maltreatment are classified as assault. Any of the assault codes may be used to indicate the external cause of any injury resulting from the confirmed abuse.

For confirmed cases of abuse, neglect and maltreatment, when the perpetrator is known, a code from Y07, Perpetrator of maltreatment and neglect, should accompany any other assault codes.

See Section I.C.19. Adult and child abuse, neglect and other maltreatment

h. Unknown or Undetermined Intent Guideline

If the intent (accident, self-harm, assault) of the cause of an injury or other condition is unknown or unspecified, code the intent as accidental intent. All transport accident categories assume accidental intent.

1) Use of undetermined intent

External cause codes for events of undetermined intent are only for use if the documentation in the record specifies that the intent cannot be determined.

i. Sequelae (Late Effects) of External Cause Guidelines

1) Sequelae external cause codes

Sequela are reported using the external cause code with the 7th character "S" for sequela. These codes should be used with any report of a late effect or sequela resulting from a previous injury.

See Section I.B.10. Sequela (Late Effects)

2) **Sequela external cause code with a related current injury**
A sequela external cause code should never be used with a related current nature of injury code.

3) **Use of sequela external cause codes for subsequent visits**
Use a late effect external cause code for subsequent visits when a late effect of the initial injury is being treated. Do not use a late effect external cause code for subsequent visits for follow-up care (e.g., to assess healing, to receive rehabilitative therapy) of the injury when no late effect of the injury has been documented.

j. **Terrorism Guidelines**

1) **Cause of injury identified by the Federal Government (FBI) as terrorism**
When the cause of an injury is identified by the Federal Government (FBI) as terrorism, the first-listed external cause code should be a code from category Y38, Terrorism. The definition of terrorism employed by the FBI is found at the inclusion note at the beginning of category Y38. Use additional code for place of occurrence (Y92.-). More than one Y38 code may be assigned if the injury is the result of more than one mechanism of terrorism.

2) **Cause of an injury is suspected to be the result of terrorism**
When the cause of an injury is suspected to be the result of terrorism a code from category Y38 should not be assigned. Suspected cases should be classified as assault.

3) **Code Y38.9, Terrorism, secondary effects**
Assign code Y38.9, Terrorism, secondary effects, for conditions occurring subsequent to the terrorist event. This code should not be assigned for conditions that are due to the initial terrorist act.

It is acceptable to assign code Y38.9 with another code from Y38 if there is an injury due to the initial terrorist event and an injury that is a subsequent result of the terrorist event.

k. **External Cause Status**
A code from category Y99, External cause status, should be assigned whenever any other external cause code is assigned for an encounter, including an Activity code, except for the events noted below. Assign a code from category Y99, External cause status, to indicate the work status of the person at the time the event occurred. The status code indicates whether the event occurred during military activity, whether a non-military person was at work, whether an individual including a student or volunteer was involved in a non-work activity at the time of the causal event.

A code from Y99, External cause status, should be assigned, when applicable, with other external cause codes, such as transport accidents and falls. The external cause status codes are not applicable to poisonings, adverse effects, misadventures or late effects.

Do not assign a code from category Y99 if no other external cause codes (cause, activity) are applicable for the encounter.

An external cause status code is used only once, at the initial encounter for treatment. Only one code from Y99 should be recorded on a medical record.

Do not assign code Y99.9, Unspecified external cause status, if the status is not stated.

21. **Chapter 21: Factors influencing health status and contact with health services (Z00-Z99)**
Note: The chapter specific guidelines provide additional information about the use of Z codes for specified encounters.

a. **Use of Z Codes in Any Healthcare Setting**
Z codes are for use in any healthcare setting. Z codes may be used as either a first-listed (principal diagnosis code in the inpatient setting) or secondary code, depending on the circumstances of the encounter. Certain Z codes may only be used as first-listed or principal diagnosis.

b. **Z Codes Indicate a Reason for an Encounter or Provide Additional Information about a Patient Encounter**
Z codes are not procedure codes. A corresponding procedure code must accompany a Z code to describe any procedure performed.

c. **Categories of Z Codes**

1) **Contact/Exposure**
Category Z20 indicates contact with, and suspected exposure to, communicable diseases. These codes are for patients who are suspected to have been exposed to a disease by close personal contact with an infected individual or are in an area where a disease is epidemic.

Category Z77, Other contact with and (suspected) exposures hazardous to health, indicates contact with and suspected exposures hazardous to health.

Contact/exposure codes may be used as a first-listed code to explain an encounter for testing, or, more commonly, as a secondary code to identify a potential risk.

2) **Inoculations and vaccinations**
Code Z23 is for encounters for inoculations and vaccinations. It indicates that a patient is being seen to receive a prophylactic inoculation against a disease. Procedure codes are required to identify the actual administration of the injection and the type(s) of immunizations given. Code Z23 may be used as a secondary code if the inoculation is given as a routine part of preventive health care, such as a well-baby visit.

3) **Status**
Status codes indicate that a patient is either a carrier of a disease or has the sequelae or residual of a past disease or condition. This includes such things as the presence of prosthetic or mechanical devices resulting from past treatment. A status code is informative, because the status may affect the course of treatment and its outcome. A status code is distinct from a history code. The history code indicates that the patient no longer has the condition.

A status code should not be used with a diagnosis code from one of the body system chapters, if the diagnosis code includes the information provided by the status code. For example, code Z94.1, Heart transplant status, should not be used with a code from subcategory T86.2, Complications of heart transplant. The status code does not provide additional information. The complication code indicates that the patient is a heart transplant patient.

For encounters for weaning from a mechanical ventilator, assign a code from subcategory J96.1, Chronic respiratory failure, followed by code Z99.11, Dependence on respirator [ventilator] status.

The status Z codes/categories are:

Z14 Genetic carrier
Genetic carrier status indicates that a person carries a gene, associated with a particular disease, which may be passed to offspring who may develop that disease. The person does not have the disease and is not at risk of developing the disease.

Z15 Genetic susceptibility to disease
Genetic susceptibility indicates that a person has a gene that increases the risk of that person developing the disease.

Codes from category Z15 should not be used as principal or first-listed codes. If the patient has the condition to which he/she is susceptible, and that condition is the reason for the encounter, the code for the current condition should be sequenced first. If the patient is being seen for follow-up after completed treatment for this condition, and the condition no longer exists, a follow-up code should be sequenced first, followed by the appropriate personal history and genetic susceptibility codes. If the purpose of the encounter is genetic counseling associated with procreative management, code Z31.5, Encounter for genetic counseling, should be assigned as the first-listed code, followed by a code from category Z15. Additional codes should be assigned for any applicable family or personal history.

Z16 Resistance to antimicrobial drugs
This code indicates that a patient has a condition that is resistant to antimicrobial drug treatment. Sequence the infection code first.

Z17 Estrogen, **and other hormones and factors** receptor status

Z18 Retained foreign body fragments

Z19 Hormone sensitivity malignancy status

Z21 Asymptomatic HIV infection status
This code indicates that a patient has tested positive for HIV but has manifested no signs or symptoms of the disease.

Z22 Carrier of infectious disease
Carrier status indicates that a person harbors the specific organisms of a disease without manifest symptoms and is capable of transmitting the infection.

Z28.3 Underimmunization status
See Section I.B.14. for underimmunization documentation by clinicians other than the patient's provider.

ICD-10-CM Official Guidelines

Z33.1 Pregnant state, incidental
This code is a secondary code only for use when the pregnancy is in no way complicating the reason for visit. Otherwise, a code from the obstetric chapter is required.

Z66 Do not resuscitate
This code may be used when it is documented by the provider that a patient is on do not resuscitate status at any time during the stay.

Z67 Blood type

Z68 Body mass index (BMI)
BMI codes should only be assigned when there is an associated, reportable diagnosis (such as obesity). Do not assign BMI codes during pregnancy.

See Section I.B.14. for BMI documentation by clinicians other than the patient's provider.

Z74.Ø1 Bed confinement status

Z76.82 Awaiting organ transplant status

Z78 Other specified health status
Code Z78.1, Physical restraint status, may be used when it is documented by the provider that a patient has been put in restraints during the current encounter. Please note that this code should not be reported when it is documented by the provider that a patient is temporarily restrained during a procedure.

Z79 Long-term (current) drug therapy
Codes from this category indicate a patient's continuous use of a prescribed drug (including such things as aspirin therapy) for the long-term treatment of a condition or for prophylactic use. It is not for use for patients who have addictions to drugs. This subcategory is not for use of medications for detoxification or maintenance programs to prevent withdrawal symptoms (e.g., methadone maintenance for opiate dependence). Assign the appropriate code for the drug use, abuse, or dependence instead.

Assign a code from Z79 if the patient is receiving a medication for an extended period as a prophylactic measure (such as for the prevention of deep vein thrombosis) or as treatment of a chronic condition (such as arthritis) or a disease requiring a lengthy course of treatment (such as cancer). Do not assign a code from category Z79 for medication being administered for a brief period of time to treat an acute illness or injury (such as a course of antibiotics to treat acute bronchitis).

Z88 Allergy status to drugs, medicaments and biological substances
Except: Z88.9, Allergy status to unspecified drugs, medicaments and biological substances status

Z89 Acquired absence of limb

Z9Ø Acquired absence of organs, not elsewhere classified

Z91.Ø- Allergy status, other than to drugs and biological substances

Z92.82 Status post administration of tPA (rtPA) in a different facility within the last 24 hours prior to admission to a current facility
Assign code Z92.82, Status post administration of tPA (rtPA) in a different facility within the last 24 hours prior to admission to current facility, as a secondary diagnosis when a patient is received by transfer into a facility and documentation indicates they were administered tissue plasminogen activator (tPA) within the last 24 hours prior to admission to the current facility.

This guideline applies even if the patient is still receiving the tPA at the time they are received into the current facility.

The appropriate code for the condition for which the tPA was administered (such as cerebrovascular disease or myocardial infarction) should be assigned first.

Code Z92.82 is only applicable to the receiving facility record and not to the transferring facility record.

Z93 Artificial opening status

Z94 Transplanted organ and tissue status

Z95 Presence of cardiac and vascular implants and grafts

Z96 Presence of other functional implants

Z97 Presence of other devices

Z98 Other postprocedural states
Assign code Z98.85, Transplanted organ removal status, to indicate that a transplanted organ has been previously removed. This code should not be assigned for the encounter in which the transplanted organ is removed. The complication necessitating removal of the transplant organ should be assigned for that encounter.
See section I.C.19. for information on the coding of organ transplant complications.

Z99 Dependence on enabling machines and devices, not elsewhere classified
Note: Categories Z89-Z9Ø and Z93-Z99 are for use only if there are no complications or malfunctions of the organ or tissue replaced, the amputation site or the equipment on which the patient is dependent.

4) **History (of)**

There are two types of history Z codes, personal and family. Personal history codes explain a patient's past medical condition that no longer exists and is not receiving any treatment, but that has the potential for recurrence, and therefore may require continued monitoring.

Family history codes are for use when a patient has a family member(s) who has had a particular disease that causes the patient to be at higher risk of also contracting the disease.

Personal history codes may be used in conjunction with follow-up codes and family history codes may be used in conjunction with screening codes to explain the need for a test or procedure. History codes are also acceptable on any medical record regardless of the reason for visit. A history of an illness, even if no longer present, is important information that may alter the type of treatment ordered.

The reason for the encounter (for example, screening or counseling) should be sequenced first and the appropriate personal and/or family history code(s) should be assigned as additional diagnos(es).

The history Z code categories are:

Z8Ø Family history of primary malignant neoplasm
Z81 Family history of mental and behavioral disorders
Z82 Family history of certain disabilities and chronic diseases (leading to disablement)
Z83 Family history of other specific disorders
Z84 Family history of other conditions
Z85 Personal history of malignant neoplasm
Z86 Personal history of certain other diseases
Z87 Personal history of other diseases and conditions
Z91.4- Personal history of psychological trauma, not elsewhere classified
Z91.5- Personal history of self-harm
Z91.81 History of falling
Z91.82 Personal history of military deployment
Z91.85 Personal history of military service
Z92 Personal history of medical treatment
Except: Z92.Ø, Personal history of contraception
Except: Z92.82, Status post administration of tPA (rtPA) in a different facility within the last 24 hours prior to admission to a current facility

5) **Screening**

Screening is the testing for disease or disease precursors in seemingly well individuals so that early detection and treatment can be provided for those who test positive for the disease (e.g., screening mammogram).

The testing of a person to rule out or confirm a suspected diagnosis because the patient has some sign or symptom is a diagnostic examination, not a screening. In these cases, the sign or symptom is used to explain the reason for the test.

A screening code may be a first-listed code if the reason for the visit is specifically the screening exam. It may also be used as an additional code if the screening is done during an office visit for other health problems. A screening code is not necessary if the screening is inherent to a routine examination, such as a pap smear done during a routine pelvic examination.

Should a condition be discovered during the screening then the code for the condition may be assigned as an additional diagnosis.

The Z code indicates that a screening exam is planned. A procedure code is required to confirm that the screening was performed.

The screening Z codes/categories:

Z11	Encounter for screening for infectious and parasitic diseases
Z12	Encounter for screening for malignant neoplasms
Z13	Encounter for screening for other diseases and disorders Except: Z13.9, Encounter for screening, unspecified
Z36	Encounter for antenatal screening for mother

6) Observation

There are three observation Z code categories. They are for use in very limited circumstances when a person is being observed for a suspected condition that is ruled out. The observation codes are not for use if an injury or illness or any signs or symptoms related to the suspected condition are present. In such cases the diagnosis/symptom code is used with the corresponding external cause code.

The observation codes are primarily to be used as a principal/first-listed diagnosis. An observation code may be assigned as a secondary diagnosis code when the patient is being observed for a condition that is ruled out and is unrelated to the principal/first-listed diagnosis. Also, when the principal diagnosis is required to be a code from category Z38, Liveborn infants according to place of birth and type of delivery, then a code from category Z05, Encounter for observation and evaluation of newborn for suspected diseases and conditions ruled out, is sequenced after the Z38 code. Additional codes may be used in addition to the observation code, but only if they are unrelated to the suspected condition being observed.

Codes from subcategory Z03.7, Encounter for suspected maternal and fetal conditions ruled out, may either be used as a first-listed or as an additional code assignment depending on the case. They are for use in very limited circumstances on a maternal record when an encounter is for a suspected maternal or fetal condition that is ruled out during that encounter (for example, a maternal or fetal condition may be suspected due to an abnormal test result). These codes should not be used when the condition is confirmed. In those cases, the confirmed condition should be coded. In addition, these codes are not for use if an illness or any signs or symptoms related to the suspected condition or problem are present. In such cases the diagnosis/symptom code is used.

Additional codes may be used in addition to the code from subcategory Z03.7, but only if they are unrelated to the suspected condition being evaluated.

Codes from subcategory Z03.7 may not be used for encounters for antenatal screening of mother. *See Section I.C.21. Screening.*

For encounters for suspected fetal condition that are inconclusive following testing and evaluation, assign the appropriate code from category O35, O36, O40 or O41.

The observation Z code categories:

Z03	Encounter for medical observation for suspected diseases and conditions ruled out
Z04	Encounter for examination and observation for other reasons Except: Z04.9, Encounter for examination and observation for unspecified reason
Z05	Encounter for observation and evaluation of newborn for suspected diseases and conditions ruled out

7) Aftercare

Aftercare visit codes cover situations when the initial treatment of a disease has been performed and the patient requires continued care during the healing or recovery phase, or for the long-term consequences of the disease. The aftercare Z code should not be used if treatment is directed at a current, acute disease. The diagnosis code is to be used in these cases. Exceptions to this rule are codes Z51.0, Encounter for antineoplastic radiation therapy, and codes from subcategory Z51.1, Encounter for antineoplastic chemotherapy and immunotherapy. These codes are to be first listed, followed by the diagnosis code when a patient's encounter is chiefly to receive radiation therapy, chemotherapy, or immunotherapy for the treatment of a neoplasm. If the reason for the encounter is more than one type of antineoplastic therapy, code Z51.0 and a code from subcategory Z51.1 may be assigned together, in which case one of these codes would be reported as a secondary diagnosis.

The aftercare Z codes should also not be used for aftercare for injuries. For aftercare of an injury, assign the acute injury code with the appropriate 7th character (for subsequent encounter).

The aftercare codes are generally first listed to explain the specific reason for the encounter. An aftercare code may be used as an additional code when some type of aftercare is provided in addition to the reason for admission and no diagnosis code is applicable. An example of this would be the closure of a colostomy during an encounter for treatment of another condition.

Aftercare codes should be used in conjunction with other aftercare codes or diagnosis codes to provide better detail on the specifics of an aftercare encounter visit, unless otherwise directed by the classification. The sequencing of multiple aftercare codes depends on the circumstances of the encounter.

Certain aftercare Z code categories need a secondary diagnosis code to describe the resolving condition or sequelae. For others, the condition is included in the code title.

Additional Z code aftercare category terms include fitting and adjustment, and attention to artificial openings.

Status Z codes may be used with aftercare Z codes to indicate the nature of the aftercare. For example, code Z95.1, Presence of aortocoronary bypass graft, may be used with code Z48.812, Encounter for surgical aftercare following surgery on the circulatory system, to indicate the surgery for which the aftercare is being performed. A status code should not be used when the aftercare code indicates the type of status, such as using Z43.Ø, Encounter for attention to tracheostomy, with Z93.Ø, Tracheostomy status.

The aftercare Z category/codes:

Z42	Encounter for plastic and reconstructive surgery following medical procedure or healed injury
Z43	Encounter for attention to artificial openings
Z44	Encounter for fitting and adjustment of external prosthetic device
Z45	Encounter for adjustment and management of implanted device
Z46	Encounter for fitting and adjustment of other devices
Z47	Orthopedic aftercare
Z48	Encounter for other postprocedural aftercare
Z49	Encounter for care involving renal dialysis
Z51	Encounter for other aftercare and medical care

8) Follow-up

The follow-up codes are used to explain continuing surveillance following completed treatment of a disease, condition, or injury. They imply that the condition has been fully treated and no longer exists. They should not be confused with aftercare codes, or injury codes with a 7th character for subsequent encounter, that explain ongoing care of a healing condition or its sequelae. Follow-up codes may be used in conjunction with history codes to provide the full picture of the healed condition and its treatment. The follow-up code is sequenced first, followed by the history code.

A follow-up code may be used to explain multiple visits. Should a condition be found to have recurred on the follow-up visit, then the diagnosis code for the condition should be assigned in place of the follow-up code.

The follow-up Z codes/categories:

ZØ8	Encounter for follow up examination after completed treatment for malignant neoplasm
ZØ9	Encounter for follow-up examination after completed treatment for conditions other than malignant neoplasm

Codes ZØ8, Encounter for follow-up examination after completed treatment for malignant neoplasm, and ZØ9, Encounter for follow up examination after completed treatment for conditions other than malignant neoplasm, may be assigned following any type of completed treatment modality (including both medical and surgical treatments).

Z39	Encounter for maternal postpartum care and examination

9) Donor

Codes in category Z52, Donors of organs and tissues, are used for living individuals who are donating blood or other body tissue. These codes are for individuals donating for others, as well as for self-donations. They are not used to identify cadaveric donations.

10) Counseling

Counseling Z codes are used when a patient or family member receives assistance in the aftermath of an illness or injury, or when support is required in coping with family or social problems.

The counseling Z codes/categories:

Z30.0-	Encounter for general counseling and advice on contraception
Z31.5	Encounter for procreative genetic counseling
Z31.6-	Encounter for general counseling and advice on procreation
Z32.2	Encounter for childbirth instruction
Z32.3	Encounter for childcare instruction
Z69	Encounter for mental health services for victim and perpetrator of abuse
Z70	Counseling related to sexual attitude, behavior and orientation
Z71	Persons encountering health services for other counseling and medical advice, not elsewhere classified Note: Code Z71.84, Encounter for health counseling related to travel, is to be used for health risk and safety counseling for future travel purposes. Code Z71.85, Encounter for immunization safety counseling, is to be used for counseling of the patient or caregiver regarding the safety of a vaccine. This code should not be used for the provision of general information regarding risks and potential side effects during routine encounters for the administration of vaccines. Code Z71.87, Encounter for pediatric-to-adult transition counseling, should be assigned when pediatric-to-adult transition counseling is the sole reason for the encounter or when this counseling is provided in addition to other services, such as treatment of a chronic condition. If both transition counseling and treatment of a medical condition are provided during the same encounter, the code(s) for the medical condition(s) treated and code Z71.87 should be assigned, with sequencing depending on the circumstances of the encounter.
Z76.81	Expectant mother prebirth pediatrician visit

11) Encounters for Obstetrical and Reproductive Services

See Section I.C.15. Pregnancy, Childbirth, and the Puerperium, for further instruction on the use of these codes.

Z codes for pregnancy are for use in those circumstances when none of the problems or complications included in the codes from the Obstetrics chapter exist (a routine prenatal visit or postpartum care). Codes in category Z34, Encounter for supervision of normal pregnancy, are always first listed and are not to be used with any other code from the OB chapter.

Codes in category Z3A, Weeks of gestation, may be assigned to provide additional information about the pregnancy. Category Z3A codes should not be assigned for pregnancies with abortive outcomes (categories O00-O08), elective termination of pregnancy (code Z33.2), nor for postpartum conditions, as category Z3A is not applicable to these conditions. The date of the admission should be used to determine weeks of gestation for inpatient admissions that encompass more than one gestational week.

The outcome of delivery, category Z37, should be included on all maternal delivery records. It is always a secondary code.

Codes in category Z37 should not be used on the newborn record.

Z codes for family planning (contraceptive) or procreative management and counseling should be included on an obstetric record either during the pregnancy or the postpartum stage, if applicable.

Z codes/categories for obstetrical and reproductive services:

Z30	Encounter for contraceptive management
Z31	Encounter for procreative management
Z32.2	Encounter for childbirth instruction
Z32.3	Encounter for childcare instruction
Z33	Pregnant state
Z34	Encounter for supervision of normal pregnancy
Z36	Encounter for antenatal screening of mother
Z3A	Weeks of gestation
Z37	Outcome of delivery
Z39	Encounter for maternal postpartum care and examination
Z76.81	Expectant mother prebirth pediatrician visit

12) Newborns and Infants

See Section I.C.16. Newborn (Perinatal) Guidelines, for further instruction on the use of these codes.

Newborn Z codes/categories:

Z76.1	Encounter for health supervision and care of foundling
ZØØ.1-	Encounter for routine child health examination
Z38	Liveborn infants according to place of birth and type of delivery

13) Routine and Administrative Examinations

The Z codes allow for the description of encounters for routine examinations, such as, a general check-up, or, examinations for administrative purposes, such as, a pre-employment physical. The codes are not to be used if the examination is for diagnosis of a suspected condition or for treatment purposes. In such cases the diagnosis code is used. During a routine exam, should a diagnosis or condition be discovered, it should be coded as an additional code. Pre-existing and chronic conditions and history codes may also be included as additional codes as long as the examination is for administrative purposes and not focused on any particular condition.

Some of the codes for routine health examinations distinguish between "with" and "without" abnormal findings. Code assignment depends on the information that is known at the time the encounter is being coded. For example, if no abnormal findings were found during the examination, but the encounter is being coded before test results are back, it is acceptable to assign the code for "without abnormal findings." When assigning a code for "with abnormal findings," additional code(s) should be assigned to identify the specific abnormal finding(s).

Pre-operative examination and pre-procedural laboratory examination Z codes are for use only in those situations when a patient is being cleared for a procedure or surgery and no treatment is given.

The Z codes/categories for routine and administrative examinations:

ZØØ	Encounter for general examination without complaint, suspected or reported diagnosis
ZØ1	Encounter for other special examination without complaint, suspected or reported diagnosis
ZØ2	Encounter for administrative examination Except: ZØ2.9, Encounter for administrative examinations, unspecified
Z32.Ø-	Encounter for pregnancy test

14) Miscellaneous Z Codes

The miscellaneous Z codes capture a number of other health care encounters that do not fall into one of the other categories. Some of these codes identify the reason for the encounter; others are for use as additional codes that provide useful information on circumstances that may affect a patient's care and treatment.

Prophylactic Organ Removal

For encounters specifically for prophylactic removal of an organ (such as prophylactic removal of breasts due to a genetic susceptibility to cancer or a family history of cancer), the principal or first-listed code should be a code from category Z4Ø, Encounter for prophylactic surgery, followed by the appropriate codes to identify the associated risk factor (such as genetic susceptibility or family history).

If the patient has a malignancy of one site and is having prophylactic removal at another site to prevent either a new primary malignancy or metastatic disease, a code for the malignancy should also be assigned in addition to a code from subcategory Z4Ø.Ø, Encounter for prophylactic surgery for risk factors related to malignant neoplasms. A Z4Ø.Ø code should not be assigned if the patient is having organ removal for treatment of a malignancy, such as the removal of the testes for the treatment of prostate cancer.

Miscellaneous Z codes/categories:

Z28	Immunization not carried out Except: Z28.3-, Underimmunization status
Z29	Encounter for other prophylactic measures
Z4Ø	Encounter for prophylactic surgery
Z41	Encounter for procedures for purposes other than remedying health state Except: Z41.9, Encounter for procedure for purposes other than remedying health state, unspecified

Z53	Persons encountering health services for specific procedures and treatment, not carried out
Z72	Problems related to lifestyle Note: These codes should be assigned only when the documentation specifies that the patient has an associated problem
Z73	Problems related to life management difficulty Note: These codes should be assigned only when the documentation specifies that the patient has an associated problem.
Z74	Problems related to care provider dependency Except: Z74.Ø1, Bed confinement status
Z75	Problems related to medical facilities and other health care
Z76.Ø	Encounter for issue of repeat prescription
Z76.3	Healthy person accompanying sick person
Z76.4	Other boarder to healthcare facility
Z76.5	Malingerer [conscious simulation]
Z91.1-	Patient's noncompliance with medical treatment and regimen
Z91.A-	Caregiver's noncompliance with patient's medical treatment and regimen
Z91.83	Wandering in diseases classified elsewhere
Z91.84-	Oral health risk factors
Z91.89	Other specified personal risk factors, not elsewhere classified

See Section I.B.14. for Z55-Z65 Persons with potential health hazards related to socioeconomic and psychosocial circumstances, documentation by clinicians other than the patient's provider

15) Nonspecific Z Codes

Certain Z codes are so non-specific, or potentially redundant with other codes in the classification, that there can be little justification for their use in the inpatient setting. Their use in the outpatient setting should be limited to those instances when there is no further documentation to permit more precise coding. Otherwise, any sign or symptom or any other reason for visit that is captured in another code should be used.

Nonspecific Z codes/categories:

ZØ2.9	Encounter for administrative examinations, unspecified
ZØ4.9	Encounter for examination and observation for unspecified reason
Z13.9	Encounter for screening, unspecified
Z41.9	Encounter for procedure for purposes other than remedying health state, unspecified
Z52.9	Donor of unspecified organ or tissue
Z86.59	Personal history of other mental and behavioral disorders
Z88.9	Allergy status to unspecified drugs, medicaments and biological substances status
Z92.Ø	Personal history of contraception

16) Z Codes That May Only be Principal/First-Listed Diagnosis

The following Z codes/categories may only be reported as the principal/first-listed diagnosis, except when there are multiple encounters on the same day and the medical records for the encounters are combined:

ZØØ	Encounter for general examination without complaint, suspected or reported diagnosis Except: ZØØ.6
ZØ1	Encounter for other special examination without complaint, suspected or reported diagnosis
ZØ2	Encounter for administrative examination
ZØ4	Encounter for examination and observation for other reasons
Z33.2	Encounter for elective termination of pregnancy
Z31.81	Encounter for male factor infertility in female patient
Z31.83	Encounter for assisted reproductive fertility procedure cycle
Z31.84	Encounter for fertility preservation procedure
Z34	Encounter for supervision of normal pregnancy
Z39	Encounter for maternal postpartum care and examination

Z38	Liveborn infants according to place of birth and type of delivery
Z4Ø	Encounter for prophylactic surgery
Z42	Encounter for plastic and reconstructive surgery following medical procedure or healed injury
Z51.Ø	Encounter for antineoplastic radiation therapy
Z51.1-	Encounter for antineoplastic chemotherapy and immunotherapy
Z52	Donors of organs and tissues Except: Z52.9, Donor of unspecified organ or tissue
Z76.1	Encounter for health supervision and care of foundling
Z76.2	Encounter for health supervision and care of other healthy infant and child
Z99.12	Encounter for respirator [ventilator] dependence during power failure

17) Social Determinants of Health

Social determinants of health (SDOH) codes describing social problems, conditions, or risk factors that influence a patient's health should be assigned when this information is documented in the patient's medical record. Assign as many SDOH codes as are necessary to describe all of the social problems, conditions, or risk factors documented during the current episode of care. For example, a patient who lives alone may suffer an acute injury temporarily impacting their ability to perform routine activities of daily living. When documented as such, this would support assignment of code Z6Ø.2, Problems related to living alone. However, merely living alone, without documentation of a risk or unmet need for assistance at home, would not support assignment of code Z6Ø.2. Documentation by a clinician (or patient-reported information that is signed off by a clinician) that the patient expressed concerns with access and availability of food would support assignment of code Z59.41, Food insecurity. Similarly, medical record documentation indicating the patient is homeless would support assignment of a code from subcategory Z59.Ø-, Homelessness.

For social determinants of health classified to chapter 21, such as information found in categories Z55-Z65, Persons with potential health hazards related to socioeconomic and psychosocial circumstances, code assignment may be based on medical record documentation from clinicians involved in the care of the patient who are not the patient's provider since this information represents social information, rather than medical diagnoses. For example, coding professionals may utilize documentation of social information from social workers, community health workers, case managers, or nurses, if their documentation is included in the official medical record.

Patient self-reported documentation may be used to assign codes for social determinants of health, as long as the patient self-reported information is signed-off by and incorporated into the medical record by either a clinician or provider.

Social determinants of health codes are located primarily in these Z code categories:

Z55	Problems related to education and literacy
Z56	Problems related to employment and unemployment
Z57	Occupational exposure to risk factors
Z58	Problems related to physical environment
Z59	Problems related to housing and economic circumstances
Z6Ø	Problems related to social environment
Z62	Problems related to upbringing
Z63	Other problems related to primary support group, including family circumstances
Z64	Problems related to certain psychosocial circumstances
Z65	Problems related to other psychosocial circumstances

See Section I.B.14. Documentation by Clinicians Other than the Patient's Provider.

22. Chapter 22: Codes for Special Purposes (UØØ-U85)

UØ7.Ø	Vaping-related disorder (see Section I.C.1Ø.e., Vaping-related disorders)
UØ7.1	COVID-19 (see Section I.C.1.g.1., COVID-19 infection)
UØ9.9	Post COVID-19 condition, unspecified (see Section I.C.1.g.1.m.)

Section II. Selection of Principal Diagnosis

The circumstances of inpatient admission always govern the selection of principal diagnosis. The principal diagnosis is defined in the Uniform Hospital Discharge Data Set (UHDDS) as "that condition established after study to be chiefly responsible for occasioning the admission of the patient to the hospital for care."

The UHDDS definitions are used by hospitals to report inpatient data elements in a standardized manner. These data elements and their definitions can be found in the July 31, 1985, Federal Register (Vol. 50, No, 147), pp. 31038-40.

Since that time, the application of the UHDDS definitions has been expanded to include all non-outpatient settings (acute care, short term, long term care and psychiatric hospitals; home health agencies; rehab facilities; nursing homes, etc.). The UHDDS definitions also apply to hospice services (all levels of care).

In determining principal diagnosis, coding conventions in the ICD-10-CM, the Tabular List and Alphabetic Index take precedence over these official coding guidelines.

(See Section I.A., Conventions for the ICD-10-CM)

The importance of consistent, complete documentation in the medical record cannot be overemphasized. Without such documentation the application of all coding guidelines is a difficult, if not impossible, task.

A. Codes for symptoms, signs, and ill-defined conditions

Codes for symptoms, signs, and ill-defined conditions from Chapter 18 are not to be used as principal diagnosis when a related definitive diagnosis has been established.

B. Two or more interrelated conditions, each potentially meeting the definition for principal diagnosis.

When there are two or more interrelated conditions (such as diseases in the same ICD-10-CM chapter or manifestations characteristically associated with a certain disease) potentially meeting the definition of principal diagnosis, either condition may be sequenced first, unless the circumstances of the admission, the therapy provided, the Tabular List, or the Alphabetic Index indicate otherwise.

C. Two or more diagnoses that equally meet the definition for principal diagnosis

In the unusual instance when two or more diagnoses equally meet the criteria for principal diagnosis as determined by the circumstances of admission, diagnostic workup and/or therapy provided, and the Alphabetic Index, Tabular List, or another coding guidelines does not provide sequencing direction, any one of the diagnoses may be sequenced first.

D. Two or more comparative or contrasting conditions

In those rare instances when two or more contrasting or comparative diagnoses are documented as "either/or" (or similar terminology), they are coded as if the diagnoses were confirmed and the diagnoses are sequenced according to the circumstances of the admission. If no further determination can be made as to which diagnosis should be principal, either diagnosis may be sequenced first.

E. A symptom(s) followed by contrasting/comparative diagnoses

GUIDELINE HAS BEEN DELETED EFFECTIVE OCTOBER 1, 2014

F. Original treatment plan not carried out

Sequence as the principal diagnosis the condition, which after study occasioned the admission to the hospital, even though treatment may not have been carried out due to unforeseen circumstances.

G. Complications of surgery and other medical care

When the admission is for treatment of a complication resulting from surgery or other medical care, the complication code is sequenced as the principal diagnosis. If the complication is classified to the T80-T88 series and the code lacks the necessary specificity in describing the complication, an additional code for the specific complication should be assigned.

H. Uncertain Diagnosis

If the diagnosis documented at the time of discharge is qualified as "probable," "suspected," "likely," "questionable," "possible," or "still to be ruled out," "compatible with," "consistent with," or other similar terms indicating uncertainty, code the condition as if it existed or was established. The bases for these guidelines are the diagnostic workup, arrangements for further workup or observation, and initial therapeutic approach that correspond most closely with the established diagnosis.

Note: This guideline is applicable only to inpatient admissions to short-term, acute, long-term care and psychiatric hospitals.

I. Admission from Observation Unit

1. Admission Following Medical Observation

When a patient is admitted to an observation unit for a medical condition, which either worsens or does not improve, and is subsequently admitted as an inpatient of the same hospital for this same medical condition, the principal diagnosis would be the medical condition which led to the hospital admission.

2. Admission Following Post-Operative Observation

When a patient is admitted to an observation unit to monitor a condition (or complication) that develops following outpatient surgery, and then is subsequently admitted as an inpatient of the same hospital, hospitals should apply the Uniform Hospital Discharge Data Set (UHDDS) definition of principal diagnosis as "that condition established after study to be chiefly responsible for occasioning the admission of the patient to the hospital for care."

J. Admission from Outpatient Surgery

When a patient receives surgery in the hospital's outpatient surgery department and is subsequently admitted for continuing inpatient care at the same hospital, the following guidelines should be followed in selecting the principal diagnosis for the inpatient admission:

- If the reason for the inpatient admission is a complication, assign the complication as the principal diagnosis.
- If no complication, or other condition, is documented as the reason for the inpatient admission, assign the reason for the outpatient surgery as the principal diagnosis.
- If the reason for the inpatient admission is another condition unrelated to the surgery, assign the unrelated condition as the principal diagnosis.

K. Admissions/Encounters for Rehabilitation

When the purpose for the admission/encounter is rehabilitation, sequence first the code for the condition for which the service is being performed. For example, for an admission/encounter for rehabilitation for right-sided dominant hemiplegia following a cerebrovascular infarction, report code I69.351, Hemiplegia and hemiparesis following cerebral infarction affecting right dominant side, as the first-listed or principal diagnosis.

If the condition for which the rehabilitation service is being provided is no longer present, report the appropriate aftercare code as the first-listed or principal diagnosis, unless the rehabilitation service is being provided following an injury. For rehabilitation services following active treatment of an injury, assign the injury code with the appropriate seventh character for subsequent encounter as the first-listed or principal diagnosis. For example, if a patient with severe degenerative osteoarthritis of the hip, underwent hip replacement and the current encounter/admission is for rehabilitation, report code Z47.1, Aftercare following joint replacement surgery, as the first-listed or principal diagnosis. If the patient requires rehabilitation post hip replacement for right intertrochanteric femur fracture, report code S72.141D, Displaced intertrochanteric fracture of right femur, subsequent encounter for closed fracture with routine healing, as the first-listed or principal diagnosis.

See Section I.C.21.c.7., Factors influencing health states and contact with health services, Aftercare.

See Section I.C.19.a., for additional information about the use of 7th characters for injury codes.

Section III. Reporting Additional Diagnoses

GENERAL RULES FOR OTHER (ADDITIONAL) DIAGNOSES

For reporting purposes, the definition for "other diagnoses" is interpreted as additional clinically significant conditions that affect patient care in terms of requiring:

clinical evaluation; or

therapeutic treatment; or

diagnostic procedures; or

extended length of hospital stay; or

increased nursing care and/or monitoring.

The UHDDS item #11-b defines Other Diagnoses as "all conditions that coexist at the time of admission, that develop subsequently, or that affect the treatment received and/or the length of stay. Diagnoses that relate to an earlier episode which have no bearing on the current hospital stay are to be excluded." UHDDS definitions apply to inpatients in acute care, short-term, long term care and psychiatric hospital setting. The UHDDS definitions are used by acute care short-term hospitals to report inpatient data elements in a standardized manner. These data elements and their definitions can be found in the July 31, 1985, Federal Register (Vol. 50, No, 147), pp. 31038-40.

Since that time, the application of the UHDDS definitions has been expanded to include all non-outpatient settings (acute care, short term, long term care and psychiatric hospitals; home health agencies; rehab facilities; nursing homes, etc.). The UHDDS definitions also apply to hospice services (all levels of care).

The following guidelines are to be applied in designating "other diagnoses" when neither the Alphabetic Index nor the Tabular List in ICD-10-CM provide direction. The listing of the diagnoses in the patient record is the responsibility of the provider.

A. Previous conditions

If the provider has included a diagnosis in the final diagnostic statement, such as the discharge summary or the face sheet, it should ordinarily be coded. Some providers include in the diagnostic statement resolved conditions or diagnoses and status-post procedures from previous admissions that have no bearing on the current stay. Such conditions are not to be reported and are coded only if required by hospital policy.

However, history codes (categories Z8Ø-Z87) may be used as secondary codes if the historical condition or family history has an impact on current care or influences treatment.

B. Abnormal findings

Abnormal findings (laboratory, x-ray, pathologic, and other diagnostic results) are not coded and reported unless the provider indicates their clinical significance. If the findings are outside the normal range and the provider has ordered other tests to evaluate the condition or prescribed treatment, it is appropriate to ask the provider whether the abnormal finding should be added.

Please note: This differs from the coding practices in the outpatient setting for coding encounters for diagnostic tests that have been interpreted by a provider.

C. Uncertain Diagnosis

If the diagnosis documented at the time of discharge is qualified as "probable,""suspected,""likely," "questionable,""possible," or "still to be ruled out,""compatible with,""consistent with," or other similar terms indicating uncertainty, code the condition as if it existed or was established. The bases for these guidelines are the diagnostic workup, arrangements for further workup or observation, and initial therapeutic approach that correspond most closely with the established diagnosis.

Note: This guideline is applicable only to inpatient admissions to short-term, acute, long-term care and psychiatric hospitals.

Section IV. Diagnostic Coding and Reporting Guidelines for Outpatient Services

These coding guidelines for outpatient diagnoses have been approved for use by hospitals/ providers in coding and reporting hospital-based outpatient services and provider-based office visits. Guidelines in Section I, Conventions, general coding guidelines and chapter-specific guidelines, should also be applied for outpatient services and office visits.

Information about the use of certain abbreviations, punctuation, symbols, and other conventions used in the ICD-10-CM Tabular List (code numbers and titles), can be found in Section IA of these guidelines, under "Conventions Used in the Tabular List." Section I.B. contains general guidelines that apply to the entire classification. Section I.C. contains chapter-specific guidelines that correspond to the chapters as they are arranged in the classification. Information about the correct sequence to use in finding a code is also described in Section I.

The terms encounter and visit are often used interchangeably in describing outpatient service contacts and, therefore, appear together in these guidelines without distinguishing one from the other.

Though the conventions and general guidelines apply to all settings, coding guidelines for outpatient and provider reporting of diagnoses will vary in a number of instances from those for inpatient diagnoses, recognizing that:

The Uniform Hospital Discharge Data Set (UHDDS) definition of principal diagnosis does not apply to hospital-based outpatient services and provider-based office visits.

Coding guidelines for inconclusive diagnoses (probable, suspected, rule out, etc.) were developed for inpatient reporting and do not apply to outpatients.

A. Selection of first-listed condition

In the outpatient setting, the term first-listed diagnosis is used in lieu of principal diagnosis.

In determining the first-listed diagnosis the coding conventions of ICD-10-CM, as well as the general and disease specific guidelines take precedence over the outpatient guidelines.

Diagnoses often are not established at the time of the initial encounter/visit. It may take two or more visits before the diagnosis is confirmed.

The most critical rule involves beginning the search for the correct code assignment through the Alphabetic Index. Never begin searching initially in the Tabular List as this will lead to coding errors.

1. **Outpatient Surgery**
   When a patient presents for outpatient surgery (same day surgery), code the reason for the surgery as the first-listed diagnosis (reason for the encounter), even if the surgery is not performed due to a contraindication.

2. **Observation Stay**
   When a patient is admitted for observation for a medical condition, assign a code for the medical condition as the first-listed diagnosis.

   When a patient presents for outpatient surgery and develops complications requiring admission to observation, code the reason for the surgery as the first reported diagnosis (reason for the encounter), followed by codes for the complications as secondary diagnoses.

B. Codes from A00.0 through T88.9, Z00-Z99, U00-U85
The appropriate code(s) from A00.0 through T88.9, Z00-Z99 and U00-U85 must be used to identify diagnoses, symptoms, conditions, problems, complaints, or other reason(s) for the encounter/visit.

C. Accurate reporting of ICD-10-CM diagnosis codes
For accurate reporting of ICD-10-CM diagnosis codes, the documentation should describe the patient's condition, using terminology which includes specific diagnoses as well as symptoms, problems, or reasons for the encounter. There are ICD-10-CM codes to describe all of these.

D. Codes that describe symptoms and signs
Codes that describe symptoms and signs, as opposed to diagnoses, are acceptable for reporting purposes when a diagnosis has not been established (confirmed) by the provider. Chapter 18 of ICD-10-CM, Symptoms, Signs, and Abnormal Clinical and Laboratory Findings Not Elsewhere Classified (codes R00-R99) contain many, but not all codes for symptoms.

E. Encounters for circumstances other than a disease or injury
ICD-10-CM provides codes to deal with encounters for circumstances other than a disease or injury. The Factors Influencing Health Status and Contact with Health Services codes (Z00-Z99) are provided to deal with occasions when circumstances other than a disease or injury are recorded as diagnosis or problems.

See Section I.C.21. Factors influencing health status and contact with health services.

F. Level of Detail in Coding

1. **ICD-10-CM codes with 3, 4, 5, 6 or 7 characters**
   ICD-10-CM is composed of codes with 3, 4, 5, 6 or 7 characters. Codes with three characters are included in ICD-10-CM as the heading of a category of codes that may be further subdivided by the use of fourth, fifth, sixth or seventh characters to provide greater specificity.

2. **Use of full number of characters required for a code**
   A three-character code is to be used only if it is not further subdivided. A code is invalid if it has not been coded to the full number of characters required for that code, including the 7th character, if applicable.

3. **Highest level of specificity**
   Code to the highest level of specificity when supported by the medical record documentation.

G. ICD-10-CM code for the diagnosis, condition, problem, or other reason for encounter/visit
List first the ICD-10-CM code for the diagnosis, condition, problem, or other reason for encounter/visit shown in the medical record to be chiefly responsible for the services provided. List additional codes that describe any coexisting conditions. In some cases, the first-listed diagnosis may be a symptom when a diagnosis has not been established (confirmed) by the provider.

H. Uncertain diagnosis
Do not code diagnoses documented as "probable", "suspected," "questionable," "rule out," "compatible with," "consistent with," or "working diagnosis" or other similar terms indicating uncertainty. Rather, code the condition(s) to the highest degree of certainty for that encounter/visit, such as symptoms, signs, abnormal test results, or other reason for the visit.

Please note: This differs from the coding practices used by short-term, acute care, long-term care and psychiatric hospitals.

I. Chronic diseases
Chronic diseases treated on an ongoing basis may be coded and reported as many times as the patient receives treatment and care for the condition(s)

J. Code all documented conditions that coexist

Code all documented conditions that coexist at the time of the encounter/visit and that require or affect patient care, treatment or management. Do not code conditions that were previously treated and no longer exist. However, history codes (categories Z80-Z87) may be used as secondary codes if the historical condition or family history has an impact on current care or influences treatment.

K. Patients receiving diagnostic services only

For patients receiving diagnostic services only during an encounter/visit, sequence first the diagnosis, condition, problem, or other reason for encounter/visit shown in the medical record to be chiefly responsible for the outpatient services provided during the encounter/visit. Codes for other diagnoses (e.g., chronic conditions) may be sequenced as additional diagnoses.

For encounters for routine laboratory/radiology testing in the absence of any signs, symptoms, or associated diagnosis, assign Z01.89, Encounter for other specified special examinations. If routine testing is performed during the same encounter as a test to evaluate a sign, symptom, or diagnosis, it is appropriate to assign both the Z code and the code describing the reason for the non-routine test.

For outpatient encounters for diagnostic tests that have been interpreted by a physician, and the final report is available at the time of coding, code any confirmed or definitive diagnosis(es) documented in the interpretation. Do not code related signs and symptoms as additional diagnoses.

Please note: This differs from the coding practice in the hospital inpatient setting regarding abnormal findings on test results.

L. Patients receiving therapeutic services only

For patients receiving therapeutic services only during an encounter/visit, sequence first the diagnosis, condition, problem, or other reason for encounter/visit shown in the medical record to be chiefly responsible for the outpatient services provided during the encounter/visit. Codes for other diagnoses (e.g., chronic conditions) may be sequenced as additional diagnoses.

The only exception to this rule is that when the primary reason for the admission/encounter is chemotherapy or radiation therapy, the appropriate Z code for the service is listed first, and the diagnosis or problem for which the service is being performed listed second.

M. Patients receiving preoperative evaluations only

For patients receiving preoperative evaluations only, sequence first a code from subcategory ZØ1.81, Encounter for pre-procedural examinations, to describe the pre-op consultations. Assign a code for the condition to describe the reason for the surgery as an additional diagnosis. Code also any findings related to the pre-op evaluation.

N. Ambulatory surgery

For ambulatory surgery, code the diagnosis for which the surgery was performed. If the postoperative diagnosis is known to be different from the preoperative diagnosis at the time the diagnosis is confirmed, select the postoperative diagnosis for coding, since it is the most definitive.

O. Routine outpatient prenatal visits

See Section I.C.15. Routine outpatient prenatal visits.

P. Encounters for general medical examinations with abnormal findings

The subcategories for encounters for general medical examinations, Z00.0- and encounter for routine child health examination, Z00.12-, provide codes for with and without abnormal findings. Should a general medical examination result in an abnormal finding, the code for general medical examination with abnormal finding should be assigned as the first-listed diagnosis. An examination with abnormal findings refers to a condition/diagnosis that is newly identified or a change in severity of a chronic condition (such as uncontrolled hypertension, or an acute exacerbation of chronic obstructive pulmonary disease) during a routine physical examination. A secondary code for the abnormal finding should also be coded.

Q. Encounters for routine health screenings

See Section I.C.21. Factors influencing health status and contact with health services, Screening

Appendix I. Present on Admission Reporting Guidelines

Introduction

These guidelines are to be used as a supplement to the *ICD-10-CM Official Guidelines for Coding and Reporting* to facilitate the assignment of the Present on Admission (POA) indicator for each diagnosis and external cause of injury code reported on claim forms (UB-04 and 837 Institutional).

These guidelines are not intended to replace any guidelines in the main body of the *ICD-10-CM Official Guidelines for Coding and Reporting*. The POA guidelines are not intended to provide guidance on when a condition should be coded, but rather, how to apply the POA indicator to the final set of diagnosis codes that have been assigned in accordance with Sections I, II, and III of the official coding guidelines. Subsequent to the assignment of the ICD-10-CM codes, the POA indicator should then be assigned to those conditions that have been coded.

As stated in the Introduction to the *ICD-10-CM Official Guidelines for Coding and Reporting*, a joint effort between the healthcare provider and the coder is essential to achieve complete and accurate documentation, code assignment, and reporting of diagnoses and procedures. The importance of consistent, complete documentation in the medical record cannot be overemphasized. Medical record documentation from any provider involved in the care and treatment of the patient may be used to support the determination of whether a condition was present on admission or not. In the context of the official coding guidelines, the term "provider" means a physician or any qualified healthcare practitioner who is legally accountable for establishing the patient's diagnosis.

These guidelines are not a substitute for the provider's clinical judgment as to the determination of whether a condition was/was not present on admission. The provider should be queried regarding issues related to the linking of signs/symptoms, timing of test results, and the timing of findings.

Please see the CDC website for the detailed list of ICD-10-CM codes that do not require the use of a POA indicator **(https://www.cdc.gov/nchs/icd/icd-1Ø-cm/files.html)**. The codes and categories on this exempt list are for circumstances regarding the healthcare encounter or factors influencing health status that do not represent a current disease or injury or that describe conditions that are always present on admission.

General Reporting Requirements

All claims involving inpatient admissions to general acute care hospitals or other facilities that are subject to a law or regulation mandating collection of present on admission information.

Present on admission is defined as present at the time the order for inpatient admission occurs -- conditions that develop during an outpatient encounter, including emergency department, observation, or outpatient surgery, are considered as present on admission.

POA indicator is assigned to principal and secondary diagnoses (as defined in Section II of the Official Guidelines for Coding and Reporting) and the external cause of injury codes.

Issues related to inconsistent, missing, conflicting or unclear documentation must still be resolved by the provider.

If a condition would not be coded and reported based on UHDDS definitions and current official coding guidelines, then the POA indicator would not be reported.

Reporting Options

- Y – Yes
- N – No
- U – Unknown
- W – Clinically undetermined
- Unreported/Not used – (Exempt from POA reporting)

Reporting Definitions

- Y = present at the time of inpatient admission
- N = not present at the time of inpatient admission
- U = documentation is insufficient to determine if condition is present on admission
- W = provider is unable to clinically determine whether condition was present on admission or not

Timeframe for POA Identification and Documentation

There is no required timeframe as to when a provider (per the definition of "provider" used in these guidelines) must identify or document a condition to be present on admission. In some clinical situations, it may not be possible for a provider to make a definitive diagnosis (or a condition may not be recognized or reported by the patient) for a period of time after admission. In some cases, it may be several days before the provider arrives at a definitive diagnosis. This does not mean that the condition was not present on admission. Determination of whether the condition was present on admission or not will be based on the applicable POA guideline as identified in this document, or on the provider's best clinical judgment.

If at the time of code assignment the documentation is unclear as to whether a condition was present on admission or not, it is appropriate to query the provider for clarification.

Assigning the POA Indicator

Condition is on the "Exempt from Reporting" list

Leave the "present on admission" field blank if the condition is on the list of ICD-10-CM codes for which this field is not applicable. This is the only circumstance in which the field may be left blank.

POA Explicitly Documented

Assign Y for any condition the provider explicitly documents as being present on admission.

Assign N for any condition the provider explicitly documents as not present at the time of admission.

Conditions diagnosed prior to inpatient admission

Assign "Y" for conditions that were diagnosed prior to admission (example: hypertension, diabetes mellitus, asthma)

Conditions diagnosed during the admission but clearly present before admission

Assign "Y" for conditions diagnosed during the admission that were clearly present but not diagnosed until after admission occurred.

Diagnoses subsequently confirmed after admission are considered present on admission if at the time of admission they are documented as suspected, possible, rule out, differential diagnosis, or constitute an underlying cause of a symptom that is present at the time of admission.

Condition develops during outpatient encounter prior to inpatient admission

Assign Y for any condition that develops during an outpatient encounter prior to a written order for inpatient admission.

Documentation does not indicate whether condition was present on admission

Assign "U" when the medical record documentation is unclear as to whether the condition was present on admission. "U" should not be routinely assigned and used only in very limited circumstances. Coders are encouraged to query the providers when the documentation is unclear.

Documentation states that it cannot be determined whether the condition was or was not present on admission

Assign "W" when the medical record documentation indicates that it cannot be clinically determined whether or not the condition was present on admission.

Chronic condition with acute exacerbation during the admission

If a single code identifies both the chronic condition and the acute exacerbation, see POA guidelines pertaining to codes that contain multiple clinical concepts.

If a single code only identifies the chronic condition and not the acute exacerbation (e.g., acute exacerbation of chronic leukemia), assign "Y."

Conditions documented as possible, probable, suspected, or rule out at the time of discharge

If the final diagnosis contains a possible, probable, suspected, or rule out diagnosis, and this diagnosis was based on signs, symptoms or clinical findings suspected at the time of inpatient admission, assign "Y."

If the final diagnosis contains a possible, probable, suspected, or rule out diagnosis, and this diagnosis was based on signs, symptoms or clinical findings that were not present on admission, assign "N".

Conditions documented as impending or threatened at the time of discharge

If the final diagnosis contains an impending or threatened diagnosis, and this diagnosis is based on symptoms or clinical findings that were present on admission, assign "Y".

If the final diagnosis contains an impending or threatened diagnosis, and this diagnosis is based on symptoms or clinical findings that were not present on admission, assign "N".

Acute and Chronic Conditions

Assign "Y" for acute conditions that are present at time of admission and N for acute conditions that are not present at time of admission.

Assign "Y" for chronic conditions, even though the condition may not be diagnosed until after admission.

If a single code identifies both an acute and chronic condition, see the POA guidelines for codes that contain multiple clinical concepts.

Codes That Contain Multiple Clinical Concepts

Assign "N" if at least one of the clinical concepts included in the code was not present on admission (e.g., COPD with acute exacerbation and the exacerbation was not present on admission; gastric ulcer that does not start bleeding until after admission; asthma patient develops status asthmaticus after admission).

Assign "Y" if all of the clinical concepts included in the code were present on admission (e.g., duodenal ulcer that perforates prior to admission).

For infection codes that include the causal organism, assign "Y" if the infection (or signs of the infection) were present on admission, even though the culture results may not be known until after admission (e.g., patient is admitted with pneumonia and the provider documents Pseudomonas as the causal organism a few days later).

Same Diagnosis Code for Two or More Conditions

When the same ICD-10-CM diagnosis code applies to two or more conditions during the same encounter (e.g. two separate conditions classified to the same ICD-10-CM diagnosis code):

Assign "Y" if all conditions represented by the single ICD-10-CM code were present on admission (e.g. bilateral unspecified age-related cataracts).

Assign "N" if any of the conditions represented by the single ICD-10-CM code was not present on admission (e.g. traumatic secondary and recurrent hemorrhage and seroma is assigned to a single code T79.2, but only one of the conditions was present on admission).

Obstetrical conditions

Whether or not the patient delivers during the current hospitalization does not affect assignment of the POA indicator. The determining factor for POA assignment is whether the pregnancy complication or obstetrical condition described by the code was present at the time of admission or not.

If the pregnancy complication or obstetrical condition was present on admission (e.g., patient admitted in preterm labor), assign "Y".

If the pregnancy complication or obstetrical condition was not present on admission (e.g., 2nd degree laceration during delivery, postpartum hemorrhage that occurred during current hospitalization, fetal distress develops after admission), assign "N".

If the obstetrical code includes more than one diagnosis and any of the diagnoses identified by the code were not present on admission assign "N". (e.g., Category O11, Pre-existing hypertension with pre-eclampsia)

Perinatal conditions

Newborns are not considered to be admitted until after birth. Therefore, any condition present at birth or that developed in utero is considered present at admission and should be assigned "Y". This includes conditions that occur during delivery (e.g., injury during delivery, meconium aspiration, exposure to streptococcus B in the vaginal canal).

Congenital conditions and anomalies

Assign "Y" for congenital conditions and anomalies except for categories QØØ-Q99, Congenital anomalies, which are on the exempt list. Congenital conditions are always considered present on admission.

External cause of injury codes

Assign "Y" for any external cause code representing an external cause of morbidity that occurred prior to inpatient admission (e.g., patient fell out of bed at home, patient fell out of bed in emergency room prior to admission)

Assign "N" for any external cause code representing an external cause of morbidity that occurred during inpatient hospitalization (e.g., patient fell out of hospital bed during hospital stay, patient experienced an adverse reaction to a medication administered after inpatient admission).

Obstetrical Conditions

Congenital conditions and anomalies

External cause of injury codes

Appendix C. 2025 ICD-10-PCS Official Guidelines for Coding and Reporting

Narrative changes effective October 1, 2024 appear in **bold** text.

Narrative changes effective April 1, 2024 appear in shaded text.

The Centers for Medicare and Medicaid Services (CMS) and the National Center for Health Statistics (NCHS), two departments within the U.S. Federal Government's Department of Health and Human Services (DHHS) provide the following guidelines for coding and reporting using the International Classification of Diseases, 10th Revision, Procedure Coding System (ICD-10-PCS). These guidelines should be used as a companion document to the official version of the ICD-10-PCS as published on the CMS website. The ICD-10-PCS is a procedure classification published by the United States for classifying procedures performed in hospital inpatient health care settings.

These guidelines have been approved by the four organizations that make up the Cooperating Parties for the ICD-10-PCS: the American Hospital Association (AHA), the American Health Information Management Association (AHIMA), CMS, and NCHS.

These guidelines are a set of rules that have been developed to accompany and complement the official conventions and instructions provided within the ICD-10-PCS itself. They are intended to provide direction that is applicable in most circumstances. However, there may be unique circumstances where exceptions are applied. The instructions and conventions of the classification take precedence over guidelines. These guidelines are based on the coding and sequencing instructions in the Tables, Index and Definitions of ICD-10-PCS, but provide additional instruction. Adherence to these guidelines when assigning ICD-10-PCS procedure codes is required under the Health Insurance Portability and Accountability Act (HIPAA). The procedure codes have been adopted under HIPAA for hospital inpatient healthcare settings. A joint effort between the healthcare provider and the coder is essential to achieve complete and accurate documentation, code assignment, and reporting of diagnoses and procedures. These guidelines have been developed to assist both the healthcare provider and the coder in identifying those procedures that are to be reported. The importance of consistent, complete documentation in the medical record cannot be overemphasized. Without such documentation accurate coding cannot be achieved.

Conventions

A1. ICD-10-PCS codes are composed of seven characters. Each character is an axis of classification that specifies information about the procedure performed. Within a defined code range, a character specifies the same type of information in that axis of classification.

Example:
The fifth axis of classification specifies the approach in sections Ø through 4 and 7 through 9 of the system.

A2. One of 34 possible values can be assigned to each axis of classification in the seven-character code: they are the numbers Ø through 9 and the alphabet (except I and O because they are easily confused with the numbers 1 and Ø). The number of unique values used in an axis of classification differs as needed.

Example:
Where the fifth axis of classification specifies the approach, seven different approach values are currently used to specify the approach.

A3. The valid values for an axis of classification can be added to as needed.

Example:
If a significantly distinct type of device is used in a new procedure, a new device value can be added to the system.

A4. As with words in their context, the meaning of any single value is a combination of its axis of classification and any preceding values on which it may be dependent.

Example:
The meaning of a body part value in the Medical and Surgical section is always dependent on the body system value. The body part value Ø in the Central Nervous body system specifies Brain and the body part value Ø in the Peripheral Nervous body system specifies Cervical Plexus.

A5. As the system is expanded to become increasingly detailed, over time more values will depend on preceding values for their meaning.

Example:
In the Lower Joints body system, the device value 3 in the root operation Insertion specifies Infusion Device and the device value 3 in the root operation Replacement specifies Ceramic Synthetic Substitute.

A6. The purpose of the alphabetic index is to locate the appropriate table that contains all information necessary to construct a procedure code. The PCS Tables should always be consulted to find the most appropriate valid code.

A7. It is not required to consult the index first before proceeding to the tables to complete the code. A valid code may be chosen directly from the tables.

A8. All seven characters must be specified to be a valid code. If the documentation is incomplete for coding purposes, the physician should be queried for the necessary information.

A9. Within a PCS table, valid codes include all combinations of choices in characters 4 through 7 contained in the same row of the table. In the example below, ØJHT3VZ is a valid code, and ØJHW3VZ is *not* a valid code.

Section: Ø **Medical and Surgical**
Body System: J **Subcutaneous Tissue and Fascia**
Operation: H **Insertion** Putting in a nonbiological appliance that monitors, assists, performs, or prevents a physiological function but does not physically take the place of a body part

Body Part	Approach	Device	Qualifier
S Subcutaneous Tissue and Fascia, Head and Neck **V** Subcutaneous Tissue and Fascia, Upper Extremity **W** Subcutaneous Tissue and Fascia, Lower Extremity	**Ø** Open **3** Percutaneous	**1** Radioactive Element **3** Infusion Device **Y** Other Device	**Z** No Qualifier
T Subcutaneous Tissue and Fascia, Trunk	**Ø** Open **3** Percutaneous	**1** Radioactive Element **3** Infusion Device **V** Infusion Pump **Y** Other Device	**Z** No Qualifier

A1Ø. "And," when used in a code description, means "and/or," except when used to describe a combination of multiple body parts for which separate values exist for each body part (e.g., Skin and Subcutaneous Tissue used as a qualifier, where there are separate body part values for "Skin" and "Subcutaneous Tissue").

Example:
Lower Arm and Wrist Muscle means lower arm and/or wrist muscle.

A11. Many of the terms used to construct PCS codes are defined within the system. It is the coder's responsibility to determine what the documentation in the medical record equates to in the PCS definitions. The physician is not expected to use the terms used in PCS code descriptions, nor is the coder required to query the physician when the correlation between the documentation and the defined PCS terms is clear.

Example:
When the physician documents "partial resection" the coder can independently correlate "partial resection" to the root operation Excision without querying the physician for clarification.

Medical and Surgical Section Guidelines (section Ø)

B2. Body System

General guidelines

B2.1a. The procedure codes in Anatomical Regions, General, Anatomical Regions, Upper Extremities and Anatomical Regions, Lower Extremities can be used when the procedure is performed on an anatomical region rather than a specific body part, or on the rare occasion when no information is available to support assignment of a code to a specific body part.

Examples:
Chest tube drainage of the pleural cavity is coded to the root operation Drainage found in the body system Anatomical Regions, General.

Suture repair of the abdominal wall is coded to the root operation Repair in the body system Anatomical Regions, General.

Amputation of the foot is coded to the root operation Detachment in the body system Anatomical Regions, Lower Extremities.

B2.1b. Where the general body part values "upper" and "lower" are provided as an option in the Upper Arteries, Lower Arteries, Upper Veins, Lower Veins, Muscles and Tendons body systems, "upper" or "lower" specifies body parts located above or below the diaphragm respectively.

Example:
Vein body parts above the diaphragm are found in the Upper Veins body system; vein body parts below the diaphragm are found in the Lower Veins body system.

B3. Root Operation

General guidelines

B3.1a. In order to determine the appropriate root operation, the full definition of the root operation as contained in the PCS Tables must be applied.

B3.1b. Components of a procedure specified in the root operation definition or explanation as integral to that root operation are not coded separately. Procedural steps necessary to reach the operative site and close the operative site, including anastomosis of a tubular body part, are also not coded separately.

Examples:
Resection of a joint as part of a joint replacement procedure is included in the root operation definition of Replacement and is not coded separately.

Laparotomy performed to reach the site of an open liver biopsy is not coded separately.

In a resection of sigmoid colon with anastomosis of descending colon to rectum, the anastomosis is not coded separately.

Multiple procedures

B3.2. During the same operative episode, multiple procedures are coded if:

a. The same root operation is performed on different body parts as defined by distinct values of the body part character.

   Examples:
   Diagnostic excision of liver and pancreas are coded separately.

   Excision of lesion in the ascending colon and excision of lesion in the transverse colon are coded separately.

b. The same root operation is repeated in multiple body parts, and those body parts are separate and distinct body parts classified to a single ICD-10-PCS body part value.

   Examples:
   Excision of the sartorius muscle and excision of the gracilis muscle are both included in the upper leg muscle body part value, and multiple procedures are coded.

   Extraction of multiple toenails are coded separately.

c. Multiple root operations with distinct objectives are performed on the same body part.

   Example:
   Destruction of sigmoid lesion and bypass of sigmoid colon are coded separately.

d. The intended root operation is attempted using one approach but is converted to a different approach.

   Example:
   Laparoscopic cholecystectomy converted to an open cholecystectomy is coded as percutaneous endoscopic Inspection and open Resection.

Discontinued or incomplete procedures

B3.3. If the intended procedure is discontinued or otherwise not completed, code the procedure to the root operation performed. If a procedure is discontinued before any other root operation is performed, code the root operation Inspection of the body part or anatomical region inspected.

Example:
A planned aortic valve replacement procedure is discontinued after the initial thoracotomy and before any incision is made in the heart muscle, when the patient becomes hemodynamically unstable. This procedure is coded as an open Inspection of the mediastinum.

Biopsy procedures

B3.4a. Biopsy procedures are coded using the root operations Excision, Extraction, or Drainage and the qualifier Diagnostic.

Examples:
Fine needle aspiration biopsy of fluid in the lung is coded to the root operation Drainage with the qualifier Diagnostic.

Biopsy of bone marrow is coded to the root operation Extraction with the qualifier Diagnostic.

Lymph node sampling for biopsy is coded to the root operation Excision with the qualifier Diagnostic.

Biopsy followed by more definitive treatment

B3.4b. If a diagnostic Excision, Extraction, or Drainage procedure (biopsy) is followed by a more definitive procedure, such as Destruction, Excision or Resection at the same procedure site, both the biopsy and the more definitive treatment are coded.

Example:
Biopsy of breast followed by partial mastectomy at the same procedure site, both the biopsy and the partial mastectomy procedure are coded.

Overlapping body layers

B3.5. If root operations such as Excision, Extraction, Repair or Inspection are performed on overlapping layers of the musculoskeletal system, the body part specifying the deepest layer is coded.

Example:
Excisional debridement that includes skin and subcutaneous tissue and muscle is coded to the muscle body part.

Bypass procedures

B3.6a. Bypass procedures are coded by identifying the body part bypassed "from" and the body part bypassed "to." The fourth character body part specifies the body part bypassed from, and the qualifier specifies the body part bypassed to.

Example:
Bypass from stomach to jejunum, stomach is the body part and jejunum is the qualifier.

B3.6b. Coronary artery bypass procedures are coded differently than other bypass procedures as described in the previous guideline. Rather than identifying the body part bypassed from, the body part identifies the number of coronary arteries bypassed to, and the qualifier specifies the vessel bypassed from.

Example:
Aortocoronary artery bypass of the left anterior descending coronary artery and the obtuse marginal coronary artery is classified in the body part axis of classification as two coronary arteries, and the qualifier specifies the aorta as the body part bypassed from.

B3.6c. If multiple coronary arteries are bypassed, a separate procedure is coded for each coronary artery that uses a different device and/or qualifier.

Example:
Aortocoronary artery bypass and internal mammary coronary artery bypass are coded separately.

Control vs. more specific root operations

B3.7. The root operation Control is defined as, "Stopping, or attempting to stop, postprocedural or other acute bleeding." Control is the root operation coded when the procedure performed to achieve hemostasis, beyond what would be considered integral to a procedure, utilizes techniques (e.g. cautery, application of substances or pressure, suturing or ligation or clipping of bleeding points at the site) that are not described by a more specific root operation definition, such as Bypass, Detachment, Excision, Extraction, Reposition, Replacement, or Resection. If a more specific root operation definition applies to the procedure performed, then the more specific root operation is coded instead of Control.

Example:
Silver nitrate cautery to treat acute nasal bleeding is coded to the root operation Control.

Example:
Liquid embolization of the right internal iliac artery to treat acute hematoma by stopping blood flow is coded to the root operation Occlusion.

Example:
Suctioning of residual blood to achieve hemostasis during a transbronchial cryobiopsy is considered integral to the cryobiopsy procedure and is not coded separately.

Excision vs. Resection

B3.8. PCS contains specific body parts for anatomical subdivisions of a body part, such as lobes of the lungs or liver and regions of the intestine. Resection of the specific body part is coded whenever all of the body part is cut out or off, rather than coding Excision of a less specific body part.

Example:
Left upper lung lobectomy is coded to Resection of Upper Lung Lobe, Left rather than Excision of Lung, Left.

Excision for graft

B3.9. If an autograft is obtained from a different procedure site in order to complete the objective of the procedure, a separate procedure is coded, except when the seventh character qualifier value in the ICD-10-PCS table fully specifies the site from which the autograft was obtained.

Examples:
Coronary bypass with excision of saphenous vein graft, excision of saphenous vein is coded separately.

Replacement of breast with autologous deep inferior epigastric artery perforator (DIEP) flap, excision of the DIEP flap is not coded separately. The seventh character qualifier value Deep Inferior Epigastric Artery Perforator Flap in the Replacement table fully specifies the site of the autograft harvest.

Fusion procedures of the spine

B3.1Øa. The body part coded for a spinal vertebral joint(s) rendered immobile by a spinal fusion procedure is classified by the level of the spine (e.g. thoracic). There are distinct body part values for a single vertebral joint and for multiple vertebral joints at each spinal level.

Example:
Body part values specify Lumbar Vertebral Joint, Lumbar Vertebral Joints, 2 or More and Lumbosacral Vertebral Joint.

B3.1Øb. If multiple vertebral joints are fused, a separate procedure is coded for each vertebral joint that uses a different device and/or qualifier.

Example:
Fusion of lumbar vertebral joint, posterior approach, anterior column and fusion of lumbar vertebral joint, posterior approach, posterior column are coded separately.

B3.1Øc. Combinations of devices and materials are often used on a vertebral joint to render the joint immobile. When combinations of devices are used on the same vertebral joint, the device value coded for the procedure is as follows:

- If an interbody fusion device is used to render the joint immobile (containing bone graft or bone graft substitute), the procedure is coded with the device value Interbody Fusion Device
- If bone graft is the *only* device used to render the joint immobile, the procedure is coded with the device value Nonautologous Tissue Substitute or Autologous Tissue Substitute
- If a mixture of autologous and nonautologous bone graft (with or without biological or synthetic extenders or binders) is used to render the joint immobile, code the procedure with the device value Autologous Tissue Substitute

Examples:
Fusion of a vertebral joint using a cage style interbody fusion device containing morsellized bone graft is coded to the device Interbody Fusion Device.

Fusion of a vertebral joint using a bone dowel interbody fusion device made of cadaver bone and packed with a mixture of local morsellized bone and demineralized bone matrix is coded to the device Interbody Fusion Device.

Fusion of a vertebral joint using both autologous bone graft and bone bank bone graft is coded to the device Autologous Tissue Substitute.

Inspection procedures

B3.11a. Inspection of a body part(s) performed in order to achieve the objective of a procedure is not coded separately.

Example:
Fiberoptic bronchoscopy performed for irrigation of bronchus, only the irrigation procedure is coded.

B3.11b. If multiple tubular body parts are inspected, the most distal body part (the body part furthest from the starting point of the inspection) is coded. If multiple non-tubular body parts in a region are inspected, the body part that specifies the entire area inspected is coded.

Examples:
Cystoureteroscopy with inspection of bladder and ureters is coded to the ureter body part value.

Exploratory laparotomy with general inspection of abdominal contents is coded to the peritoneal cavity body part value.

B3.11c. When both an Inspection procedure and another procedure are performed on the same body part during the same episode, if the Inspection procedure is performed using a different approach than the other procedure, the Inspection procedure is coded separately.

Example:
Endoscopic Inspection of the duodenum is coded separately when open Excision of the duodenum is performed during the same procedural episode.

Occlusion vs. Restriction for vessel embolization procedures

B3.12. If the objective of an embolization procedure is to completely close a vessel, the root operation Occlusion is coded. If the objective of an embolization procedure is to narrow the lumen of a vessel, the root operation Restriction is coded.

Examples:
Tumor embolization is coded to the root operation Occlusion, because the objective of the procedure is to cut off the blood supply to the vessel.

Embolization of a cerebral aneurysm is coded to the root operation Restriction, because the objective of the procedure is not to close off the vessel entirely, but to narrow the lumen of the vessel at the site of the aneurysm where it is abnormally wide.

Release procedures

B3.13. In the root operation Release, the body part value coded is the body part being freed and not the tissue being manipulated or cut to free the body part.

Example:
Lysis of intestinal adhesions is coded to the specific intestine body part value.

Release vs. Division

B3.14. If the sole objective of the procedure is freeing a body part without cutting the body part, the root operation is Release. If the sole objective of the procedure is separating or transecting a body part, the root operation is Division.

Examples:
Freeing a nerve root from surrounding scar tissue to relieve pain is coded to the root operation Release.

Severing a nerve root to relieve pain is coded to the root operation Division.

Reposition for fracture treatment

B3.15. Reduction of a displaced fracture is coded to the root operation Reposition and the application of a cast or splint in conjunction with the Reposition procedure is not coded separately. Treatment of a nondisplaced fracture is coded to the procedure performed.

Examples:
Casting of a nondisplaced fracture is coded to the root operation Immobilization in the Placement section.

Putting a pin in a nondisplaced fracture is coded to the root operation Insertion.

Transplantation vs. Administration

B3.16. Putting in a mature and functioning living body part taken from another individual or animal is coded to the root operation Transplantation. Putting in autologous or nonautologous cells is coded to the Administration section.

Example:
Putting in autologous or nonautologous bone marrow, pancreatic islet cells or stem cells is coded to the Administration section.

Transfer procedures using multiple tissue layers

B3.17. The root operation Transfer contains qualifiers that can be used to specify when a transfer flap is composed of more than one tissue layer, such as a musculocutaneous flap. For procedures involving transfer of multiple tissue layers including skin, subcutaneous tissue, fascia or muscle, the procedure is coded to the body part value that describes the deepest tissue layer in the flap, and the qualifier can be used to describe the other tissue layer(s) in the transfer flap.

Example:
A musculocutaneous flap transfer is coded to the appropriate body part value in the body system Muscles, and the qualifier is used to describe the additional tissue layer(s) in the transfer flap.

Excision/Resection followed by replacement

B3.18. If an excision or resection of a body part is followed by a replacement procedure, code both procedures to identify each distinct objective, except when the excision or resection is considered integral and preparatory for the replacement procedure.

Examples:
Mastectomy followed by reconstruction, both resection and replacement of the breast are coded to fully capture the distinct objectives of the procedures performed.

Maxillectomy with obturator reconstruction, both excision and replacement of the maxilla are coded to fully capture the distinct objectives of the procedures performed.

Excisional debridement of tendon with skin graft, both the excision of the tendon and the replacement of the skin with a graft are coded to fully capture the distinct objectives of the procedures performed.

Esophagectomy followed by reconstruction with colonic interposition, both the resection and the transfer of the large intestine to function as the esophagus are coded to fully capture the distinct objectives of the procedures performed.

Examples:
Resection of a joint as part of a joint replacement procedure is considered integral and preparatory for the replacement of the joint and the resection is not coded separately.

Resection of a valve as part of a valve replacement procedure is considered integral and preparatory for the valve replacement and the resection is not coded separately.

Detachment procedures of extremities

B3.19. The root operation Detachment contains qualifiers that can be used to specify the level where the extremity was amputated. These qualifiers are dependent on the body part value in the "upper extremities" and "lower extremities" body systems. For procedures involving the detachment of all or part of the upper or lower extremities, the procedure is coded to the body part value that describes the site of the detachment.

Example:
An amputation at the proximal portion of the shaft of the tibia and fibula is coded to the Lower leg body part value in the body system Anatomical Regions, Lower Extremities, and the qualifier High is used to specify the level where the extremity was detached.

The following definitions were developed for the Detachment qualifiers

Body Part	Qualifier	Definition
Upper arm and upper leg	1	High: Amputation at the proximal portion of the shaft of the humerus or femur
	2	Mid: Amputation at the middle portion of the shaft of the humerus or femur
	3	Low: Amputation at the distal portion of the shaft of the humerus or femur
Lower arm and lower leg	1	High: Amputation at the proximal portion of the shaft of the radius/ulna or tibia/fibula
	2	Mid: Amputation at the middle portion of the shaft of the radius/ulna or tibia/fibula
	3	Low: Amputation at the distal portion of the shaft of the radius/ulna or tibia/fibula
Hand and Foot	0	Complete*
	4	Complete 1st Ray
	5	Complete 2nd Ray
	6	Complete 3rd Ray
	7	Complete 4th Ray
	8	Complete 5th Ray
	9	Partial 1st Ray
	B	Partial 2nd Ray
	C	Partial 3rd Ray
	D	Partial 4th Ray
	F	Partial 5th Ray
Thumb, finger, or toe	0	Complete: Amputation at the metacarpophalangeal/metatarsal-phalangeal joint
	1	High: Amputation anywhere along the proximal phalanx
	2	Mid: Amputation through the proximal interphalangeal joint or anywhere along the middle phalanx
	3	Low: Amputation through the distal interphalangeal joint or anywhere along the distal phalanx

*When coding amputation of Hand and Foot, the following definitions are followed:

- Complete: Amputation through the carpometacarpal joint of the hand, or through the tarsal-metatarsal joint of the foot.
- Partial: Amputation anywhere along the shaft or head of the metacarpal bone of the hand, or of the metatarsal bone of the foot.

B4. Body Part

General guidelines

B4.1a. If a procedure is performed on a portion of a body part that does not have a separate body part value, code the body part value corresponding to the whole body part.

Example:
A procedure performed on the alveolar process of the mandible is coded to the mandible body part.

B4.1b. If the prefix "peri" is combined with a body part to identify the site of the procedure, and the site of the procedure is not further specified, then the procedure is coded to the body part named. This guideline applies only when a more specific body part value is not available.

Examples:
A procedure site identified as perirenal is coded to the kidney body part when the site of the procedure is not further specified.

A procedure site described in the documentation as peri-urethral, and the documentation also indicates that it is the vulvar tissue and not the urethral tissue that is the site of the procedure, then the procedure is coded to the vulva body part.

A procedure site documented as involving the periosteum is coded to the corresponding bone body part.

B4.1c. If a single vascular procedure is performed on a continuous section of an arterial or venous body part, code the body part value corresponding to the anatomically most proximal (closest to the heart) portion of the arterial or venous body part.

Example:
A procedure performed on a continuous section of artery from the femoral artery to the external iliac artery with the point of entry at the femoral artery is coded to the external iliac body part.

A procedure performed on a continuous section of artery from the femoral artery to the external iliac artery with the point of entry at the external iliac artery is also coded to the external iliac artery body part.

Branches of body parts

B4.2. Where a specific branch of a body part does not have its own body part value in PCS, the body part is typically coded to the closest proximal branch that has a specific body part value. In the cardiovascular body systems, if a general body part is available in the correct root operation table, and coding to a proximal branch would require assigning a code in a different body system, the procedure is coded using the general body part value.

Examples:
A procedure performed on the mandibular branch of the trigeminal nerve is coded to the trigeminal nerve body part value.

Occlusion of the bronchial artery is coded to the body part value Upper Artery in the body system Upper Arteries, and not to the body part value Thoracic Aorta, Descending in the body system Heart and Great Vessels.

Bilateral body part values

B4.3. Bilateral body part values are available for a limited number of body parts. If the identical procedure is performed on contralateral body parts, and a bilateral body part value exists for that body part, a single procedure is coded using the bilateral body part value. If no bilateral body part value exists, each procedure is coded separately using the appropriate body part value.

Examples:
The identical procedure performed on both fallopian tubes is coded once using the body part value Fallopian Tube, Bilateral.

The identical procedure performed on both knee joints is coded twice using the body part values Knee Joint, Right and Knee Joint, Left.

Coronary arteries

B4.4. The coronary arteries are classified as a single body part that is further specified by number of arteries treated. One procedure code specifying multiple arteries is used when the same procedure is performed, including the same device and qualifier values.

Examples:
Angioplasty of two distinct coronary arteries with placement of two stents is coded as Dilation of Coronary Artery, Two Arteries with Two Intraluminal Devices.

Angioplasty of two distinct coronary arteries, one with stent placed and one without, is coded separately as Dilation of Coronary Artery, One Artery with Intraluminal Device, and Dilation of Coronary Artery, One Artery with no device.

Tendons, ligaments, bursae and fascia near a joint

B4.5. Procedures performed on tendons, ligaments, bursae and fascia supporting a joint are coded to the body part in the respective body system that is the focus of the procedure. Procedures performed on joint structures themselves are coded to the body part in the joint body systems.

Examples:
Repair of the anterior cruciate ligament of the knee is coded to the knee bursa and ligament body part in the bursae and ligaments body system.

Knee arthroscopy with shaving of articular cartilage is coded to the knee joint body part in the Lower Joints body system.

Skin, subcutaneous tissue and fascia overlying a joint

B4.6. If a procedure is performed on the skin, subcutaneous tissue or fascia overlying a joint, the procedure is coded to the following body part:

- Shoulder is coded to Upper Arm
- Elbow is coded to Lower Arm
- Wrist is coded to Lower Arm
- Hip is coded to Upper Leg
- Knee is coded to Lower Leg
- Ankle is coded to Foot

Fingers and toes

B4.7. If a body system does not contain a separate body part value for fingers, procedures performed on the fingers are coded to the body part value for the hand. If a body system does not contain a separate body part value for toes, procedures performed on the toes are coded to the body part value for the foot.

Example:
Excision of finger muscle is coded to one of the hand muscle body part values in the Muscles body system.

Upper and lower intestinal tract

B4.8. In the Gastrointestinal body system, the general body part values Upper Intestinal Tract and Lower Intestinal Tract are provided as an option for the root operations such as Change, Insertion, Inspection, Removal and Revision. Upper Intestinal Tract includes the portion of the gastrointestinal tract from the esophagus down to and including the duodenum, and Lower Intestinal Tract includes the portion of the gastrointestinal tract from the jejunum down to and including the rectum and anus.

Example:
In the root operation Change table, change of a device in the jejunum is coded using the body part Lower Intestinal Tract.

B5. Approach

Open approach with percutaneous endoscopic assistance

B5.2a. Procedures performed using the open approach with percutaneous endoscopic assistance are coded to the approach Open.

Example:
Laparoscopic-assisted sigmoidectomy is coded to the approach Open.

Percutaneous endoscopic approach with hand-assistance or extension of incision

B5.2b. Procedures performed using the percutaneous endoscopic approach, with hand-assistance, or with an incision or extension of an incision to assist in the removal of all or a portion of a body part, or to anastomose a tubular body part with or without the temporary exteriorization of a body structure, are coded to the approach value Percutaneous Endoscopic.

Examples:
Hand-assisted laparoscopic sigmoid colon resection with exteriorization of a segment of the colon for removal of specimen with return of colon back into abdominal cavity is coded to the approach value percutaneous endoscopic.

Laparoscopic sigmoid colectomy with extension of stapling port for removal of specimen and direct anastomosis is coded to the approach value percutaneous endoscopic.

Laparoscopic nephrectomy with midline incision for removing the resected kidney is coded to the approach value percutaneous endoscopic.

Robotic-assisted laparoscopic prostatectomy with extension of incision for removal of the resected prostate is coded to the approach value percutaneous endoscopic.

External approach

B5.3a. Procedures performed within an orifice on structures that are visible without the aid of any instrumentation are coded to the approach External.

Example:
Resection of tonsils is coded to the approach External.

B5.3b. Procedures performed indirectly by the application of external force through the intervening body layers are coded to the approach External.

Example:
Closed reduction of fracture is coded to the approach External.

Percutaneous procedure via device

B5.4. Procedures performed percutaneously via a device placed for the procedure are coded to the approach Percutaneous.

Example:
Fragmentation of kidney stone performed via percutaneous nephrostomy is coded to the approach Percutaneous.

B6. Device

General guidelines

B6.1a. A device is coded only if a device remains after the procedure is completed. If no device remains, the device value No Device is coded. In limited root operations, the classification provides the qualifier values Temporary and Intraoperative, for specific procedures involving clinically significant devices, where the purpose of the device is to be utilized for a brief duration during the procedure or current inpatient stay. If a device that is intended to remain after the procedure is completed requires removal before the end of the operative episode in which it was inserted, both the insertion and removal of the device should be coded.

B6.1b. Materials such as sutures, ligatures, radiological markers and temporary post-operative wound drains are considered integral to the performance of a procedure and are not coded as devices.

B6.1c. Procedures performed on a device only and not on a body part are specified in the root operations Change, Irrigation, Removal and Revision, and are coded to the procedure performed.

Example:
Irrigation of percutaneous nephrostomy tube is coded to the root operation Irrigation of indwelling device in the Administration section.

Drainage device

B6.2. A separate procedure to put in a drainage device is coded to the root operation Drainage with the device value Drainage Device.

Obstetric Section Guidelines (section 1)

C. Obstetrics Section

Products of conception

C1. Procedures performed on the products of conception are coded to the Obstetrics section. Procedures performed on the pregnant female other than the products of conception are coded to the appropriate root operation in the Medical and Surgical section.

Examples:
Amniocentesis is coded to the products of conception body part in the Obstetrics section.

Repair of obstetric urethral laceration is coded to the urethra body part in the Medical and Surgical section.

Procedures following delivery or abortion

C2. Procedures performed following a delivery or abortion for curettage of the endometrium or evacuation of retained products of conception are all coded in the Obstetrics section, to the root operation Extraction and the body part Products of Conception, Retained.

Diagnostic or therapeutic dilation and curettage performed during times other than the postpartum or post-abortion period are all coded in the Medical and Surgical section, to the root operation Extraction and the body part Endometrium.

Radiation Therapy Section Guidelines (section D)

D. Radiation Therapy Section

Brachytherapy

D1.a. Brachytherapy is coded to the modality Brachytherapy in the Radiation Therapy section. When a radioactive brachytherapy source is left in the body at the end of the procedure, it is coded separately to the root operation Insertion with the device value Radioactive Element.

Example:
Brachytherapy with implantation of a low dose rate brachytherapy source left in the body at the end of the procedure is coded to the applicable treatment site in section D, Radiation Therapy, with the modality Brachytherapy, the modality qualifier value Low Dose Rate, and the applicable isotope value and qualifier value. The implantation of the brachytherapy source is coded separately to the device value Radioactive Element in the appropriate Insertion table of the Medical and Surgical section. The Radiation Therapy section code identifies the specific modality and isotope of the brachytherapy, and the root operation Insertion code identifies the implantation of the brachytherapy source that remains in the body at the end of the procedure.

Exceptions:
Implantation of Cesium-131 brachytherapy seeds embedded in a collagen matrix to the treatment site after resection of brain tumor is coded to the root operation Insertion with the device value Radioactive Element, Cesium-131 Collagen

Implant. Similarly, implantation of Palladium-103 brachytherapy seeds embedded in a collagen matrix to the treatment site after resection of brain tumor is coded to the root operation Insertion with the device value Radioactive Element, Palladium-103 Collagen Implant. These procedures are coded to the root operation Insertion only, because the device value identifies both the implantation of the radioactive element and a specific brachytherapy isotope.

D1.b. A separate procedure to place a temporary applicator for delivering the brachytherapy is coded to the root operation Insertion and the device value Other Device.

Examples:
Intrauterine brachytherapy applicator placed as a separate procedure from the brachytherapy procedure is coded to Insertion of Other Device, and the brachytherapy is coded separately using the modality Brachytherapy in the Radiation Therapy section.

Intrauterine brachytherapy applicator placed concomitantly with delivery of the brachytherapy dose is coded with a single code using the modality Brachytherapy in the Radiation Therapy section.

New Technology Section Guidelines (section X)

E. New Technology Section

General guidelines

E1.a. Section X codes fully represent the specific procedure described in the code title, and do not require additional codes from other sections of ICD-10-PCS. When section X contains a code title which fully describes a specific new technology procedure, and it is the only procedure performed, only the section X code is reported for the procedure. There is no need to report an additional code in another section of ICD-10-PCS.

Example:
XWØ43A6 Introduction of Cefiderocol Anti-infective into Central Vein, Percutaneous Approach, New Technology Group 6, can be coded to indicate that Cefiderocol Anti-infective was administered via a central vein. A separate code from table 3EØ in the Administration section of ICD-10-PCS is not coded in addition to this code.

E1.b. When multiple procedures are performed, New Technology section X codes are coded following the multiple procedures guideline.

Examples:
Dual filter cerebral embolic filtration used during transcatheter aortic valve replacement (TAVR), X2A5312 Cerebral Embolic Filtration, Dual Filter in Innominate Artery and Left Common Carotid Artery, Percutaneous Approach, New Technology Group 2, is coded for the cerebral embolic filtration, along with an ICD-10-PCS code for the TAVR procedure.

An extracorporeal flow reversal circuit for embolic neuroprotection placed during a transcarotid arterial revascularization procedure, a code from table X2A, Assistance of the Cardiovascular System is coded for the use of the extracorporeal flow reversal circuit, along with an ICD-10-PCS code for the transcarotid arterial revascularization procedure.

F. Selection of Principal Procedure

The following instructions should be applied in the selection of principal procedure and clarification on the importance of the relation to the principal diagnosis when more than one procedure is performed:

1. Procedure performed for definitive treatment of both principal diagnosis and secondary diagnosis
   a. Sequence procedure performed for definitive treatment most related to principal diagnosis as principal procedure.
2. Procedure performed for definitive treatment and diagnostic procedures performed for both principal diagnosis and secondary diagnosis.
   a. Sequence procedure performed for definitive treatment most related to principal diagnosis as principal procedure
3. A diagnostic procedure was performed for the principal diagnosis and a procedure is performed for definitive treatment of a secondary diagnosis.
   a. Sequence diagnostic procedure as principal procedure, since the procedure most related to the principal diagnosis takes precedence.
4. No procedures performed that are related to principal diagnosis; procedures performed for definitive treatment and diagnostic procedures were performed for secondary diagnosis
   a. Sequence procedure performed for definitive treatment of secondary diagnosis as principal procedure, since there are no procedures (definitive or nondefinitive treatment) related to principal diagnosis.

Appendix D. Abnormal EKGs

This section lists commonly overlooked abnormal findings on EKG reports that may have potential to affect MS-DRG assignment. To assist the coder in determining if a CC or MCC condition exists, possible conditions associated with the abnormality, signs and symptoms that may be present, and drugs that may be used to treat the condition are included in this section. According to coding guidelines, the CCs and MCCs must affect patient care in terms of requiring clinical evaluation; therapeutic treatment; further evaluation by diagnostic studies, procedures, or consultation; extended length of stay; or increased nursing care; and/or monitoring for reporting purposes.

Abnormal Tracing Documentation

Atrioventricular (AV) block, complete Third degree AV block.	**Definition:** Electrical impulses passing from the atria to the ventricles are blocked at the AV node. The atria and ventricles become completely dissociated and beat independently of one another. Also referred to as complete AV block, complete heart block, complete atrioventricular dissociation, third degree AV block. **Signs and Symptoms:** Lethargy, postural hypotension, shortness of breath, syncope, dizziness, or acute heart failure. Complete heart block usually results from infections; rheumatic fever, fibrosis, or scarring from a myocardial infarction, digitalis toxicity, or congenital abnormalities. **Treatment:** Discontinuation of digitalis when the underlying cause is due to digitalis toxicity, atropine, or artificial pacemaker for temporary or permanent use.
Mobitz (type) II atrioventricular block Incomplete atrioventricular block: Mobitz (type) II second degree, Mobitz (type) II	**Definition:** Every second, third, or fourth electrical impulse from the atria to the ventricles is blocked at the AV node. **Signs and Symptoms:** Lethargy, postural hypotension, shortness of breath, syncope, or dizziness. Second degree heart block often occurs in arteriosclerotic heart disease, and sometimes results from digitalis toxicity. **Treatment:** Discontinuation of digitalis when the underlying cause is due to digitalis toxicity, atropine, or artificial pacemaker for temporary or permanent use.
Other bilateral bundle branch block Bifascicular block NOS Bilateral bundle branch block NOS Right bundle branch with left bundle branch block [incomplete] [main stem]	**Definition:** Disturbance in the electrical system (branches of the bundle of HIS) in the ventricles of the heart. The electrical impulses do not pass through the electrical system because of a block in the right or left bundle branch, resulting in the impulse traveling through the ventricular heart muscle itself. Associated abbreviations are RBB, LBB, BBB. **Signs and Symptoms:** Bundle branch block overall is considered a benign arrhythmia and usually doesn't cause symptoms. The underlying cause may be myocardial fibrosis or digitalis toxicity. The patient may exhibit signs of digitalis toxicity, i.e., anorexia, nausea, vomiting, headache, lethargy, irritability, or photophobia. Left bundle branch block is associated with left ventricular disease and has a poorer prognosis. **Treatment:** Discontinuation of digitalis when the underlying cause is due to digitalis toxicity, otherwise they require no direct treatment.
Trifascicular block	**Definition:** A form of bifascicular block, as well as a first-degree heart block. **Signs and Symptoms:** Syncope, dizziness, lightheadedness, chest pain, shortness of breath. **Treatment:** Prophylactic ventricular pacemaker or treatment of the underlying cause(s).
Other specified conduction disorders Dissociation: atrioventricular [AV] interference isorhythmic Nonparoxysmal AV nodal tachycardia	**Definition:** Electrical impulses are following an abnormal pathway, within the atrioventricular node or beside it. **Signs and Symptoms:** Palpitations are common. **Treatment:** Treatment varies but may include digoxin, ß-blockers, calcium blockers, some patients are candidates for Valsalva maneuver, carotid massage, IV verapamil, electrical conversion, or pathway ablation.
Paroxysmal supraventricular tachycardia Paroxysmal tachycardia: atrial [PAT] atrioventricular [AV] junctional nodal	**Definition:** Sudden, or abrupt, onset of an abnormal rapid heart beat that originates above the ventricles of the heart, specifically in the atrium, atrioventricular node, or atrioventricular junction. **Signs and Symptoms:** Patients may be asymptomatic, or they may present with minor palpitations, or more severe symptoms such as palpitations, dizziness, chest pain, fatigue, syncope, diaphoresis, or nausea. **Treatment:** Treatment may include intravenous adenosine or calcium channel blockers, vagal maneuvers, carotid massage, or cardioversion.

Paroxysmal ventricular tachycardia Ventricular tachycardia [paroxysmal]	**Definition:** Sudden, or abrupt, onset of an abnormal rapid heart beat that originates in the ventricles of the heart and produces a heart rate of at least 12Ø beats per minute. **Signs and Symptoms:** Palpitations; in sustained ventricular tachycardia pressure will fall and heart failure may follow. **Treatment:** Treatment occurs when ventricular tachycardia causes symptoms or when episodes last more than 3Ø seconds even without causing symptoms. If the blood pressure starts to fall, cardioversion is immediately required. Commonly used drugs are lidocaine, procainamide, and amiodarone. In some cases, radiofrequency ablation may be performed to destroy the small abnormal area in the ventricles or open-heart surgery. If other therapy is ineffective, an automatic defibrillator may be implanted.
Atrial flutter	**Definition:** Rapid, regular atrial rhythm that may result in a heart rate over 1ØØ heart beats per minute. **Signs and Symptoms:** Symptoms are dependent on the heart rate. If the heart rate is less than 12Ø beats per minute and regular there may be no symptoms. Higher heart rates can result in palpitations, dizziness, and syncope. **Treatment:** Treatment is geared toward slowing the ventricular response vs. correcting, or restoring, the sinus rhythm. Digoxin, verapamil, quinidine, procainamide, flecainide, ß-blockers, and intravenous ibutilide may be used, as well as cardioversion and RF ablation.
Ventricular fibrillation	**Definition:** Rapid, irregular ventricular rhythm. The heart's lower chambers are contracting in a rapid and unsynchronized way. The underlying cause is usually severe myocardial damage, or may be the result of drug toxicity, i.e. digitalis, quinidine, or epinephrine. **Signs and Symptoms:** The heart pumps little or no blood and death results within minutes if treatment is not immediate. **Treatment:** DC countershock and drug therapy i.e., intravenous lidocaine and ß-blockers, insertion of an implantable cardioverter-defibrillator.
Ventricular flutter	**Definition:** Rapid, irregular ventricular rhythm. The heart's lower chambers are contracting in a rapid and unsynchronized way. The underlying cause is usually severe myocardial damage, or may be the result of drug toxicity, i.e., digitalis, quinidine, or epinephrine. **Signs and Symptoms:** The heart pumps little or no blood and death results within minutes if treatment is not immediate. **Treatment:** DC countershock and drug therapy i.e., intravenous lidocaine and ß-blockers, insertion of an implantable cardioverter-defibrillator.

Appendix E. Abnormal Laboratory Values

This section provides a reference range of normal laboratory values and associated conditions that may function as an MCC/CC condition should the laboratory values be abnormal. To assist the coder in determining if an MCC/CC condition exists, signs and symptoms, and treatments associated with abnormal labs are listed. According to coding guidelines, these MCC/CCs must affect patient care in terms of requiring clinical evaluation; therapeutic treatment; further evaluation by diagnostic studies, procedures, or consultation; extended length of stay; or increased nursing care; and/or monitoring for reporting purposes.

Note: Reference ranges provided in Appendix E are from a combination of established official medical sources and national diagnosis foundations; be sure to reference your own hospital-approved or facility-approved reference range for each lab value.

Acetones or Ketones—Blood—Increased Level

Reference Range: 0.3-2.0 mg/dL Negative (A); 2-4 mg/dL Negative (K)

Condition	Signs & Symptoms	Treatment
Ketoacidosis	Excessive thirst, polyuria, irritability, weakness, coma, stupor, dehydration, fruity breath odor	Restricted diet, monitoring of blood sugar levels
Ketosis, alcoholic	Vomiting and dehydration in association with other symptoms of alcoholism such as delirium tremens and cirrhosis	Intravenous infusion of normal saline and glucose

Acid Phosphatase—Blood—Increased Level

Reference Range: 0-0.8 Units/L

Condition	Signs & Symptoms	Treatment
Failure, renal, chronic, Stage IV, V ESRD	Bruising, dyspnea, lethargy, weakness, anorexia, polyuria, hematuria	Fluid restrictions, dialysis, transfusion(s) of blood and blood components

Albumin—Blood—Decreased Level

Reference Range: 3.5-5.0 g/dL

Condition	Signs & Symptoms	Treatment
Burns, by extent of body surface involved	Can result from thermal, electrical, or chemical injuries; severity is determined by the size and depth of the burn	Reverse isolation, skin grafts, intravenous fluids, invasive monitoring, high protein/high calorie diet
Syndrome, nephrotic	Edema, lethargy, anorexia, orthostatic hypotension	Diuretics, steroid therapy, sodium-restricted high protein diet, frequent urine protein monitoring

Aldosterone—Blood—Increased Level

Reference Range: 8.1-15.5 ng/dL.

Condition	Signs & Symptoms	Treatment
Failure, heart, congestive, all forms except unspecified	Peripheral edema, shortness of breath; cyanosis is present on occasion; heart rate is irregular; moist rales at base of lungs with productive cough; confusion is usually present	Sodium-restricted diet, digitalis regulation, O_2 therapy, diuretics

Alkaline Phosphatase—Blood—Increased Level

Reference Range: 30-120 Units/L

Condition	Signs & Symptoms	Treatment
Calculus of bile duct	Epigastric pain, nausea and vomiting, jaundice	Intravenous fluids and medications, surgery
Cancer of liver	Weakness, fever, weight loss, right upper quadrant mass, pain	Chemotherapy, radiation, surgery
Leukemia	Weight loss, anorexia, pain in extremities, listlessness	Chemotherapy, intravenous fluids, transfusion(s) of blood and blood components, antibiotic therapy
Embolism, pulmonary	Dyspnea, rales in lungs, sudden onset of substernal pain, dizziness, pallor	Heparin, diuretics

Amylase—Blood—Increased Level

Reference Range: 0-130 Units/L

Condition	Signs & Symptoms	Treatment
Pancreatitis, acute	Epigastric pain, nausea, vomiting, fever, sweats, dizziness, confusion	Intravenous fluids, pain medication, replacement of calcium and magnesium, if indicated
Failure, renal, acute, unspecified	Thirst, dyspnea, lethargy, weakness, anorexia, nausea	Management of diet, fluid, and electrolytes; possible dialysis
Failure, renal, chronic, Stage IV, V ESRD	Bruising, dyspnea, lethargy, weakness, anorexia, polyuria, hematuria	Fluid restrictions, dialysis, transfusion(s) of blood and blood components
Ketoacidosis	Excessive thirst, polyuria, irritability, weakness, coma, stupor, dehydration, fruity breath odor	Restricted diet, monitoring of blood sugar levels

Arterial Blood Gases (ABGs)—Bicarbonate (HCO_3)—Decreased Level

Reference Range: 24-28 mEq/L

Condition	Signs & Symptoms	Treatment
Acidosis, metabolic	Hypotension, weakness, pallor, pulmonary edema	Fluid balance, electrolyte monitoring
Failure, renal, chronic, Stage IV, V ESRD	Bruising, dyspnea, lethargy, weakness, anorexia, polyuria, hematuria	Fluid restrictions, dialysis, transfusion(s) of blood and blood components
Infarction, myocardial, acute	Severe chest pain, gallop rhythm and other cardiac arrhythmias, shortness of breath, diaphoresis	Continuous monitoring, O_2 therapy, pain medication, intravenous fluids, intravenous medications, possible resuscitation
Ketoacidosis	Excessive thirst, polyuria, irritability, weakness, coma, stupor, dehydration, fruity breath odor	Restricted diet, monitoring of blood sugar levels

ABGs—pCO_2—Decreased Level

Reference Range: 35-45 mm Hg

Condition	Signs & Symptoms	Treatment
Acidosis, metabolic	Hypotension, weakness, pallor, pulmonary edema	Fluid balance, electrolyte monitoring
Alkalosis, respiratory	Retention of CO_2 and increasing pCO_2; hypoventilation, dyspnea, drowsiness, weakness, malaise, and nausea due to conditions such as spinal cord injury, pulmonary disease, or drugs such as narcotics	Sedation, prevention of further hyperventilation

ABGs—pCO_2—Increased Level

Reference Range: 35-45 mm Hg

Condition	Signs & Symptoms	Treatment
Alkalosis, metabolic	Nausea, vomiting, anorexia	Administration of aluminum chloride, respiratory therapy
Alkalosis, respiratory	Decrease in CO_2; hyperventilation; confusion; lightheadedness; muscle twitching or spasms; nausea; vomiting; tremors in hands; numbness or tingling in hands, feet, or face Due to conditions such as fever, lack of oxygen, liver disease, lung disease, aspirin poisoning, high altitudes	Breathe into paper bag, oxygen, chemical loss correction such as chloride/potassium
Disease, chronic obstructive pulmonary with acute exacerbation or acute bronchitis or asthma	Wheezing, productive cough, shortness of breath	Intermittent positive pressure breathing (IPPB) therapy, intravenous fluids, bronchodilators, antibiotics, physical therapy, artificial ventilation

ABGs—pH—Decreased Level

Reference Range: 7.35-7.45

Condition	Signs & Symptoms	Treatment
Acidosis, metabolic	Hypotension, weakness, pallor, pulmonary edema	Fluid balance, electrolyte monitoring
Acidosis, respiratory	Retention of CO_2 and increasing pCO_2; hypoventilation, dyspnea, drowsiness, weakness, malaise, and nausea due to conditions such as spinal cord injury, pulmonary disease, or drugs such as narcotics	Establishment of airway, O_2 therapy, artificial ventilation, bicarbonate administration
Ketoacidosis	Excessive thirst, polyuria, irritability, weakness, coma, stupor, dehydration, fruity breath odor	Restricted diet, monitoring of blood sugar levels, fluid replacement, insulin administration

ABGs—pO_2—Decreased Level

Reference Range: 75-100 mm Hg

Condition	Signs & Symptoms	Treatment
Disease, chronic obstructive pulmonary with acute exacerbation or acute bronchitis or asthma	Wheezing, productive cough, shortness of breath	IPPB therapy, intravenous fluids, bronchodilators, antibiotics, physical therapy, artificial ventilation
Cor pulmonale, acute	Wheezing, marked fatigue, persistent cough, dyspnea	IPPB therapy, bronchodilators
Edema, pulmonary acute	Increased respiration and pulse rate, shortness of breath, cough, anxiety, cyanosis, diaphoresis	Decreased rate of intravenous fluids, diuretics, intake and output monitoring, O_2 therapy, mechanical ventilation

A1C (Hemoglobin A1C)—Increased Level

Reference Range: <5.7% (5.7%–6.4% indicates prediabetes; 6.5% or higher indicates diabetes)

Condition	Signs & Symptoms	Treatment
Prediabetes or diabetes	Blurry vision, fatigue, increased urination, increased thirst, slow healing, frequent infections	Diabetic medication(s), dietary restrictions, monitoring of blood sugar levels, weight management

Bilirubin—Indirect—Increased Level

Reference Range: 0.1-1.0 mg/dL

Condition	Signs & Symptoms	Treatment
Anemia, hemolytic	Vomiting, anorexia, weight loss	Transfusion(s) of blood and blood components, chemotherapy, iron therapy, O_2 therapy
Failure, heart, congestive, all forms except unspecified	Peripheral edema, shortness of breath; cyanosis is present on occasion; heart rate is irregular; moist rales at base of lungs with productive cough; confusion is usually present	Sodium-restricted diet, digitalis regulation, O_2 therapy, diuretics

Bilirubin—Total/Direct—Increased Level

Reference Range: 0.1-0.5 mg/dL (D); 0.1-1.2 mg/dL (T)

Condition	Signs & Symptoms	Treatment
Calculus of bile duct	Epigastric pain, nausea and vomiting, jaundice	Intravenous fluids and medications, surgery
Cancer of liver	Weakness, fever, weight loss, right upper quadrant mass, pain	Chemotherapy, radiation, surgery
Hepatitis, acute	Jaundice, anorexia, dark urine, pruritus, light-colored stools	Rest, force fluids, antiemetics for nausea, isolation precautions for blood and other body fluids

Bleeding Time—Increased Level

Reference Range: 2-10 minutes

Condition	Signs & Symptoms	Treatment
Anemia, aplastic	Weakness, fatigue, shortness of breath, bruising, nosebleeds	Reverse isolation, transfusion(s) of blood and blood components
Disseminated intravascular coagulation (DIC)	Occurs as a complication of other conditions such as infection, neoplastic disease, burns, and obstetric complications. Characterized by abnormal bleeding such as from the gastrointestinal tract and small wounds such as intravenous sites. Bruising is also present.	Transfusion of plasma or platelets; intravenous heparin administration; intake and output monitoring
Disease, Von Willebrand	Bruising, menorrhagia, epistaxis and possible hemorrhage as a result of surgery	Increased level of factor viii through infusion of cryoprecipitate or fresh frozen plasma prior to surgery or during bleeding episodes

Blood Urea Nitrogen (BUN)—Blood—Increased Level

Reference Range: 9-22 mg/dL

Condition	Signs & Symptoms	Treatment
Infarction myocardial, acute	Severe chest pain, gallop rhythm and other cardiac arrhythmias, shortness of breath, diaphoresis	Continuous monitoring, O_2 therapy, pain medication, intravenous fluids, intravenous medications, possible resuscitation
Failure, renal, acute, unspecified	Thirst, dyspnea, lethargy, weakness, anorexia, nausea	Transfusion(s) of blood and blood components, dialysis, fluid restrictions
Shock, cardiogenic	Rapidly developing mental confusion, physical weakness, cold extremities, moist and cool skin, rapid and weak pulse, oliguria, pulmonary edema, hypotension	Fluid balance, O_2 therapy, cardiac monitoring

Brain Natriuretic Peptide (BNP)—Increased Level

Reference Range: <100 pg/mL

Condition	Signs & Symptoms	Treatment
Embolism, pulmonary	Dyspnea, rales in lungs, sudden onset of substernal pain, dizziness, pallor	Heparin, diuretics
Failure, heart, congestive, all forms	Peripheral edema, shortness of breath; cyanosis is present on occasion; heart rate is irregular; moist rales at base of lungs with productive cough; confusion is usually present	Sodium-restricted diet, digitalis regulation, O2 therapy, diuretics
Failure, renal, acute, unspecified	Thirst, dyspnea, lethargy, weakness, anorexia, nausea	Transfusion(s) of blood and blood components, dialysis, fluid restrictions
Hypertension, pulmonary	Chest pain, cough, dizziness and fainting, edema, fatigue, shortness of breath, palpitations	O2 therapy, physical exercise, anticoagulation, diuretics, vasodilators
Sepsis	Confusion, delirium, fever, tachypnea, tachycardia, mottled skin, hypotension, chills, flushing, fatigue, organ dysfunction	Treat underlying infection, antibiotics, IV fluids, vasoconstrictors, blood pressure support, steroids, mechanical ventilation

Calcium—Blood—Increased Level

Reference Range: 8.5-10.5 mg/dL

Condition	Signs & Symptoms	Treatment
When cancer such as breast or prostate cancer metastasizes to bones, causing them to break and leak calcium into bloodstream	Extreme drowsiness/fatigue, weakness, anorexia, constipation, confusion, and loss of interest	Surgery, chemotherapy, radiation therapy
Failure, renal, acute, unspecified	Thirst, dyspnea, lethargy, weakness, anorexia, nausea	Transfusion(s) of blood and blood components, dialysis, fluid restriction

Carbon Dioxide (CO_2)—Decreased Level

Reference Range: 22-30 mEq/L

Condition	Signs & Symptoms	Treatment
Acidosis, metabolic	Hypotension, weakness, pallor, pulmonary edema	Fluid balance, electrolyte monitoring
Ketoacidosis	Excessive thirst, polyuria, irritability, weakness, coma, stupor, dehydration, fruity breath odor	Restricted diet, monitoring of blood sugar levels

Complete Blood Count (CBC)— Hematocrit (Hct)—Decreased Level

Reference Range: Male 40-54%; Female 36-46%

Condition	Signs & Symptoms	Treatment
Anemia, aplastic	Weakness, fatigue, shortness of breath, bruising, nosebleeds	Reverse isolation, transfusion(s) of blood and blood components
Anemia, due to acute blood loss	Tingling of extremities, dyspnea, bleeding	Iron therapy, transfusion(s) of blood and blood components, O_2 therapy
Failure, renal, chronic, Stage IV, V ESRD	Bruising, dyspnea, lethargy, weakness, anorexia, polyuria, hematuria	Sodium-restricted diet, digitalis regulation, O_2 therapy, diuretics
Leukemia	Weight loss, anorexia, pain in extremities, listlessness	Chemotherapy, intravenous fluids, transfusion(s) of blood and blood components, antibiotic therapy

CBC—Hematocrit (Hct) Increased Level

Reference Range: Male 40-54%; Female 36-46%

Condition	Signs & Symptoms	Treatment
Disease, chronic obstructive pulmonary with acute exacerbation or acute bronchitis or asthma	Wheezing, productive cough, shortness of breath	IPPB therapy, intravenous fluids, bronchodilators, antibiotics, physical therapy, artificial ventilation
Shock, hypovolemic	Cold clammy skin, tachycardia, shallow respirations, hypotension, weak thready pulse, confusion	Intravenous therapy, frequent monitoring of vital signs, intake and output monitoring

CBC—Hemoglobin (Hgb)—Decreased Level

Reference Range: Male 13.5-18 g/dL; Female 12-16 g/dL

Hospital Range:______________

Condition	Signs & Symptoms	Treatment
Anemia, aplastic	Weakness, fatigue, shortness of breath, bruising, nosebleeds	Reverse isolation, transfusion(s) of blood and blood components
Anemia, due to acute blood loss	Tingling of extremities, dyspnea, bleeding	Iron therapy, transfusion(s) of blood and blood components, O_2 therapy
Cancer: Large intestine Liver Rectum Small intestine	Pain, change in bowel or bladder habit, diarrhea, constipation melena, weight loss, clay-colored stools, digestive disturbances, pain, incomplete bowel movement, bleeding of rectum, weight loss, vomiting, fever, chills	Chemotherapy, radiation therapy, surgery
Failure, renal, chronic, Stage IV, V ESRD	Bruising, dyspnea, lethargy, weakness, anorexia, polyuria, hematuria	Fluid restrictions, dialysis, transfusion(s) of blood and blood components
Leukemia	Weight loss, anorexia, pain in extremities, listlessness	Chemotherapy, intravenous fluids, transfusion(s) of blood and blood components, antibiotic therapy

CBC—Hemoglobin (Hgb)—Increased Level

Reference Range: Male 13.5-18 g/dL; Female 12-16 g/dL

Condition	Signs & Symptoms	Treatment
Disease, chronic obstructive pulmonary with acute exacerbation or acute bronchitis or asthma	Wheezing, productive cough, shortness of breath	IPPB therapy, intravenous fluids, bronchodilators, antibiotics, physical therapy, artificial ventilation
Failure, heart, congestive, all forms except unspecified	Peripheral edema, shortness of breath; cyanosis is present on occasion; heart rate is irregular; moist rales at base of lungs with productive cough; confusion is usually present; paroxysmal nocturnal dyspnea, wheezing	Sodium-restricted diet, digitalis regulation, O_2 therapy, diuretics

CBC—Mean Corpuscular Hemoglobin (MCH)—Decreased Level

Reference Range: 27-31 pg

Condition	Signs & Symptoms	Treatment
Anemia, due to acute blood loss	Tingling of extremities, dyspnea, bleeding	Iron therapy, transfusion(s) of blood and blood components, O_2 therapy

CBC—Mean Corpuscular Hemoglobin Concentration (MCHC)—Decreased Level

Reference Range: 32-36%

Condition	Signs & Symptoms	Treatment
Anemia, due to acute blood loss	Tingling of extremities, dyspnea, bleeding	Iron therapy, transfusion(s) of blood and blood components, O_2 therapy

CBC—Mean Corpuscular Volume (MCV)—Decreased Level

Reference Range: Male 80-94 μm^3; Female 78-97 μm^3

Condition	Signs & Symptoms	Treatment
Anemia, due to acute blood loss	Tingling of extremities, dyspnea, bleeding	Iron therapy, transfusion(s) of blood and blood components, O_2 therapy
Failure, renal, chronic, Stage IV, V ESRD	Bruising, dyspnea, lethargy, weakness, anorexia, polyuria, hematuria	Fluid restrictions, dialysis, transfusion(s) of blood and blood components

CBC—Red Blood Count (RBC)—Decreased Level

Reference Range: Male 4.4-6.0 $10^6/mm^3$; Female 4.2-5.5 $10^6/mm^3$

Condition	Signs & Symptoms	Treatment
Anemia, aplastic	Weakness, fatigue, shortness of breath	Reverse isolation, transfusion(s) of blood and blood components
Anemia, acute posthemorrhagic	Weight loss, weakness, pain, anorexia	B12, folic acid supplement, iron therapy, transfusion(s) of blood and blood components
Failure, renal, chronic, Stage IV, V ESRD	Bruising, dyspnea, lethargy, weakness, anorexia, polyuria, hematuria	Fluid restrictions, dialysis, transfusion(s) of blood and blood components

CBC—RBC—Increased Level

Reference Range: Male 4.4-6.0 $10^6/mm^3$; Female 4.2-5.5 $10^6/mm^3$

Condition	Signs & Symptoms	Treatment
Cor pulmonale, acute	Wheezing, marked fatigue, persistent cough, dyspnea	IPPB therapy, bronchodilators

CBC—White Blood Count (WBC)—Above 10,000

Reference Range: 5,000-10,000 cells/µL

Condition	Signs & Symptoms	Treatment
Failure, renal, chronic, Stage IV, V ESRD	Bruising, dyspnea, lethargy, weakness, anorexia, polyuria	Fluid restrictions, dialysis, transfusion(s) of blood and blood components
Embolism, pulmonary	Dyspnea, rales in lungs, sudden onset of substernal pain, dizziness, pallor, hemoptysis	Heparin, diuretics
Failure, renal, acute, unspecified	Thirst, dyspnea, lethargy, weakness, anorexia, nausea and vomiting	Management of diet, fluid, electrolytes. Possible dialysis
Infarction, myocardial acute	Severe chest pain, gallop rhythm and other cardiac arrhythmias, shortness of breath, diaphoresis	Continuous monitoring, O_2 therapy, pain medication, intravenous fluids, intravenous medications, possible resuscitation, drug therapy
Infections, acute	Fever, malaise, chills	Intravenous fluids, antibiotic therapy
Leukemia	Weight loss, anorexia, pain in extremities, listlessness	Chemotherapy, intravenous fluids, transfusion(s) of blood and blood components, antibiotic therapy
Pneumonia	Dyspnea, chills, chest pain, cough, fever, headache	Intravenous fluids, O_2 therapy, antibiotic therapy
Pneumonia, aspiration	Cyanosis, cough, dyspnea	Intravenous fluids, O_2 therapy, antibiotic therapy
Pneumonia, pneumococcal 481	Cough, severe chest pain, shortness of breath	Intravenous fluids, O_2 therapy, antibiotic therapy
Pneumonia, E. coli/proteus	Chest pain, shortness of breath, malaise	Intravenous fluids, O_2 therapy, antibiotic therapy
Pneumonia, staphylococcal	Headache, chest pain, cough	Intravenous fluids, O_2 therapy, antibiotic therapy
Pyelonephritis	Nausea and vomiting, frequency of urination, dysuria, flank pain, chills	Sulfonamides, intravenous fluids, force fluids, antibiotic therapy
Urinary tract infection	Fever, dysuria, frequency, burning on urination, hematuria	Urinary antiseptics, antibiotic therapy, intravenous fluids, force fluids

CBC—WBC—Below 5,000

Reference Range: 5,000-10,000 cells/µL

Condition	Signs & Symptoms	Treatment
Anemia, aplastic	Weakness, fatigue, shortness of breath, bruising, nosebleeds	Reverse isolation, transfusion(s) of blood and blood components

Chloride (Cl)—Blood, Electrolytes—Decreased Level

Reference Range: 95-105 mEq/L

Condition	Signs & Symptoms	Treatment
Burns, by extent of body surface involved	Can result from thermal, electrical, or chemical injuries; severity is determined by the size and depth of the burn	Reverse isolation, skin grafts, intravenous fluids, invasive monitoring, high protein/high calorie diet
Hyponatremia	Weakness, muscle cramps and spasms, confusion, irritability	Intravenous fluids, sodium concentrate
Ketoacidosis	Excessive thirst, polyuria, irritability, weakness, coma, stupor, dehydration, fruity breath odor	Restricted diet, monitoring of blood sugar levels

Chloride (Cl)—Blood, Electrolytes—Increased Level

Reference Range: 95-105 mEq/L

Condition	Signs & Symptoms	Treatment
Acidosis, metabolic	Hypotension, weakness, pallor, pulmonary edema	Fluid balance, electrolyte monitoring
Failure, renal, acute, unspecified	Thirst, dyspnea, lethargy, weakness, anorexia, nausea	Management of diet, fluid and electrolytes; possible dialysis
Hypernatremia	Poor skin turgor, dry mucous membranes, confusion, stupor, coma	Intravenous fluids, force fluids, administration of H_2O

Cholesterol—Increased Level

Reference Range: 150-250 mg/dL

Condition	Signs & Symptoms	Treatment
Calculus of bile duct	Epigastric pain, nausea and vomiting, jaundice	Intravenous fluids and medications, surgery
Diabetes mellitus, with ketoacidosis hyperosmolarity, other coma	Excessive thirst, polyuria, irritability, weakness	Restricted diet, monitoring of blood sugar levels, treatment for symptomatology
Failure, renal, acute, unspecified	Thirst, dyspnea, lethargy, weakness, anorexia, nausea	Transfusion(s) of blood and blood components, dialysis, fluid restriction
Infarction, myocardial acute	Severe chest pain, gallop rhythm and other cardiac arrhythmias, shortness of breath, diaphoresis	Continuous monitoring, O_2 therapy, pain medication, intravenous fluids, intravenous medications, possible resuscitation

Cold Agglutinins—Increased Level

Reference Range: 1: 15 Titer or less

Condition	Signs & Symptoms	Treatment
Anemia, hemolytic	Vomiting, anorexia, weight loss	Transfusion(s) of blood and blood components, chemotherapy, iron and O_2 therapy
Hepatitis, acute	Jaundice, anorexia, dark urine, pruritus, light-colored stools	Rest, force fluids, antiemetics for nausea, isolation precautions for blood and other body fluids
Pneumonia	Dyspnea, chills, chest pain, cough, fever, headache	Intravenous fluids, O_2 therapy, antibiotic therapy

Cortisol—Decreased Level

Reference Range: 5–25 mcg/dL (morning or am labs); 3–10 mcg/dL (afternoon or pm labs)

Condition	Signs & Symptoms	Treatment
Problem with pituitary gland (hypopituitarism) or adrenal gland (Addison's disease)	Abdominal pain, dehydration, hypoglycemia, hypotension, hyperkalemia, nausea, vomiting, diarrhea, muscle weakness, weight loss	Replace cortisol and aldosterone, hydration

Cortisol—Increased Level

Reference Range: 5–25 mcg/dL (morning or am labs); 3–10 mcg/dL (afternoon or pm labs)

Condition	Signs & Symptoms	Treatment
Cushing syndrome, inflammation	Hypertension, bone loss, type 2 diabetes, rounded face, weight gain, delayed wound healing	Medications to manage cortisol levels, surgery/radiation to treat pituitary or adrenal tumors, anti-inflammatory diet

C-reactive protein (CRP)—Increased Level

Reference Range: < 0.9 mg/dL (1–10 mg/dL is moderately elevated; >10 mg/dL is marked elevation; >50mg/dL is severe elevation)

Condition	Signs & Symptoms	Treatment
Infection, inflammation, sepsis, arthritis, osteomyelitis, autoimmune disease, pregnancy	Fever, chills, tachypnea, tachycardia, nausea, vomiting, achy joints	Management of infection or underlying disease, antimicrobial medication, anti-inflammatory medication

Creatinine—Blood—Increased Level

Reference Range: 0.6-1.2 mg/dL

Condition	Signs & Symptoms	Treatment
Failure, renal, acute, unspecified	Thirst, dyspnea, lethargy, weakness, anorexia, nausea	Management of diet, fluid and electrolytes; possible dialysis
Glomerulonephritis, acute	Hypertension, hematuria, azotemia, fatigue	Diuretics, dietary restrictions, antibiotics, dialysis or surgical transplantation
Urinary tract infection	Fever, dysuria, frequency, burning on urination, hematuria	Urinary antiseptics, antibiotic therapy, intravenous fluids, force fluids

Creatinine Phosphokinase (CPK) (CK)—Blood—Increased Level

Reference Range: 0-150 Units/L

Condition	Signs & Symptoms	Treatment
Infarction, myocardial, acute	Severe chest pain, gallop rhythm and other cardiac arrhythmias, shortness of breath, diaphoresis	Continuous monitoring, O_2 therapy, pain medication, intravenous fluids, intravenous medications, possible resuscitation
Muscular dystrophy	Predominant symptom is weakness; as disease progresses, muscle atrophy, abnormal gait, and cardiac symptoms, such as tachycardia appear	Physical therapy, orthopaedic appliances, surgery to release contractures
Embolism, pulmonary	Dyspnea, rales in lungs, sudden onset of substernal pain, dizziness, pallor	Heparin, diuretics

Creatinine Phosphokinase MB—Fraction (CPK-MB) (CK-MB)—Increased Level

Reference Range: < 3%

Condition	Signs & Symptoms	Treatment
Infarction, myocardial, acute	Severe chest pain, gallop rhythm and other cardiac arrhythmias, shortness of breath, diaphoresis	Continuous monitoring, O_2 therapy, pain medication, intravenous fluids, intravenous medications, possible resuscitation
Muscular dystrophy	Predominant symptom is weakness; as disease progresses, muscle atrophy, abnormal gait, and cardiac symptoms, such as tachycardia appear	Physical therapy, orthopaedic appliances, surgery to release contractures

Differential (WBC-DIFF)—Basophils—Increased Level

Reference Range: 0.4-1%

Condition	Signs & Symptoms	Treatment
Anemia, hemolytic	Vomiting, anorexia, weight loss	Transfusion(s) of blood and blood components, chemotherapy, iron therapy, O_2 therapy
Leukemia	Weight loss, anorexia, pain in extremities, listlessness	Chemotherapy, intravenous fluids, transfusion(s) of blood and blood components, antibiotic therapy

Differential (WBC-DIFF)—Eosinophils—Increased Level

Reference Range: 1-3%

Condition	Signs & Symptoms	Treatment
Cancer, lung	Cough, dyspnea, chest and shoulder pain, fever, weight loss, hemoptysis	Surgery, chemotherapy, radiation therapy
Disease, Addison's	Features of crisis include anorexia, headache, weakness, nausea, vomiting, apprehension, diarrhea, abdominal pain, and syncope; chronic Addison's disease may show indications resembling hypoglycemia (i.e., hunger, sweating, irritability, nervousness, depression)	Glucocorticoid and mineralocorticoid replacement
Leukemia	Weight loss, anorexia, pain in extremities, listlessness	Chemotherapy, intravenous fluids, transfusion(s) of blood and blood components, antibiotic therapy
Reaction, allergic (Extravasation)	Can assume a variety of forms from contact dermatitis to anaphylactic shock; most reactions occur on the skin or in the respiratory or gastrointestinal tract	Maintenance of airway, epinephrine, aminophylline

Differential (WBC-DIFF)—Lymphocytes—Decreased Level

Reference Range: 25-35%

Condition	Signs & Symptoms	Treatment
Anemia, aplastic	Weakness, fatigue, shortness of breath, bruising, nosebleeds	Reverse isolation, transfusion(s) of blood and blood components
Burns, by extent of body surface involved	Can result from thermal, electrical or chemical injuries; severity is determined by depth and size of burn	Reverse isolation, skin grafts, intravenous fluids, invasive monitoring, high protein/high-calorie diet
Disease, Hodgkin's	Lymphadenopathy, infections, purpura, fatigue	Reverse isolation, radiation therapy, chemotherapy

Differential (WBC-DIFF)—Lymphocytes—Increased Level

Reference Range: 25-35%

Condition	Signs & Symptoms	Treatment
Leukemia	Weight loss, anorexia, pain in extremities, listlessness	Chemotherapy, intravenous fluids, transfusion(s) of blood and blood components, antibiotic therapy
Leukemia, acute lymphoblastic	Lymphadenopathy, infections, purpura, fatigue	Reverse isolation, chemotherapy, bone marrow transplantation
Pneumonia	Dyspnea, chills, chest pain, cough, fever, headache	Intravenous fluids, O_2 therapy, antibiotic therapy

Differential (WBC-DIFF)—Segmented Neutrophils (Segs)—Decreased Level

Reference Range: 51-67%

Condition	Signs & Symptoms	Treatment
Anemia, aplastic	Weakness, fatigue, shortness of breath, bruising, nosebleeds	Reverse isolation, transfusion(s) of blood and blood components
Disease, Addison's	Features of crisis include anorexia, headache, weakness, nausea, vomiting, apprehension, diarrhea, abdominal pain, and syncope; chronic Addison's disease may show indications resembling hypoglycemia (i.e., hunger, sweating, irritability, nervousness, depression)	Glucocorticoid and mineralocorticoid replacement

Differential (WBC-DIFF)—Segmented Neutrophils (Segs)—Increased Level

Reference Range: 51-67%

Condition	Signs & Symptoms	Treatment
Infarction, acute myocardial	Severe chest pain, gallop rhythm and other cardiac arrhythmias, shortness of breath, diaphoresis	Continuous monitoring, O_2 therapy, pain medication, intravenous fluids, intravenous medications, possible resuscitation
Leukemia	Weight loss, anorexia, pain in extremities, listlessness	Chemotherapy, intravenous fluids, transfusion(s) of blood and blood components, antibiotic therapy
Pneumonia	Dyspnea, chills, chest pain, cough, fever, headache	Intravenous fluids, O_2 therapy, antibiotic therapy

Ejection fraction (EF)—Decreased Level

Reference Range: 55–70%

Condition	Signs & Symptoms	Treatment
Heart failure with reduced ejection fraction (HFrEF), systolic heart failure	Dyspnea, lower extremity edema, weakness, fatigue, heart palpitations, confusion	Management of cardiac disease and diabetes, diuresis, weight management, ACE inhibitors, beta blockers

Ejection fraction (EF)—Increased Level

Reference Range: 55–70%

Condition	Signs & Symptoms	Treatment
Hypertrophic cardiomyopathy	Arrhythmia, fatigue, heart fluttering, dizziness or fainting, shortness of breath, lower extremity edema	Pacemaker or ICD, septal ablation or myectomy, CABG, heart transplant, beta blockers, calcium channel blockers, anticoagulants

Erythrocyte Sedimentation Rate (ESR)—Increased Level

Reference Ranges:
- Male < 50 years old: ≤15 mm/hr
- Male > 50 years old: ≤20 mm/hr
- Female < 50 years old: ≤ 20 mm/hr
- Female > 50 years old: ≤30 mm/hr
- Child: ≤ 10 mm/hr
- Newborn: 0–2 mm/hr

Condition	Signs & Symptoms	Treatment
Infection, inflammation, sepsis	Fever, loss of appetite, nausea, vomiting, achy joints and muscles, weight loss, anemia	Management of infection or underlying disease, antimicrobial medication, anti-inflammatory medication

Gamma Glutamyl Transferase (GT, GGT)—Increased Level

Reference Range: 0-30 Units/L

Condition	Signs & Symptoms	Treatment
Calculus of bile duct	Epigastric pain, nausea and vomiting, jaundice	Intravenous fluids and medications, surgery
Pancreatitis, acute	Epigastric pain, nausea, vomiting, fever, sweats, dizziness, confusion	Intravenous fluids, pain medication, replacement of calcium and magnesium, if indicated

Glucose (Fasting Blood Sugar [FBS])—Blood—Decreased Level

Reference Range: 70-115 mg/dL

Condition	Signs & Symptoms	Treatment
Cancer of pancreas	Diarrhea, weight loss, abdominal pain, jaundice, nausea, anorexia	Surgery, chemotherapy, radiation therapy
Failure, renal, chronic, Stage IV, V ESRD	Bruising, dyspnea, lethargy, weakness, anorexia, polyuria, hematuria	Fluid restrictions, dialysis, transfusion(s) of blood and blood components
Hepatitis, acute	Jaundice, anorexia, dark urine, pruritus, light-colored stools	Rest, force fluids, antiemetics for nausea, isolation precautions for blood and other body fluids
Reaction, hypoglycemia	Sudden onset of sweating, pale skin, blurred vision, possible loss of consciousness	Withhold insulin, food or juice given with sugar, glucose injection

Glucose (FBS)—Blood—Increased Level

Reference Range: 70-115 mg/dL

Condition	Signs & Symptoms	Treatment
Diabetes mellitus, with ketoacidosis, hyperosmolarity, or other coma	Excessive thirst, polyuria, irritability, weakness	Diet restriction, monitoring of blood sugar, treatment for symptomatology
Failure, heart, congestive, all forms except unspecified	Peripheral edema, shortness of breath; cyanosis is present on occasion; heart rate is irregular, moist rales at base of lungs with productive cough; confusion is usually present	Sodium-restricted diet, digitalis regulation, O_2 therapy, diuretics
Failure, renal, acute, unspecified	Thirst, dyspnea, lethargy, weakness, anorexia, nausea	Transfusion(s) of blood and blood components, dialysis, fluid restrictions
Infarction, myocardial, acute	Severe chest pain, gallop rhythm, and other cardiac arrhythmias, shortness of breath, diaphoresis	Continuous monitoring, O_2 therapy, pain medication, intravenous fluids, intravenous medications, possible resuscitation
Infections (acute)	Fever, malaise, chills	Intravenous fluids, antibiotic therapy
Ketoacidosis	Excessive thirst, polyuria, irritability, weakness, coma, stupor, dehydration, fruity breath odor	Restricted diet, monitoring of blood sugar levels

International Normalized Ratio (INR)—Increased Level

Reference Range: 0.8–1.1

Therapeutic Range: 2.0–3.5

Condition	Signs & Symptoms	Treatment
Poisoning or adverse effect of anticoagulants, drug interactions	Bleeding (such as from the GI or urinary tract), hemorrhage, bruising, headache	Anticoagulant adjustment or cessation, vitamin K, fresh frozen plasma transfusion

Lactate Dehydrogenase (LDH) (LD)—Increased Level

Reference Range: 50-150 Units/L

Condition	Signs & Symptoms	Treatment
Failure, heart, congestive, all forms except unspecified	Peripheral edema, shortness of breath; cyanosis is present on occasion; heart rate is irregular; moist rales at base of lungs with productive cough; confusion is usually present	Sodium-restricted diet, digitalis regulation, O_2 therapy, diuretics
Anemia, hemolytic	Vomiting, anorexia, weight loss	Transfusion(s) of blood and blood components, chemotherapy, iron therapy, O_2 therapy
Infarction, myocardial, acute	Severe chest pain, gallop rhythm and other cardiac arrhythmias, shortness of breath, diaphoresis	Continuous monitoring, O_2 therapy, pain medication, intravenous fluids, intravenous medications, possible resuscitation
Embolism, pulmonary	Dyspnea, rales in lungs, sudden onset of substernal pain, dizziness, pallor	Heparin, diuretics

Lipase—Increased Level

Reference Range: 0-1.5 Units/dL

Condition	Signs & Symptoms	Treatment
Failure, renal, acute, unspecified	Thirst, dyspnea, lethargy, weakness, anorexia, nausea	Management of diet, fluid and electrolytes; possible dialysis
Pancreatitis, acute	Epigastric pain, nausea, vomiting, fever, sweats, dizziness, confusion	Intravenous fluids, pain medication, replacement of calcium and magnesium, if indicated

Magnesium—Blood—Increased Level

Reference Range: 1.5-2.5 mmol/L

Condition	Signs & Symptoms	Treatment
Failure, renal, chronic, Stage IV, V ESRD	Bruising, dyspnea, lethargy, weakness, anorexia, polyuria, hematuria	Fluid restrictions, dialysis, transfusion(s) of blood and blood components
Leukemia	Weight loss, anorexia, pain in extremities, listlessness	Chemotherapy, intravenous fluids, transfusion(s) of blood and blood components, antibiotic therapy

N-Terminal Pro B-Type Natriuretic Peptide (NT-proBNP)—Increased Level

Reference Range: < 125 pg/mL for adults 75 years or younger; < 450 pg/mL for adults over age 75

Condition	Signs & Symptoms	Treatment
Embolism, pulmonary	Dyspnea, rales in lungs, sudden onset of substernal pain, dizziness, pallor	Heparin, diuretics
Failure, heart, congestive, all forms	Peripheral edema, shortness of breath; cyanosis is present on occasion; heart rate is irregular; moist rales at base of lungs with productive cough; confusion is usually present	Sodium-restricted diet, digitalis regulation, O2 therapy, diuretics
Failure, renal, acute, unspecified	Thirst, dyspnea, lethargy, weakness, anorexia, nausea	Transfusion(s) of blood and blood components, dialysis, fluid restrictions
Hypertension, pulmonary	Chest pain, cough, dizziness and fainting, edema, fatigue, shortness of breath, palpitations	O2 therapy, physical exercise, anticoagulation, diuretics, vasodilators
Sepsis	Confusion, delirium, fever, tachypnea, tachycardia, mottled skin, hypotension, chills, flushing, fatigue, organ dysfunction	Treat underlying infection, antibiotics, IV fluids, vasoconstrictors, blood pressure support, steroids, mechanical ventilation

Osmolality—Blood—Decreased Level

Reference Range: 280-300 mOsm/kg

Condition	Signs & Symptoms	Treatment
Cancer of bronchus	Productive cough, shortness of breath, dyspnea	Chemotherapy, intravenous fluids
Cancer of lung	Congestion, shortness of breath, productive cough	Chemotherapy, intravenous fluids, surgery, radiation therapy
Deficiency, ADH	Polydipsia, polyuria, headaches, fatigue	Antidiuretic hormone replacement therapy, intake and output monitoring, daily weights
Hyponatremia	Weakness, muscle cramps and spasms, confusion, anorexia, nausea	Intravenous fluids, sodium concentrate

Osmolality—Blood—Increased Level

Reference Range: 280-300 mOsm/kg

Condition	Signs & Symptoms	Treatment
Hypernatremia	Irritability, lethargy, weakness, confusion, stupor, coma	Intravenous fluids, force fluids, administration of H_2O

Platelet Count—Decreased Level

Reference Range: 150,000-400,000 cells/μL

Condition	Signs & Symptoms	Treatment
Anemia, aplastic	Weakness, fatigue, shortness of breath, bruising, nosebleeds	Reverse isolation, transfusion(s) of blood and blood components
Leukemia	Weight loss, anorexia, pain in extremities, listlessness	Chemotherapy, intravenous fluids, transfusion(s) of blood and blood components, antibiotic therapy

Platelet Count—Increased Level

Reference Range: 150,000-400,000 cells/μL

Condition	Signs & Symptoms	Treatment
Infections (acute)	Fever, malaise, chills	Intravenous fluids, antibiotic therapy

Potassium (K)—Blood—Decreased Level

Reference Range: 3.5-5.0 mEq/L

Condition	Signs & Symptoms	Treatment
Failure, renal, acute, unspecified	Thirst, dyspnea, lethargy, weakness, anorexia, nausea	Management of diet, fluid and electrolytes; possible dialysis
Ketoacidosis	Excessive thirst, polyuria, irritability, weakness, coma, stupor, dehydration, fruity breath odor	Restricted diet, monitoring of blood sugar levels
Leukemia	Weight loss, anorexia, pain in extremities, listlessness	Chemotherapy, intravenous fluids, transfusion(s) of blood and blood components, antibiotic therapy

Potassium (K)—Blood—Increased Level

Reference Range: 3.5-5.0 mEq/L

Condition	Signs & Symptoms	Treatment
Anemia, hemolytic	Vomiting, anorexia, weight loss	Transfusion(s) of blood and blood components, chemotherapy, iron therapy, O_2 therapy
Disease, Addison's	Features of crisis include anorexia, headache, weakness, dizziness, nausea, vomiting, apprehension, diarrhea, abdominal pain, and syncope; chronic Addison's disease may show indications resembling hypoglycemia (i.e., hunger, sweating, irritability, nervousness and depression)	Glucocorticoid and mineralocorticoid replacement
Failure, renal, acute, unspecified	Thirst, dyspnea, lethargy, weakness, anorexia, nausea	Management of diet, fluid and electrolytes; possible dialysis

Protein—Blood—Decreased Level

Reference Range: 6.0-8.5 g/dL

Condition	Signs & Symptoms	Treatment
Burns, by extent of body surface involved	Can result from thermal, electrical, or chemical injuries; severity is determined by the size and depth of the burn	Reverse isolation, skin grafts, intravenous fluids, invasive monitoring, high protein/high-calorie diet
Hypernatremia	Irritability, lethargy, weakness, confusion, stupor, coma	Intravenous fluids, force fluids, administration of H_2O
Malnutrition, severe, moderate, mild, other, and unspecified	Can be due to a number of diseases and can be a result of socioeconomic factors; symptoms include muscle and fat wasting, edema, and electrolyte imbalances	Nutritional therapy including oral dietary supplements and total parenteral nutrition (TPN)

Prothrombin Time—Increased Level

Reference Range: 11-13 seconds or 70-100%

Condition	Signs & Symptoms	Treatment
Disseminated intravascular coagulation (DIC)	Occurs as a complication of other conditions such as infection, neoplastic disease, burns, and obstetric complications; characterized by abnormal bleeding such as from the gastrointestinal tract and small wounds such as intravenous sites; bruising is also present	Transfusion of plasma or platelets; intravenous heparin administration; intake and output monitoring
Failure, heart, congestive, all forms except unspecified	Peripheral edema, shortness of breath; cyanosis is present on occasion; heart rate is irregular; moist rales at base of lungs with productive cough; confusion is usually present	Sodium-restricted diet, digitalis regulation, O_2 therapy, diuretics
Acquired hemophilia	Symptoms range from asymptomatic to severe bleeding as a result of minor trauma; bleeding into joints and muscles can occur, with resultant swelling and pain	Nonaspirin oral analgesia for pain; deficient factor replacement required prior to even minor surgical procedures

Reticulocyte Count—Decreased Level

Reference Range: 0.5-1.5%

Condition	Signs & Symptoms	Treatment
Anemia, aplastic.	Weakness, fatigue, shortness of breath, bruising, nosebleeds	Reverse isolation, transfusion(s) of blood and blood components
Anemia, hemolytic	Vomiting, anorexia, weight loss	Transfusion(s) of blood and blood components, chemotherapy, iron therapy, O_2 therapy
Anemia, due to acute blood loss	Tingling of extremities, dyspnea, bleeding	Iron therapy, transfusion(s) of blood and blood components, O_2 therapy

Reticulocyte Count—Increased Level

Reference Range: 0.5-1.5%

Condition	Signs & Symptoms	Treatment
Anemia, aplastic	Weakness, fatigue, shortness of breath, bruising, nosebleeds	Reverse isolation, transfusion(s) of blood and blood components
Anemia, hemolytic	Vomiting, anorexia, weight loss	Transfusion(s) of blood and blood components, chemotherapy, iron therapy, O_2 therapy
Anemia, due to acute blood loss	Tingling of extremities, dyspnea, bleeding	Iron therapy, transfusion(s) of blood and blood components, O_2 therapy

Sedimentation Rate—Increased Level

Reference Range: Male 0-20 mm/hr; Female 0-30 mm/hr

Condition	Signs & Symptoms	Treatment
Cancer of stomach	Weakness, constipation, abdominal pain, anorexia, weight loss, hematemesis, melena	Chemotherapy, radiation therapy, surgery, pain medications
Endocarditis, bacterial	Skin lesions, weight loss, weakness, sweating, fever, heart murmur	Intravenous fluids, antibiotic therapy
Infarction, myocardial, acute	Severe chest pain, gallop rhythm and other cardiac arrhythmias, shortness of breath, diaphoresis	Continuous monitoring, O_2 therapy, pain medication, intravenous fluids, intravenous medications, possible resuscitation
Infections (acute)	Fever, malaise, chills	Intravenous fluids, antibiotic therapy

Serum Glutamic—Oxaloacetic Transaminase (SGOT)—Increased Level

Reference Range: 0-35 Units/L

Condition	Signs & Symptoms	Treatment
Embolism, pulmonary	Dyspnea, rales in lungs, sudden onset of substernal pain, dizziness, pallor	Heparin, diuretics
Failure, heart, congestive, all forms except unspecified	Peripheral edema, shortness of breath; cyanosis is present on occasion; heart rate is irregular; moist rales at base of lungs with productive cough; confusion is usually present	Sodium-restricted diet, digitalis regulation, O_2 therapy, diuretics
Infarction, myocardial, acute	Severe chest pain, gallop rhythm and other cardiac arrhythmias, shortness of breath, diaphoresis	Continuous monitoring, O_2 therapy, pain medication, intravenous fluids, intravenous medications, possible resuscitation

Serum Glutamic—Pyruvic Transaminase (SGPT) (ALT)—Increased Level

Reference Range: 0-35 Units/L

Condition	Signs & Symptoms	Treatment
Infarction, myocardial, acute	Severe chest pain, gallop rhythm and other cardiac arrhythmias, shortness of breath, diaphoresis	Continuous monitoring, O_2 therapy, pain medication, intravenous fluids, intravenous medications, possible resuscitation
Failure, heart, congestive, all forms except unspecified	Peripheral edema, shortness of breath; cyanosis is present on occasion; heart rate is irregular; moist rales at base of lungs with productive cough; confusion is usually present	Sodium-restricted diet, digitalis regulation, O_2 therapy, diuretics

Sodium (Na)—Blood, Electrolytes—Decreased Level

Reference Range: 135-145 mEq/L

Condition	Signs & Symptoms	Treatment
Disease, Addison's	Features of crisis include anorexia, headache, weakness, dizziness, nausea, vomiting, apprehension, diarrhea, abdominal pain, and syncope; chronic Addison's disease may show indications resembling hypoglycemia (i.e., hunger, sweating, irritability, nervousness and depression)	Glucocorticoid and mineralocorticoid replacement
Failure, renal, chronic, Stage IV, V ESRD	Bruising, dyspnea, lethargy, weakness, anorexia, polyuria, hematuria	Fluid restrictions, dialysis, transfusion(s) of blood and blood components
Hyponatremia	Weakness, muscle cramps and spasms, confusion, irritability	Intravenous fluids, sodium concentrate
Ketoacidosis	Excessive thirst, polyuria, irritability, weakness, coma, stupor, dehydration, fruity breath odor	Restricted diet, monitoring of blood sugar levels

Sodium (Na)—Blood, Electrolytes—Increased Level

Reference Range: 135-145 mEq/L

Condition	Signs & Symptoms	Treatment
Failure, heart, congestive, all forms except unspecified	Peripheral edema, shortness of breath; cyanosis is present on occasion; heart rate is irregular; moist rales at base of lungs with productive cough; confusion is usually present	Sodium-restricted diet, digitalis regulation, O_2 therapy, diuretics
Failure, renal, acute, unspecified	Thirst, dyspnea, lethargy, weakness, anorexia, nausea	Management of diet, fluid and electrolytes; possible dialysis
Hypernatremia	Poor skin turgor, dry mucous membranes, confusion, stupor, coma	Intravenous fluids, force fluids, administration of H_2O

Sodium (Na)—Urine—Decreased Level

Reference Range: 40-220 mEq/24 hr

Condition	Signs & Symptoms	Treatment
Failure, heart, congestive, all forms except unspecified	Peripheral edema, shortness of breath; cyanosis is present on occasion; heart rate is irregular; moist rales at base of lungs with productive cough; confusion is usually present	Sodium-restricted diet, digitalis regulation, O_2 therapy, diuretics
Failure, renal, chronic, Stage IV, V ESRD	Bruising, dyspnea, lethargy, weakness, anorexia, polyuria, hematuria	Fluid restrictions, dialysis, transfusion(s) of blood and blood components

Sodium (Na)—Urine—Increased Level

Reference Range: 40-220 mEq/24 hr

Condition	Signs & Symptoms	Treatment
Disease, Addison's	Features of crisis include anorexia, headache, weakness, dizziness, nausea, vomiting, apprehension, diarrhea, abdominal pain, and syncope; chronic Addison's disease may show indications resembling hypoglycemia (i.e., hunger, sweating, irritability, nervousness and depression)	Glucocorticoid and mineralocorticoid replacement

Total Iron Binding Capacity (TIBC)—Decreased Level

Reference Range: 220-370 µg/dL

Condition	Signs & Symptoms	Treatment
Anemia, aplastic	Weakness, fatigue, shortness of breath, bruising, nosebleeds	Reverse isolation, transfusion(s) of blood and blood components
Anemia, sickle cell with crisis	Enlarged heart, tachycardia, heart murmurs, fatigue, dyspnea, joint and bone pain	Supportive care such as rest, analgesics, warm compresses. Transfusion of packed red blood cells may be necessary
Failure, renal, chronic, Stage IV, V ESRD	Bruising, dyspnea, lethargy, weakness, anorexia, polyuria, hematuria	Fluid restriction, dialysis, transfusion(s) of blood and blood components

Total Iron Binding Capacity (TIBC)—Increased Level

Reference Range: 220-370 µg/dL

Condition	Signs & Symptoms	Treatment
Anemia, due to acute blood loss	Tingling of extremities, dyspnea, bleeding	Iron therapy, transfusion(s) of blood and blood components, O_2 therapy

Uric Acid—Blood—Decreased Level

Reference Range: 3-7 mg/dL

Condition	Signs & Symptoms	Treatment
Burns, by extent of body surface involved	Can result from thermal, electrical, or chemical injuries; severity is determined by the size and depth of the burn	Reverse isolation, skin grafts, intravenous fluids, invasive monitoring, high-protein/high-calorie diet

Uric Acid—Blood—Increased Level

Reference Range: 3-7 mg/dL

Condition	Signs & Symptoms	Treatment
Failure, renal, acute, unspecified	Thirst, dyspnea, lethargy, fatigue, anorexia, nausea	Management of diet, fluid and electrolytes; possible dialysis
Infarction, myocardial, acute	Severe chest pain, gallop rhythm and other cardiac arrhythmias, shortness of breath, diaphoresis	Continuous monitoring, O_2 therapy, pain medication, intravenous fluids, intravenous medications, possible resuscitation
Leukemia, myelogenous, chronic	Anorexia, weight loss, weakness, fatigue, bruising, epistaxis, low-grade fever	Chemotherapy is primary treatment; other treatments may include allopurinol to prevent increased uric acid and antibiotics for infections

Urinalysis—Bile—Increased Level

Reference Range: Negative

Condition	Signs & Symptoms	Treatment
Calculus of bile duct	Epigastric pain, nausea and vomiting, jaundice	Intravenous fluids and medications, surgery
Hepatitis, acute	Jaundice, anorexia, dark urine, pruritus, light-colored stools	Rest, force fluids, antiemetics for nausea, isolation precautions for blood and other body fluids

Urinalysis—Ketones or Acetones—Increased Level

Reference Range: Negative

Condition	Signs & Symptoms	Treatment
Ketoacidosis	Excessive thirst, polyuria, irritability, weakness, coma, stupor, dehydration, fruity breath odor	Restricted diet, monitoring of blood sugar levels
Ketosis, alcoholic	Vomiting and dehydration in association with other symptoms of alcoholism such as delirium tremens and cirrhosis	Intravenous infusion of normal saline and glucose

Urinalysis—pH—Decreased Level

Reference Range: 4.5-8

Condition	Signs & Symptoms	Treatment
Acidosis, metabolic	Hypotension, weakness, pallor, pulmonary edema	Fluid balance, electrolyte monitoring
Acidosis, respiratory	Retention of CO_2 and increasing pCO_2; hypoventilation, dyspnea, drowsiness, weakness, malaise, nausea	Establishment of airway, O_2 therapy, artificial ventilation

Urinalysis—pH—Increased Level

Reference Range: 4.5-8

Condition	Signs & Symptoms	Treatment
Failure, renal, chronic, Stage IV, V ESRD	Bruising, dyspnea, lethargy, weakness, anorexia, polyuria, hematuria	Fluid restrictions, dialysis, transfusion(s) of blood and blood components
Urinary tract infection	Fever, dysuria, frequency, burning on urination, hematuria	Urinary antiseptics, antibiotic therapy, intravenous fluids, force fluids

Urinalysis—Protein (Albumin)—Increased Level

Reference Range: Negative.

Condition	Signs & Symptoms	Treatment
Disease, renal acute, tubular	Fatigue, vomiting, anorexia, polyuria	Fluid restrictions, dialysis
Urinary tract infection	Fever, dysuria, frequency, burning on urination, hematuria	Urinary antiseptics, antibiotic therapy, intravenous fluids, force fluids
Toxemia of pregnancy	Develops in the late second trimester or third trimester of pregnancy; symptoms include hypertension, edema, and weight gain; in severe eclampsia, seizures and coma can occur	Sedatives, bed rest, frequent monitoring of blood pressure, intake and output, daily weight; cesarean section or induction of labor may be necessary

Urinalysis—Specific Gravity—Decreased Level

Reference Range: 1.005-1.030

Condition	Signs & Symptoms	Treatment
Disease, renal acute, tubular	Fatigue, vomiting, anorexia, polyuria	Fluid restrictions, dialysis

Urinalysis—Specific Gravity—Increased Level

Reference Range: 1.005-1.030

Condition	Signs & Symptoms	Treatment
Failure, heart, congestive, all forms except unspecified	Peripheral edema, shortness of breath; cyanosis is present on occasion; heart rate is irregular; moist rales at base of lungs with productive cough; confusion is usually present	Sodium-restricted diet, digitalis regulation, O_2 therapy, diuretics

Urinalysis—Urobilinogen—Increased Level

Reference Range: 0-4.0 mg/24 hr

Condition	Signs & Symptoms	Treatment
Anemia, hemolytic	Vomiting, anorexia, weight loss	Transfusion(s) of blood and blood components, chemotherapy, iron therapy, O_2 therapy

Urinalysis—Microscopic Exam—Cast Hyaline—Increased Level

Reference Range: 0-4/lp

Condition	Signs & Symptoms	Treatment
Failure, heart, congestive, all forms except unspecified	Peripheral edema, shortness of breath; cyanosis is present on occasion; heart rate is irregular; moist rales at base of lungs with productive cough; confusion is usually present	Sodium-restricted diet, digitalis regulation, O_2 therapy, diuretics
Disease, renal acute, tubular	Fatigue, vomiting, anorexia, polyuria	Fluid restrictions, dialysis

Urinalysis—Microscopic Exam—White Blood Cells (WBCs)—Increased Level

Reference Range: 0-4/hpf

Condition	Signs & Symptoms	Treatment
Pyelonephritis	Nausea and vomiting, frequency of urination, dysuria, flank pain, chills	Antibiotic therapy, urinary analgesics, surgery if obstruction is present, force fluids
Urinary tract infection	Fever, dysuria, frequency, burning on urination, hematuria	Urinary antiseptics, antibiotic therapy, intravenous fluids, force fluids

Urine Culture—Presence of Pathogens

Reference Range: Negative

Condition	Signs & Symptoms	Treatment
Urinary tract infection	Fever, dysuria, frequency, burning on urination, hematuria	Urinary antiseptics, antibiotic therapy, intravenous fluids, force fluids

Appendix F. Pharmacology List

This section enables the coder to quickly review drugs, drug actions, and indications that are often associated with overlooked or undocumented diagnoses. The coder should review the patient's medication record and know what condition the physician is treating with the prescribed medication based on documentation in the medical record. When documentation is lacking, the coder can reference this section to locate the drug, determine the drug action, confirm drug indications, and when necessary query the physician. When applicable, some of the drugs provided in this resource have also been mapped to their appropriate Z code for long-term drug use.

This section enables the coder to quickly review drugs, drug actions, and indications that are often associated with overlooked or undocumented diagnoses. The coder should review the patient's medication record and know what condition the physician is treating with the prescribed medication based on documentation in the medical record. When documentation is lacking, the coder can reference this section to locate the drug, determine the drug action, confirm drug indications, and when necessary query the physician.

Drug	Z Code	Drug Action/Classification	Indications
5-fluorouracil (5-FU) [fluorouracil]	Z79.631	Antimetabolite agent	Skin, colorectal, breast, stomach, and pancreas cancer
6-mercaptopurine (6-MP) [mercaptopurine]	Z79.631	Antimetabolite agent	Acute lymphoblastic leukemia
Abilify [aripiprazole]		Antipsychotic	Depression; bipolar I disorder; schizophrenia; autism symptoms
Acarbose [acarbose]	Z79.84	Oral hypoglycemic	Diabetes mellitus
Acetaminophen with codeine [acetaminophen/codeine phosphate]	Z79.891	Analgesic, narcotic	Moderate to severe pain
Aclasta [zoledronic acid]	Z79.83	Bisphosphonate	Osteoporosis in postmenopausal women; Paget's disease
Actemra [tocilizumab]	Z79.620	Immunosuppressive biologic/monoclonal antibody	Rheumatoid arthritis; systemic sclerosis-associated interstitial lung disease; giant cell arteritis; polyarticular or systemic juvenile idiopathic arthritis; cytokine release syndrome; COVID-19 for certain pediatric and adult populations
Actimmune [interferon gamma-1b]	Z79.69	Other immunosuppressant/immunomodulator	Chronic granulomatous disease; malignant osteopetrosis
Activella [estradiol/norethindrone acetate]	Z79.890	Estrogen therapy	Menopause symptoms; vaginal and vulvar atrophy; osteoporosis prevention
Actonel [risedronate sodium]	Z79.83	Bisphosphonate	Osteoporosis; Paget's disease
Actoplus Met [metformin hydrochloride/pioglitazone hydrochloride]	Z79.84	Oral hypoglycemic	Diabetes mellitus
Actos [pioglitazone hydrochloride]	Z79.84	Oral hypoglycemic	Diabetes mellitus
Aczone [dapsone]		Acne agent, topical	Acne vulgaris
Adderall XR [amphetamine aspartate and sulfate/dextroamphetamine saccharate and sulfate]		CNS stimulant	Attention deficit hyperactivity disorder (ADHD)
Adlarity [donepezil hydrochloride]		Acetylcholinesterase/cholinesterase inhibitors	Dementia due to Alzheimer's
Admelog [insulin lispro]	Z79.4	Insulin	Diabetes mellitus
Advair [fluticasone propionate/salmeterol xinafoate]	Z79.51	Corticosteroid – inhaled/antiasthmatic	Prophylaxis and treatment of asthma and COPD
Advil [ibuprofen]	Z79.1	Nonsteroidal anti-inflammatory drug (NSAID)	Pain or fever relief
Afrezza [human insulin recombinant]		Insulin – inhaled	Diabetes mellitus
Agamree [vamorolone]	Z79.52	Corticosteroid	Duchenne muscular dystrophy

Pharmacology List

Drug	Z Code	Drug Action/Classification	Indications
Aggrastat [tirofiban hydrochloride]	Z79.02	Antiplatelet	Unstable angina; heart attacks
Aimovig [erenumab-aooe]	Z79.620	Immunosuppressive biologic/monoclonal antibody	Migraine headache prevention
AirDuo RespiClick [fluticasone propionate/salmeterol xinafoate]	Z79.51	Corticosteroid – inhaled/antiasthmatic	Asthma
Aklief [trifarotene]		Acne agent, topical	Acne vulgaris
Aldactone [spironolactone]		Cardiovascular agent; antihypertensive agent; diuretic; electrolytic and renal agent	Severe heart failure; ascites associated with cirrhosis; hypokalemia; hypertension; fluid retention in heart failure, cirrhosis, and nephrotic syndrome
Aleve [naproxen sodium]	Z79.1	Nonsteroidal anti-inflammatory drug (NSAID)	Reduction of temporary aches and pains
Allegra allergy [fexofenadine hydrochloride]		Antihistamine	Seasonal allergic rhinitis
Allopurinol [allopurinol]		Antigout	Gouty arthritis; renal calculus; hyperuricemia; hyperuricemia secondary to leukemia; hyperuricemia secondary to lymphoma
Alora [estradiol]	Z79.890	Estrogen therapy	Menopause symptoms
Alphagan P [brimonidine tartrate]		Antiglaucoma agent (ophthalmic); antihypertensive, ocular	Open angle glaucoma or another condition in which pressure in the eye is too high (ocular hypertension)
Alprazolam [alprazolam]		Antianxiety; sedative/hypnotic	Anxiety and panic disorders
Altabax [retapamulin]	Z79.2	Antibiotic, topical	Skin infections
Altace [ramipril]		ACE inhibitor	Heart failure; hypertension
Alvesco [ciclesonide]	Z79.51	Corticosteroid – inhaled; antiasthmatic	Prophylaxis and treatment of asthma
Amaryl [glimepiride]	Z79.84	Oral hypoglycemic	Diabetes mellitus
Ambien [zolpidem tartrate]		CNS depressant; anxiolytic/sedative/hypnotic	Insomnia
Amikacin [amikacin sulfate]	Z79.2	Antibiotic	Gram-negative bacterial infections such as Pseudomonas, Escherichia coli (E. coli), Proteus, Klebsiella-Enterobacter-Serratia
Amitriptyline HCl [amitriptyline hydrochloride]		Antidepressant	Depression
Amoxicillin [amoxicillin]	Z79.2	Antibiotic	Treatment of infections with a broad spectrum of bactericidal activity against many gram-positive and gram-negative microorganisms; otitis media, gonorrhea, skin, respiratory, gastrointestinal, and genitourinary infections
Ampicillin [ampicillin sodium]	Z79.2	Antibiotic	Bacterial infections
Ampyra [dalfampridine]		Potassium channel blocker	Improvement in walking in patients with multiple sclerosis
Amrix [cyclobenzaprine hydrochloride]			Adjunct to rest and physical therapy for muscle spasms
Anaprox DS [naproxen sodium]	Z79.1	Nonsteroidal anti-inflammatory drug (NSAID)	Pain, inflammation or fever relief
Anastrozole [anastrozole]	Z79.811	Aromatase inhibitor	Postmenopausal breast cancer
Androderm [testosterone]	Z79.890	Testosterone therapy – topical	Primary hypogonadism; hypogonadotropic hypogonadism
AndroGel [testosterone]	Z79.890	Testosterone therapy – topical	Primary hypogonadism; hypogonadotropic hypogonadism
Angeliq [drospirenone/estradiol]	Z79.890	Estrogen therapy	Menopause symptoms
Angiomax [bivalirudin]	Z79.02	Antithrombotic	Prevention of blood clots
Antineoplastic/chemotherapy		Antineoplastic	Cancer
Aphexda [motixafortide]		Immunostimulant	Multiple myeloma

Drug	Z Code	Drug Action/Classification	Indications
Apidra [insulin glulisine recombinant]	Z79.4	Insulin	Diabetes mellitus
Aranelle [ethinyl estradiol/norethindrone]	Z79.3	Contraceptive	Prevention of pregnancy; acne
Aranesp [darbepoetin alfa]		Erythropoiesis-stimulating agent (ESA)	Treatment of anemia in disorders such as CKD and neoplasms
Aredia [pamidronate disodium]	Z79.83	Bisphosphonate	Osteoporosis
Argatroban [argatroban]	Z79.Ø2	Antithrombotic	Prophylaxis and treatment of venous thrombosis in thrombocytopenia patients
Aricept [donepezil hydrochloride]		Acetylcholinesterase/cholinesterase inhibitors	Dementia due to Alzheimer's
Arimidex [anastrozole]	Z79.811	Aromatase inhibitor; antineoplastic	Postmenopausal breast cancer
Arixtra [fondaparinux sodium]	Z79.Ø1	Anticoagulant	Venous thrombosis and pulmonary embolism
Arnuity Ellipta [fluticasone furoate]	Z79.51	Corticosteroid – inhaled; antiasthmatic	Prophylaxis and treatment of asthma
Aromasin [exemestane]	Z79.811	Aromatase inhibitor	Postmenopausal breast cancer
Arthrotec [diclofenac sodium/misoprostol]	Z79.1	Nonsteroidal anti-inflammatory drug (NSAID)-prostaglandin combo	Treatment of patients with osteoarthritis or rheumatoid arthritis who may develop stomach ulcers from taking nonsteroidal anti-inflammatory drugs (NSAIDs) alone
Asmanex [mometasone furoate]	Z79.51	Corticosteroid – inhaled; antiasthmatic	Prophylaxis and treatment of asthma
Astagraf XL [tacrolimus]	Z79.621	Calcineurin inhibitor; immunosuppressant	Prophylaxis of organ transplant rejection
Atelvia [risedronate sodium]	Z79.83	Bisphosphonate	Osteoporosis
Atenolol [atenolol]		Beta blocker	Angina pectoris; hypertension; acute myocardial infarction
Ativan [lorazepam]		Antianxiety; sedative/hypnotic	Anxiety disorder associated with depressive symptoms; controls tension, agitation, irritability, and insomnia
Atripla [efavirenz/emtricitabine/tenofovir disoproxil fumarate]		Antiretroviral	HIV
Atrovent HFA [ipratropium bromide]		Antiasthmatic/bronchodilator	Chronic bronchitis, emphysema; bronchial asthma
Augmentin [amoxicillin/clavulanate potassium]	Z79.2	Antibiotic	Bacterial infections of the middle ear, lower respiratory, sinus, skin and skin structures; urinary tract infections
Augtyro [repotrectinib]		Kinase inhibitor	ROS1-Positive non-small cell lung cancer
Avapro [irbesartan]		Antihypertensive	Hypertension
Avelox [moxifloxacin hydrochloride]	Z79.2	Antibiotic	Bacterial infections of the skin, sinuses, lungs, or stomach; plague
Aviane-28 [ethinyl estradiol/levonorgestrel]	Z79.3	Contraceptive	Prevention of pregnancy
Avonex [interferon beta-1a]	Z79.69	Other immunosuppressant/immunomodulator	Treatment of relapsing multiple sclerosis
Axid AR [nizatidine]		Histamine H2-receptor antagonist	Acid/peptic disorder; gastroesophageal reflux; duodenal, gastric, and peptic ulcers
Ayvakit [avapritinib]		Multikinase inhibitor	Unresectable or metastatic gastrointestinal stromal tumor (GIST); advanced systemic mastocytosis
Azactam [aztreonam]	Z79.2	Antibiotic	Severe bacterial infections
Azithromycin [azithromycin]	Z79.2	Antibiotic	Bacterial infections

Drug	Z Code	Drug Action/Classification	Indications
Azstarys [serdexmethylphenidate and dexmethylphenidate]		CNS stimulant	Attention deficit hyperactivity disorder (ADHD)
Bactrim [sulfamethoxazole/trimethoprim]	Z79.2	Antibiotic	Urinary tract infections; acute otitis media; acute exacerbation of chronic bronchitis; shigellosis; Pneumocystis carinii infections
Basaglar [insulin glargine]	Z79.4	Insulin	Diabetes mellitus
Bayer [acetylsalicylic acid]	Z79.82	Aspirin	Prophylaxis and treatment of heart attacks, angina or strokes; reduction of fever, pain, and inflammation
Benztropine mesylate [benztropine mesylate]		Anticholinergic antiparkinson agent	Parkinson's disease
Betaseron [interferon beta-1b]	Z79.69	Other immunosuppressant/immunomodulator	Treatment of relapsing multiple sclerosis
Betoptic [betaxolol hydrochloride]		Beta blocker; ophthalmic glaucoma agent	Lowering of intraocular pressure; also used for treatment of ocular hypertension and chronic open-angle glaucoma
Beyaz [drospirenone/ethinyl estradiol/levomefolate calcium]	Z79.3	Contraceptive	Prevention of pregnancy; acne vulgaris
Beyfortus [nirsevimab-alip]	Z79.62Ø	Immunostimulant; monoclonal antibody	Lower respiratory tract disease (LRTD) caused by RSV
Biaxin XL [clarithromycin]	Z79.2	Antibiotic	Acid/peptic disorder or ulcer; acute exacerbation chronic bronchitis; human immunodeficiency virus; lower and upper respiratory tract infection; sinus infection; prophylaxis mycobacterium avium complex; pharyngitis; pneumonia; tonsillitis
Bijuva [estradiol/progesterone]	Z79.89Ø	Estrogen/progesterone therapy	Menopausal symptoms
Biktarvy [bictegravir sodium/emtricitabine/ tenofovir alafenamide fumarate]		Antiretroviral	HIV
Biltricide [praziquantel]		Antiparasitic	Infections from Schistosoma species and liver flukes
Bimzelx [bimekizumab]	Z79.69	Other immunosuppressant/immunomodulator	Plaque psoriasis
Binosto [alendronate sodium]	Z79.83	Bisphosphonate	Osteoporosis
Bleomycin [bleomycin]	Z79.632	Antitumor antibiotic	Squamous cell carcinoma; Hodgkin's disease; non-Hodgkin's lymphoma; malignant pleural effusion; testicular cancer
Brenzavvy [bexagliflozin]	Z79.84	Oral hypoglycemic	Diabetes mellitus
Breo Ellipta [fluticasone furoate/vilanterol trifenatate]	Z79.51	Corticosteroid – inhaled; antiasthmatic	Asthma and COPD
Brexafemme [ibrexafungerp]		Antifungal	Vulvovaginal candidiasis
Briellyn [ethinyl estradiol/norethindrone]	Z79.3	Contraceptive	Prevention of pregnancy
Brilinta [ticagrelor]	Z79.Ø2	Antiplatelet	Unstable angina; heart attacks; prevention of blood clots
Brisdelle [paroxetine mesylate]		Selective serotonin reuptake inhibitor (SSRI)	Vasomotor symptoms related to menopause
Briumvi [ublituximab-xiiy]	Z79.62Ø	Immunosuppressive biologic; monoclonal antibody	Multiple sclerosis
Bufferin [aspirin]	Z79.82	Aspirin	Pain, reduce fever or inflammation; prophylaxis and treatment of heart attack, stroke, angina
Buprenorphine HCl and Naloxone HCl [buprenorphine hydrochloride/naloxone hydrochloride]	Z79.891	Analgesic, narcotic	Opioid addiction

Drug	Z Code	Drug Action/Classification	Indications
Buspirone HCl [buspirone hydrochloride]		Antianxiety	Generalized anxiety disorder
Busulfex [busulfan]	Z79.630	Chemotherapeutic alkylating agent	Chronic myelogenous leukemia
Butrans [buprenorphine]	Z79.891	Analgesic, narcotic	Chronic pain
Bydureon bcise [exenatide]	Z79.85	Antidiabetic – non-insulin injectable	Diabetes mellitus
Byetta [exenatide]	Z79.85	Antidiabetic – non-insulin injectable	Diabetes mellitus
Caldolor [ibuprofen]	Z79.1	Nonsteroidal anti-inflammatory drug (NSAID)	Pain or fever relief
Cambia [diclofenac potassium]	Z79.1	Nonsteroidal anti-inflammatory drug (NSAID)	Migraine headache
Camila [norethindrone]	Z79.3	Contraceptive	Prevention of pregnancy; menstrual disorders
Camptosar [irinotecan]	Z79.634	Topoisomerase inhibitor	Metastatic colon or rectal cancer
Camzyos [mavacamten]		Cardiovascular agent	Symptomatic obstructive hypertrophic cardiomyopathy (HCM)
Caplyta [lumateperone]		Antipsychotic	Schizophrenia
Cardizem CD [diltiazem hydrochloride]		Calcium channel blocker	Chronic stable angina; angina due to coronary artery spasm; hypertension
Cardura [doxazosin mesylate]		Antiadrenergic; antihypertensive	Benign prostatic hyperplasia; hypertension
Carmustine [carmustine]	Z79.630	Chemotherapeutic alkylating agent	Brain tumors; Hodgkin's disease; multiple myeloma; non-Hodgkin's lymphoma
Cefazolin sodium [cefazolin sodium]	Z79.2	Antibiotic	Bacterial infections
Cefepime hydrochloride [cefepime hydrochloride]	Z79.2	Antibiotic	Bacterial infections
Cefprozil [cefprozil]	Z79.2	Antibiotic	Bacterial infections
Ceftriaxone [ceftriaxone sodium]	Z79.2	Antibiotic	Bacterial infections
Cefuroxime sodium [cefuroxime sodium]	Z79.2	Antibiotic	Bacterial infections
Celebrex [celecoxib]	Z79.1	Nonsteroidal anti-inflammatory drug (NSAID)	Osteoarthritis; rheumatoid arthritis; juvenile rheumatoid arthritis; ankylosing spondylitis; acute pain; primary dysmenorrhea
Celestone Soluspan [betamethasone acetate/betamethasone sodium phosphate]	Z79.52	Corticosteroid; antiasthmatic	Asthma; severe inflammation
Celexa [citalopram hydrobromide]		Antidepressant	Depression
CellCept [mycophenolate mofetil]	Z79.624	Inhibitors of nucleotide synthesis; immunosuppressant	Prophylaxis of organ transplant rejection
Centany [mupirocin]	Z79.2	Antibiotic, topical	Bacterial skin infections
Cephalexin [cephalexin]	Z79.2	Antibiotic	Bacterial infections
Cerubidine [daunorubicin hydrochloride]	Z79.632	Antitumor antibiotic	Leukemia
Chlorambucil [chlorambucil]	Z79.630	Chemotherapeutic alkylating agent	Chronic lymphocytic leukemia; malignant lymphoma
Cibinqo [abrocitinib]	Z79.622	Janus kinase (JAK) inhibitor	Atopic dermatitis
Cimduo [lamivudine/tenofovir disoproxil fumarate]		Antiretroviral	HIV
Cipro [ciprofloxacin hydrochloride]	Z79.2	Antibiotic	Cystitis; infectious diarrhea; gonorrhea; bone and joint infection; gastrointestinal tract infection; lower and upper respiratory tract infection; sinus infection; urinary tract infection; nosocomial pneumonia; chronic prostatitis
Ciprofloxacin [ciprofloxacin]	Z79.2	Antibiotic	Bacterial infections
Cisplatin [cisplatin]	Z79.630	Chemotherapeutic alkylating agent	Cancer

Pharmacology List

Drug	Z Code	Drug Action/Classification	Indications
Clarithromycin [clarithromycin]	Z79.2	Antibiotic	Skin and respiratory bacterial infections; stomach ulcers caused by Helicobacter pylori
Claritin [loratadine]		Antihistamine	Seasonal allergic rhinitis; chronic idiopathic urticaria
Cleocin [clindamycin phosphate]	Z79.2	Antibiotic	Bacterial infections
Climara [estradiol]	Z79.890	Estrogen therapy	Osteoporosis; menopausal symptoms; vaginal and vulvar atrophy; hypoestrogenism; ovarian failure
Clindamycin [clindamycin phosphate]	Z79.2	Antibiotic	Bacterial infections
Clonazepam [clonazepam]		Anticonvulsant	Absence, akinetic, and myoclonic epilepsy; Lennox-Gastaut syndrome; panic disorders
Clonidine HCl [clonidine hydrochloride]		Antihypertensive	Hypertension
Clopidogrel bisulfate [clopidogrel bisulfate]	Z79.02	Antiplatelet	Unstable angina; heart attacks; prevention of blood clots
Codeine [codeine sulfate]	Z79.891	Analgesic, narcotic	Mild to moderate pain
Colace [docusate sodium]		Gastrointestinal agent; laxative, stool softener	Constipation
Colazal [balsalazide]		Anti-inflammatory	Ulcerative colitis
Colocort [hydrocortisone]	Z79.52	Corticosteroid	Inflammation of the colon
Columvi [glofitamab-gxbm]	Z79.620	Monoclonal antibody	Large B-cell lymphoma
CombiPatch [ethinyl estradiol/norethindrone acetate]	Z79.890	Estrogen therapy	Menopause symptoms; vaginal and vulvar atrophy; osteoporosis prevention
Combivent Respimat [ipratropium bromide/albuterol sulfate]		Antiasthmatic/bronchodilator	Chronic bronchitis, emphysema; bronchial asthma
Compro [prochlorperazine]		Antiemetic; antipsychotic	Nausea and vomiting; manic phase of bipolar syndrome or schizophrenia
Copaxone [glatiramer acetate]	Z79.69	Other immunosuppressant/immunomodulator	Multiple sclerosis
Coreg [carvedilol]		Beta blocker	Hypertension; chronic heart failure; left ventricular dysfunction following myocardial infarction
Coreg CR [carvedilol phosphate]		Beta blocker	Hypertension; chronic heart failure; left ventricular dysfunction following myocardial infarction
Cortef [hydrocortisone]	Z79.52	Corticosteroid	Severe inflammation
Cortenema [hydrocortisone]	Z79.52	Corticosteroid	Inflammation of the colon
Cortifoam [hydrocortisone acetate]	Z79.52	Corticosteroid	Colon and rectum inflammation
Cosentyx [secukinumab]	Z79.620	Immunosuppressive biologic; monoclonal antibody	Plaque psoriasis; psoriatic arthritis; ankylosing spondylitis
Cozaar [losartan potassium]		Antihypertensive	Hypertension
Crestor [rosuvastatin calcium]		HMG-CoA reductase inhibitor (statin)	Hypercholesterolemia; hyperlipidemia; hyperproteinemia
Cyclosporine [cyclosporine]	Z79.621	Calcineurin inhibitor	Prophylaxis of organ transplant rejection
Cyltezo [adalimumab-abdm]	Z79.620	Immunosuppressive biologic; monoclonal antibody	Rheumatoid arthritis; juvenile idiopathic arthritis; psoriatic arthritis; Crohn's disease; ulcerative colitis; plaque psoriasis
Cymbalta [duloxetine hydrochloride]		Antidepressant, serotonin and norepinephrine reuptake inhibitor (SNRI)	Major depressive disorder; general anxiety disorder; fibromyalgia; diabetic peripheral neuropathy; chronic musculoskeletal pain
Cytarabine [cytarabine]	Z79.631	Antimetabolite agent	Leukemia
Cytomel [liothyronine sodium]		Thyroid hormone	Hypothyroidism or prevention of euthyroid goiters
Cytoxan [cyclophosphamide]	Z79.630	Chemotherapeutic alkylating agent	Cancer

Drug	Z Code	Drug Action/Classification	Indications
Daptomycin [daptomycin]	Z79.2	Antibiotic	Bacterial infections of the skin, underlying tissues, and bloodstream
Daybue [trofinetide]		CNS agent	Rett syndrome
Daypro [oxaprozin]	Z79.1	Nonsteroidal anti-inflammatory drug (NSAID)	Osteoarthritis; rheumatoid arthritis; juvenile rheumatoid arthritis
Daysee [ethinyl estradiol/levonorgestrel]	Z79.3	Contraceptive	Prevention of pregnancy
Defencath [taurolidine, heparin]	Z79.Ø1	Antimicrobial; anticoagulant	Catheter-related bloodstream infections
Delestrogen [estradiol valerate]	Z79.89Ø	Estrogen therapy	Menopause symptoms
Demerol [meperidine hydrochloride]	Z79.891	Analgesic, narcotic	Moderate to severe pain
Depakote [divalproex sodium]		Anticonvulsant	Bipolar affective disorder; complex absence, complex partial and mixed pattern epilepsy; migraine headache
Depo-Medrol [methylprednisolone acetate]	Z79.52	Corticosteroid	Arthritis; joint disorders
Depo-Provera [medroxyprogesterone acetate]	Z79.3	Contraceptive	Prevention of pregnancy
Depo-SubQ Provera [medroxyprogesterone acetate]	Z79.3	Contraceptive	Prevention of pregnancy; menstrual disorder pain
Descovy [emtricitabine/tenofovir alafenamide]		Antiretroviral	HIV
Desogestrel/ethinyl estradiol [desogestrel/ethinyl estradiol]	Z79.3	Contraceptive	Prevention of pregnancy
Detrol [tolterodine tartrate]		Muscarinic receptor antagonist	Overactive bladders in patients with urinary frequency, urgency, or urge incontinence
Dexamethasone Intensol [dexamethasone]	Z79.52	Corticosteroid	Arthritis; allergic disorders; breathing disorders; inflammation; lupus
Dexilant [dexlansoprazole]		Proton pump inhibitor	Erosive esophagitis; heartburn; nonerosive gastroesophageal reflux disease
DiaBeta [glyburide]	Z79.84	Oral hypoglycemic	Diabetes mellitus
Diclegis [doxylamine succinate/pyridoxine hydrochloride]		Antiemetic	Nausea/vomiting in pregnancy
Dificid [fidaxomicin]	Z79.2	Antibiotic	Clostridium difficile
Diflucan [fluconazole]		Antifungal	Oropharyngeal and esophageal candidiasis; cryptococcal meningitis in AIDS patients; vaginal candidiasis
Digoxin [digoxin]		Antiarrhythmic; inotropic agent	Heart failure; atrial flutter; atrial fibrillation; supraventricular tachycardia
Dilantin [phenytoin sodium]		Anticonvulsant	Grand mal and psychomotor seizures
Dilaudid [hydromorphone hydrochloride]	Z79.891	Analgesic, narcotic	Moderate to severe pain
Diovan [valsartan]		Antihypertensive	Hypertension; heart failure; post-myocardial infarction
Diskets [methadone hydrochloride]		Opioid agonist	Treatment of opioid addiction
Disulfiram [disulfiram]		Alcohol treatment	Alcoholism
Divigel [estradiol]	Z79.89Ø	Estrogen therapy – topical	Menopause symptoms
Dovato [dolutegravir sodium/lamivudine]		Antiretroviral	HIV
Doxorubicin [doxorubicin]	Z79.632	Antitumor antibiotic	Hodgkin lymphoma; non-Hodgkin lymphoma; specific types of cancers and leukemias
Doxycycline [doxycycline]	Z79.2	Antibiotic	Bacterial infections; acne

Drug	Z Code	Drug Action/Classification	Indications
Duavee [bazedoxifene acetate/conjugated estrogens]	Z79.890	Estrogen therapy	Menopause symptoms; osteoporosis
Duetact [glimepiride/pioglitazone hydrochloride]	Z79.84	Oral hypoglycemic	Diabetes mellitus
Duexis [famotidine/ibuprofen]	Z79.1	Nonsteroidal anti-inflammatory drug (NSAID)	Osteoarthritis and rheumatoid arthritis; reduce risk of upper gastrointestinal ulcers
Dulera [formoterol fumarate/mometasone furoate]	Z79.51	Corticosteroid – inhaled; antiasthmatic	Asthma
Dupixent [dupilumab]	Z79.620	Immunosuppressive biologic; monoclonal antibody	Atopic dermatitis; asthma; chronic rhinosinusitis with nasal polys; eosinophilic esophagitis; prurigo nodularis
Duramorph PF [morphine sulfate]	Z79.891	Analgesic, narcotic	Moderate to severe pain
Durlaza [aspirin]	Z79.82	Aspirin	Pain; inflammation; prevention of heart attack, stroke, angina
Dymista [azelastine/fluticasone]		Corticosteroid – intranasal	Seasonal allergies
E.E.S. [erythromycin ethylsuccinate]	Z79.2	Antibiotic	Bacterial infections
Efavirenz (efavirenz)		Antiretroviral	HIV
Effexor XR [venlafaxine hydrochloride]		Antidepressant, serotonin and norepinephrine reuptake inhibitors (SNRIs)	Major depressive disorder; social anxiety disorder; panic disorder
Effient [prasugrel hydrochloride]	Z79.02	Antiplatelet	Reduce risk of heart attack or stroke
Elestrin [estradiol]	Z79.890	Estrogen therapy	Menopause symptoms
Elfabrio [pegunigalsidase alfa-iwxj]		Enzyme replacement therapy	Fabry disease
Eligard [leuprolide acetate]	Z79.818	Agents affecting estrogen receptors and estrogen levels	Palliative treatment of prostate cancer symptoms
Eliquis [apixaban]	Z79.01	Anticoagulant	Venous thrombosis
Elrexfio [elranatamab-bcmm]	Z79.620	Monoclonal antibody	Multiple myeloma
Enbrel [etanercept]	Z79.620	Immunosuppressive biologic; antirheumatic	Rheumatoid arthritis; polyarticular juvenile idiopathic arthritis; psoriatic arthritis; ankylosing spondylitis; plaque psoriasis
Enjaymo [sutimlimab-jome]	Z79.69	Other immunosuppressant/immunomodul ator	Decreases need for red blood cell transfusion due to breakdown of red blood cells (hemolysis) in adults with cold agglutinin disease (CAD)
Enpresse-28 [ethinyl estradiol/levonorgestrel]	Z79.3	Contraceptive	Prevention of pregnancy
Entocort EC [budesonide]	Z79.52	Corticosteroid	Crohn's disease; ulcerative colitis
Entresto [sacubitril/valsartan]		Angiotensin II receptor blocker; neprilysin inhibitor	Chronic heart failure
Entyvio [vedolizumab]	Z79.620	Immunosuppressive biologic; monoclonal antibody	Crohn's disease; ulcerative colitis
Envarsus XR [tacrolimus]	Z79.621	Calcineurin inhibitor	Prophylaxis of organ transplant rejection
Epinephrine [epinephrine]		Bronchodilator, cardiotonic	Hypotension associated with septic shock; anaphylaxis
Epivir, Epivir-HBV [lamivudine]		Antiretroviral	HIV; chronic hepatitis B
Epkinly [epcoritamab-bysp]	Z79.620	Monoclonal antibody	Large B-cell lymphoma; high-grade B-cell lymphoma
Eptifibatide [eptifibatide]	Z79.02	Antiplatelet	Unstable angina; heart attacks; prevention of blood clots
Erelzi [etanercept-szzs]	Z79.620	Immunosuppressive biologic	Rheumatoid arthritis; polyarticular juvenile idiopathic arthritis; psoriatic arthritis; ankylosing spondylitis
Ertapenem [ertapenem sodium]	Z79.2	Antibiotic	Bacterial infections of the stomach, urinary tract, pelvis, skin, and lung
ERYC [erythromycin]	Z79.2	Antibiotic	Respiratory tract infections

Drug	Z Code	Drug Action/Classification	Indications
Erygel [erythromycin]	Z79.2	Antibiotic, topical	Bacterial skin infections
EryPed [erythromycin ethylsuccinate]	Z79.2	Antibiotic	Bacterial infections; rheumatic fever attacks
Ery-Tab [erythromycin]	Z79.2	Antibiotic	Bacterial infections
Erythrocin [erythromycin lactobionate]	Z79.2	Antibiotic	Bacterial infections
Erythromycin [erythromycin]	Z79.2	Antibiotic	Respiratory tract infections
Estrace [estradiol]	Z79.890	Estrogen therapy	Vaginal cream for treatment of vaginal and vulvar atrophy
EstroGel [estradiol]	Z79.890	Estrogen therapy – topical	Menopause symptoms
Etoposide [etoposide]	Z79.634	Topoisomerase inhibitor	Small cell lung cancer
Evista [raloxifene hydrochloride]	Z79.810	Selective estrogen receptor modulator (SERM)	Osteoporosis in postmenopausal women
Exemestane [exemestane]	Z79.811	Aromatase inhibitor	Postmenopausal breast cancer
Exxua [gepirone]		Antidepressant	Major depressive disorder
Fareston [toremifene citrate]	Z79.810	Selective estrogen receptor modulator (SERM)	Postmenopausal breast cancer
Farxiga [dapagliflozin propanediol]	Z79.84	Oral hypoglycemic	Diabetes mellitus
Faslodex [fulvestrant]	Z79.818	Agents affecting estrogen receptors and estrogen levels	Hormone-related breast cancer; metastatic breast cancer
Feldene [piroxicam]	Z79.1	Nonsteroidal anti-inflammatory drug (NSAID)	Treatment of pain and inflammation due to arthritis
Femara [letrozole]	Z79.811	Aromatase inhibitor	Postmenopausal breast cancer
Femhrt [ethinyl estradiol/norethindrone acetate]	Z79.3, Z79.890	Contraceptive; estrogen therapy	Prevention of pregnancy; menopause symptoms; osteoporosis prevention
Femring [estradiol acetate]	Z79.890	Estrogen therapy	Osteoporosis prevention; menopausal symptoms; hypoestrogenism; ovarian failure
Fentanyl citrate [fentanyl citrate]	Z79.891	Analgesic, narcotic	Postprocedural or chronic pain
Fentora [fentanyl citrate]	Z79.891	Analgesic, narcotic	Breakthrough cancer pain
Fetroja [cefiderocol]	Z79.2	Antibiotic	Complicated urinary tract infections; hospital-acquired bacterial pneumonia; ventilator-associated bacterial pneumonia
Fiasp [insulin aspart]	Z79.4	Insulin	Diabetes mellitus
Filspari [sparsentan]		Endothelin and angiotensin II receptor antagonist	Primary immunoglobulin A nephropathy (IgAN)
Fioricet with codeine [acetaminophen/ butalbital/caffeine/codeine phosphate]	Z79.891	Analgesic, narcotic	Tension headaches
Firmagon [degarelix]	Z79.890	Hormone therapy	Prostate cancer
Flagyl [metronidazole]	Z79.2	Antibiotic	Bacterial infections
Flavoxate HCl [flavoxate hydrochloride]		Urinary antispasmodic	Relief of dysuria, urgency, nocturia, suprapubic pain, frequency, and incontinence associated with cystitis, prostatitis, urethritis, and urethrocystitis/urethrotrigonitis
Flomax [tamsulosin hydrochloride]		Antiadrenergic	Benign prostatic hyperplasia
Flonase allergy relief [fluticasone propionate]		Corticosteroid – intranasal	Perennial and seasonal allergic rhinitis
Flovent HFA [fluticasone propionate]	Z79.51	Corticosteroid – inhaled; antiasthmatic	Asthma
Fosamax [alendronate sodium]	Z79.83	Bisphosphonate	Osteoporosis; Paget's disease

Pharmacology List

Drug	Z Code	Drug Action/Classification	Indications
Fosinopril sodium [fosinopril sodium]		ACE inhibitor	Hypertension; heart failure
Fosrenol [lanthanum carbonate]		Phosphate binder	End-stage renal disease (ESRD)
Fragmin [dalteparin sodium]	Z79.Ø1	Anticoagulant	Venous thrombosis
Fruzaqla [fruquintinib]		Kinase inhibitor	Colorectal cancer
Gengraf [cyclosporine]	Z79.621	Calcineurin inhibitor	Prophylaxis of organ transplant rejection
Gentamicin sulfate [gentamicin sulfate]	Z79.2	Antibiotic	Severe bacterial infections
Gildagia [ethinyl estradiol/norethindrone]	Z79.3	Contraceptive	Prevention of pregnancy
Gildess 24 FE [ethinyl estradiol/norethindrone acetate]	Z79.3	Contraceptive	Prevention of pregnancy
Glimepiride [glimepiride]	Z79.84	Oral hypoglycemic	Diabetes mellitus
Glucotrol XL [glipizide]	Z79.84	Oral hypoglycemic	Diabetes mellitus
Glumetza [metformin hydrochloride]	Z79.84	Oral hypoglycemic	Diabetes mellitus
Glyburide (micronized) [glyburide]	Z79.84	Oral hypoglycemic	Diabetes mellitus
Glynase [glyburide]	Z79.84	Oral hypoglycemic	Diabetes mellitus
Glyset [miglitol]	Z79.84	Oral hypoglycemic	Diabetes mellitus
Harvoni [ledipasvir/sofosbuvir]		Antiviral	Chronic hepatitis C
Heparin sodium [heparin sodium]	Z79.Ø1	Anticoagulant	Prophylaxis and treatment of venous thrombosis, pulmonary embolism; prevention of cerebral thrombosis; treatment of consumptive coagulopathies
Hiprex [methenamine]	Z79.2	Antibiotic	Recurring bladder infection
Humalog [insulin lispro recombinant]	Z79.4	Insulin	Diabetes mellitus
Humira [adalimumab]	Z79.62Ø	Immunosuppressive biologic; monoclonal antibody	Rheumatoid arthritis; juvenile idiopathic arthritis; psoriatic arthritis; Crohn's disease; ulcerative colitis; plaque psoriasis; hidradenitis suppurativa; uveitis
Humulin R [insulin recombinant]	Z79.4	Insulin	Diabetes mellitus
Hycamtin [topotecan hydrochloride]	Z79.634	Topoisomerase inhibitor	Ovarian cancer; small cell lung cancer; cervical cancer
Hydrocodone [acetaminophen/hydrocodone bitartrate]	Z79.891	Analgesic, narcotic	Moderate to severe pain
Hydrocodone bitartrate and acetaminophen [acetaminophen/hydrocodone bitartrate]	Z79.891	Analgesic, narcotic	Moderate to severe pain
Hydrocortisone [hydrocortisone]	Z79.52	Corticosteroid	Addison's disease; arthritis; immune disorders; allergies; breathing problems
Hydromorphone HCl [hydromorphone hydrochloride]	Z79.891	Analgesic, narcotic	Moderate to severe pain
Hydroxyurea [hydroxyurea]	Z79.64	Myelosuppressive agent	Pain related to sickle cell disease; chronic myeloid leukemia; ovarian cancer; skin cancer
Hyrimoz [adalimumab-adaz]	Z79.62Ø	Immunosuppressive biologic; monoclonal antibody	Rheumatoid arthritis; juvenile idiopathic arthritis; psoriatic arthritis; Crohn's disease; ulcerative colitis; plaque psoriasis; ankylosing spondylitis
Hyzaar [hydrochlorothiazide/losartan potassium]		Antihypertensive	Hypertension
Ibsrela [tenapanor hydrochloride]		NHE-3 inhibitor	Irritable bowel syndrome with constipation (IBS-C)
Ibuprofen [ibuprofen]	Z79.1	Nonsteroidal anti-inflammatory drug (NSAID)	Pain or fever relief

Drug	Z Code	Drug Action/Classification	Indications
Imitrex [sumatriptan succinate]		Antimigraine	Migraine headache
Imjudo [tremelimumab]	Z79.620	Immunosuppressive biologic; monoclonal antibody	Unresectable hepatocellular carcinoma
Imuran [azathioprine]	Z79.624	Inhibitors of nucleotide synthesis; antirheumatic; immunosuppressant	Rheumatoid arthritis; prophylaxis of organ transplant rejection
Indocin [indomethacin]	Z79.1	Nonsteroidal anti-inflammatory drug (NSAID)	Treatment of pain and inflammation
Inpefa [sotagliflozin]		Cardiovascular agent	Heart failure
Intron A [interferon alfa 2-b]	Z79.69	Other immunosuppressant/immunomodulator	Cancer; hepatitis
Invanz [ertapenem sodium]	Z79.2	Antibiotic	Bacterial infections of the stomach, urinary tract, pelvis, skin, and lung
Invokamet [canagliflozin/metformin hydrochloride]	Z79.84	Oral hypoglycemic	Diabetes mellitus
Invokana [canagliflozin]	Z79.84	Oral hypoglycemic	Diabetes mellitus
Isoniazid [isoniazid]	Z79.2	Antibiotic	Tuberculosis
Isoproterenol hydrochloride [isoproterenol hydrochloride]		Adrenergic agent/catecholamine	Shock; cardiac arrest; heart failure; bronchospasm
Isopto Carpine [pilocarpine hydrochloride]		Cholinergic parasympathomimetic agent	Reduction of intraocular pressure in open-angle glaucoma or ocular hypertension; management of acute angle-closure glaucoma
Isordil Titradose [isosorbide dinitrate]		Smooth muscle relaxant	Acute anginal attacks
Isturisa [osilodrostat]		Cortisol synthesis inhibitor	Cushing's disease in adults
Ixempra [ixabepilone]	Z79.633	Mitotic inhibitor	Advanced breast cancer
Izervay [avacincaptad pegol]		Anti-angiogenic ophthalmic agent	Geographic atrophy due to age-related macular degeneration
Jantoven [warfarin sodium]	Z79.01	Anticoagulant	Venous thrombosis, pulmonary embolism; prevention of cerebral thrombosis; treatment of consumptive coagulopathies
Janumet [metformin hydrochloride/sitagliptin phosphate]	Z79.84	Oral hypoglycemic	Diabetes mellitus
Januvia [sitagliptin phosphate]	Z79.84	Oral hypoglycemic	Diabetes mellitus
Jaypirca [pirtobrutinib]		Kinase inhibitor	Mantle cell lymphoma
Jentadueto [linagliptin/metformin hydrochloride]]	Z79.84	Oral hypoglycemic	Diabetes mellitus
Jesduvroq [daprodustat]		Erythropoiesis-stimulating agent (ESA)	Treatment of anemia in CKD patients on dialysis
Junel [ethinyl estradiol/norethindrone acetate]	Z79.3	Contraceptive	Prevention of pregnancy
Katerzia [amlodipine benzoate]		Antihypertensive	Hypertension; coronary artery disease (CAD); chronic stable angina; prinzmetal's angina; variant angina
Kazano [alogliptin benzoate/metformin hydrochloride]	Z79.84	Oral hypoglycemic	Diabetes mellitus
Kenalog-10; Kenalog-40 [triamcinolone acetonide]	Z79.52	Corticosteroid	Gouty arthritis; bursitis; tenosynovitis; epicondylitis; rheumatoid arthritis; synovitis; osteoarthritis
Keytruda [pembrolizumab]	Z79.620	Immunosuppressive biologic; monoclonal antibody	Unresectable or metastatic melanoma
Kimmtrak [tebentafusp-tebn]		Antineoplastic	Uveal melanoma
Klaron [sulfacetamide sodium]	Z79.2	Antibiotic, topical	Acne vulgaris

Pharmacology List

Drug	Z Code	Drug Action/Classification	Indications
Klonopin [clonazepam]		Anticonvulsant; CNS depressant	Epilepsy; seizures; panic disorder
Klor-Con [potassium chloride]		Mineral; electrolyte	Hypokalemia
Kombiglyze [metformin hydrochloride/saxagliptin hydrochloride]	Z79.84	Oral hypoglycemic	Diabetes mellitus
K-Tab [potassium chloride]		Mineral; electrolyte	Hypokalemia
Lamisil [terbinafine hydrochloride]		Antifungal	Tinea cruris (jock itch); T. pedis (athlete's foot); T. corporis (ringworm)
Lanoxin [digoxin]		Antiarrhythmic; inotropic agent	Heart failure; chronic atrial fibrillation
Lantus [insulin glargine recombinant]	Z79.4	Insulin	Diabetes mellitus
Lasix [furosemide]		Antihypertensive; diuretic	Hypertension; edema associated with heart failure and renal disease
Leqembi [lecanemab-irmb]		Amyloid beta-directed antibody	Dementia due to Alzheimer's
Lescol XL [fluvastatin sodium]		HMG-CoA reductase inhibitor (statin)	Hypercholesterolemia; hyperlipidemia; hyperlipoproteinemia
Letrozole [letrozole]	Z79.811	Aromatase inhibitor; antineoplastic	Postmenopausal breast cancer
Leukeran [chlorambucil]	Z79.63Ø	Chemotherapeutic alkylating agent	Cancer
Levemir [insulin detemir recombinant]	Z79.4	Insulin	Diabetes mellitus
Levonest [levonorgestrel/ethinyl estradiol]	Z79.3	Contraceptive	Prevention of pregnancy; menstrual disorders; acne
Levoxyl [levothyroxine sodium]	Z79.89Ø	Thyroid hormone	Hypothyroidism; pituitary thyrotropin suppression
Lexapro [escitalopram oxalate]		Antidepressant, selective serotonin reuptake inhibitor (SSRI)	Depression; anxiety
Lialda [mesalamine]		Anti-inflammatory	Ulcerative colitis
Lidocaine HCl [lidocaine hydrochloride]		Antiarrhythmic	Management of ventricular arrhythmias or during cardiac manipulation, such as cardiac surgery
Liletta [levonorgestrel]	Z79.3	Contraceptive	Intrauterine device to prevent pregnancy
Lincocin [lincocin hydrochloride]	Z79.2	Antibiotic	Severe bacterial infections
Lipitor [atorvastatin calcium]		HMG-CoA reductase inhibitor (statin)	Hypercholesterolemia; hyperlipidemia; hyperproteinemia
Lisinopril [lisinopril]		ACE inhibitor	Heart failure; hypertension
Litfulo [ritlecitinib]		Multikinase inhibitor	Alopecia areata
Lithium carbonate [lithium carbonate]		Antimanic	Control of manic episodes in bipolar disorders
Livtencity [maribavir]		Antiviral	Post-transplant CMV infection/disease
Lo Loestrin Fe [ethinyl estradiol/norethindrone acetate]	Z79.3	Contraceptive	Prevention of pregnancy
Locoid [hydrocortisone butyrate]	Z79.52	Corticosteroid – topical	Atopic dermatitis; other dermatoses
Lomotil [diphenoxylate hydrochloride/atropine sulfate]		Antidiarrheal	Symptoms of chronic and functional diarrhea
Lopid [gemfibrozil]		Lipid regulating agent	Hypercholesterolemia; hyperlipidemia; hyperlipoproteinemia; hypertriglyceridemia
Lopressor [metoprolol tartrate]		Beta blocker	Angina pectoris; hypertension; acute myocardial infarction
Loqtorzi [toripalimab-tpzi]	Z79.62Ø	Monoclonal antibody	Nasopharyngeal carcinoma
Lorazepam [lorazepam]		Antianxiety; sedative/hypnotic; anticonvulsant; antiemetic	Anxiety disorder associated with depressive symptoms; controls tension, agitation, irritability, and insomnia
Loryna [drospirenone/ethinyl estradiol]	Z79.3	Contraceptive	Prevention of pregnancy

Pharmacology List

Drug	Z Code	Drug Action/Classification	Indications
LoSeasonique [ethinyl estradiol/levonorgestrel]	Z79.3	Contraceptive	Prevention of pregnancy
Lotensin [benazepril hydrochloride]		ACE inhibitor	Hypertension
Lotrel [amlodipine besylate/benazepril hydrochloride]		Antihypertensive	Hypertension
Lovastatin [lovastatin]		HMG-CoA reductase inhibitor (statin)	Hypercholesterolemia; hyperlipidemia; hyperlipoproteinemia
Lovenox [enoxaparin sodium]	Z79.Ø1	Anticoagulant	Venous thrombosis and pulmonary embolism
Low-Ogestrel-28 [norgestrel/ethinyl estradiol]	Z79.3	Contraceptive	Prevention of pregnancy
Lupkynis [voclosporin]	Z79.621	Calcineurin inhibitor; immunosuppressant	Lupus nephritis
Lupron Depot [leuprolide acetate]	Z79.818	Agents affecting estrogen receptors and estrogen levels; antineoplastic	Endometriosis symptoms; uterine fibroids; symptoms of prostate cancer
Macrobid [nitrofurantoin]	Z79.2	Antibiotic	Urinary tract infections
Macrodantin [nitrofurantoin]	Z79.2	Antibiotic	Urinary tract infections
Meclizine hydrochloride [meclizine hydrochloride]		Antihistamine; antiemetic	Nausea, vomiting, and dizziness associated with motion sickness; symptoms of vertigo
Medrol [methylprednisolone]	Z79.52	Corticosteroid	Allergic and edematous states; collagen disorders
Megace ES [megestrol acetate]	Z79.818	Agents affecting estrogen receptors and estrogen levels; progestin; antineoplastic	Endometrial or advanced breast cancers; weight loss due to AIDS
Menest [esterified estrogens]	Z79.89Ø	Estrogen therapy	Menopause symptoms; ovarian failure
Menostar [estradiol]	Z79.89Ø	Estrogen therapy	Menopause symptoms; osteoporosis prevention
Mepron [atovaquone]	Z79.2	Antibiotic	Pneumonia due to Pneumocystis jirovecii
Merrem [meropenem]	Z79.2	Antibiotic	Bacterial infections of skin or stomach; bacterial meningitis
Mesalamine [mesalamine]		Anti-inflammatory	Ulcerative colitis
Metformin [metformin hydrochloride]	Z79.84	Oral hypoglycemic	Diabetes mellitus
Methadone HCl [methadone hydrochloride]	Z79.891	Analgesic, narcotic; opioid agonist	Pain; treatment of opioid addiction
Methadose [methadone hydrochloride]	Z79.891	Analgesic, narcotic; opioid agonist	Acute and chronic pain
Methergine [methylergonovine maleate]		Oxytocic agent	Routine management of postpartum hemorrhage after delivery of placenta
Methotrexate sodium [methotrexate sodium]	Z79.631	Antimetabolite agent	Cancer
Methylprednisolone [methylprednisolone]	Z79.52	Corticosteroid	Inflammatory disorders
Metronidazole [metronidazole]	Z79.2	Antibiotic	Bacterial infections
Miacalcin [calcitonin salmon]		Calcitonin	Hypercalcemia; osteoporosis; Paget's disease
Miebo [perfluorhexyloctane]		Ophthalmic anti-inflammatory agent	Dry eye disease
Minivelle [estradiol]	Z79.89Ø	Estrogen therapy	Menopause symptoms; osteoporosis prevention
Minocin [minocycline hydrochloride]	Z79.2	Antibiotic	Bacterial infections; acne
Mirena [levonorgestrel]	Z79.3	Contraceptive	Intrauterine device for prevention of pregnancy; menstrual disorders
Mitomycin [mitomycin]	Z79.632	Antitumor antibiotic; antineoplastic	Stomach and pancreas cancer
Mobic [meloxicam]	Z79.1	Nonsteroidal anti-inflammatory drug (NSAID)	Treatment of pain and inflammation due to osteoarthritis and rheumatoid arthritis

Drug	Z Code	Drug Action/Classification	Indications
Monoclonal antibodies	Z79.620	Immunosuppressive biologic	Cancer; prophylaxis of organ transplant rejection
Monodox [doxycycline]	Z79.2	Antibiotic	Bacterial infections; acne
Mono-Linyah [norgestimate/ethinyl estradiol]	Z79.3	Contraceptive	Prevention of pregnancy; menstrual disorders; acne
Monurol [fosfomycin tromethamine]	Z79.2	Antibiotic	Bacterial bladder infections
Morphine sulfate [morphine sulfate]	Z79.891	Analgesic, narcotic	Moderate to severe pain
Motrin IB [ibuprofen]	Z79.1	Nonsteroidal anti-inflammatory drug (NSAID)	Pain or fever relief
Mounjaro [tirzepatide]	Z79.85	Antidiabetic – non-insulin injectable	Diabetes mellitus
MS Contin [morphine sulfate]	Z79.891	Analgesic, narcotic	Moderate to severe pain
Multaq [dronedarone hydrochloride]		Antiarrhythmic	Atrial fibrillation; atrial flutter
Mycobutin [rifabutin]	Z79.2	Antibiotic	Mycobacterium avium complex (MAC) prophylactic in HIV patients
Mytesi [crofelemer]		Antidiarrheal	Diarrhea occurring in HIV/AIDs patient's on anti-retroviral therapy
Nabumetone [nabumetone]	Z79.1	Nonsteroidal anti-inflammatory drug (NSAID)	Osteoarthritis and rheumatoid arthritis
Nalfon [fenoprofen calcium]	Z79.1	Nonsteroidal anti-inflammatory drug (NSAID)	Pain or inflammation relief; osteoarthritis; rheumatoid arthritis
Namzaric [memantine/donepezil hydrochlorides]		Acetylcholinesterase/cholinesterase inhibitors	Dementia due to Alzheimer's
Naprelan [naproxen sodium]	Z79.1	Nonsteroidal anti-inflammatory drug (NSAID)	Pain or inflammation relief
Naprosyn [naproxen]	Z79.1	Nonsteroidal anti-inflammatory drug (NSAID)	Rheumatoid, gouty arthritis and osteoarthritis; ankylosing spondylitis; bursitis; dysmenorrhea; pain, mild to moderate; tendonitis
Natazia [estradiol valerate/dienogest]	Z79.3	Contraceptive	Prevention of pregnancy; menstrual disorders
Nebupent [pentamidine isethionate]	Z79.2	Antibiotic; antifungal	Fungal infections; Pneumocystis jirovecii (carinii) pneumonia in HIV patients
Nefazodone HCl [nefazodone hydrochloride]		Antidepressant	Depression
Nembutal sodium [pentobarbital sodium]		Sedative/hypnotic	Insomnia; adjunct medication in diagnostic procedures or for emergency use with convulsive disorders
NeoProfen [ibuprofen lysine]	Z79.1	Nonsteroidal anti-inflammatory drug (NSAID)	Pain or fever relief in premature infants
Neoral [cyclosporine]	Z79.621	Calcineurin inhibitor	Prophylaxis of organ transplant rejection; rheumatoid arthritis; psoriasis
Neosporin [bacitracin, neomycin]	Z79.2	Antibiotic, topical	Bacterial skin infections
Neurontin [gabapentin]		Anticonvulsant	Postherpetic neuralgia; partial onset seizures
Nexium [esomeprazole magnesium]		Proton pump inhibitor	Gastroesophageal reflux disease (GERD); erosive esophagitis
Nexletol [bempedoic acid]		Antihyperlipidemic	Heterozygous familial hypercholesterolemia; established atherosclerotic cardiovascular disease requiring additional lowering of LDL-C
Nexplanon [etonogestrel]	Z79.3	Contraceptive	Implantable device used for prevention of pregnancy
Ngenla [somatrogon-ghla]		Growth hormone	Growth failure
Nitrofurantoin [nitrofurantoin]	Z79.2	Antibiotic	Bacterial urinary tract infections

Drug	Z Code	Drug Action/Classification	Indications
Nitrostat [nitroglycerin]		Muscle relaxant; antianginal; antihypertensive; coronary vasodilator	Angina pectoris; heart failure associated with myocardial infarction; hypertension, perioperative; surgery, adjunct
Norpace [disopyramide phosphate]		Antiarrhythmic	Coronary artery disease; prevention, recurrence, and control of unifocal, multifocal, and paired PVCs
Norvasc [amlodipine besylate]		Antihypertensive	Hypertension; coronary artery disease (CAD); chronic stable angina; prinzmetal's angina; variant angina
Novolin [insulin recombinant]	Z79.4	Insulin	Diabetes mellitus
Novolog [insulin aspart recombinant]	Z79.4	Insulin	Diabetes mellitus
Nucynta [tapentadol hydrochloride]	Z79.891	Analgesic, narcotic	Moderate to severe pain
NuvaRing [etonogestrel/ethinyl estradiol]	Z79.3	Contraceptive	Vaginal ring to prevent pregnancy
Ogsiveo [nirogacestat]		Antineoplastic	Desmoid tumors
Ojjaara [momelotinib]	Z79.622	Janus kinase (JAK) inhibitor	Myelofibrosis
Olumiant [baricitinib]	Z79.622	Janus kinase (JAK) inhibitor	Rheumatoid arthritis
Omvoh [mirikizumab-mrkz]	Z79.620	Monoclonal antibody	Ulcerative colitis
Opdualag [nivolumab and relatlimab-rmbw]		Antineoplastic combination	Unresectable or metastatic melanoma
Oracea [doxycycline]	Z79.2	Antibiotic	Rosacea
Orapred ODT [prednisolone sodium phosphate]	Z79.52	Corticosteroid	Inflammatory disorders
Orbactiv [oritavancin diphosphate]	Z79.2	Antibiotic	Bacterial skin infections
Orencia [abatacept]	Z79.69	Other immunosuppressant/immunomodulator	Rheumatoid arthritis; polyarticular juvenile idiopathic arthritis; psoriatic arthritis; prophylaxis of acute graft versus host disease (aGVHD)
Orilissa [elagolix]	Z79.890	Hormone therapy	Pain associated with endometriosis
Orphenadrine citrate [orphenadrine citrate]		Muscle relaxant	Acute spasms, tension, and post-trauma cases
Orserdu [elacestrant]	Z79.818	Agents affecting estrogen receptors and estrogen levels	Advanced or metastatic breast cancer
Oseni [alogliptin benzoate/pioglitazone hydrochloride]	Z79.84	Oral hypoglycemic	Diabetes mellitus
Osphena [ospemifene]	Z79.810	Selective estrogen receptor modulator (SERM)	Postmenopausal dyspareunia due to vaginal atrophy; osteoporosis; menopausal symptoms
Otezla [apremilast]	Z79.61	Immunomodulator; antirheumatic	Psoriatic arthritis; plaque psoriasis; oral ulcers associated with Behcet's disease
Oxazepam [oxazepam]		Antianxiety	Anxiety, tension, and withdrawal from alcohol
Oxbryta [voxelotor]		Hemoglobin S polymerization inhibitor	Sickle cell disease
Oxycodone HCl [oxycodone hydrochloride]	Z79.891	Analgesic, narcotic	Moderate to severe pain
OxyContin [oxycodone hydrochloride]	Z79.891	Analgesic, narcotic	Moderate to severe pain
Ozempic [semaglutide]	Z79.85	Antidiabetic – non-insulin injectable	Diabetes mellitus
Paclitaxel [paclitaxel]	Z79.633	Mitotic inhibitor	Cancer of the breast, ovaries, and lung; AIDS-related Kaposi's sarcoma
Paxil [paroxetine hydrochloride]		Antidepressant; selective serotonin reuptake inhibitor (SSRI)	Obsessive-compulsive disorder; major depressive disorder; panic disorder; social anxiety disorder; generalized anxiety disorder; posttraumatic stress disorder

Pharmacology List

Drug	Z Code	Drug Action/Classification	Indications
Paxlovid [nirmatrelvir, ritonavir]		Antiviral	COVID-19
PediaPred [prednisolone sodium phosphate]	Z79.52	Corticosteroid	Inflammatory disorders
PegIntron [peginterferon alfa-2b]	Z79.69	Other immunosuppressant/immunomodulator; antiviral	Hepatitis C
Penicillin-VK [penicillin V potassium]	Z79.2	Antibiotic	Chorea, prevention; endocarditis, prevention, secondary to tooth extraction; erysipelas; infections of the skin, skin structures, and upper respiratory tract; rheumatic fever, prophylaxis; scarlet fever; Vincent's gingivitis; Vincent's pharyngitis
Pentam [pentamidine isethionate]	Z79.2	Antibiotic; antifungal	Severe bacterial lung infections; fungal infections; Pneumocystis jirovecii (carinii) pneumonia
Pentasa [mesalamine]		Anti-inflammatory	Crohn's disease; ulcerative colitis
Pepcid AC [famotidine]		Histamine H2-receptor inhibitor	Acid/peptic disorder; adenoma, secretory; gastroesophageal reflux; duodenal and gastric ulcer; Zollinger-Ellison syndrome
Percocet [oxycodone hydrochloride/acetaminophen]	Z79.891	Analgesic, narcotic	Moderate to severe pain
Persantine [dipyridamole]	Z79.Ø2	Antiplatelet	Prevention of blood clots after heart valve surgery
Pfizerpen [penicillin g potassium]	Z79.2	Antibiotic	Severe bacterial infections
Phenobarbital [phenobarbital sodium]		Anticonvulsant	Grand mal epilepsy; sedative
Piqray [alpelisib]		Kinase inhibitor	Postmenopausal advanced or metastatic breast cancer
Pitocin [oxytocin]		Uterotonic	Induction or stimulation of labor at term; control of bleeding after childbirth
Plan B One-Step [levonorgestrel]	Z79.3	Contraceptive	Prevention of pregnancy
Plavix [clopidogrel bisulfate]	Z79.Ø2	Antiplatelet	Lessening of the chance of heart attack or stroke
Pluvicto [lutetium Lu 177 vipivotide tetraxetan]		Radioligand therapeutic agent	Metastatic castration-resistant prostate cancer (mCRPC)
Pomalyst [pomalidomide]	Z79.61	Immunomodulator; antineoplastic	Multiple myeloma; Kaposi sarcoma
Pombiliti [cipaglucosidase alfa-atga]		Lysosomal enzyme	Pompe disease
Ponstel [mefenamic acid]	Z79.1	Nonsteroidal anti-inflammatory drug (NSAID)	Mild to moderate pain; primary dysmenorrhea
Ponvory [ponesimod]	Z79.69	Other immunosuppressant/immunomodulator	Relapsing forms of multiple sclerosis (MS)
Pradaxa [dabigatran etexilate mesylate]	Z79.Ø1	Anticoagulant	Prophylaxis and treatment of blood clots in patients with atrial fibrillation
Prasugrel [prasugrel hydrochloride]	Z79.Ø2	Antiplatelet	Lessening the chance of heart attack or stroke
Pravastatin sodium [pravastatin sodium]		HMG-CoA reductase inhibitor (statin)	Hypercholesterolemia; hyperlipidemia; hyperlipoproteinemia
Prednisolone [prednisolone]	Z79.52	Corticosteroid	Inflammatory disorders
Prednisone [prednisone]	Z79.52	Corticosteroid	Immunosuppressant effects; relief of inflammation; used in arthritis, polymyositis and other systemic diseases
Pregnyl [chorionic gonadotropin]		Gonadotropic hormone	Prepubertal cryptorchidism; hypogonadism; corpus luteum insufficiency and infertility
Prempro [conjugated estrogens/medroxyprogesterone acetate]	Z79.89Ø	Estrogen/progesterone therapy	Menopause symptoms; osteoporosis; atrophic vaginitis

Drug	Z Code	Drug Action/Classification	Indications
Prevacid [lansoprazole]		Proton pump inhibitor	Acid/peptic disorder; erosive esophagitis; duodenal ulcer; Zollinger-Ellison syndrome
Prezcobix [darunavir/cobicistat]		Antiretroviral	HIV
Prezista [darunavir]		Antiretroviral	HIV
Priftin [rifapentine]	Z79.2	Antibiotic	Tuberculosis
Prilosec [omeprazole magnesium]		Proton pump inhibitor	Acid/peptic disorder; endocrine adenoma; erosive esophagitis; systemic mastocytosis; gastroesophageal reflux; duodenal, peptic and gastric ulcer; Zollinger-Ellison syndrome
Primaxin [cilastatin sodium/imipenem]	Z79.2	Antibiotic	Bacterial septicemia; endocarditis; bacterial infections of the skin, lower respiratory tract, intra-abdomen, bones, and joints
Pristiq [desvenlafaxine]		Antidepressant; serotonin and norepinephrine reuptake inhibitor (SNRI)	Major depressive disorder
Procardia [nifedipine]		Calcium channel blocker	Vasospastic angina; chronic stable angina; hypertension
Prograf [tacrolimus]	Z79.621	Calcineurin inhibitor	Prophylaxis of organ transplant rejection
Prolia [denosumab]	Z79.620	Immunosuppressive biologic; monoclonal antibody	Osteoporosis
Promethazine hydrochloride [promethazine hydrochloride]		Anesthesia, adjunct to; antiemetic; antihistamine; antitussive/expectorant; sedative/hypnotic; vertigo/motion sickness/vomiting	Anesthesia; adjunct; angioedema; conjunctivitis; dermographism; hypersensitivity, motion sickness; pain; perennial, seasonal, and allergic rhinitis; sedation, obstetrical; urticaria
Propranolol hydrochloride [propranolol hydrochloride]		Beta blocker	Angina pectoris; hypertension; cardiac arrhythmias
Protonix [pantoprazole sodium]		Proton pump inhibitor	Short-term treatment and maintenance therapy of erosive esophagitis associated with gastroesophageal reflux disease (GERD)
Protopic [tacrolimus]	Z79.621	Calcineurin inhibitor	Atomic dermatitis (eczema)
Proventil-HFA [albuterol sulfate]		Antiasthmatic/bronchodilator	Asthma
Provera [medroxyprogesterone acetate]	Z79.3, Z79.890	Contraceptive; progestin; antineoplastic	Prevention of pregnancy; amenorrhea; carcinoma, endometrium, adjunct; carcinoma, renal; hemorrhage
Prozac [fluoxetine hydrochloride]		Selective serotonin reuptake inhibitor (SSRI)	Bulimia nervosa; depression; obsessive-compulsive disorder
Pulmicort [budesonide]	Z79.51	Corticosteroid – inhaled; antiasthmatic	Prophylaxis and treatment of asthma
Qalsody [tofersen]		CNS agent	Amyotrophic lateral sclerosis
Qelbree [viloxazine hydrochloride]		Selective norepinephrine reuptake inhibitor	Attention deficit hyperactivity disorder (ADHD)
Qnasl [beclomethasone dipropionate]		Corticosteroid – intranasal	Perennial and seasonal allergies; vasomotor rhinitis
Qtern [dapagliflozin/saxagliptin]	Z79.84	Oral hypoglycemic	Diabetes mellitus
Quinapril hydrochloride [quinapril hydrochloride]		ACE inhibitor	Hypertension; heart failure
Qulipta [atogepant]		Calcitonin gene-related peptide inhibitor	Migraine headache prevention
Quviviq [daridorexant hydrochloride]		CNS depressant	Insomnia
Qvar Redihaler [beclomethasone dipropionate]	Z79.51	Corticosteroid – inhaled; antiasthmatic	Prophylaxis and treatment of asthma
Raloxifene HCl [raloxifene hydrochloride]	Z79.810	Selective estrogen receptor modulator (SERM)	Osteoporosis in postmenopausal women
Rapaflo [silodosin]		Antiadrenergic	Benign prostatic hyperplasia

Pharmacology List

Drug	Z Code	Drug Action/Classification	Indications
Rapamune [sirolimus]	Z79.623	Mammalian target of rapamycin (mTOR) inhibitor	Prophylaxis of organ transplant rejection
Rayos [prednisone]	Z79.52	Corticosteroid; antiasthmatic	Arthritis; blood disorders; allergies; asthma
Rebif [interferon beta-1a]	Z79.69	Other immunosuppressant/immunomodulator	Treatment of relapsing multiple sclerosis
Reclast [zoledronic acid]	Z79.83	Bisphosphonate	Osteoporosis; Paget's disease; bone cancer
Relenza [zanamivir]		Antiviral	Treat and prevent influenza A and B
Relyvrio [sodium phenylbutyrate/taurursodiol]		Central nervous system agent	Amyotrophic lateral sclerosis (ALS)
Remicade [infliximab]	Z79.620	Immunosuppressive biologic; monoclonal antibody	Ankylosing spondylitis; psoriatic arthritis; rheumatoid arthritis; Crohn's disease; ulcerative colitis
Renvela [sevelamer carbonate]		Phosphate binder	Chronic kidney disease (CKD) on dialysis
Repaglinide [repaglinide]	Z79.84	Oral hypoglycemic	Diabetes mellitus
Restasis [cyclosporine ophthalmic emulsion]	Z79.621	Calcineurin inhibitor	Ocular inflammation due to keratoconjunctivitis sicca
Restoril [temazepam]		Sedative/hypnotic	Insomnia
Retrovir [zidovudine]		Antiretroviral	HIV
Revlimid [lenalidomide]	Z79.61	Immunomodulator; antineoplastic	Multiple myeloma following autologous stem cell transplant; myelodysplastic syndromes; mantle cell lymphoma
Reyvow [lasmiditan]		Antimigraine	Migraine headache
Rezzayo [rezafungin]		Antifungal	Candidemia; invasive candidiasis
Rifadin [rifampin]	Z79.2	Antibiotic	Tuberculosis
Rimactane [rifampin]	Z79.2	Antibiotic	Tuberculosis
Rinvoq [upadacitinib]	Z79.622	Janus kinase (JAK) inhibitor	Rheumatoid arthritis; psoriatic arthritis; ankylosing spondylitis; ulcerative colitis
Risperdal [risperidone]		Antipsychotic/antimanic	Schizophrenia; bipolar I disorder
Ritalin [methylphenidate hydrochloride]		CNS stimulant	Attention deficit hyperactivity disorder (ADHD); narcolepsy
Rituxan [rituximab]	Z79.620	Immunosuppressive biologic; monoclonal antibody	Non-Hodgkin's lymphoma; chronic lymphocytic leukemia; rheumatoid arthritis; granulomatosis with polyangiitis; pemphigus vulgaris
Roxicodone [oxycodone hydrochloride]	Z79.891	Analgesic, narcotic	Pain relief
Rukobia [fostemsavir tromethamine]		Antiretroviral	HIV
Rybelsus [semaglutide]	Z79.84	Oral hypoglycemic	Diabetes mellitus
Rystiggo [rozanolixizumab-noli]		Antineoplastic	Myasthenia gravis
Ryzneuta [efbemalenograstim alfa-vuxw]		Immunostimulant	Neutropenia
Sabril [vigabatrin]		Anticonvulsant	Refractory complex partial seizures
Sandimmune [cyclosporine]	Z79.621	Calcineurin inhibitor	Prophylaxis of organ transplant rejection
Savaysa [edoxaban tosylate]	Z79.01	Anticoagulant	Prophylaxis and treatment of venous thrombosis, pulmonary embolism; prevention of blood clots due to atrial fibrillation
Scemblix [asciminib hydrochloride]		Kinase inhibitor	Philadelphia chromosome-positive chronic myeloid leukemia
Seasonale [levonorgestrel/ethinyl estradiol]	Z79.3	Contraceptive	Prevention of pregnancy
Seasonique [ethinyl estradiol/levonorgestrel]	Z79.3	Contraceptive	Prevention of pregnancy

Drug	Z Code	Drug Action/Classification	Indications
Septra [sulfamethoxazole trimethoprim]	Z79.2	Antibiotic	Urinary tract infections; acute otitis media; acute exacerbations of chronic bronchitis; shigellosis
Serevent [salmeterol xinafoate]		Bronchodilator	Asthma
Seromycin [cycloserine]	Z79.2	Antibiotic	Tuberculosis; urinary tract infections
Seroquel XR [quetiapine fumarate]		Antipsychotic	Schizophrenia; bipolar disorder; major depressive disorder
Silvadene [silver sulfadiazine]	Z79.2	Antibiotic, topical	Wound sepsis due to second/third degree burns
Simulect [basiliximab]	Z79.620	Immunosuppressive biologic; monoclonal antibody	Prophylaxis of organ transplant rejection
Sinemet [carbidopa/levodopa]		Antiparkinsonism	Parkinson's disease
Singulair [montelukast sodium]		Antiasthmatic	Asthma; exercise-induced bronchoconstriction; perennial and seasonal allergic rhinitis
Sirolimus [sirolimus]	Z79.623	Mammalian target of rapamycin (mTOR) inhibitor	Prophylaxis of organ transplant rejection
Sitagliptin [sitagliptin/metformin hydrochloride]	Z79.84	Oral hypoglycemic	Diabetes mellitus
Sivextro [tedizolid phosphate]	Z79.2	Antibiotic	Skin infections including MRSA
Skyclarys [omaveloxolone]		CNS stimulant	Friedrich's ataxia
Skyla [levonorgestrel]	Z79.3	Contraceptive	Intrauterine device to prevent pregnancy
Skyrizi [risankizumab]	Z79.620	Immunosuppressive biologic; monoclonal antibody	Plaque psoriasis
Sodium nitroprusside [sodium nitroprusside]		Vasodilator	Hypertensive crisis; control surgical bleeding; acute congestive heart failure
Soliqua [insulin glargine/lixisenatide]	Z79.4	Insulin	Diabetes mellitus
Solodyn [minocycline hydrochloride]	Z79.2	Antibiotic	Bacterial infections
Solosec [secnidazole]	Z79.2	Antibiotic	Bacterial vaginal inflammation; trichomoniasis
Soltamox [tamoxifen citrate]	Z79.810	Selective estrogen receptor modulator (SERM)	Breast cancer
Solu-Cortef [hydrocortisone sodium succinate]	Z79.52	Corticosteroid; antiasthmatic	Asthma; severe inflammation; allergic reactions
Solu-Medrol [methylprednisolone sodium succinate]	Z79.52	Corticosteroid	Anti-inflammatory and antiallergenic for shock and ulcerative colitis
Sotyktu [deucravacitinib]		Multikinase inhibitor	Plaque psoriasis
Spiriva [tiotropium bromide]		Antiasthmatic/bronchodilator	Chronic obstructive pulmonary disease (COPD); asthma
Sprintec [norgestimate/ethinyl estradiol]	Z79.3	Contraceptive	Prevention of pregnancy
Stelara [ustekinumab]	Z79.620	Immunosuppressive biologic; monoclonal antibody	Plaque psoriasis; psoriatic arthritis; Crohn's disease; ulcerative colitis
Strattera [atomoxetine hydrochloride]		CNS stimulant	Attention deficit hyperactivity disorder (ADHD)
Streptomycin sulfate [streptomycin sulfate]	Z79.2	Antibiotic	Severe bacterial infections
Suboxone [buprenorphine/naloxone]		Opioid agonist	Treatment of opioid addiction
Sunlenca [lenacapavir]		Antiretroviral	HIV
Supprelin LA [histrelin acetate]	Z79.818	Agents affecting estrogen receptors and estrogen levels	Precocious puberty
Suprax [cefixime]	Z79.2	Antibiotic	Bacterial infections

Pharmacology List

Drug	Z Code	Drug Action/Classification	Indications
Sylatron [peginterferon alfa-2b]	Z79.69	Other immunosuppressant/immunomodulator	Prevention of recurrent malignant melanoma
Symbicort [budesonide/formoterol fumarate dihydrate]	Z79.51	Corticosteroid – inhaled; antiasthmatic	Prophylaxis and treatment of asthma and COPD
Symbyax [olanzapine/fluoxetine]		Antidepressant	Acute depressive episodes associated with bipolar I disorder; treatment-resistant depression
Symlin [pramlintide]	Z79.85	Antidiabetic – non-insulin injectable	Diabetes mellitus
Symtuza [darunavir/cobicistat/emtricitabine/tenofovir alafenamide]		Antiretroviral	HIV
Synarel [nafarelin acetate]	Z79.818	Agents affecting estrogen receptors and estrogen levels	Endometriosis symptoms; precocious puberty
Synercid [dalfopristin/quinupristin]	Z79.2	Antibiotic	Severe blood infections
Synjardy [empagliflozin/metformin hydrochloride]	Z79.84	Oral hypoglycemic	Diabetes mellitus
Synthroid [levothyroxine sodium]	Z79.890	Thyroid hormone	Hypothyroidism
Tacrolimus [tacrolimus]	Z79.621	Calcineurin inhibitor	Prophylaxis of organ transplant rejection
Talicia [omeprazole magnesium/amoxicillin/rifabutin]	Z79.2	Combination antibiotic	Helicobacter pylori
Taltz [ixekizumab]	Z79.620	Immunosuppressive biologic; monoclonal antibody	Plaque psoriasis; psoriatic arthritis; ankylosing spondylitis; axial spondyloarthritis
Talvey [talquetamab-tgvs]		Antineoplastic	Multiple myeloma
Tamiflu [oseltamivir phosphate]		Antiviral	Treatment and prevention of influenza A and B
Tamoxifen citrate [tamoxifen citrate]	Z79.810	Selective estrogen receptor modulator (SERM)	Metastatic breast cancer in postmenopausal women
Tavneos [avacopan]	Z79.69	Other immunosuppressant/immunomodulator	ANCA-associated vasculitis
Taxotere [docetaxel]	Z79.633	Mitotic inhibitor	Cancer
Tazicef [ceftazidime]	Z79.2	Antibiotic	Confirmed or suspected bacterial infections
Teflaro [ceftaroline fosamil]	Z79.2	Antibiotic	Bacterial skin infections; pneumonia
Tegretol [carbamazepine]		Anticonvulsant; analgesic	Epilepsy, especially with complex symptomatology; specific analgesic for trigeminal neuralgia
Temozolomide [temozolomide]	Z79.630	Chemotherapeutic alkylating agent	Chronic myelogenous leukemia
Tenormin [atenolol]		Beta blocker	Angina pectoris; hypertension; acute myocardial infarction
Terazosin HCl [terazosin hydrochloride]		Antiadrenergic	Benign prostatic hypertrophy; hypertension
Terlivaz [terlipressin]		Antidiuretic hormone	Kidney function in hepatorenal syndrome
Testim [testosterone]	Z79.890	Testosterone therapy – topical	Primary hypogonadism
Tetracycline [tetracycline]	Z79.2	Antibiotic	Bacterial infections
Thalomid [thalidomide]	Z79.61	Immunomodulator	Multiple myeloma; erythema nodosum leprosum
Tiazac [diltiazem hydrochloride]		Calcium channel blocker	Chronic stable angina; atrial fibrillation; atrial flutter; hypertension; paroxysmal supraventricular tachycardia
Tobradex [tobramycin/dexamethasone]		Aminoglycoside ocular anti-infective; anti-inflammatory	Infectious conjunctivitis; dermatosis, corticosteroid-responsive with secondary infection; foreign body in eye; corneal inflammation; uveitis
Tobramycin [dexamethasone/tobramycin]	Z79.2	Antibiotic	Bacterial eye infections

Drug	Z Code	Drug Action/Classification	Indications
Topamax [topiramate]		Anticonvulsant	Epilepsy; primary generalized tonic-clonic seizures; seizures associated with Lennox-Gastaut syndrome; migraine headache
Toprol-XL [metoprolol succinate]		Beta blocker	Angina pectoris; hypertension
Toremifene citrate [toremifene citrate]	Z79.810	Selective estrogen receptor modulator (SERM)	Metastatic breast cancer in postmenopausal women
Torisel [temsirolimus]	Z79.623	Mammalian target of rapamycin (mTOR) inhibitor	Renal cell carcinoma
Toujeo Solostar [insulin glargine recombinant]	Z79.4	Insulin	Diabetes mellitus
Tradjenta [linagliptin]	Z79.84	Oral hypoglycemic	Diabetes mellitus
Trazodone HCl [trazodone hydrochloride]		Antidepressant	Depression
Trelegy Ellipta [fluticasone furoate/umeclidinium bromide/vilanterol trifenatate]	Z79.51	Corticosteroid – inhaled; antiasthmatic	COPD
Trelstar [triptorelin pamoate]	Z79.818	Agents affecting estrogen receptors and estrogen levels	Palliative treatment of prostate cancer symptoms
Tremfya [guselkumab]	Z79.620	Immunosuppressive biologic; monoclonal antibody	Plaque psoriasis
Tresiba [insulin degludec]	Z79.4	Insulin	Diabetes mellitus
Triamterene and hydrochlorothiazide [triamterene/hydrochlorothiazide]		Antihypertensive; diuretic	Edema; hypertension
Trijardy XR [empagliflozin/linagliptin/metformin hydrochloride]	Z79.84	Oral hypoglycemic	Diabetes mellitus
Tri-Lo-Estarylla [ethinyl estradiol/norgestimate]	Z79.3	Contraceptive	Prevention of pregnancy
Tri-Lo-Sprintec [ethinyl estradiol/norgestimate]	Z79.3	Contraceptive	Prevention of pregnancy
Trimethoprim [trimethoprim]	Z79.2	Antibiotic	Acute exacerbation chronic bronchitis; travelers' diarrhea; infections of the middle, lower respiratory tract, and urinary tract; pneumonia, pneumocystis; shigellosis
Triptodur [triptorelin]	Z79.818	Agents affecting estrogen receptors and estrogen levels	Precocious puberty
Tri-Sprintec [ethinyl estradiol/norgestimate]	Z79.3	Contraceptive	Prevention of pregnancy; acne
Trokendi XR [topiramate]		Anticonvulsant	Epilepsy; primary generalized tonic clonic seizures; seizures associated with Lennox-Gastaut syndrome; migraine headache
Trulicity [dulaglutide]	Z79.85	Antidiabetic – non-insulin injectable	Diabetes mellitus
Truqap [capivasertib]		Antineoplastic; kinase inhibitor	Breast cancer
Truvada [emtricitabine/tenofovir disoproxil fumarate]		Antiretroviral	HIV
Turalio [pexidartinib]		Kinase inhibitor	Symptomatic tenosynovial giant cell tumor
Tygacil [tigecycline]	Z79.2	Antibiotic	Bacterial skin or digestive system infections; pneumonia
Tzield [teplizumab-mzwv]	Z79.85	Antidiabetic – non-insulin injectable	Delay onset of stage 3 type 1 diabetes
Ubrelvy [ubrogepant]		Calcitonin gene-related peptide inhibitor	Migraine headache
Unasyn [ampicillin sodium/sulbactam sodium]	Z79.2	Antibiotic	Bacterial infections

Drug	Z Code	Drug Action/Classification	Indications
Vabomere [meropenem; vaborbactam]	Z79.2	Antibiotic	Complicated urinary tract infections; pyelonephritis
Vabysmo [faricimab-svoa]		Anti-angiogenic ophthalmic agent	Neovascular age-related macular degeneration; diabetic macular edema
Vagifem [estradiol]	Z79.890	Estrogen therapy	Menopause symptoms
Valium [diazepam]		Antianxiety; muscle relaxant; anticonvulsant	Anxiety, tension, withdrawal from alcohol; muscle spasms and anticonvulsant therapy; epilepsy, generalized tonic-clonic; status epilepticus; stiff-person syndrome; tetanus
Vancocin HCl [vancomycin hydrochloride]	Z79.2	Antibiotic	Severe bacterial infections
Vancomycin HCl [vancomycin hydrochloride]	Z79.2	Antibiotic	Severe bacterial infections
Vanflyta [quizartinib]		Kinase inhibitor	Acute myeloid leukemia
Varenicline tartrate [varenicline tartrate]		Smoking cessation aid	Nicotine addiction; smoking
Vasotec [enalaprilat maleate]		ACE inhibitor	Heart failure; hypertension
Velivet [desogestrel/ethinyl estradiol]	Z79.3	Contraceptive	Prevention of pregnancy
Velsipity [etrasimod]		Anti-inflammatory	Ulcerative colitis
Venlafaxine HCl [venlafaxine hydrochloride]		Antidepressant, serotonin and norepinephrine reuptake inhibitor (SNRI)	Major depressive disorder; social anxiety disorder; panic disorder
Ventolin HFA [albuterol sulfate]		Antiasthmatic/bronchodilator	Asthma
Veozah [fezolinetant]		CNS agent	Menopause symptoms
Verapamil HCL [verapamil hydrochloride]		Calcium channel blocker	Angina pectoris; chronic stable angina; atrial fibrillation; atrial flutter; paroxysmal supraventricular tachycardia; ventricular arrhythmia; hypertension
Viagra [sildenafil citrate]		Phosphodiesterase-5 (PDE5) inhibitor	Erectile dysfunction
Vibativ [telavancin hydrochloride]	Z79.2	Antibiotic	Pneumonia; severe bacterial skin infections
Vibramycin [doxycycline calcium]	Z79.2	Antibiotic	Bacterial infections
Victoza [liraglutide]	Z79.85	Antidiabetic – non-insulin injectable	Diabetes mellitus
Vinblastine sulfate [vinblastine sulfate]	Z79.633	Mitotic inhibitor	Cancer
Vincristine sulfate PFS [vincristine sulfate]	Z79.633	Mitotic inhibitor	Cancer
Virazole [ribavirin]		Antiviral	Respiratory syncytial virus (RSV)
Viread [tenofovir disoproxil fumarate]		Antiretroviral	HIV; chronic hepatitis B
Voltaren Arthritis Pain [diclofenac sodium]	Z79.1	Nonsteroidal anti-inflammatory drug (NSAID)	Treatment of pain, inflammation, and joint stiffness due to arthritis
Vonjo [pacritinib]		Multikinase inhibitor	Treats intermediate or high-risk primary or secondary myelofibrosis in adults with low platelets
Voquezna [vonoprazan, amoxicillin, and clarithromycin]	Z79.2	Antibiotic, antimicrobial; potassium-competitive acid blocker	Helicobacter pylori
Vtama [tapinarof]		Topical antipsoriatic	Plaque psoriasis
Vumerity [diroximel fumarate]	Z79.69	Other immunosuppressant/immunomodulator	Relapsing forms of multiple sclerosis (MS)
Vytorin [ezetimibe/simvastatin]		HMG-CoA reductase inhibitor (statin); cholesterol absorption inhibitor	Hyperlipidemia; hypercholesterolemia
Wakix [pitolisant hydrochloride]		CNS stimulant	Narcolepsy

Drug	Z Code	Drug Action/Classification	Indications
Warfarin sodium [warfarin sodium]	Z79.Ø1	Anticoagulant	Prophylaxis and treatment of venous thrombosis; treatment of atrial fibrillation with embolization (pulmonary embolism), arrhythmias, myocardial infarction, and stroke prevention
Wellbutrin SR, Wellbutrin XL [bupropion hydrochloride]		Antidepressant	Depression
Xacduro [sulbactam, durlobactam]	Z79.2	Antibiotic	Hospital-acquired bacterial pneumonia and ventilator-associated bacterial pneumonia caused by Acinetobacter baumannii-calcoaceticus complex
Xalatan [latanoprost]		Prostaglandin F2? analogue	Glaucoma, open-angle; ocular hypertension
Xanax, Xanax XR [alprazolam]		Antianxiety; sedative/hypnotic	Anxiety disorders with panic disorder and depression
Xarelto [rivaroxaban]	Z79.Ø1	Anticoagulant	Prophylaxis and treatment of venous thrombosis, pulmonary embolism; prevention of blood clots due to atrial fibrillation
Xdemvy [lotilaner]		Antiparasitic	Demodex blepharitis
Xeljanz, Xeljanz XR [tofacitinib citrate]	Z79.622	Janus kinase (JAK) inhibitor	Rheumatoid arthritis; psoriatic arthritis
Xeloda [capecitabine]	Z79.631	Antimetabolite agent	Cancer of the breast, colon, colorectal
Xelstrym [dextroamphetamine]		CNS stimulant	Attention deficit hyperactivity disorder (ADHD)
Xenleta [lefamulin acetate]	Z79.2	Antibiotic	Community-acquired bacterial pneumonia
Xgeva [denosumab]	Z79.62Ø	Immunosuppressive biologic; monoclonal antibody	Treatment and prevention of bone resorption and prevention of bone fracture
Xifaxan [rifaximin]	Z79.2	Antibiotic	E. coli diarrhea
Xigduo XR [dapagliflozin/metformin hydrochloride]	Z79.84	Oral hypoglycemic	Diabetes mellitus
Xpovio [selinexor]		Antineoplastic	Multiple myeloma in adults
Xulane [ethinyl estradiol/norelgestromin]	Z79.3	Contraceptive	Prevention of pregnancy
Xultophy 1ØØ/3.6 [insulin degludec/liraglutide]	Z79.4	Insulin	Diabetes mellitus
Xyrem [sodium oxybate]		CNS depressant; anxiolytic/sedative/hypnotic	Cataplexy and/or excessive daytime sleepiness in narcolepsy
Xyzal Allergy 24Hr [levocetirizine dihydrochloride]		Antihistamine	Perennial allergic rhinitis; chronic idiopathic urticaria
Yasmin [drospirenone/ethinyl estradiol]	Z79.3	Contraceptive	Prevention of pregnancy
Yaz [drospirenone/ethinyl estradiol]	Z79.3	Contraceptive	Prevention of pregnancy; menstrual disorders
Zavzpret [zavegepant]		Calcitonin gene-related peptide inhibitor	Migraine headache
Zerbaxa [ceftolozane sulfate/tazobactam sodium]	Z79.2	Antibiotic	Complicated urinary tract and intra-abdominal infections
Zestoretic [lisinopril/hydrochlorothiazide]		ACE inhibitor	Heart failure; hypertension
Zestril [lisinopril]		ACE inhibitor	Heart failure; hypertension
Zetia [ezetimibe]		Antihyperlipidemic	Hypercholesterolemia; sitosterolemia
Ziac [bisoprolol fumarate/ hydrochlorothiazide]		Antihypertensive	Hypertension
Zilbrysq [zilucoplan]	Z79.69	Other immunosuppressant/immunomodulator	Myasthenia gravis
Zipsor [diclofenac potassium]	Z79.1	Nonsteroidal anti-inflammatory drug (NSAID)	Pain and inflammation relief

Drug	Z Code	Drug Action/Classification	Indications
Zithromax [azithromycin]	Z79.2	Antibiotic	Infections of the cervix, lower respiratory tract, skin and skin structures, urethra, nongonococcal; mycobacterium avium complex; pharyngitis, streptococcal pneumonia; tonsillitis
Zocor [simvastatin]		HMG-CoA reductase inhibitor (statin)	Hypercholesterolemia; hyperlipidemia; hyperlipoproteinemia; hypertriglyceridemia
Zoladex [goserelin acetate]	Z79.818	Agents affecting estrogen receptors and estrogen levels	Palliative treatment of prostate cancer and breast cancer symptoms; endometriosis
Zoloft [sertraline hydrochloride]		Antidepressant	Anxiety with panic disorder and depression; obsessive-compulsive disorder
Zometa [zoledronic acid]	Z79.83	Bisphosphonate	Multiple myeloma; Paget's disease
Zortress [everolimus]	Z79.623	Mammalian target of rapamycin (mTOR) inhibitor	Prophylaxis of organ transplant rejection
Zovia 1/5ØE-28 [ethinyl estradiol/ethynodiol diacetate]	Z79.3	Contraceptive	Prevention of pregnancy
Zovirax [acyclovir]		Antiviral	Genital herpes and herpes zoster infections
Zubsolv [buprenorphine/naloxone]		Opioid agonist	Treatment of opioid addiction
Zurzuvae [zuranolone]		CNS agent	Postpartum depression
Zyloprim [allopurinol]		Antigout	Gouty arthritis; renal calculus; hyperuricemia; hyperuricemia secondary to leukemia; hyperuricemia secondary to lymphoma
Zynyz [retifanlimab-dlwr]	Z79.6Ø	Immune checkpoint inhibitor; immunosuppressant	Merkel cell carcinoma
Zyprexa [olanzapine]		Antipsychotic/antimanic	Psychotic disorders; schizophrenia
Zyrtec allergy [cetirizine hydrochloride]		Antihistamine	Perennial and seasonal allergic rhinitis; chronic urticaria
Zyvox [linezolid]	Z79.2	Antibiotic	Severe bacterial infections

Appendix G. Organisms

This section lists by specimen site normal flora and possible pathogens to help the coder differentiate between what is normal and what is an indication of an abnormal situation that may be overlooked as an MCC/CC condition. According to coding guidelines, these MCC/CCs must affect patient care in terms of requiring clinical evaluation; therapeutic treatment; further evaluation by diagnostic studies, procedures, or consultation; extended length of stay; or increased nursing care; and/or monitoring for reporting purposes.

Specimen Site	Normal Flora/Possible Pathogens
Bladder	**Normal Condition of Flora:** Specimen is normally sterile and free of organism growth. **Possible Pathogens:** Any organism; common contaminants are *Enterobacter, Escherichia coli (E. coli), Klebsiella,* and *Staphylococcus epidermidis.*
Blood (multiple cultures usually performed)	**Normal Condition of Flora:** Specimen is normally sterile and free of organism growth. **Possible Pathogens:** Any organism; common contaminant is Staphylococcus epidermidis. Most common pathogens are *Bacteroides species, Haemophilus influenzae (H. influenzae), Staphylococcus aureus* and *Streptococcus pyogenes, E. coli, Pseudomonas, Streptococcus pneumoniae*. Opportunistic fungi include *Candida, Nocardia, Blastomyces dermatitidis, Histoplasma capsulatum*.
Cerebrospinal fluid	**Normal Condition of Flora:** Specimen is normally sterile and free of organism growth. **Possible Pathogens:** Any organism; common contaminant is Staphylococcus epidermidis. Pathogens include *Haemophilus influenzae, E. coli, Neisseria meningitidis* and *Streptococci agalactiae*. Viruses include coxsackie A and B, echovirus, HSV, mumps, HIV, adenovirus. Fungi include *Histoplasma capsulatum, Cryptococcus neoformans, Coccidioides immitis*.
Cervix	**Normal Condition of Flora:** Diphtheroids, *E. coli*, lactobacilli, nonhemolytic *Streptococcus*, and *Staphylococcus epidermidis*. **Possible Pathogens:** *Candida albicans* (in large numbers), *Gardnerella vaginalis, Neisseria gonorrhoeae*, and *Trichomonas,* human papilloma virus (HPV).
External ear	**Normal Condition of Flora:** Bacillus species, diphtheroids, *Saprophytic fungi*, alpha hemolytic streptococci, and *Staphylococcus epidermis.* **Possible Pathogens:** *Streptococcus pneumoniae* is the most significant. *Candida albicans, Haemophilus influenzae, Proteus* species, *Pseudomonas* species, *Staphylococcus aureus*, and *Papovavirus.*
Middle ear	**Normal Condition of Flora:** Specimen is normally sterile and free of organism growth. **Possible Pathogens:** Acute otitis media common contaminants include *H. influenzae, Streptococcus pneumoniae*, beta-hemolytic streptococci. Chronic otitis media common contaminants include *Staphylococcus aureus, Pseudomonas, Proteus*, and influenza virus.
Eye	**Normal Condition of Flora:** Diphtheroids, *Moraxella* species, *Neisseria* species, and *Staphylococcus epidermis.* **Possible Pathogens:** Any organisms; common pathogens include *H. influenzae, Staphylococcus aureus*, and *Streptococcus viridans.*
Joints	**Normal Condition of Flora:** Specimen is normally sterile and free of organism growth. **Possible Pathogens:** Common contaminants include *Staphylococcus aureus, Staphylococcus epidermidis, Streptococcus pneumoniae, H. influenzae*, group B, *Klebsiella pneumoniae*. Viruses include mumps, rubella, parvovirus. Fungi include *Candida, Blastomyces dermatitidis, Coccidioides immitis.*
Kidney	**Normal Condition of Flora:** Specimen is normally sterile and free of organism growth. **Possible Pathogens:** Any organism; most common are *Staphylococcus* and streptococci.
Large intestine, colon and rectum	**Normal Condition of Flora:** *Aspergillus, Bacillus subtilis, Bacteroides, Candida, Clostridium species*, diphtheroids, *Enterobacter*, enterococci, *E. coli, Fusobacterium, Klebsiella*, lactobacilli, *Peptococcus, Peptostreptococcus, Proteus* species, *Pseudomonas* species, staphylococci, and yeasts. **Possible Pathogens:** *Campylobacter species, Chlamydia, Neisseria gonorrhoeae, Candida albicans* in large numbers, *Salmonella* species, *Shigella* species, *Vibrio cholera*, and *Yersinia* species. Viruses include rotavirus, CMV.
Lower ileum	**Normal Condition of Flora:** *Clostridium perfringens, Enterococcus*, occasionally *E. coli*, lactobacilli, staphylococci, *Streptococcus* of viridans group. **Possible Pathogens:** *Salmonella* species and *Shigella* species.

Specimen Site	Normal Flora/Possible Pathogens
Mouth	**Normal Condition of Flora:** (After newborn period) bacteroids, *Branhamella catarrhalis*, *Candida albicans*, diphtheroids, *E. coli*, *Haemophilus* species, *Neisseria mucosa*, *Peptostreptococcus lactobacillus*, *Staphylococcus epidermidis* and *Streptococcus* of viridans group. **Possible Pathogens**: *Candida albicans* in large numbers, *Haemophilus influenzae* and *Haemophilus parainfluenzae*, *Staphylococcus aureus* (in large numbers), *Streptococcus* group A.
Nasal passages	**Normal Condition of Flora:** Diphtheroids, *Enterobacteriaceae* species, gram-positive bacilli, *Klebsiella* species, *Staphylococcus* species and *Streptococcus* species. **Possible Pathogens**: *H. influenzae*; acute sinusitis common contaminants include *Staphylococcus aureus*, *Streptococcus pneumoniae*, *Klebsiella*, *Enterobacter*, alpha hemolytic streptococci, *Moraxella catarrhalis*; chronic sinusitis common contaminants include *Staphylococcus aureus*, *Streptococcus pneumoniae*, alpha hemolytic streptococci, *Mucor*, *Aspergillus*.
Nasopharynx	**Normal Condition of Flora**: (Sterile at birth) Bacteroids, diphtheroids, *E. coli*, gram-positive bacilli, *H. influenzae*, *Neisseria* species, staphylococci, streptococci, *Streptococcus pneumoniae* and *Proteus* species. Marked predominance of any of these organisms may be clinically significant even if it is a normal inhabitant. **Possible Pathogens**: *Bordetella pertussis*, *Corynebacterium diphtheriae*; in large numbers: *E. coli*, gram-negative bacilli, *Haemophilus* species, *Proteus* species, *Pseudomonas* species, *Staphylococcus aureus*, and *Streptococcus pneumoniae*.
Pericardium	**Normal Condition of Flora**: Specimen is usually sterile and free of organism growth. **Possible Pathogens:** Any organism; common contaminants are *Staphylococcus aureus*, *Streptococcus pneumoniae*, *Enterobacteriaceae*, *Pseudomonas*, *H. influenzae*, *Candida*, *Actinomyces*.
Peritoneal fluid	**Normal Condition of Flora:** Specimen is usually sterile and free of organism growth. **Possible Pathogens:** Any organism; common contaminants are *E. coli*, enterococci, *Streptococcus pneumoniae*, *Clostridium*, *Staphylococcus aureus*, alpha hemolytic streptococci.
Pleural fluid	**Normal Condition of Flora:** Specimen is usually sterile and free of organism growth. **Possible Pathogens:** Any organism; common contaminants are *Staphylococcus aureus*, *Staphylococcus epidermidis*, *Streptococcus pneumoniae*, *H. influenzae*, *E. coli*, *Klebsiella pneumoniae*.
Skin	**Normal Condition of Flora**: *Acinetobacter*, alpha hemolytic streptococci, *Candida albicans*, diphtheroids, enterococci, enterococci propionibacterium, *Proteus*, *Staphylococcus epidermidis*, and *Staphylococcus* species. **Possible Pathogens**: *Clostridium* species, *Corynebacterium* diphtheriae, *E. coli*, *Klebsiella*, *Neisseria*, *Staphylococcus aureus*, *Staphylococcus pyogenes*. Viruses include papillomavirus, varicella-simplex. Fungi include: *Trichophyton*, *Actinomyces*, *Nocardia*, *Microsporum*.
Sputum	**Normal Condition of Flora:** Specimen is normally free of organism growth. **Possible Pathogens:** Any organism; common contaminants are oral bacteria. The greater the number of squamous epithelial cells, the greater the contamination by oral-pharynx materials. Most common pathogens include gram negative bacilli or *Staphylococcus aureus*. Others are *H. influenzae* and *Streptococcus pneumoniae*.
Stomach, small Intestine	**Normal Condition of Flora:** Specimen is normally free of organism growth. Scant bacteria in two-thirds to include *E. coli*, *Klebsiella*, *Enterobacteriaceae*, enterococci, alpha hemolytic streptococci, *Staphylococcus epidermidis*, diphtheroids. **Possible Pathogens:** *Helicobacter pylori*, *Campylobacter jejuni*.
Stool, feces	**Normal Condition of Flora:** Bacteroids, *Clostridium albicans* (in large numbers), diphtheroids, *Enterobacter* species, *E. coli*, *Fusobacterium*, *Klebsiella* species, *Lactobacillus* species, *Peptococcus* species, *Peptostreptococcus* species, *Proteus* species, *Pseudomonas* species, *Staphylococcus* species, *Streptococcus* species, and yeast. **Possible Pathogens:** *Campylobacter* species, *Candida albicans* (in large numbers), *Salmonella* species, *Shigella* species, *Vibrio cholera*, and *Yersinia* species. *Candida albicans* can be pathogenic when preceded by antibiotic therapy.
Throat	**Normal Condition of Flora**: Diphtheroids, *E. coli*, *Haemophilus* species, *Staphylococcus* species, *Streptococcus* species. **Possible Pathogens:** *Bordetella pertussis*, *Corynebacterium* diphtheria, *Haemophilus* species; in large numbers: *E. coli*, *Proteus* species, *Pseudomonas* species, *Staphylococcus aureus*, *Streptococcus pneumoniae*, *Streptococcus pyogenes* group A.

Specimen Site	Normal Flora/Possible Pathogens
Trachea, bronchi, lungs, sinus cavities	**Normal Condition of Flora**: Specimen is normally sterile and free of organism growth. **Possible Pathogens:** *Candida albicans*, *Coccidioides*, *E. coli* or *Proteus mirabilis*, *H. influenzae*, *Klebsiella*, *Mycoplasma pneumoniae*, parainfluenza virus, Pneumocystis, Pseudomonas, *Salmonella*, staphylococci, *Streptococcus pneumoniae*; viruses include influenza, rhinovirus, coronavirus, adenovirus
Ureter	**Normal Condition of Flora**: Specimen is normally sterile and free of organism growth. **Possible Pathogens:** Any organism; most common pathogen is *E. coli.*, *Proteus*, *Pseudomonas*, and *Staphylococcus aureus*.
Urethra	**Normal Condition of Flora:** Diphtheroids, *Enterococcus*, *Mycoplasma*, *Staphylococcus epidermidis.* **Possible Pathogens:** Common contaminants for males are *Neisseria gonorrhoeae*, *Chlamydia*, *Gardnerella vaginalis*, *E. coli*, and *Klebsiella*, *Enterobacteriaceae*. Common contaminants for females include *Candida albicans*, *Neisseria gonorrhoeae*, *Trichomonas*, *Clostridium perfringens*, *Gardnerella vaginalis*, *Chlamydia*, and yeasts.
Urine, clean catch	**Normal Condition of Flora:** Specimen is normally sterile and free of organism growth. **Possible Pathogens:** Any organism count greater than 100,000 organisms per milliliter. Chronic infection may have repeatedly lower colony counts. Common contaminant is *Staphylococcus epidermidis*. Most common pathogen is *E. coli*. Others include *Proteus*, *Pseudomonas*, *Staphylococcus aureus*, *Klebsiella*, *Enterobacteriaceae*, *Candida albicans*, beta-hemolytic streptococci.
Vagina	**Normal Condition of Flora:** (Adult) *Candida albicans*, *Clostridium sporogenes*, diphtheroids, *E. coli*, lactobacilli, nonhemolytic and alpha hemolytic *Streptococcus* species, *Staphylococcus epidermidis*, and yeasts. **Possible Pathogens:** *Candida albicans* (in large numbers), *Gardnerella vaginalis*, *Neisseria gonorrhoeae*, and *Trichomonas*.
Wound or abscess	**Normal Condition of Flora:** Specimen is normally sterile and free of organism growth. **Possible Pathogens:** *Clostridium* species, *E. coli*, *Pseudomonas* species, *Proteus* species, *Staphylococcus aureus*, *Streptococcus pyogenes* group A; a common contaminant is *Staphylococcus epidermidis*.

Organisms

Appendix H. Noninvasive Diagnostic Test Outcomes

This section links noninvasive diagnostic tests with signs and symptoms that may have been the reason for the physician to order the test, as well as diagnostic outcomes. This information will assist the coder to conduct a record review for clinical clues that may affect DRG assignment. According to coding guidelines, MCC/CCs must affect patient care in terms of requiring clinical evaluation; therapeutic treatment; further evaluation by diagnostic studies, procedures, or consultation; extended length of stay; or increased nursing care; and/or monitoring for reporting purposes.

Cardiology Procedures

Myocardial perfusion imaging (pharmacologic stress testing)	**Signs and Symptoms:** Chest pain suspected to be of cardiac origin (to include tightness, pressure and discomfort), evaluation of the results of coronary bypass or balloon angioplasty, syncope, abnormal exercise EKG, abnormal cardiovascular function study, dyspnea, shortness of breath **Diagnostic Outcomes:** Acute myocardial infarction, ischemic heart disease, ventricular arrhythmia, cardiomyopathy, cardioembolic strokes, postmyocardial infarction, cardiomegaly, angina pectoris, coronary atherosclerosis, heart failure, aortic aneurysm, peripheral angiography, status post heart transplant evaluation, coronary artery bypass or balloon angioplasty
Transesophageal echocardiography (TEE)	**Signs and Symptoms:** Syncope and collapse, fever, shock, persistent febrile state, pre-existent valvular pathology, inadequate defined volume status for ventilator patients, heart mass **Diagnostic Outcomes:** Mitral, tricuspid, and aortic valve disorders; endocarditis; aneurysm of heart; myocarditis; cardiomyopathy; acquired cardiac septal defect; cerebral embolism; cerebrovascular disease; coarctation of aorta; volume depletion; fluid overload; mechanical complication cardiac device; implant or graft (including cardiac pacemaker or heart valve prosthesis); status post heart transplant or valve replacement; malignant or secondary neoplasm of heart; thoracic aorta disruption after blunt trauma; monitor heart function during cardiac surgery; evaluation of left atrial thrombosis and masses; in the evaluation of bacterial endocarditis and its complications; and in the evaluation of intracardiac shunts
Transthoracic echocardiography (TTE)	**Signs and Symptoms:** Syncope and collapse, chest pain, heart murmur, abnormal heart sounds, bacteremia, fever, shock, dyspnea, and shortness of breath **Diagnostic Outcomes:** Hypertensive heart disease, pulmonary hypertension, endocarditis, acute cor pulmonale, atrial fibrillation, pulmonary embolism and infarction, myocarditis, cardiomyopathy, heart failure, systemic lupus erythematosus, acute myocardial infarction, acquired septal defect, angina pectoris, cerebral embolism, poisoning by chemotherapy and immunosuppressive drugs, mechanical complication of cardiac device, implant or graft (including cardiac pacemaker or heart valve prosthesis), malignant or secondary neoplasm of heart

Neurology Procedures

Electromyography (EMG)	**Signs and Symptoms:** Muscle spasms, pain in limb, abnormal involuntary movements, abnormality in gait, lack of coordination, changes in skin sensation (tingling, numbness, burning, or prickling sensation), voice disturbances **Diagnostic Outcomes:** Intervertebral disc disorders, muscular dystrophy, neuropathy, systemic lupus, sarcoidosis, myalgia, neuralgia, neuritis, radiculitis, acquired spondylolisthesis, cervical spinal cord injury, botulism, diabetes with neurogenic manifestations, peripheral nervous system disorders, chronic renal failure, injury to peripheral nerves, malignant neoplasm of spinal cord and meninges, anesthesia and paresthesia, especially of the extremities
Nerve conduction testing (amplitude, latency/velocity, F-wave study)	**Signs and Symptoms:** Muscle spasms, pain in limb, abnormal involuntary movements, abnormality in gait, lack of coordination, changes in skin sensation (tingling, numbness, burning, or prickling sensation), voice disturbances **Diagnostic Outcomes:** Myopathy, radiculopathy, intervertebral disc disorders, myalgia, neuralgia, neuritis, neuropathy, radiculitis, acquired spondylolisthesis, spinal cord injuries, diabetes with neurological manifestations, chronic renal failure, malignant neoplasms of spinal cord and meninges